Principles & Te

Patient

D0435345

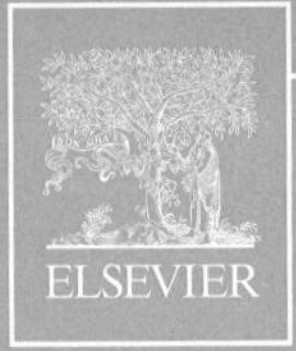

evolve

The Latest Evolution in Learning.

Evolve provides online access to free learning resources and activities designed specifically for the textbook you are using in your class. The resources will provide you with information that enhances the material covered in the book and much more.

Visit the Web address listed below to start your learning evolution today!

LOGIN: http://evolve.elsevier.com/Pierson/

Evolve provides online access to free learning resources designed specifically for the textbook you are using. These resources will give you the information you need to quickly and successfully learn the topics covered in Principles and Techniques of Patient Care 3E and more.

Evolve Free Resources:

Instructor: The instructor learning resources include everything for the student, and:

- Teaching Tips-thoughts and advise from the author on teaching course content.
- Content updates
- Case Studies

Student:

- Weblinks-an exciting resource that lets you link to hundreds of websites carefully chosen to supplement the content of the textbook. The weblinks are regularly updated with new ones added as they develop.
- Content updates
- Case studies

Think outside the book...evolve.

Principles & Techniques of Patient Care

Frank M. Pierson, MA, PT
Assistant Professor Emeritus
The Ohio State University
Columbus, Ohio

Sheryl L. Fairchild, BS, PT
Consultant
Stoneham, Massachusetts

Third Edition

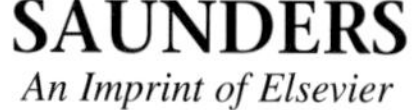

SAUNDERS
An Imprint of Elsevier

Saunders
An Imprint of Elsevier

The Curtis Center
Independence Square West
Philadelphia, Pennsylvania 19106

PRINCIPLES AND TECHNIQUES OF PATIENT CARE ISBN 0-7216-9379-2
Copyright © 2002, Elsevier (USA). All rights reserved.

No part of this publication may be reproduced or transmitted in any form or by any means, electronic, mechanical, including photocopying, recording, or any information storage and retrieval system, without prior permission in writing from the publisher.

Permissions may be sought directly from Elsevier's Health Sciences Rights Department in Philadelphia, USA: phone: (+1)215-238-7869, fax: (+1)215-238-2239, email: healthpermissions@elsevier.com. You may also complete your request on-line via the Elsevier Science homepage (http://www.elsevier.com), by selecting 'Customer Support' and then 'Obtaining Permissions'.

Previous editions copyrighted 1999, 1994

Library of Congress Cataloging-in-Publication Data

Pierson, Frank M.
Principles and techniques of patient care / Frank M. Pierson, Sheryl L. Fairchild.—3rd ed.
p. ; cm.
Includes bibliographical references and index.
ISBN 0-7216-9379-2
1. Patients—Care. 2. Nursing. 3. Allied health personnel. I. Fairchild, Sheryl L. II. Title.
[DNLM: 1. Physical Therapy Techniques—methods. 2. Patient Care Planning. WB 460 P624p 2002]
RT42 .P48 2002
615.8′2—dc21

2002066885

Editor: Andrew Allen
Developmental Editor: Peg Waltner
Publishing Services Manager: Catherine Jackson
Project Manager: Mary Stueck
Designer: Amy Buxton

TG/KPT

Printed in the United States of America.

Last digit is the print number: 9 8 7 6 5 4 3

Acknowledgments

This third edition could not have been planned, prepared, produced, published, and distributed without the support, assistance, and guidance of many persons, organizations, and institutions. Therefore we sincerely appreciate and are grateful for the involvement of Theron Ellinger, Senior Medical Photographer, Biomedical Communication Services, School of Allied Medical Professions, The Ohio State University, for his skill and commitment to producing high-quality photographs, and Sheryl L. Fairchild for her photographic contributions.

The persons who willingly served as subjects or participated in the new photographs used in this edition were: Helene Lamp, Melissa Roberto, Rosalind Kiley, Adeline Joyce, Joyce Shaw, Marcia Orlowski, Jillian LeBrun, Kathleen Barnes, Stephanie Pavoni, Timothy Byram, Kerry Melville, Kristen Grotke, James Capbell, Greg Wenger, Paul Schumacher, Christina Ferraro, Theresa Skybo, James Rishel, Thomas Rountree, Robert Baker, and Bette Holloway.

These persons served as primary resource contact to facilities, equipment, or subjects: Kathleen Barnes, MS, PT, Chair PTA Program; Joyce Shaw, MS, PT, Clinical Coordinator, Physical Therapy faculty, Endicott College, Beverly, Massachusetts; Patti Reid, Director, Clinical Laboratory, School of Nursing, The Ohio State University; Michelle Graf, PT, Acute Rehabilitation Team Leader, The Ohio State University Medical Center; Pat Kulich, RN, CIC, Department of Epidemiology, The Ohio State University Medical Center; Theresa Berner, OTR/L, Rehabilitation Team Leader, The Ohio State University Medical Center; Barbara Bostic, PT, Director of Out-Patient Rehabilitation Services, The Ohio State University Medical Center; and Melissa Roberto, MS, PT, LATC, Site Manager, Malden Medical Center, Hallmark Health, Malden, Massachusetts.

We also extend appreciation to: Hallmark Health at Malden Medical Center, Malden, Massachusetts; Physical Therapy Program, Endicott College, Beverly, Massachusetts; Juzo, Cuyahoga Falls, Ohio; Epidemiology Department, The Ohio State University Medical Center; Rehabilitation Services Department, The Ohio State University Medical Center; Acute Rehabilitation Services Floor, The Ohio State University Medical Center; and the Clinical Laboratory, School of Nursing, The Ohio State University, for granting access to materials, equipment, or facilities; Peg Waltner, Developmental Editor, for her excellent editorial skills and suggestions, her assistance with the final review and preparation of the manuscript, and her support throughout the length of the project; Andrew M. Allen, Editor; Suzanne Honscharik, Senior Editorial Assistant; Jamie Lyn Thornton, Project Manager; Amy Buxton, Designer; and the other staff members of Elsevier Science involved with this edition for their support and assistance with the production, distribution, and sales of the book.

Finally, we extend our gratitude to our family members and friends, especially Barbara and Sally, who made it possible for us to spend the time necessary to plan, prepare, and submit the manuscript. Their understanding of our needs and encouragement during the course of the project was greatly appreciated.

We dedicate this edition to
our families, loved ones, and previous and future patients.

Preface

Because of the positive response of the students, faculty, and practitioners who used the second edition of this text as a teaching-learning resource, W.B. Saunders Company requested that a third edition be prepared. To add a more extensive clinical base to the content, Sheryl L. Fairchild, BS, PT, was invited to be a coauthor. Ms. Fairchild's background as a clinician and Administrative Director at Malden Hospital, Malden, Massachusetts, as well as her experience as Director of Clinical Operations of Hallmark Health, for more than 23 years enabled her to provide a new dimension to the content of the book. Her suggestions and recommendations for revisions of previously published material and for the addition of new material have been extremely beneficial. The users of this edition will benefit from her clinical insights and competence and her professional knowledge and expertise. She has been a valuable asset to the planning, development, preparation, and review of the manuscript before its submission. Some excellent suggestions, recommendations, and, in some instances, corrections to the second edition provided by persons who have used this book were reviewed and many of them have been incorporated into this edition.

We are especially grateful to those persons who formally reviewed and critiqued the second edition for their valuable feedback. Each chapter of the second edition was reviewed carefully and the content of the majority of them was revised to ensure the material reflected current principles and techniques of patient care. Furthermore, the sequence of the chapters was reordered to more closely follow the sequence of events or activities a caregiver should perform before and during the provision of patient care. Important revisions or additions occurred in several chapters and one previous chapter was divided into two chapters to reorganize and present the material more clearly. The first chapter was revised to improve the introduction of the caregiver-to-patient interaction, communication, assessment, examination, evaluation, and documentation. Brief sections about the advantages of patient cotreatment by two or more caregivers and the need to be aware of cultural differences that exist among persons were added.

A new chapter specifically related to infection control has become Chapter 2. Information provided in it reflects the concepts of the use of Standard and Transmission-Based Precautions, hand-washing techniques, and the use of protective garments. The chapter was positioned early in the book to emphasize the importance of the material and to prepare the reader to use proper techniques when providing patient care. The assessment and measurement of vital signs is now Chapter 3 and assessment of pain has been included as a fifth vital sign. The section on body composition assessment has been deleted, except for the girth and volume measurement techniques of the extremities. Those techniques were transposed to the new Chapter 11, where they complement the information presented in the chapter. New photographs related to body mechanics depict the use of a normal lumbar lordosis during lifting activities, which has supportive evidence indicating that it is the safest and most effective position to use. Minor revisions were made to the content and photographs related to positioning and draping, basic exercise, and transfers. Additional photographs showing independent wheelchair activities (that is, performing a "wheelie," ascending and descending a curb, stairs, escalator) and some new wheelchair features appear in Chapter 8. A new chapter related to basic wound care, management of lymphedema, and manual techniques to improve respiratory function was developed. It includes current information about girth and volumetric measurements of the extremities, intermittent compression pumps, and compression garments. Other revisions or additions, such as new or replacement photography and redesigned or new information boxes, procedure outlines, and tables, were provided in the majority of the chapters to improve the content and assist the reader's comprehension of the material.

We believe the changes and additions have enhanced the quality of the third edition. Our intent was to incorporate the concepts, procedures, and techniques of patient care that were acceptable and used in clinical practice at the time the manuscript was prepared. Although it is probable that some changes in the acceptance or use of some of these concepts, procedures, or techniques may occur by the time this text is available for use, it is believed the majority of the content will continue to describe safe and effective approaches to patient care. A review of the Acknowledgments will indicate those persons, organizations, and institutions that were involved with this project. We are indebted to them for their contributions and we extend our sincere gratitude and appreciation to each of them. Furthermore, we recognize that the amount of success this edition may experience will be, in large measure, attributable to their support and assistance.

Sheryl L. Fairchild
Frank M. Pierson

Contents

CHAPTER 1

Introduction to Patient Care Activities

objectives *After studying this chapter, the reader will be able to:*

- Describe a process for the examination and evaluation of a patient.
- List the four components of a problem-oriented status note.
- Identify information that would be classified as "subjective" and information that would be classified as "objective."
- Describe how subjective and objective information could be obtained through an evaluation.
- Discuss the importance of examining and evaluating each patient before establishing a plan of care.
- Describe the major components or categories of the patient management process.
- List five barriers to communications and describe how you would overcome them.
- Describe five guidelines to use to communicate with a person with a disability.
- Describe the major components of a written home program.

key terms

Assessment The measurement or quantification of a variable or the placement of a value on something. Assessment should not be confused with examination or evaluation.

Caregiver The person who is treating or working with the patient; examples are the therapist, therapist assistant, aide, or family member.

Communication The exchange of information through verbal (oral), written, or nonverbal (visual) means.

Documentation Written or printed matter conveying authoritative information, records, or evidence.

Electrodiagnosis The use of an electrical current to assist with the diagnosis of a patient's condition.

Evaluation A dynamic process in which the practitioner makes clinical judgments based on data gathered during the examination.

Examination The process of obtaining a history, performing relevant systems reviews, and selecting and administering specific tests and measures.

Goniometry The measurement of the range of motion of a joint of the body.

Kinesthesia The sense by which position, weight, and movement are perceived.

Orthosis An orthopedic appliance used to support, align, prevent, or correct deformities or to replace the function of parts of the body; a brace or splint is an example of an orthosis.

Outcome measure A quantifiable or objective means to determine the effectiveness of treatment or performance that is usually expressed with the use of functional terms.

Problem-oriented medical record (POMR) A system developed to organize a medical record that uses a common list of patient problems as its base.

Proprioception Perception mediated by proprioceptors or proprioceptive testing; sensation and awareness about the movements and position of body parts or the body.

Prosthesis The artificial replacement of an absent body part; an artificial limb is an example of a prosthesis.

Radiograph An image or a record produced on exposed or processed film through radiography; a roentgenogram.

SOAP An acronym, the letters of which identify each section of a patient's status. *Note:* S, subjective; O, objective; A, assessment; P, plan.

Stereognosis The ability to recognize the form (shape) of an object by touch.

Two-point discrimination The ability to recognize or differentiate two blunt points when they are simultaneously applied to the skin.

INTRODUCTION

This book has been prepared to assist persons responsible for and involved with patient care in providing safe and effective care. The term *caregiver* rather than therapist, nurse, health care practitioner, therapist assistant, technologist, technician, aide, or family member will be used to designate the person who is treating or working with the patient or client. It is recognized that the term "client" is sometimes more appropriate to describe a person who receives treatment. Furthermore, the term "consumer" may be used to describe the receiver of care. However, for consistency, the term "patient" is used throughout this text to describe the person who receives treatment. Similarly, the term "intervention" may be used rather than the term "treatment," but for consistency the term "treatment" is used in this text. The procedures and techniques contained in the text were selected because they can be applied or adapted for use for a variety of patients to assist them to fulfill their functional needs or goals. The knowledgeable and experienced practitioner will realize that there are alternative techniques or procedures that provide safe and effective ways to perform many of the patient activities described in the text.

It is anticipated and expected that the health care practitioner or caregiver will modify or adjust any technique or procedure to benefit the patient or better suit a specific situation or environment. The safety of the patient and the persons involved with providing care must be maintained at all times. The patient should be encouraged to perform maximally whenever his or her active participation is desired.

The caregiver will need to guide, direct, and instruct each patient. For many patients, a brief demonstration of an activity or the use of equipment by the caregiver or another patient will enable the person to understand his or her role better. Verbal, written, and nonverbal communication (NVC) between the caregiver, the patient, and family members will be necessary. The purpose of each activity, its expected outcome, and the method of performance should be explained to the patient.

No activity should be attempted unless sufficient personnel and equipment are available to accomplish the task safely. All persons who assist with the patient's care must be trained and competent; the equipment must function properly and be safe and stable; and the patient must be evaluated to determine the capacity to assist with or perform a particular activity.

Patient examination and *evaluation*, patient safety, and communication between the caregiver and the patient are required to promote quality patient care. Lack of attention to any one of these areas will usually adversely affect the quality of care the patient receives.

INTERPROFESSIONAL COLLABORATION

A team of caregivers from different professions who review a patient's condition, determine the problems amenable to treatment, discuss potential treatment solutions, and make decisions to resolve the problems is used by many organizations. This interprofessional collaboration approach is particularly useful for the patient with complex medical, social, economic, or other problems. To be successful, interprofessional collaboration requires the team members to meet collectively and periodically to problem solve and reach decisions about management of the patient. Collaboration, coordination, and communication are the important factors used by the team to assist the patient to effectively fulfill goals or needs. The interprofessional team members must be competent professionals who are willing to function interdependently to maximally benefit the patient. Team members must be prepared to recognize and accept the value of other members' professional knowledge, skills, and expertise; work through role conflicts that may develop as a result of overlapping roles of the members; understand the basic components of each member's profession; be able to communicate effectively with each other; and participate in leadership. The interprofessional team approach must be patient centered rather than profession centered, and so team members must be able to provide advice, counsel, and recommendations based on each member's knowledge and expertise that will lead to the best outcome for the patient. Group members need to be adept in the application of group process skills; therefore it is recommended that a portion of their formal education be devoted to an introduction to and practice of techniques, skills, and activities associated with group interaction. Furthermore, the opportunity to collaborate with students from various professional programs (such as medicine, social work, nursing, law, theology, allied health professions) to discuss and resolve complex case-study patient scenarios would be beneficial in preparation for future interprofessional team collaboration. Table 1-1 presents rationales for the support of and opposition to the use of interprofessional collaboration from the perspective of the patient and the participating professional.

PROFESSIONAL COLLABORATION

Another concept used in patient care is professional team work or, more specifically, cotreatment. This method of treatment is particularly important for professions that have levels or types of caregivers. Examples are medicine, physician/physician's assistant; nursing, registered nurse/licensed practical nurse/nurse's aide; occupational therapy, occupational therapist/occupational therapist assistant; and physical therapy, physical therapist/physical therapist assistant/aide. In these professions, the assistant functions with direction, guidance and, in some situations, direct supervision by the more responsible or primary caregiver in accordance with statutory, professional, or ethical requirements. In addition, the patient's limitations, condition, needs, response to treatment, and the environment where the treatment is provided may influence or affect the relationship between the two caregivers.

An ideal relationship exists when the two caregivers cotreat the patient. In such a relationship, the two persons

Table 1-1 **Interprofessional Collaboration**

Rationale for Client/Patient	Rationale for Professional	Rationale Against Client/Patient	Rationale Against Professional
Comprehensive approach	Opportunity for members to better understand the skills, expertise, and roles of other professionals	Process may overwhelm the patient	May have personal and professional identity reduced; may lose professional autonomy
Reduction in duplication or fragmentation of professional services and activities	Opportunity for members to become more aware of and effective in own professional role and application of professional expertise and knowledge	May not produce better quality care	Reduces personal decision making
Team is better able to address complex problems	Enhances ability and provides opportunity to network and refer to other professionals	May not result in best decisions due to professional role conflicts	Takes time away from other patients; is time-consuming process
Team decision making is better due to input from different professionals	Broadens interaction with other professionals; leads to professional development	Apt to be more costly (time, money, effort)	Causes separation from professionals, peers, and colleagues
Results in interventions for complex problems that exceed what an individual could accomplish		May reduce the one-on-one relationship between the patient and individual professionals	Interprofessional collaboration may not be a value of the profession; professional becomes reluctant to participate

cooperatively establish the roles and activities each will perform. The primary caregiver evaluates the patient, provides a plan of care, determines the therapeutic interventions to be used, assigns tasks and responsibilities for the assistant to follow, establishes the goals or desired outcome of treatment, and periodically evaluates the results of the treatment and the patient's responses to the treatment. The assistant performs the treatment activities for which he or she is qualified and communicates frequently, orally and in writing, with the primary caregiver. Changes in the patient's condition, outcomes of the therapeutic procedures used, and observations by the assistant assist the primary caregiver to alter or adjust the plan of care. The primary caregiver will eventually perform the activities necessary to terminate the treatment and discharge the patient from services.

It is imperative for the primary caregiver to be aware of the activities of the assistant and for the assistant to understand the rationale for the interventions performed and inform the primary caregiver of the patient's response to treatment. Furthermore, the cotreatment approach to patient care depends on the cooperation, collaboration, and coordination of the activities performed by the two caregivers to maximize the effectiveness of patient care.

ORIENTATION

Before providing any form of treatment, including an *examination* and evaluation, the caregiver must initially orient the patient. This orientation comprises a personal introduction; informing the patient of the treatment goals, desired outcome, and potential risks; interviewing the patient (as part of the examination and evaluation) to obtain information; and instructing the patient regarding participation.

In a treatment setting, the caregiver should greet and identify the patient, state his or her own name clearly, and indicate the type of professional or technical status. The patient should be informed why he or she has been referred to the service unit, the type of treatment to be received, and any serious risks or adverse effects associated with the proposed treatment. At this time the patient should have the opportunity to ask questions, obtain additional information, and agree to or decline treatment. During the interview the caregiver should confirm the patient's name and medical diagnosis and then progress to the *assessment*, examination, and evaluation of the patient. Next, the caregiver should instruct the patient more specifically about the treatment and the patient's role or expected level of performance. After the plan of care and objectives have been determined with the patient, treatment sessions can commence. During subsequent treatment sessions, several of the steps can be eliminated or modified as the patient becomes more familiar with the treatment process. However, the caregiver should always discuss each treatment activity with the patient and instruct or guide the person's performance (Procedure 1-1).

PROCEDURE 1-1

Orientation of the Patient

Introduce yourself by name and title or professional designation.
Verify or confirm patient information you have received such as name, diagnosis, purpose of treatment, and referral source.
Interview the patient to obtain relevant information; be alert for culturally different norms or traditions.
Perform assessment, examination, and evaluation activities to establish the patient's capabilities, condition, problems, needs, and goals.
Establish treatment goals and functional outcomes with patient input.
Inform the patient of the treatment plan and techniques selected to fulfill outcome goals; include information about risks or adverse effects associated with the treatment.
Encourage the patient to ask questions to obtain information to enable the person to consent to or decline treatment.
Request the patient to sign an informed consent document or record the oral consent in the medical record.

AWARENESS OF CULTURAL DIVERSITY

Today a caregiver is more likely to treat persons whose cultural or religious foundations vary greatly from what is often considered to be "mainstream" or "traditional." In preparation, the caregiver should be aware of his or her own personal biases, prejudices, attitudes, and values to better understand the effect these beliefs may exert on a patient if they are applied injudiciously. The caregiver should learn about or research the cultural norms and traditions associated with different ethnic or religious groups before treatment to be able to exhibit desirable behavior toward those individuals and their family members. Differences in language, both verbal and nonverbal; cultural or religious norms or traditions; and personal bias or prejudice can create problems between the caregiver and the patient (Table 1-2).

Understanding the cultural norms of a patient can assist the caregiver to enhance the effectiveness of the treatment by improving *communication* and developing respect between the two individuals. A judgment by the caregiver about a patient, based on cultural or religious bias of the caregiver, may affect the patient's care if the caregiver believes the patient's behavior is "unusual" when compared with the caregiver's concept of "normal" behavior. It is suggested that the caregiver begin being culturally aware by becoming knowledgeable of the basic cultural norms and traditions of the Native American, African American, Hispanic, and Asian cultures and the basic norms and traditions of the Protestant, Roman Catholic, Jewish, Muslim, and Buddhist religions. Other cultures and religions may need to be investigated depending on the potential for exposure to patients from those cultures and religions.

Table 1-2 Glossary of Terms Related to Cultural Diversity

CULTURE
The shared values, norms, traditions, customs, arts, history, folklore, and institutions of a group of people.

CULTURAL COMPETENCE
A set of academic and interpersonal skills that allow individuals to increase their understanding and appreciation of cultural differences and similarities within, among, and between groups. This requires a willingness and ability to draw on knowledgeable persons of and from the community in developing focused interventions, communications, and other supports.

CULTURAL DIVERSITY
Differences in race, ethnicity, language, nationality, or religion among various groups within a community, organization, or nation. A city is said to be culturally diverse if its residents include members of different groups.

CULTURAL SENSITIVITY
An awareness of the nuances of one's own and other cultures.

CULTURALLY APPROPRIATE
Demonstrating both sensitivity to cultural differences and similarities and effectiveness in using cultural symbols to communicate.

ETHNIC
Belonging to a common group often linked by race, nationality, and language with a common cultural heritage or derivation.

RACE
A socially defined population that is derived from distinguishable physical characteristics that are genetically transmitted.

Because of their cultural or religious norms and traditions, some patients may rely on spiritual healing, family remedies, "folk" or "faith" healers, or supernatural power of healing more than traditional health care treatment. Herbal medicines, medicinal amulets, poultices, acupuncture, magnetic forces, and prayer vigils may be forms of alternative treatment used by persons from certain cultures and should be recognized by the caregiver as treatment adjuncts.

Furthermore, cultural norms may explain why some patients arrive late for an appointment or why some patients may not appear at all or why some patients discontinue treatment before all sessions have been completed. The caregiver should be aware that gestures used by one culture may have a derogatory or offensive meaning or a meaning different from the one intended when a person of a different culture views it. Therefore it is important to clarify the meaning or intent of the gesture when it is used initially. At times an interpreter may be needed so communication can be meaningful and appropriate relationships can be established. In some situations the interpreter may be a family member or friend and at other times a professional translator may be needed. A family member may insist on observing the treatment or remaining with the patient throughout the treatment session.

The intent of this section is to encourage the caregiver to become more knowledgeable about cultural and religious differences among patients and to be prepared to adapt to those differences when necessary to promote quality care. The words one uses and the actions exhibited should convey respect for differences in the age, gender, race or ethnicity, abilities, and sexual orientation of each person. Only a few examples of cultural or religious norms or traditions have been presented and you will need to investigate other sources for further information about this topic. Many rights of persons who are culturally diverse are protected by the Americans with Disabilities Act (ADA) and the Civil Rights Act of 1964. In addition, these or similar rights may be contained in institutional personnel policies, patient rights statements, and governmental documents.

INFORMED CONSENT

Before the initial treatment of a patient, the caregiver has the responsibility to inform the person about the proposed treatment, some of the alternative treatments available, and associated primary known risks. The patient then has the right to consent to or reject the proposed treatment. This is the process of informed consent.

To ensure that the patient is properly informed, the caregiver must provide sufficient information about the proposed treatment and any alternative treatment appropriate for the person's condition to permit the person to arrive at an intelligent and knowledgeable decision. The patient must be able to understand the information so it must be presented using terms and language that are comprehendable. A translator or an interpreter may be required for persons who do not speak or comprehend English.

Known or potential primary risks associated with the treatment should be explained and the person should have an opportunity to ask questions and receive responses to them about any aspect of the proposed treatment. The caregiver should provide responses that are within the level of knowledge, training, and competence and based on expected or anticipated results or outcomes. The caregiver should not state or imply that certain results or outcomes will occur and he or she should not offer any indication to guarantee that specific results or outcomes will be attained.

If the patient has not reached the legal age of consent or has been judged to be mentally confused or incompetent to participate in the informed consent decision-making process, it probably will be necessary to obtain consent from a legally qualified surrogate, such as a parent, guardian, family member, or court-appointed advocate.

Box 1-1 Elements of the Informed Consent Process

Description of the patient's condition, diagnosis, or evaluative data and information

Description or outline of the proposed, recommended treatment plan, techniques, or procedures

Primary, known, anticipated, or potential risks; complications; and precautions associated with the proposed treatment

Expected prognosis or outcome of the proposed treatment without a stated or implied guarantee of results (that is, decrease or absence of pain, specific functional improvement, specific flexibility or strength gain)

Alternative forms of treatment appropriate for the person's condition with potential risks, complications, and precautions and the expected prognosis of the alternative treatment

Questions from the patient and responses from the caregiver that are thorough and honest; if you are unsure of or do not know the response to a question, indicate that to the patient, but attempt to locate the information or refer the patient to a qualified resource (that is, nurse, physician, social worker, pharmacist)

Explain the potential or possible consequence of no treatment if the patient refuses or rejects treatment

Document that you provided the patient with the opportunity for informed consent before initiation of treatment and his or her decision to consent to or refuse treatment

The caregiver should document that the process of informed consent was performed in accordance with preestablished, written policies and procedures of the service unit (that is, department, rehabilitation unit, office) or agency with which the caregiver is associated (that is, hospital department, school system, home health agency, outpatient facility, skilled nursing facility, or subacute care facility). In some situations, it may be prudent to have the patient or a surrogate sign a document to indicate the person has been informed of the proposed treatment and that consent to the treatment is authorized. The caregiver will need to use judgment and follow the recommendations of the facility or agency, risk manager, or legal counsel to determine whether each patient should be required to sign an informed consent authorization for treatment. If signed documents are not used, policies and procedures of the facility or agency must be specific and clearly indicate the process each caregiver is to use when discussing informed consent decisions with the patient. Failure by the caregiver to fully inform a patient about the proposed treatment before the initiation of treatment and obtain his or her consent to receive treatment can, in some situations, constitute professional negligence. Informed consent is a right to which each patient is entitled; therefore the caregiver has the obligation to inform the patient of the proposed treatment, its alternatives, and its foreseeable risks before initiation of treatment (Box 1-1).

PRINCIPLES OF DOCUMENTATION

The *documentation* of patient care is an important component of the written record maintained for each patient. Physicians, nurses, therapists, social workers, and many other persons involved with providing patient care perform documentation. Lawrence Weed developed the concept of the *problem-oriented medical record* (POMR) in the 1960s. This system has been accepted for use by many health care facilities throughout the United States, some of which have developed their own variations. This system is based on a list of patient problems, a database, and a series of status (progress) notes designated as the "initial," "interim," and "discharge" notes. When all departments or service units of a given facility use the POMR approach to record keeping, a higher quality of patient care may be anticipated, better communication between and among the caregivers is more likely to occur, and better decisions about the patient's treatment can be made. Information about the patient and the plan of care is contained in the status notes, which are written in the following format: subjective, objective, assessment, and plan, or SOAP.

Problem-Oriented Medical Record Description

The POMR has four phases: formation of a database (current and past information about the patient); development of a specific, current problem list (problems to be treated by various practitioners); identification of a specific treatment plan (developed by each caregiver); and assessment of the effectiveness of the treatment plans. When the POMR system is used, each practitioner adds evaluations, treatment planning, and treatment decision-making information and data to the patient's database and problem list.

The SOAP notes should contain important, relevant information about the patient; they should indicate and clearly reflect the patient's condition and subsequent changes in the condition; and they should be written frequently so information is reported promptly and regularly. The method used to gather the information and the development of the examination and evaluation and planning phases are described in the section related to the patient management process. The relationship of the SOAP notes to the decision-making process and the purposes of documentations are described in several articles and textbooks. Excellent resources for information about the POMR and SOAP notes are listed in the Bibliography.

Some suggestions of ways to improve the quality and meaningfulness of documentation are listed in Box 1-2.

Entry Corrections Occasionally it may be necessary to correct an entry. Careful and proper correction of an entry will help avoid accusations of tampering, changing the entry for self-serving reasons or intent, or capricious alteration of the medical record, especially if litigation is involved or being considered. Standard procedures should be followed when you are correcting a note:

- Draw a single line through the inaccurate information, but be certain the material remains legible.
- Date and initial the correction and add a note in the margin stating why the correction was necessary.
- Enter the corrected statement in the chronologic sequence of the record and be certain it is clear which entry the correction replaces.
- Use black ink for all corrections and entries.

In some situations it may be beneficial to have the corrected statement witnessed by a colleague. Avoid alterations that create the appearance of tampering (such as erasing or writing over a word or phrase to improve legibility). Never attempt to obliterate material in the record by using a felt marker, correction fluid, a typewriter overstrike, or an eraser. Improper alteration of an entry can create many problems for the practitioner if the entry is questioned or used as evidence during litigation. The practitioner's credibility, honesty, and intent will be challenged, which may lead to charges of incompetence, negligent behavior, or poor judgment. Many errors of judgment are not negligent acts, but any attempt to hide them can create serious problems for the practitioner. Never enter a note or sign an entry for someone else and do not ask someone else to perform such acts for you. During litigation or when questions arise about the patient's care, the medical record is the primary source of information about the care a patient received and the response to treatment; therefore accurate, timely, and proper documentation is important. Failure to maintain proper documentation and records can delay or cause denial of reimbursement, lead to dismissal or disciplinary action against the practitioner, affect the accreditation status of the facility, weaken the defense of the defendant during litigation, or cause improper or poor quality treatment to be delivered. A basic principle to follow is this: maintain the record so that, if all the persons who were originally treating a patient were to disappear suddenly, the next group of practitioners could immediately continue to provide the best quality treatment by using only the information from the record.

Documentation is becoming more and more important as a means to assess or measure the quality of care received by the patient so the caregiver or facility will be more likely to receive payment from a third-party payer (such as Medicare or an insurance company). Persons who review claims and make reimbursement and treatment-related decisions have focused on indicators of functional outcomes of treatment contained in the caregiver's documentation. This process can be expected to continue; therefore the caregiver must be aware of the need to provide accurate, current, function-oriented documentation. In addition, the use of function-oriented, objective, and measurable data in the documentation process will result in the greatest likelihood of obtaining a favorable reimbursement response to submitted claims

Box 1-2 Ways to Improve Documentation

Avoid general statements and provide specific, concise, clarifying information. Instead of stating that "The patient is uncooperative," state "the patient refused to perform active assistive exercise."

Use objective statements. Instead of stating that "Patient ambulates," state that "Patient ambulates 25 feet in 1 minute using bilateral axillary crutches on a level surface, with assistance, using a three-point pattern for three repetitions, with a 5-minute rest period between ambulations." Functional outcome measure statements will more accurately describe the patient's condition and assist with obtaining reimbursement for the services provided.

Be complete with your statements; record the significant or important information about the patient's condition, progress, or response to treatment. *Remember:* if an activity is not documented, it may be considered as not having occurred. If an unusual activity or procedure is used, document why it was selected and used. Unusual incidents and the action taken after the incident should be recorded. An objective description of the patient's condition or reaction after the incident should be recorded. An incident report should be filed with the risk manager or similar individual and it may be necessary to document that it was prepared and filed.

Provide continuity with your status (that is, progress) notes; be certain to indicate why or how you reached a particular decision about the care or treatment you provided, particularly if it deviated from the usual, acceptable care or treatment. Programs or treatment plans designed for the patient to follow at home should be well documented and should include precautions. Your documentation should indicate how you determined (or the steps taken to ensure) the patient or family member understood and could comply with the instructions.

Identify that you informed the patient of the treatment to be provided and its risks or hazards, the information was understood by the patient, and consent to treatment was given. If a consent form is used by the service unit, a copy signed by the patient should be in the medical record.

Be prompt and timely with your entries and be certain your writing is legible, including your signature and professional or staff designation; be certain the information is accurate and there is consistency between entries; investigate and clarify contradictory information. For example, is it the right hip or the left hip that requires treatment?

Use abbreviations that have been standardized or accepted and approved by the facility or the profession.

Be certain there are no empty or open lines between entries and that there are no open spaces within the notes; use the format approved by the human information systems department or used by the facility or profession.

Outline the major elements of the notes in your mind or on paper before you enter it in the record to avoid having to make a correction or a change in the notes. Avoid omissions, such as the date of initial or subsequent treatments, a change in treatment, or a discharge summary.

Properly countersign the entries of other persons according to state statutes and facility requirements; read the entry before countersigning it. In many cases it will be prudent to review the proposed entry before it is placed in the record to be certain it is accurate and complete.

and gaining approval to continue treatment from the third-party payer. Furthermore, it seems reasonable to anticipate that a patient will have more motivation to accomplish a functional goal or task that is meaningful to the person than to strive to attain a given strength or range-of-motion value. In addition, well-organized, accurate, relevant, and prompt documentation improves communication among the persons providing care.

When a caregiver documents the treatment provided or supervised, it is necessary to indicate the functional outcome or outcomes attained by the patient. Through the use of objective and measurable terms, language, or data, the documentation must report the extent of change in the patient's condition that resulted from the treatment. The results of initial and repeated muscle strength tests, *goniometry* measurements, and vital signs data are examples of objective, measurable information. However, it is also necessary to provide objective information that indicates the patient's ability or capacity to perform functional activities that are related to the activities in the home, workplace, and community and during recreation. Strength and range-of-motion data could be linked to the person's functional ability to perform dressing, feeding, and personal hygiene tasks at home; reaching, lifting, and carrying objects or use of office equipment at work; transfer and mobility activities in the community; and various sport or recreational activities. The reader is encouraged to propose other examples that would associate treatment techniques with functional outcomes. The caregiver should be certain the functional outcomes relate directly to the preestablished treatment goals or *outcome measures* stated in the treatment plan.

PRINCIPLES OF PATIENT MANAGEMENT

Before the initial treatment of a patient, the caregiver must develop and follow a process of gathering information and data so a quality plan of care can be developed and implemented. Major components of the process include examination of the patient, evaluation of the examination information and data, postulation of a diagnosis and prognosis, development of a plan of care, and the selection of intervention activities and techniques best suited to alter or change the patient's condition to attain desired functional outcomes (Procedure 1-2). The plan of care and the interventions should be derived from the diagnosis and prognosis. The caregiver should focus the plan of care so it will lead to the desired outcomes, which are usually expressed as short- or long-term objectives and functional goals. Inherent in the process is the frequent reevaluation of the patient's condition and the response to treatment, which may result in a change in the interventions used or the modification of the functional goals. To complete the process, planning and preparing for the termination of treatment, which could occur as early as the first or second treatment session, a reevaluation must be performed. Refer to the Appendix at the end of this chapter for examples of forms used to document patient care.

It is important to understand the examination establishes a baseline of data and information that describes the patient's current condition and level of function and can be used to measure the patient's progress and response to treatment. Barriers to treatment (that is, a person with receptive aphasia or a mental, psychologic, or social impairment) should be determined by the examination and documented in the medical record. The evaluation assists in establishing a functional diagnosis and prognosis for the patient, setting outcome goals, and developing the plan of care.

The plan of care, developed from decisions the caregiver makes in accordance with the diagnosis and prognosis, should contain treatment procedures, techniques, and activities that will be most effective to fulfill the established goals and anticipated outcomes. The sequence and frequency of the program and the need for equipment and level of assistance required by the patient must be determined. Consideration should be given at this time to planning for the termination of treatment. Because of the cost-containment requirements of most third-party payers, many patients will receive only a few treatment sessions from a qualified caregiver. Therefore the caregiver must plan and prepare a program for treatment activities to be performed at home or other site after the patient's formal treatment program is terminated. Equipment needs, financial assistance, family education and training, referral procedures, and follow-up or extended care may need to be considered as alternate treatment plans are developed.

Implementation of the procedures, techniques, and activities selected by the caregiver should be performed using the sequence and frequency determined previously. The caregiver must frequently and consistently reevaluate and measure the patient's progress and response to treatment. The extent to which the patient fulfills the short- and long-term goals and accomplishes the functional outcomes must be measured and documented. It is not sufficient, for example, to document that a patient's active range of motion of shoulder flexion has increased from 90 to 120 degrees. Reporting a functional outcome, such as the independent application and removal of clothing over the head, should be a component of the documentation. The caregiver must be prepared to continue, revise, or modify the treatment plan or the individual components of the treatment program based on the patient's progress and response to the treatment. Attention will need to be given to the plan and program for treatment at home if the caregiver determines that it will be necessary. Education and training of the patient and a family member should be provided, as well as the opportunity to practice the activities to be performed at home.

When the treatment program is to be terminated, the caregiver should evaluate and measure the patient's functional outcomes and compare them with the expected outcomes and the home treatment program should be reviewed

PROCEDURE 1-2

Patient Management Process

Examination of the patient to gather subjective and objective information and data and perform tests and measures to determine the patient's current condition and functional abilities.

Evaluate the information and data to make clinical judgments and decisions.

Postulate a clinical diagnosis and prognosis based on the results of the evaluation.

Form a plan of care based on the prognosis.

- Identify and select the intervention activities and techniques projected to be most effective to attain functional outcomes.
- Establish the sequence, frequency, and duration of the plan.
- Consider termination of treatment, including the development of a home treatment program if it becomes necessary.

Implement the plan.

- Apply techniques, activities, or procedures selected to accomplish functional outcomes.
- Revise or modify the plan depending on the patient's response or progress.
- Evaluate and document the patient's response frequently; determine his or her progress toward functional outcomes.

Terminate the plan.

- Evaluate the patient's functional activities to determine the need for further treatment elsewhere.
- If appropriate, instruct family members or home caregiver and provide time for them to practice.
- Provide a written home program and place a copy in the patient's medical record; document the patient's functional outcomes; document the date and time for reevaluation if necessary.

and finalized. The written or printed program should be given to the patient or family member and a copy should be placed in the medical record or maintained in a separate file.

A summary of the patient's condition and the functional outcomes and goals accomplished, future treatment plans, and any reevaluation or follow-up care appointments should be documented in the medical record.

Additional information about the patient management process can be found in several of the resources listed in the Bibliography.

PRINCIPLES OF PATIENT EXAMINATION AND EVALUATION

Examination guidelines are presented in Box 1-3. The patient's emotional response or reaction to the condition, family unit interactions, the support system available, the potential for improvement or regression of the condition, and the goals or expectations the person has for the treatment program should also be considered. The patient should be informed of the findings or results of the examination and evaluation and should be consulted and asked to assist with

Box 1-3 Guidelines for Patient Examination

Gather subjective and objective information and data.

- Subjective information and data can be obtained through interviews with the patient, family members, relatives, friends, or other caregivers and the medical record. Effective interview techniques and active listening skills are necessary to elicit beneficial responses. Information to obtain patient data includes the following:
  - Concept of the primary problem or complaint and its effect on function
  - Description of the progression or regression of the condition during the time it has existed
  - Description of the primary cause of the condition, problem, or complaint
  - Description of the results of any previous treatment for the same or similar condition, including medications used
  - Description of the current activities, life-style, occupation, social interactions, goals (support system), and needs
  - Concept of the severity, location, persistence, and effect of pain (obtain a thorough pain assessment)
  - Description of current medication
- Objective information and data can be obtained through interviews, the medical record, observation, and specific tests and measures. Observations of the patient should include the following:
  - General appearance, body build, and any deformities or absent body parts
  - Skin appearance and condition (that is, color, lesions, scars, texture)
  - Standing and sitting posture
  - Ambulation activities such as abnormal patterns, posture, use of aids, ability to perform functional tasks (that is, stairs, inclines, uneven surfaces), and level of independence
  - Mobility and flexibility (that is, bending, reaching, changing position)
  - Balance, stability, coordination, equilibrium, and motor control when sitting, standing, ambulating, or performing functional tasks
  - Application of assistive devices including *orthosis, prosthesis,* splints, or bandages
- Palpate the patient's:
  - Skin and subcutaneous tissue to determine texture, temperature, flexibility, laxity, firmness, and composition (that is, nodules, edema, erythema, pliability)
  - Muscles, tendons, ligaments to determine tone, pain response, bulk, composition, stability, laxity
  - Joints to determine swelling, shape, response to pain, joint space, crepitus, laxity
  - Bony features to locate landmarks, pain response, alignment
  - Arterial pulses to determine presence, rate, rhythm, and force
- Tests and measures should include:
  - Muscle strength and endurance using manual or mechanical methods
  - Joint motion and range tested actively and passively with goniometer
  - Joint integrity using manual or mechanical methods
  - Sensory mechanisms
    - Protective reactions to pain, temperature, pressure
    - Discriminatory reactions of *kinesthesia,* proprioception, *stereognosis, two-point discrimination,* touch-feel (that is, texture, shape)
    - Reflexes related to tissue stretch, posture, gross and fine motor skills
    - Automatic reactions (such as "righting," equilibrium, synergies)
- Cardiopulmonary function should include:
  - Vital signs at rest and after activity
  - Results of special pulmonary and cardiac function tests
- Functional capacity and ability to perform daily tasks should include:
  - Transfer activities, bed mobility, positional changes
  - Personal care and hygiene activities
  - Application, removal, and use of assistive devices and equipment
  - Ambulation and mobility activities with and without assistive aids
  - Mental and cognitive functions
- Other tests and reports if available should include:
  - *Radiograph* films, scans, reports
  - Laboratory reports
  - *Electrodiagnosis* tests (that is, electromyography)
  - Biopsy reports
  - Speech, hearing, language, and vision tests
  - Psychologic tests or evaluations

the development of the goals and outcomes of the treatment.

Goals of treatment should be established cooperatively with the patient and the caregiver. These goals are usually designated as interim, or short term, and terminal, or long term. Short-term goals are usually a specific component or lead-in activity for a long-term goal. An example of a short-term goal is: "The patient will be able to perform a sitting push-up in a wheelchair 10 times in 1 minute within 2 weeks." This would lead to the long-term goal of: "The patient will be able to perform an independent sitting transfer from the bed to a wheelchair within 2 minutes and return to the bed within 2 minutes in not more than 3 weeks." Goals must be stated in objective, measurable terms and should indicate who will perform the activity, by what means the goal will be accomplished, the need for equipment or assistance, the time frame in which to accomplish the goal, and the functional outcome expected. Goals should be modified or revised depending on the patient's performance and progress. Finally, goals and outcomes should be realistic and attainable for each patient.

The material in Box 1-3 is intended to be a guide to the areas that could be considered during the examination. Not all of the activities will be necessary or appropriate for each patient and the selection of the proper tests or procedures is the responsibility of the caregiver. However, for many patients, specific tests and measures will be required to obtain the data needed to develop the best plan of care (Fig. 1-1). The purpose of the examination and evaluation is to identify the patient's abilities, the problems to be treated, and the person's needs and goals so that outcomes can be established. The plan of care should result from the clinical diagnosis and prognosis determined by the caregiver and should include the intervention activities and techniques best suited to fulfill the goals and outcomes of the prognosis. The sequence, frequency, and duration of the plan of care must be established. Implementation of the plan of care, using preselected intervention procedures and techniques, provides the means to fulfill the treatment objectives, goals, and outcomes (Box 1-4).

The caregiver must be vigilant and conscientiously reexamine and reevaluate the patient frequently to maintain quality care. Failure to revise or adjust the treatment program, based on the patient's response to the program, may delay the patient's recovery or limit the extent of improvement of functional skills and independence. In summary, it is necessary to examine and evaluate the findings of the examination to form a basis for the development and implementation of the plan of care. Frequent examinations and evaluations must be performed to measure the patient's progress toward the treatment objectives, goals, and outcomes.

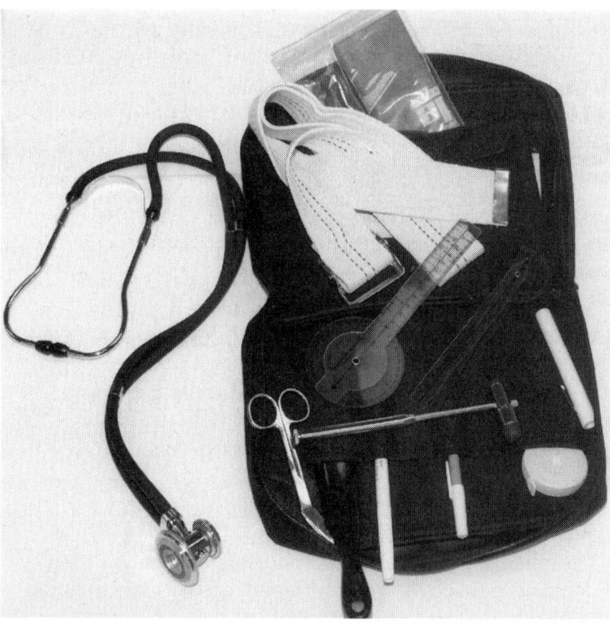

Fig. 1-1 Equipment used for patient examination.

Box 1-4 Principles of Patient Examination and Evaluation

- Initiates the process prior to any treatment; reexamine and reevaluate the patient frequently.
- Establishes a baseline of the patient's condition and functional status.
- Provides data and information to: develop the treatment plan and program; measure the patient's progress and response to treatment; determine the need to revise or modify the plan of care, goals, or functional outcomes.
- Measures the patient's attainment of goals or functional outcomes.
- Provides data and information for use by other persons.

PATIENT AND FAMILY EDUCATION

The public continues to demonstrate an interest in and desire to become better informed about medical and health care in general and about the specific medical and health care that individuals receive. Patients and family members expect to be consulted and informed about the care they receive. Questions related to the need for, efficacy of, and expected results or outcome of treatment are routinely asked. The practitioner must be prepared to provide appropriate and accurate responses without expressing or implying a guarantee or promise that a specific outcome or result will be achieved. The patient must be informed, with language and terminology that is understandable, about the treatment to be received so an informed decision about its value and safety can be made.

The caregiver has the responsibility to educate the patient and family about the treatment program and activities, but patient confidentiality must be respected and have the patient's permission before sharing information with the family. Goals of treatment should be established cooperatively by the patient and caregiver once the patient has been informed of the various possibilities for his or her care.

These goals should be stated in objective, measurable terms, which should include a time frame, how or by what means the goals will be accomplished, the need for equipment or assistive aids, and an indication of the expected functional outcome.

Interim, or short-term, goals and terminal, or long-term, goals must be developed and agreed upon. After the goals have been established, the caregiver can provide an overview or explanation of techniques or procedures that will be used to accomplish the goals. The effectiveness of the treatment program is measured by the accomplishment of the goals and subsequent patient outcomes. Goals can be revised when it is apparent the goal was an underestimate or overestimate of the patient's ability or progress (Box 1-5).

Another component of patient and family education is instruction for a home program. Many patients will require assistance from others to perform exercises and other activities in the environment of a home, health club, school, or other nonmedical facility. Ideally, the home program should be performed by the patient before termination of treatment, with a family member present and under the direction of the caregiver. The family member must be instructed about the responsibilities and level of assistance required of them. The patient and family member should practice the specific activities included in the home program while the caregiver observes and corrects improper performance. The home program should be printed or written and given to the patient for future reference. A copy is maintained with the patient's medical record or documentation materials at the treatment facility.

Instructions should include an outline of the exercises or activities, frequency of performance of the program, number of repetitions for each exercise, precautions or contraindications for each exercise, required equipment or supplies, specific instructions and diagrams to guide and direct the patient, caregiver's name and telephone number, and any scheduled reevaluation or reappointment sessions (Procedure 1-3). Finally, information about when or whether to terminate the program should be provided.

Information about the health care delivery system or resources in the community may need to be provided to assist the patient or family member to contact a particular agency or to obtain available benefits.

Box 1-5 Goal Statements

General concepts
- Objective terms are used
- Measurable outcomes are stated
- Realistic, attainable outcomes are identified
- Statements are oriented to the person involved, performance expected, time frame anticipated, functional outcome expected, and equipment or assistive aids needed

Short-term (interim) goals
- Preparatory component of long-term goal
- Lead-in activity for long-term goal
- Sequential activities that produce cumulative effect
- Support and promote functional outcome

Long-term (terminal) goal
- Evolves from short-term goals
- Describes maximal performance or outcome desired
- Describes functional outcome as a necessary component
- May be revised or modified based on the patient's progress and performance

PROCEDURE 1-3

Home Program Components

Determine the need or value for the patient to continue treatment after the formal treatment concludes.

Determine the environment and assistance available: home (family member), health club (health care practitioner), school (friend), or other.

Prepare the program before termination of the scheduled treatment sessions.

Instruct and supervise the patient and the assistant as they practice the program activities before termination of scheduled treatment sessions.

Provide a written (typed or printed) program with specific instructions, which is individualized for each patient.
- Outline and describe the activities, exercises, and positions to be used; provide diagrams as necessary.
- State goals and expected results, as necessary.
- Provide objective indicators of performance (that is, repetitions, distance, time) and the frequency and duration of the program.
- Provide indicators of successful completion, fulfillment, or accomplishment of goals, functional outcomes, or activities.
- List equipment and supplies that will be needed.
- Indicate precautions or contraindications associated with the exercises or activities.
- Provide the date, time, and location of scheduled reevaluation or reappointment if appropriate or necessary.
- Inform the patient when or whether to terminate the program.
- Provide the caregiver's name, telephone number, and address.

Document the preparation and assignment of the home program and maintain a copy in the medical record or patient's file.

Education can be performed through direct contact between the patient and family members and the caregiver, printed materials, slides or videotapes, and demonstrations. The specific instructional methods selected should coincide with the social, economic, mental, and physical factors manifested by or available to the patient and family members.

COMMUNICATION

Communication among persons is a primary function of life. For the caregiver, communication with patients, family members, other practitioners, and coworkers is a necessity. The caregiver should recognize that different forms of communication, such as verbal, nonverbal, and attentive listening, may be required depending on the purpose or situation related to the communication. Various barriers to communication should be recognized, documented, and avoided whenever possible. Patient-caregiver rapport can be established quickly through the use of effective communication or delayed by the lack of it. The information presented in this chapter is designed to provide guidelines or reminders for the caregiver and should not be considered all-encompassing or complete.

Instructions and information can be presented to the patient verbally, nonverbally, and with various audiovisual methods. Oral communication is the most prevalent style used. When you communicate orally, terms and concepts should be presented in language the listener understands. Lay language is the most satisfactory for most patients and family members. For example, use "bend" rather than "flex," "turn" or "twist" rather than "rotate," and "straighten" rather than "extend" when instructing the patient or family. Directions should guide the patient to perform or act and should be brief and concise. Functional terms or phrases such as "push," "stand," "sit," "turn toward me," and "reach to the left" are more effective than nonfunctional terms such as "Now, the first thing I want you to do is. . ." or "The next thing I want you to do is. . . ." However, it is necessary to provide some transitional terms and phrases, such as "Push with your hands on the armrests," "Straighten your hips and knees," or "Move your right crutch and left leg forward." The patient should be given time to process the message and the time required for processing will vary from person to person.

The tone, volume, and inflection of your voice can detract from or add to your message. You can either stimulate or calm a patient with your voice and behavior. For example, consider the mixed message you may give to a patient if you scowl or grimace while telling the patient that he or she performed well. When you desire to encourage or stimulate a patient to act quickly, use a louder than normal volume and a sharper tone to your voice as you say, "Stand up, now!" and simultaneously clap your hands. For the nervous or apprehensive patient you can use a lower than normal volume and a softer tone as you speak. It may also help assure the patient if you sit next to him or her or rest a hand on a shoulder while you talk. Think of other examples how the volume, tone, and inflection of your voice, along with your nonverbal cues, can add to or detract from your message.

Observation of the patient's reaction to the message will help you to determine whether the person understands it, has questions, or is puzzled by it. Maintaining eye contact between yourself and the patient allows both persons to relate to nonverbal cues and maintain better interaction. For example, when you are working with a patient's foot and ankle and he or she is supine or sitting, be certain to look at the patient's face rather than at the foot as you give your instructions.

It will be helpful to provide an overview or a description of the total activity and its components before giving specific instructions or directions. The specific responsibilities or activities expected of the patient can be presented and emphasized later. Many caregivers find it helpful to have the patient repeat the instructions to determine the ability to comprehend and retain the information and to estimate preparedness to perform. It is not sufficient to ask, "Do you understand what you are to do?" or "Do you understand the instructions?" because many patients will respond affirmatively even when they do not understand. Listen for the appropriate sequence and completeness of the repeated instructions. You may request the patient to demonstrate certain activities, such as prepositioning an extremity or the body or performing wheelchair tasks such as locking or unlocking the wheels, swinging away the front rigging, or positioning other equipment. These activities, when performed properly, will assist the caregiver to assess the patient's level of comprehension and readiness to function.

The NVC makes up the majority of human communication and may be even more effective than verbal communication. It is done through facial expressions, posture, gestures, body movements, or changes in body responses. Some forms of NVC are planned, whereas other forms are spontaneous, uncontrollable, or involuntary (Table 1-3). Most of us have been in embarrassing or stressful situations and have sensed a change in the color or temperature of our skin or experienced an increase in perspiration. These are examples of spontaneous, uncontrolled, or involuntary NVC. Facial expressions tend to be spontaneous, but at times they are planned for a specific effect. A frown or smile will indicate a negative or positive response to a patient's performance. When we use specific hand gestures or pantomime or demonstrate activities, we are using planned NVC. The skilled caregiver will know when and how to best use these various forms of NVC.

The caregiver should also observe the patient to identify how NVC is used. Often, more information and a more accurate estimation of the patient's response or reaction to instructions can be obtained through NVC.

Table 1-3 Forms of Nonverbal Communication

Form	Examples
Appearance	Dress, grooming, cleanliness
Body movements	Abrupt, slow, threatening, caring
Body positions	Sitting, standing, walking
Facial expressions	Smiling, frowning, grimacing
Gestures	Using hands and arms to guide or direct
Pantomime	Demonstrating the activity
Posture	Erect, slouched
Touch	Therapeutic, caring, directive, guiding
Spontaneous response to stress	Blushing, perspiring, trembling

The use of touch by the caregiver is another form of NVC that can add to the communication process. A brief hug, a hand squeeze, or a pat on the back can convey a message to a patient that cannot be sent as effectively orally. However, touch must be used in a therapeutic, caring way, and the caregiver must avoid any suggestion of sexual implications. Examples of improper and unacceptable forms of touch include patting, slapping, or stroking a patient's buttocks; squeezing the thigh; or stroking various body parts, except during a therapeutic massage or exercise activity. You must demonstrate care when you grasp, handle, or touch the patient, especially during massage and exercise when sensitive body areas are touched. The perineum and buttocks of all patients and the breasts of women and sometimes men should be draped as described in Chapter 5. When it is therapeutically necessary to massage, grasp, hold, or touch a potentially sensitive area, it may be prudent to state the reason the area is being touched or handled. In some situations, it may be wise to have another person observe or assist as you perform a particular treatment to protect yourself and to demonstrate your concern for the patient. Because touch may be construed to have a sexual implication by any patient, regardless of how careful the caregiver has been, any indication of impropriety must be avoided.

Written communication should follow guidelines similar to those listed for verbal communication. It should be brief, concise, and specific and should use language the reader will be most likely to understand. The guidelines previously given for the development of home programs are applicable here. Typed or printed instructions are more easily read than handwritten ones. Diagrams, drawings, or photographs are extremely useful to show specific positions or the sequence of movements. Films, videotapes, and slides are other forms of communication that can be useful to educate or instruct a patient or the family.

Box 1-6 Barriers to Effective Communication

Distance between the sender and receiver; excessive distance decreases effectiveness.
Noise and environmental confusion interfere with and may distort the message.
Inability of the receiver to comprehend the message.
Inability of the receiver to interpret or understand technical, medical, and professional terms, language, or abbreviations.
Inadequate amount of feedback occurs between the receiver and sender.
Complex messages may be difficult to interpret and comprehend.
Sender and receiver may interpret the message differently.
Cultural, gender, or age differences between the sender and receiver may affect the interpretation or comprehension of the message.
Illegible writing affects the accuracy and comprehension of the message.

The use of consistent language and the manner in which oral or written instructions or directions are given to a patient should enhance the patient's level of understanding and capacity to learn. This concept is particularly important when complex activities are being taught and when a patient's mental capacities have been altered. Repetition and practice of activities that require motor control or coordination usually will enhance the patient's skill and ensure a safer performance. A complex activity should be performed consistently in the same or a very similar manner, regardless of the person assisting or guiding the patient.

There are many barriers that can adversely affect verbal and NVC between a caregiver and the patient. A noisy treatment area, an excessive distance between the two persons, distractions in the treatment area, the language used by the caregiver (that is, technical language instead of lay language), the position of furniture or equipment and of the persons who are communicating, the time available to communicate, and the individual values or biases of each person are some examples of deterrents and potential barriers to verbal and NVC. The astute caregiver will be aware of and be able to identify these factors and avoid, eliminate, or reduce them. This awareness and the subsequent action to overcome these conditions or factors are important keys to effective communication (Box 1-6).

Being an attentive listener is another communication skill the caregiver should develop. Evaluating the patient's tone of voice; observing the nonverbal cues provided by listening for the main theme of the message; focusing on the content of the message rather than on the way the message is communicated; and providing verbal feedback to clarify understanding of the message are examples of being an attentive listener. This aspect of communication may be overlooked or slighted by the caregiver and the result may be a loss of information.

COMMUNICATING WITH A PERSON WITH A DISABILITY

Caregivers must become aware of their responsibility to communicate appropriately with a person with a disability. You should first and foremost maintain the person's self-esteem by considering the person first in your words and thoughts. The person's disability should be described accurately, if it needs to be included in the message, but it is more important to emphasize the person's abilities rather than disability. For example, the statement "John, who has a spinal cord injury, uses a wheelchair for mobility" is more appropriate than "Because he has a broken back, John is confined to a wheelchair." The use of the term "person with a disability" is preferable to the term "disabled person" to promote the person's self-esteem and recognition as a person first.

Some suggestions to improve your communications with persons with disabilities are in Box 1-7. You should speak directly with the person rather than with a companion and should be prepared to shake hands. In some instances you may need to grasp the person's forearm or use your left hand rather than your right hand as you meet or greet the person. *Note:* some cultures may not permit the use of a handshake as a means of greeting and some cultures may use variations of the traditional handshake as their form of greeting.

Box 1-7 Guidelines for Communicating with Persons with Disabilities

- Speak and interact directly with the person with the disability.
- Greet the person as you would greet persons without a disability; shake hands or forearm or use your left hand as appropriate.
- Identify yourself and other persons in a group to the person who is visually impaired.
- Stoop or squat to communicate with a person in a wheelchair; position yourself in front and at eye level.
- Avoid leaning or sitting on a person's wheelchair; use care when handling assistive aids.
- Avoid statements, gestures, or actions that patronize; interact in the same manner you would interact with persons who do not have a disability.
- Tactilely or visually cue the person who is hearing impaired to indicate your presence.
- Be patient and listen carefully when interacting with a person who has difficulty speaking; use questions that require brief responses.
- Determine whether the person desires assistance before assisting him or her; wait for instructions.

The person who is visually impaired will appreciate knowing who is speaking, so you should identify yourself, similar to the way in which you identify yourself when using a telephone. It will be necessary to identify each individual in a group and each individual should identify himself or herself when speaking. Remember it is not necessary to increase the volume of your voice when speaking with a person who is visually impaired. When speaking with a person who is seated, stoop or squat and position yourself in front of and at eye level with the person.

A person who is hearing impaired will need to have tactile (touch, tap) or visual (hand wave, gesture) cueing from you before you begin speaking. If the person is able to lip read, you should stand so that the person can see your lips clearly, speak slowly, and enunciate carefully. Some hearing impaired may communicate using sign language (Fig. 1-2). Again, increasing the volume of your voice is unnecessary in most communication situations.

When you communicate with a person who has difficulty speaking, intensify your listening skills and provide feedback to the individual to indicate your understanding of the message. Avoid correcting, interrupting, anticipating what the person will be said, or speaking for him or her. Be patient during the conversation and wait for confirmation

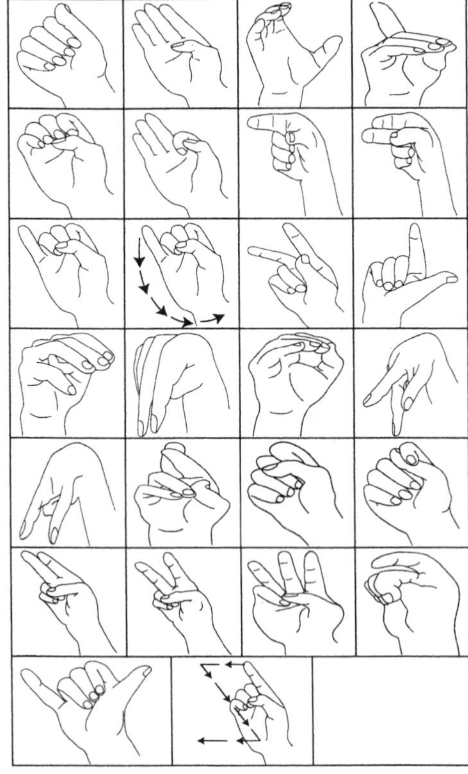

Fig. 1-2 American Hand Alphabet for the Deaf. (Courtesy of the Deaf Services Center, Worthington, OH, 2001.)

of your feedback before continuing. The use of questions that require brief responses or that can be answered by a head nod or shake may assist this person. At times you may sense or realize that a person with a disability will require assistance to perform a task or activity. When this occurs, you should ask the person whether assistance is desired and, if it is desired, ask for specific instructions or directions.

Occasionally, even the experienced caregiver may feel awkward or embarrassed when communicating with a person with a disability, especially if an expression related to the disability is used during the conversation. Examples are "I am looking forward to seeing you again," "I'll see you later," "Did you hear about the big fire?" and "Let's go over the plan one step at time." In most instances the person with a disability will recognize these statements as expressions and components of the usual communication pattern, so there is no need to apologize or bring attention to the statement, but you may want to consider how you can limit the use of these expressions and others in the future. You should avoid the use of terms such as "victim," "stricken," and "afflicted" because they tend to indicate an unhealthy status.

Being aware of and applying these suggestions will enable you to communicate with persons with a disability appropriately, to maintain their self-esteem, and to recognize them as persons with abilities rather than to stereotype them as being "disabled."

Communication between the caregiver and the patient is a critical aspect of patient care. The caregiver will be challenged to be aware of the importance of communication and to make every effort to communicate effectively. This can be accomplished through proper use of verbal, nonverbal, visual, and written communication.

SAFETY CONSIDERATIONS

The caregiver bears primary responsibility for the safety of each patient, regardless of the treatment provided and, in some situations, who provides it. Patient transfers, changes in position, exercise activities, and the transport of equipment or patients have the potential to cause injury; therefore the caregiver must maintain a safe environment and equipment that functions properly. Family members must be instructed how to assist the patient safely and should be informed of any specific precautions related to the patient's care. The patient also has to assume some responsibility to maintain personal safety. Proper hygiene, skin care, changes in position, proper handling techniques, bowel and bladder management procedures, and transfer patterns may have to be performed or directed by the patient. The patient frequently knows what is the best approach and the caregiver should listen and follow the patient's suggestions if they are reasonable and safe. Patients must be informed that they share responsibility for their health and safety within the limitations of their condition and abilities.

Incidents leading to patient injuries can be linked to the use of improperly functioning or poorly maintained equipment, a physical setting with hazardous obstacles or congested space, an excessive number of patients in the treatment area in relation to the personnel available to treat them, and the limited availability of personnel (as in the early morning or late afternoon or during lunch). In addition, information about the various products used for treatment and equipment maintenance should be maintained in a notebook or manual (that is, Material Safety Data Sheets Manual [MSDS] for easy reference and review) (Fig. 1-3). The caregiver should be especially alert when treating a patient who is elderly, debilitated, or mentally disoriented; who is very young or has decreased mental capacity or a decreased physiologic status (such as open burns or wounds, spinal cord injury, diabetes, or cardiopulmonary deficits); or who is emotionally disturbed.

An elderly patient may experience physiologic changes that could adversely affect tolerance and ability to perform various tasks or activities. A listing of some of the common changes that occur as a result of the aging process appear in Table 1-4. It should be noted that, except for changes in vision, auditory acuity, mental capacity and tactile sense, physiologic changes may also occur in a younger person who has been immobilized for a prolonged period.

During the examination and evaluation process, the caregiver should determine which if any of these changes have occurred and what effect they could have on the patient's ability to function and tolerate treatment. Activities that place the patient at risk such as transfers, ambulation, bed positioning, and many types of exercise should be performed cautiously. Decreased bone density can be a precursor for a fracture during transfers and ambulation and decreased skin integrity may lead to skin tears during transfers, bed positioning, or exercise. The patient may need to be taught to use visual cues to compensate for the loss of *proprioception*, or kinesthetic sense. The reader is encouraged to

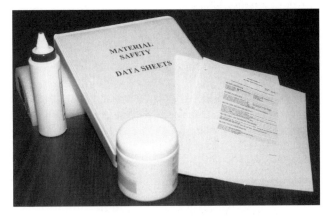

Fig. 1-3 Material Safety Data Sheets manual.

Table 1-4 Physiologic Changes Associated with Aging

Physiologic Change	Potential Problem or Deficit
Decreased skin integrity	Skin tears; poor wound healing
Loss of bone density	Fractures, especially long bones
Decreased strength	Difficulty performing motor task
Decreased physical condition	Cardiopulmonary or cardiovascular systems may not respond adequately
Decreased muscle and connective tissue elasticity	Contractures; difficulty performing daily activities
Altered visual acuity	Falls; difficulty with tasks requiring visual input
Altered hearing acuity	Difficulty with tasks requiring auditory input
Decreased balance	Falls; difficulty maintaining safe sitting, standing, or walking activities
Altered proprioception	Falls; difficulty performing motor tasks, especially ambulation
Altered kinesthesia	Falls; difficulty performing motor tasks, especially ambulation
Altered mental capacity	Difficulty with comprehension of written, oral, or visual instructions
Decreased tactile sense	Burns; lacerations; difficulty differentiating objects or materials by touch

Box 1-8 Safety Recommendations

Wash your hands before and after treating each patient to reduce cross-contamination and transmission of disease. This is the single-most important activity to prevent the spread of infection.

Maintain sufficient space to maneuver equipment or perform a task. Store equipment that is not in use so it will not interfere with patient care. Position a patient so he or she is not at risk of being struck by passing personnel or equipment.

Do not perform transfers or ambulation in an area where your view is obstructed, such as near a door or the corner of a hallway, or where space is inadequate or too congested for the activity.

Routinely evaluate equipment and be certain it functions properly; establish a maintenance program for each item.

Position equipment, furniture, and assistive aids so the items are stable, secure, and accessible when they are being used. Remove them when they are not in use so they do not interfere with patient and caregiver movements.

Keep the floor clear of electric cords, litter, loose rugs or floor mats, water, dirt, and other similar hazards.

Do not leave patients unattended, especially if they are compromised physiologically or mentally.

Protect the patient with safety straps, bed rails, or similar items when they are not closely attended, according to established agency, regulatory body, and state or federal restrictions and guidelines.

Obtain the equipment and supplies needed and prepare the treatment area before the patient arrives to avoid the need to leave the patient unattended.

Be certain the personnel who provide patient care are trained, qualified, and competent in their assigned duties.

Avoid storing potentially hazardous equipment or materials in a location where they are hidden from view or where there is a risk of a patient obtaining them. Do not store chemicals or heavy objects on a shelf above shoulder level. Clearly label the contents and weight of boxes or other containers.

consider other problems that may arise for the elderly patient who exhibits any of the changes presented. Furthermore, protective, preventive, or compensatory actions that could be taken to reduce the possibility of injury to the patient should be considered and performed.

A patient with one or more of these conditions may experience difficulty tolerating the treatment or may be more easily injured than other patients. The prudent caregiver will consider all the information related to the patient and will modify or revise the patient's treatment to reduce the likelihood of injury. The caregiver should also be aware of the need for safety and should follow established guidelines regarding body mechanics and personal health as described in Chapter 4. Some recommendations for promoting safety are listed in Box 1-8.

Accidents and subsequent injuries tend to occur when health care personnel or family members are careless, inadequately trained, inattentive, or excessively busy. Additional information and suggestions regarding patient safety are contained in the chapters on transfers (Chapter 7), ambulation (Chapter 9), and infection control (Chapter 2).

SUMMARY

It is important to inform the patient of the planned treatment and about the responsibilities or participation in the activity. The explanation should contain the anticipated or desired results or outcomes of the treatment and any potential adverse effects. The patient should have the opportunity to consent to or reject treatment based on the receipt of sufficient information to make an informed decision. The presence of the patient in the treatment area should not be assumed to be an expression of his or her consent for treatment.

A patient management process is necessary to examine and evaluate the patient, develop a clinical diagnosis and prognosis, establish a plan of care, and implement the plan. Before treating a patient, the caregiver should perform proper hand-washing techniques to reduce the transmission of pathogens from one person to another. Documentation of the examination and evaluation information and data, plan of care, and treatment goals or outcomes is necessary to provide a written record of the treatment given and the results attained by the patient and to aid in reimbursement for the services rendered by the caregiver. For many patients, it may be necessary to educate the family or other persons about further treatment or care and a home program may be prepared.

Communication between the caregiver and each patient can be improved if the caregiver reduces or avoids certain communication barriers and develops the skills associated with being an attentive listener.

The safety of the patient must be the priority of all persons involved in all treatment activities performed. The responsibility for patient safety remains with the primary caregiver, even when the patient is treated by supportive personnel whom the caregiver supervises. An important activity related to patient safety is the use of proper and frequent hand-washing techniques.

self-study ACTIVITIES

- Describe the criteria associated with short- and long-term goals.
- Describe at least three reasons a patient's family members may need to be educated by a primary caregiver and provide the rationale for each reason.
- Explain the types of communication you would use to instruct a patient to ambulate with crutches, perform a standing assisted transfer, instruct a family member to guard a patient who uses crutches, and perform active assistive exercise.
- List at least four factors you should consider related to the general aspects of patient safety.
- Explain why it is important and necessary to evaluate or assess each patient before beginning treatment or developing a treatment plan.
- Describe how each examination and evaluation component may assist you to make decisions or resolve clinical problems about the plan of care you develop with the patient.
- Explain why it is important to develop a treatment plan with the patient rather than for the patient.

problem SOLVING

1. A 43-year-old female has sustained a fracture of her right distal tibia and comes to the department directly from the emergency room. Orders are for gait training with crutches, without weight bearing on the right lower extremity. What questions would be appropriate to ask the patient concerning her home environment and what would be your discharge goals?
2. You have an inpatient in the hospital who has just refused treatment from you. What documentation in the medical record should be considered?
3. You are the moderator in a meeting with three persons; one has a severe hearing deficit, another has a severe visual deficit, and the third is in a wheelchair. How will you seat each person and what will you do to improve communications among the group members?
4. During your clinical education experience, you are treating four female patients with different cultural backgrounds: an African American, a Hispanic, a Japanese, and a Vietnamese. You are having difficulties interacting with each of them and they are not responding to your instructions and suggestions. What do you believe may be the cause for the difficulties and what will you do to improve the situation?

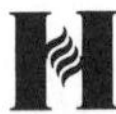

The Malden Hospital
OUTPATIENT PHYSICAL THERAPY INITIAL EVALUATION

Patient's Name:

Medical Record #:

D.O.B.:

Social History: (occupation, date out of work, support systems, cultural/spiritual . . .)

Prior Functional Status:

Hand Dominance: R/L

Barriers to Treatment: (cognitive/emotional, physical/developmental)
Resolution to Identified Barriers:
Do you feel safe at home? ❑ Yes ❑ No **If no, would you like to see a social worker?** ❑ Yes ❑ No

Past Medical History: Cancer Heart Disease Diabetes COPD HBP

Precautions/Vital Signs:	**Medications/Allergies:**
Date of Injury/Occurrence:	**Date of Surgery:**

History of Present Illness/Reason for Referral:

Prior Rehabilitation:	**Diagnostic Tests:**

Pain Assessment:

CONSTANT/INTERMITTENT
NONE WORST
1 2 3 4 5 6 7 8 9 10

Signature: ______________________ Date: ______________ Time: _____:_____ AM PM

ME5139.08 p.1 12/98

Continued

Fig. Appendix 1 Outpatient Initial Evaluation. (From Chorzewski R, Dente E, Hansen C, Roberto M: *Outpatient Initial Evaluation Form.* The Malden Hospital, Malden, MA, Nov. 2000.)

The Malden Hospital
OUTPATIENT PHYSICAL THERAPY INITIAL EVALUATION

Patient's Name:

Medical Record #:

D.O.B.:

Posture ❑ WNL

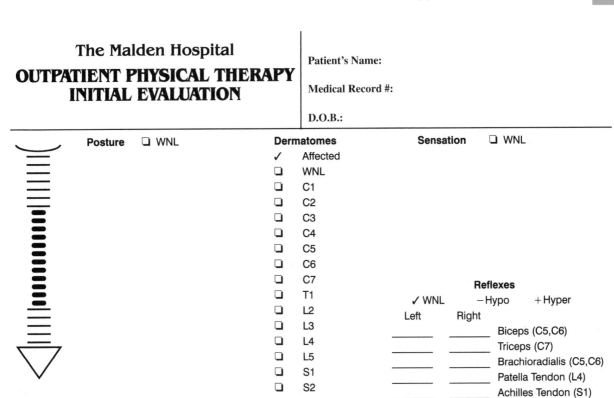

Dermatomes
✓ Affected
❑ WNL
❑ C1
❑ C2
❑ C3
❑ C4
❑ C5
❑ C6
❑ C7
❑ T1
❑ L2
❑ L3
❑ L4
❑ L5
❑ S1
❑ S2

Sensation ❑ WNL

Reflexes

✓ WNL −Hypo +Hyper

Left	Right	
______	______	Biceps (C5,C6)
______	______	Triceps (C7)
______	______	Brachioradialis (C5,C6)
______	______	Patella Tendon (L4)
______	______	Achilles Tendon (S1)

Active Movements (AM) ❑ N/A

Cervical **Lumbar**

FB
SBL SBR
RL RR
BB

FB
SBL SBR
RL RR
BB

Passive Intervertebral Movement (PIVM) ❑ N/A

Segment	FB	SBL	SBR	RL	RR	BB

AM Key:
End of ROM ●
Limited by Pain X
Deviation ➡

PIVM Mobility Key:
0 Ankylosed
1 Considerable Restriction
2 Slight Restriction
3 Normal
4 Slight Increase
5 Considerable Increase
6 Unstable

ROM and Strength ❑ WNL

	LEFT		RIGHT			LEFT		RIGHT	
SHOULDER	**A/PROM**	**MMT**	**A/PROM**	**MMT**	**HIP**	**A/PROM**	**MMT**	**A/PROM**	**MMT**
Flexion					Flexion				
Extension					Extension				
Internal Rot					Internal Rot				
External Rot					External Rot				
Abduction					Abduction				
Horiz Abduction					Adduction				
Horiz Adduction					**KNEE**				
ELBOW					Flexion				
Flexion					Extension				
Extension					**ANKLE**				
WRIST					Dorsiflexion				
Flexion					Plantarflexion				
Extension					Inversion				
Supination					Eversion				
Pronation					Ext. Hall. Long				
Grip					Flex. Hall. Long				

Signature: ______________________ Date: ______________ Time: _____:_____AM PM

ME5139.08 p.2 12/98

Continued

Fig. Appendix 1, cont'd For legend see p. 18.

The Malden Hospital
OUTPATIENT PHYSICAL THERAPY INITIAL EVALUATION

Patient's Name:

Medical Record #:

D.O.B.:

Palpation/Soft Tissue ❑ WNL

Joint Play ❑ WNL

Special Tests

Other ❑ N/A

EDUCATIONAL ASSESSMENT

1. Motivation Level - ❑ Eager ❑ Anxious ❑ Inquisitive ❑ Uncooperative ❑ Uninterested ❑ Denies need for ed.
2. Learning Style - ❑ Demonstration ❑ Visual / Written ❑ Auditory

Other: ____________________

Functional Mobility ❑ WNL

Balance ❑ WNL

Gait ❑ WNL Assistive Device: Stairs:

Gait Kinematics:

Girth/Edema ❑ N/A

	Left	Right

Signature: ____________________ Date: ____________ Time: ____:____ AM PM

ME5139.08 p.3 12/98

Fig. Appendix 1, cont'd For legend see p. 18.

The Malden Hospital

OUTPATIENT REHABILITATION INITIAL PLAN OF CARE

Patient's Name:

Medical Record #:

D.O.B.:

Problem List:

Functional LTG'S:_________Weeks

Functional STG'S: (2 Weeks):

Plan:

Frequency/Duration:

Assessment:

Patient/family stated goals/perception of treatment:
Rehabilitation potential: ❑ Excellent ❑ Good ❑ Fair ❑ Poor

Therapist's Signature/Date/Time

I have read/understand the attendance policy and my intended treatment plan and I agree to participate accordingly.

I certify that the outpatient services outlined above are required and are authorized by me with a written plan of treatment to be reviewed by me every 30 days. This patient is under my care and is in need of physical/occupational therapy.

Patient's Signature

MD'S Signature

ME 5139.08 p.4 12/98

Fig. Appendix 1, cont'd For legend see p. 18.

The Malden Hospital

Patient Home Exercise Program
Patient Education/Instruction
Family Education/Involvement

Patient's Name:

Medical Record #

D.O.B.:

Date Instructed	Date Independent	Home Exercise Program	Patient Education	Exercise/Patient Education	Handouts	Comments

ME5139.07 p.1 12/98

Fig. Appendix 2 Patient Home Exercise Program. (From Chorzewski R, Dente E, Hansen C, Roberto M: *Outpatient Initial Evaluation Form.* The Malden Hospital, Malden, MA, Nov. 2000.)

The Malden Hospital

Outpatient Physical Therapy Flowsheet

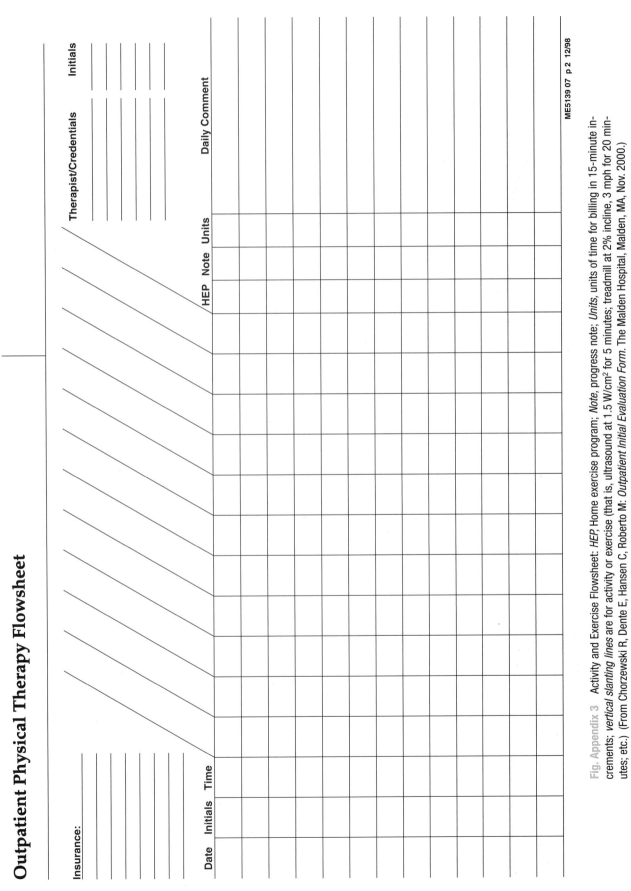

Insurance:

Therapist/Credentials	Initials

Date	Initials	Time												HEP	Note	Units	Daily Comment

ME5139 07 p 2 12/98

Fig. Appendix 3 Activity and Exercise Flowsheet: *HEP,* Home exercise program; *Note,* progress note; *Units,* units of time for billing in 15-minute increments; *vertical slanting lines* are for activity or exercise (that is, ultrasound at 1.5 W/cm^2 for 5 minutes; treadmill at 2% incline, 3 mph for 20 minutes; etc.) (From Chorzewski R, Dente E, Hansen C, Roberto M: *Outpatient Initial Evaluation Form.* The Malden Hospital, Malden, MA, Nov. 2000.)

The Malden Hospital
OUTPATIENT REHABILITATION
TWO WEEK REASSESSMENT

Patient's Name:

Medical Record #:

D.O.B.:

Room #: Allergies:

Current Treatment: See Treatment Flow Sheet for Specific Treatment Techniques

PROBLEM LIST

A/PROM:

Strength:

Soft Tissue Mobility/Integrity:

Pain/Tenderness:

Posture:

Other (SpecialTests):

Edema/Girth:

Home Exercise Program:

Gait:

Additions to Plan/Changes:

ADL's/Function:

Short Term Goals

Therapist:____________________ Date: __________ Time: _____:_____ AM PM

ME5139.06 12/98

Fig. Appendix 4 Two-Week Reassessment. (From Chorzewski R, Dente E, Hansen C, Roberto M: *Outpatient Initial Evaluation Form.* The Malden Hospital, Malden, MA, Nov. 2000.)

CHAPTER 2

Approaches to Infection Control

objectives *After studying this chapter, the reader will be able to:*

- Define asepsis, medical asepsis, surgical asepsis, and contamination.
- Describe and perform proper techniques of hand washing for clean and sterile situations.
- Describe and perform the proper application and removal of protective garments for clean and sterile situations.
- Explain the concept, use, and value of Standard and Transmission-Based Precautions.

key terms

Acquired Immunodeficiency Syndrome (AIDS) Acronym for acquired immune deficiency syndrome, which is caused by the human immunodeficiency virus (HIV).

Asepsis Absence of microorganisms that produce disease; the prevention of infection by maintaining a sterile condition.

Contamination When something is rendered unclean or unsterile; an item, surface, or field is considered to be contaminated whenever it has come into contact with anything that is not sterile.

Decontamination The use of physical or chemical means to remove, inactivate, or destroy bloodborne pathogens on a surface or item to the point where they are no longer capable of transmitting infectious particles and the surface or item is rendered safe for handling, use, or disposal.

Disinfection The destruction or removal of pathogenic organisms, but not necessarily their spores.

Hepatitis Inflammation of the liver.

Infection The production of a disease or harmful condition by the entrance of disease-producing germs into an organism.

Isolation Separation from others.

Medical asepsis Practices that help to reduce the number and spread of microorganisms.

Microorganism A tiny living animal or plant that can cause disease.

Nosocomial Pertaining to or originating in a hospital.

Pathogen A microorganism that produces disease.

Sepsis The presence of pathogenic microorganisms or their toxins in the blood or tissues.

Spore A hard, thick-walled capsule formed by some bacteria that contains only the essential parts of the protoplasm of the bacterial cell.

Sterile Containing no microorganisms; free from germs.

Sterilization A process by which all microorganisms, including spores, are destroyed.

Surgical asepsis Practices that render and keep objects and areas free of all microorganisms.

Wound A bodily injury caused by physical means, with disruption of the normal continuity of structures.

INTRODUCTION

The caregiver may be required to interact with patients who require care of open *wounds* or whose condition requires the use of medical or surgical aseptic techniques. You must remember that *microorganisms* are present on the skin, in the air, in patient wounds, and throughout the environment. Be aware of the process of *contamination* and *infection* so that you, the patient, and other persons or objects can be protected from *pathogen* microorganisms. This protection can be enhanced by the interruption of the cycle of infection.

Microorganisms move or are "communicated" or transmitted from place to place by various means in a cyclical manner. When this cycle is interrupted, the microorganism cannot grow, spread, and cause disease. This cyclic process includes a place where the microorganisms can grow and reproduce (that is, a host or reservoir). Examples of hosts are animals and human beings.

The microorganisms require a means by which they can leave the host (that is, exit the reservoir). Examples are a person's nose, mouth, throat, ear, eye, intestinal tract, urinary tract, multiple body fluids (especially blood), and wounds. Transmission of microorganisms from one person to another (that is, a vehicle of transmission) is necessary to spread the infection. Examples are the air, droplets of water (by a cough or sneeze), hands, equipment or mat pads, instruments (needles, scalpels, thermometers), eating utensils, linens, and body fluids such as blood, semen, saliva, and vaginal secretions.

To infect another person, the microorganism must be able to enter that person (that is, it must have a portal of entry). Examples of such portals are a break in the person's skin barrier, mucous membranes, mouth, nose, ears, and genitourinary tract. Finally, the person who receives the microorganisms must be susceptible to them (that is, be a susceptible host). An example of a susceptible host is a person whose body systems cannot destroy, repel, remove, or ward off the microorganisms (Box 2-1).

Some microorganisms are more difficult to destroy than are others and medications (such as, antibiotics) designed to kill or reduce the number of microorganisms are necessary to augment the protective actions of the body's systems. Some pathogens are totally resistant to medications or actions taken to reduce their numbers or prevent their growth. For example, up to now, no effective treatment (medication or vaccine) has been found to destroy or effectively reduce HIV, associated with *acquired immunodeficiency syndrome (AIDS)*.

Most microorganisms grow or proliferate best in a dark, warm, moist environment, and they are less likely to grow when they are exposed to a light, cool, dry, or extremely hot environment. Therefore steam, gas, ultraviolet rays, and dry heat are frequently used to sterilize contaminated objects. Some microorganisms require oxygen to support their growth, whereas others do not, and some produce cells called *spores* (such as anthrax, botulism, histoplasmosis). Because of the thick, hard protective walls of the spore, spores are very difficult to destroy, especially when they are located deep in a wound.

The caregiver has the responsibility to interrupt or establish barriers to the infection cycle at any stage of the process. Some barriers to infection are the use of proper hand-washing techniques, the wearing of gloves and other protective clothing, the proper removal and disposal of a contaminated dressing or bandage, and being aware of *isolation* techniques. It may not be possible nor will the objective be to completely eliminate all pathogens from an area or object to create *asepsis*. However, it is usually possible to affect the number of pathogens in an area so their concentration, influence, or capacity to create an infection is reduced by a person's immune system or by the use of medications designed to kill the remaining pathogenic microorganisms.

Box 2-1 Cycle of Cross-Contamination and Infection

Reservoir for organism and host:
(Person with staphylococcal infection)
↓
Method of exit for the organism:
(Draining wound)
↓
Method of transmission of the organism:
(Soiled dressings, exudate from the wound, soiled linen)
↓
Method of entry of the organism into a new host:
(Cut, abrasion, cuticle tear, or any break in the skin)
↓
Susceptible host:
(Person with low or limited systemic resistance to the organism)
↓
Infection develops in new host:
Barriers to interrupt the cycle include proper disposal of dressings and linen and use of standard precautions, protective clothing, gloves, and proper hand-washing techniques.

PRINCIPLES AND CONCEPTS

A caregiver may become involved in the management of wounds, with patients who have a transmissible infection, or with patients who must be protected from the environment to avoid becoming infected. Therefore he or she must understand how to protect the patient, other persons, and himself or herself from becoming contaminated or infected.

Current isolation precautions rely on the concepts of medical and *surgical asepsis* and how pathogens can be transmitted. The primary purpose of the precautions is to protect persons or objects from becoming contaminated or infected by pathogenic microorganisms. It is important that the caregiver understand the three most common means of transmission (contact, droplet, airborne) so quality care can be delivered and therapeutic procedures or activities can be applied safely.

Techniques of *medical asepsis* are designed to keep pathogens confined to a specific area, object, or person. Medical asepsis may involve isolation of a patient to protect health care workers, other patients, and other persons from the pathogenic microorganisms associated with the patient. For example, patients with tuberculosis, *hepatitis*, a staphylococcal or streptococcal infection, or another communicable or transmissible disease may be isolated in a private room. Specific care must be taken by persons who have contact with the patient, including contact with soiled dressings or articles of clothing, to reduce the possibility of becoming infected. The use of protective clothing by the caregiver will be necessary to protect the caregiver from the patient. Extreme care must be used when you remove protective clothing after treating a patient who is in isolation to reduce cross-contamination from the patient. This is referred to as a "clean approach."

Pathogens can be transmitted by coughing and sneezing and through body fluids such as tears, perspiration, urine, blood, semen, vaginal secretions, mucus, vomitus, and feces. The body has several means to provide barriers to pathogens or to rid the body of them. The primary barrier is the skin when it is intact. The skin is relatively impermeable to the absorption of external substances and to the loss of many body fluids. Cilia in the respiratory tract assist in filtering and trapping microorganisms to prevent them from entering deeply into the body. When these natural barriers are disrupted, protection is reduced, and the possibility of becoming infected is increased. Therefore when treating someone who has an infection or who is more likely to become infected, it is imperative to establish barriers other than the body's natural ones.

In the treatment area, general cleanliness of equipment, floors, and restrooms and proper control of heat, light, and air are important considerations. Proper disposal of soiled linen, gowns, protective garments (gloves, caps, masks), dressing material, bandages, and other disposable items is important. The use of appropriate techniques to maintain at least medical asepsis should be followed, especially hand-washing activities. Each employee should understand and adhere to practices and procedures that can be used to protect a specific patient, other patients, and persons such as visitors or employees, and the employee from infection or contamination.

CONTROL OF DISEASE IN THE HEALTH CARE ENVIRONMENT

There are many resources available to obtain information about the prevention of disease transmission and the spread of pathogenic microorganisms. Much of the information is not new, but in recent years a greater emphasis has been placed on the concept that each patient should be treated as if he or she had a transmissible or infectious disease. The spread of and serious consequences associated with AIDS, which is caused by HIV, and hepatitis, especially the type caused by the hepatitis B virus (HBV), have created the need for health care workers and others who may have close, personal contact with a person with one of these two diseases to use caution during contact. Both diseases are life threatening. Hepatitis B is more easily contracted, but can be prevented with a vaccine. Currently there is no vaccine to prevent or cure AIDS, but some drug regimens have demonstrated the ability to slow the disease process. Because these two life-threatening diseases have become more prevalent and are spread through contact with various body fluids, the emphasis on cleanliness and *sterile* techniques has increased. In 1985, the Centers for Disease Control and Prevention (CDC) recommended the use of Universal Precautions to protect health care workers and reduce the transmission of these diseases. Basically the precautions stated that gloves and other personal protective equipment should be used when there would be contact with any patient's blood or body fluid containing blood. The CDC now recommends the use of Standard Precautions by health care workers when they have contact with any patient's blood or body fluid, whether or not it contains blood, secretions, or excretions and Transmission-Based Precautions when in contact with special patients. The rationale for this concept is explained in greater detail in the Infection Control and Isolation Precautions sections of this chapter.

Some excellent and basic sources of information about infection control are the CDC; Occupational Safety and Health Administration (OSHA); Environmental Protection Agency (EPA); city, county, and state health departments; and the infection control department, or a similar department, of a local hospital. Furthermore, seminars and other types of continuing education programs, including hospital-based programs for employees regarding AIDS and hepatitis, are available to health care personnel. Many brochures, textbooks, pamphlets, newspapers, magazines, and visual aids contain information about these and other diseases; some of these sources are listed in the Bibliography.

Individual institutions and agencies have enacted policies and procedures to control the spread or transmission of infection and disease. The caregiver and all other persons who treat patients, handle soiled patient linen, remove wound dressings, or collect disposed items (that is, needles and other sharps) used to treat patients must become familiar with and adhere to established policies and procedures and develop proper personal habits for maximal protection.

Patients must be protected from *nosocomial* infections, which can be spread from patient to patient or to a given patient by a caregiver who is careless or does not follow accepted infection-control measures. Basic measures of prevention include frequent hand washings (before and after treatment of each patient), using proper hand-washing techniques, and the wearing of appropriate protective clothing such as gloves, gown, cap, and mask. A caregiver may try to avoid one or more of these measures because of a perceived lack of time; poor access to the items; poor location of the sink; a lack of proper-sized apparel; dermatitis as a result of frequent hand washing, a reaction to the available soap or detergent, or a reaction to latex gloves; a lack of understanding of the importance of using infection control methods for each patient; or poor motivation to comply with the policies and procedures for other reasons. Therefore it may be necessary for the employer or department supervisor to reduce as many of these factors as possible, whether they are real or perceived, to make it more convenient for the caregiver to comply with the policies and procedures.

HAND-WASHING TECHNIQUES

An especially important activity you, the caregiver, must perform before and after the treatment of each patient is to WASH YOUR HANDS. Frequent hand washing must become a habit for every caregiver to protect himself or herself and other persons and to reduce the spread of pathogens (Box 2-2). In addition, when wound care is part of the treatment, proper application and removal of protective garments and adherence to established infection control measures must be performed.

Faucet handles, towel dispensers, soap bars, and the edges and basins of sinks are considered contaminated, so avoid touching any of these items with your hands during the hand-washing process. Liquid soap that can be obtained from a hand- or foot-operated dispenser and disposable paper towels are recommended. In addition, water that splashes from the sink will contaminate your clothing. Remove jewelry, especially rings and bracelets, with stones or indentations before washing your hands and do not replace them until treatment has been completed. Females should avoid the use of false fingernails because they can harbor pathogens and cannot be cleaned satisfactorily with soap and water. Your hands will have the greatest protection from cross-contamination if access to the faucet and the water temperature controls can be accomplished with knee or foot controls. When it is necessary to use your hands to turn the water supply on and off, use a dry paper towel as a barrier between your hand and the faucet handle.

When liquid soap is used and is dispensed by a foot control or contained in an individual, one-time-use brush, greater protection against cross-contamination will be provided. Using a bar of soap that has been used by other persons increases the possibility of cross-contamination and should be avoided whenever possible. A suggested solution to this situation is to substitute liquid soap dispensers for bar soap. If these dispensers are operated by hand, the area you touch to release the soap or detergent should be considered contaminated. For self-protection, use a dry towel to operate the dispenser.

Be certain to properly care for your hands by washing them with water that is warm, not hot or cold. Dry your hands completely after each washing, apply a skin moisturizer occasionally during the day, and be cautious when you have torn cuticles, skin irritations, and other skin lesions.

Hand washing is used to remove or reduce the number of pathogenic microorganisms on the skin of your hands, wrists, and forearms. Many of these microorganisms may not be troublesome or dangerous to the person with an intact and fully functioning immune system and whose other barriers to infection function normally. However, these same microorganisms may produce an infection in a patient if they enter a wound, when the patient's immune system has been disrupted, or when the patient's condition is a debilitating one. The caregiver may transmit pathogenic microorganisms obtained from one patient to another patient with the hands, causing an infection to develop in the second patient. This is one example of how a nosocomial infection can be transmitted. Other methods include soiled linen or clothing; air movement or circulation; improperly cleansed eating utensils, instruments, or equipment; and through moisture droplets.

Box 2-2 Criteria for Hand Washing

- Before and after patient contact
- Before and after contact with wounds, dressings, specimens, bed linen, and protective clothing
- After contact with secretions or excretions
- Before and after toileting
- After sneezing, coughing, or nose blowing
- After removing gloves
- Before and after eating

Friction is a very important component of hand washing and is used to cleanse the creases and wrinkles of the fingers and loosen soil and pathogens that have collected on the skin. The use of a brush to cleanse the wrinkles and creases of your knuckles is recommended before you treat a patient who is highly susceptible to infection and as a part of surgical asepsis. A disposable wooden probe, or "orange stick," can be used to clean under the fingernails.

Various types of soap or detergent may be used as a cleanser. In some settings an antimicrobial or germicidal agent (that is, 2% chlorhexidine gluconate [CHG]) may be added to the cleansing medium, but these additives may produce an allergic skin reaction on some people's hands. The lather produced by the cleansing medium helps to lift the soil and microorganisms from the skin and hold them in the lather so they will be removed when you rinse your hands.

The principle regarding hand washing is to wash your hands before and immediately after treatment of a patient. The more likely it is that the patient is contaminated or has an infection, the more important it is that you wash your hands before and after providing treatment. If the caregiver's hands are not soiled grossly from contact with the patient it may be acceptable to perform a handrub, using a hand-sanitizing product rather than performing hand washing. These products contain a high concentration of ethyl alcohol with an emollient and are highly effective as antiseptic solutions. A potential disadvantage of these products is they may cause more skin dryness than when soap and water are used. When a hand cream is used to replenish moisture to the skin, care must be taken because the dispenser may become contaminated and pathogens can be transported in the hand cream. When you are required to expose a wound or change a dressing, you should apply gloves after you wash your hands and then wash your hands after the gloves are removed. You should also avoid placing your fingers in your nose, eyes, ears, or mouth after patient care. It is also important to perform hand washing after toileting.

There are several techniques that can be used to wash your hands. Regardless of the method you use, it is important to cleanse your hands thoroughly and frequently (Procedures 2-1 and 2-2). Avoid touching any potentially contaminated surface during or at the conclusion of the hand-washing process. If gloves and other protective clothing are to be applied, they should be applied at this time.

PROCEDURE 2-1

Hand Washing for Medical Asepsis

1. Remove all jewelry (an exception may be made for a smooth, band-type ring); approach the wash area, but avoid touching the sink and other nearby objects with your clothing or hands.
2. Turn on the water and mix it to a warm temperature to allow the soap to lather easily and to cause the least harm to your skin.
3. Wet your wrists and hands with your fingers directed downward, but do not touch the sink rim or basin.
4. Apply the soap and begin to wash your hands using friction and rotatory or rubbing motions (Fig. 2-1, *A* and *B*).
5. Wash for at least 30 seconds; wash longer if you have treated a patient known to have an infection.
   a. Wash the palm and dorsum of each hand at least 10 seconds each, using friction and rotatory motions.
   b. Interlace your fingers and wash between them for at least 10 seconds, being certain to wash the web or interspace between each finger (Fig. 2-1, *C*).
   c. Use a soft brush to wash the creases of each finger and its cuticle and under the fingernails, or you may use a pointed, disposable wood probe ("orange stick") to clean under each fingernail, discarding the probe after use (Fig. 2-1, *D* and *E*).

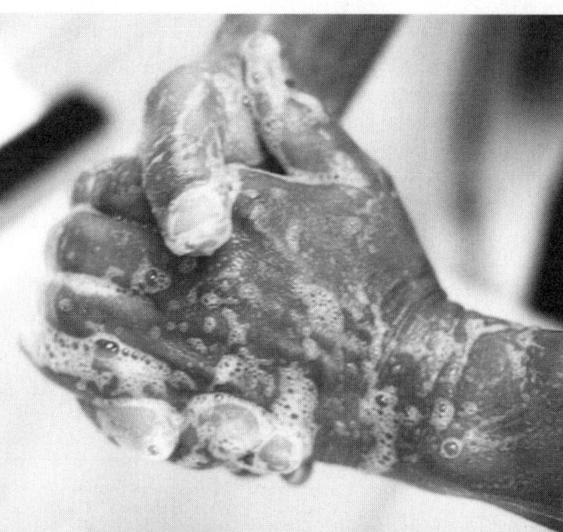

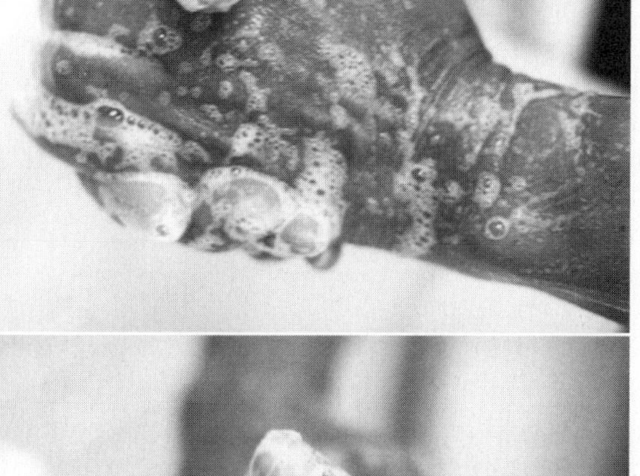

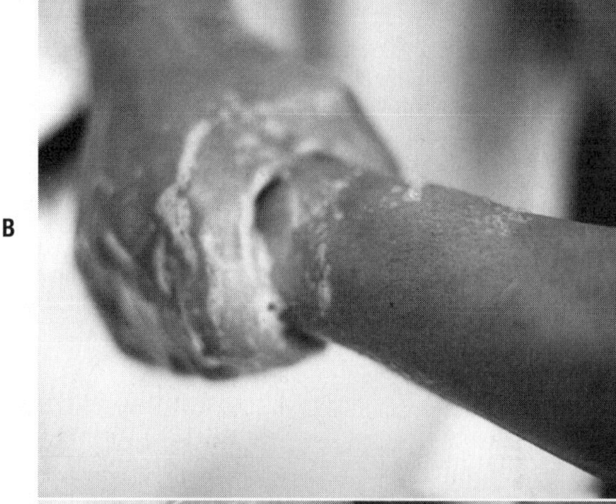

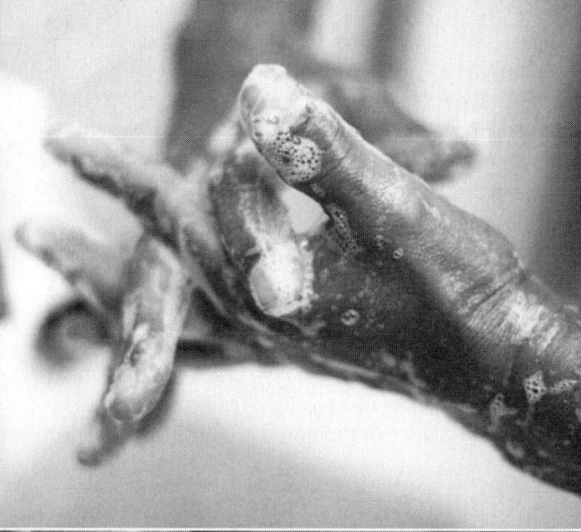

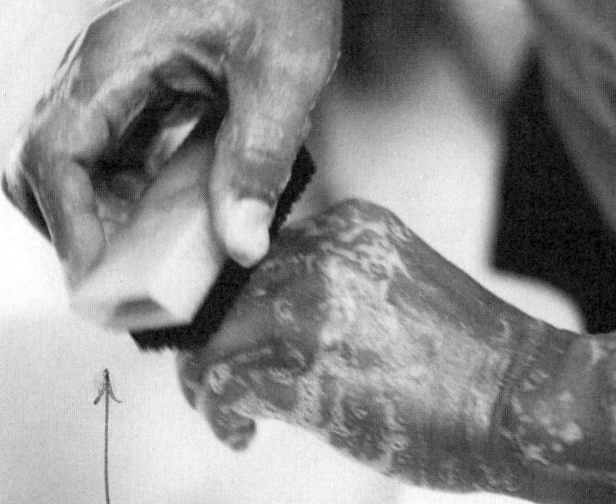

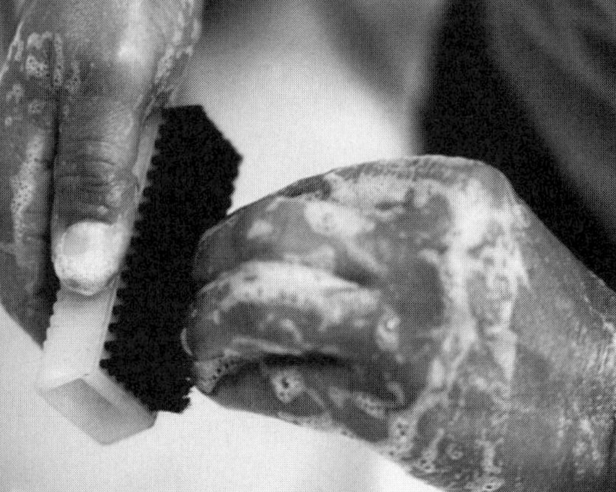

FIG. 2-1 Hand washing for medical asepsis.

where does one get the brush? Is it sanitary?

Continued

PROCEDURE 2-1

Hand Washing for Medical Asepsis—cont'd

d. Wash your wrist and the lower 2 to 3 inches of the distal end of your forearm using friction and rotatory motions.

6. Rinse your hands from the wrist to the fingers with the fingers directed downward, but do not rinse the area of skin proximal to where it was washed. If you have just treated a patient or removed a dressing from a patient with a known infection, wash your wrist and lower forearm again for 30 seconds and rinse as described previously; repeat steps 4 through 7 for a total of approximately 60 seconds and do a final rinse as described previously (Fig. 2-1, *F*).
7. Dry your hands thoroughly with a disposable towel. (The towel may be paper or cloth, but must be disposed of after use.) Allow the water to flow from the tap as you dry your hands. Use a dry paper or cloth towel to turn off a hand-operated faucet and then discard all towels in an appropriate container.

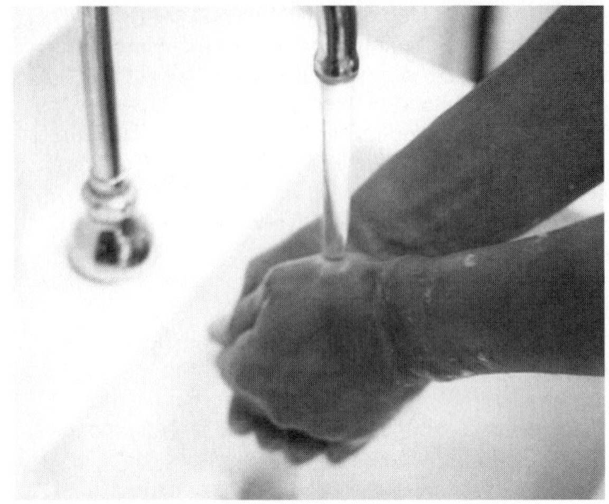
F

PROCEDURE 2-2

Hand Washing for Surgical Asepsis

1. Remove all jewelry from your hands, neck, and ears and approach the wash area with your arms exposed to approximately 3 inches above the elbow. Avoid touching the sink and other nearby objects with your clothing or hands.
2. Turn on the water and mix it to a warm temperature; follow the directions given previously for turning on the water if the faucet is hand operated.
3. Wet your hands and apply the soap or detergent according to the previous directions.
4. Wash your hands as outlined for medical asepsis, except that you will have to wash your entire forearm to approximately 3 inches above your elbow. This process will require approximately 7 minutes (Fig. 2-2, *A*).
5. Rinse your hands by holding them with your fingers upward so that the rinse water flows from a clean to an unclean area (that is, from your fingers to your elbows). Do not allow your hands, forearms, or upper arms to contact the sink or your body (Fig. 2-2, *B*).
6. Clean your fingernails, cuticles, and skin creases with a brush using vigorous strokes; you may use a pointed, disposable wood probe ("orange stick") to clean under each fingernail, discarding the probe after use.
7. Perform a final rinse with your hands directed upward (Fig. 2-2, *C*).

A
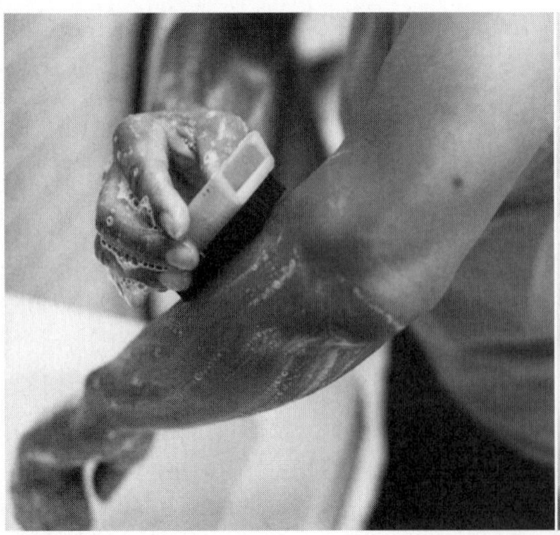

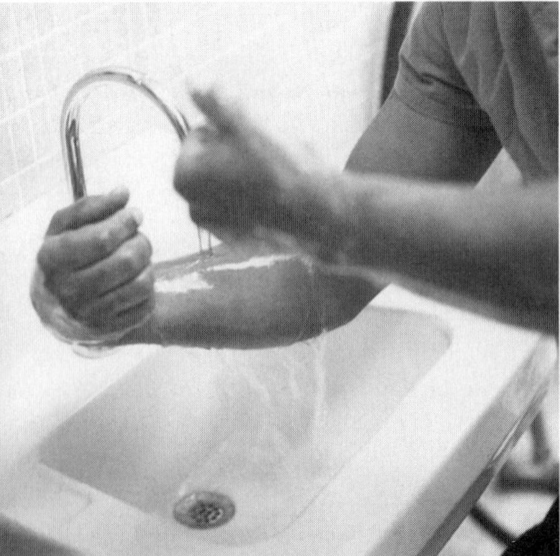
B

Fig. 2-2 Hand washing for surgical asepsis.

PROCEDURE 2-2

Hand Washing for Surgical Asepsis—cont'd

8. Dry your hands, forearms, and the distal area of your upper arms thoroughly using a sterile towel or air dryer. Avoid contact between the towel and your clothing and between your washed skin and your clothing or other nonsterile areas. Wrap your hands and forearms in a dry, sterile towel before applying protective clothing or gloves; hold your hands above waist level and slightly away from your body until you begin your treatment or patient care activities.

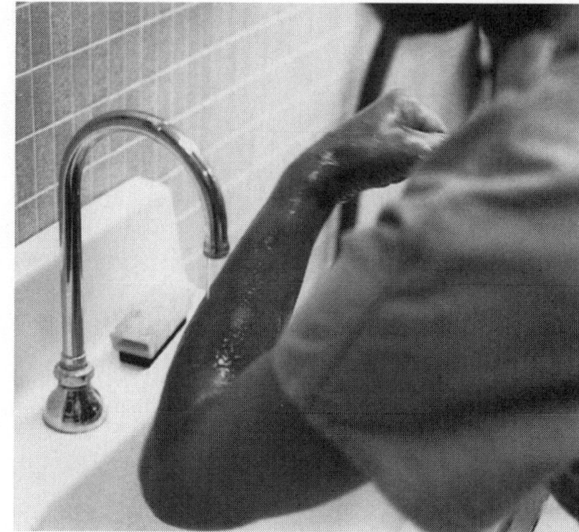

C

Box 2-3 Standard Precautions

Standard Precautions represent a system of infection control in which it is assumed that every direct contact with a patient's body fluids is potentially infectious.

Barriers
- Gloves
- Protective clothing
- Eye protection
- Face shield
- Mask
- Mouthpiece, intubation device, resuscitation bag during cardiopulmonary resuscitation (CPR)

Hand care
- Avoid wearing artificial fingernails; they may separate from the real nail, producing a pocket for pathogen growth.
- Always wear gloves when treating a patient who places you at risk to contact a body fluid, especially blood; avoid contact with the outer surface of the gloves when they are removed.
- Thoroughly wash your hands before and after patient care, especially if your hands were in contact with a body fluid.

Sharps (needles, scalpel blades)
- Dispose all sharps in a puncture-proof container immediately after their use.
- Do not uncap or expose needles until they are needed.
- Use caution when you handle and dispose of the item to avoid wounding yourself.

Miscellaneous
- Avoid eating, drinking, smoking, applying cosmetics or lip balm, and handling contact lenses in a patient care area.
- Avoid hand contact with mucous membranes of your eyes, nose, mouth, or ears.
- Handle all linen carefully, especially linen soiled by a patient's body fluid or waste; dispose and transport it in the proper bag, hamper, or container.
- Avoid unnecessary contact with a patient who places you at risk to contact a body fluid or waste product, especially the blood.
- Report incidents of contact with a patient's body fluid or waste product on an unprotected area of your body; seek immediate assistance if a direct blood-to-blood contact occurs between you and a patient.

Infection Control

The CDC has revised the previous information about the use of Universal Precautions and has developed a two-tiered approach to infection and isolation precautions termed "Standard Precautions and Transmission-Based Precautions."

The more important of the two approaches are the Standard Precautions, which are designed to protect health care workers and patients in a hospital regardless of their diagnosis or infection status; these precautions are considered to be the best means to control nosocomial infections. These precautions apply to blood; all body fluids, secretions, and excretions except sweat, regardless whether they contain visible blood; nonintact skin; and mucous membranes. Standard Precautions synthesizes the major components associated with Universal Precautions and applies to all bodily fluids, secretions, and excretions of any patient. Use of these precautions decreases the risk of transmission of pathogens from moist body substances and protects against the transmission of undiagnosed and diagnosed infections (Box 2-3).

The Transmission-Based Precautions are designed to protect the caregiver from specialized patients with highly transmissible pathogens who are known or suspected to be infected by epidemiologically important pathogens that can be spread by direct contact with dry skin or contaminated surfaces, droplets of moisture, or airborne particles.

The caregiver must follow proper infection control procedures, which include hand washing; using gloves or a gown when in contact with blood, body fluids, secretions, and excretions; contaminated patient's skin or linen and personal items; and using a mask, eye protection, or shield when fluid sprays or splashes are anticipated.

ISOLATION PRECAUTIONS

Current isolation precaution guidelines are linked to the method by which pathogens are transmitted and hence are termed "Transmission-Based Precautions." This system relies on the concepts and principles associated with medical and surgical asepsis to protect a person or object from becoming contaminated or infected by transmissible pathogens.

A patient may be isolated from other patients and the hospital environment because he or she has a disease or infection that is transmissible. The person may be placed in a private room with another patient with the same disease. When the person is in isolation, specific actions designed to interrupt the route of transmission of pathogens from the patient must be followed by any person who enters the patient's environment. The use of proper hand-washing techniques and the use of personal protective equipment (that is, gloves, gowns, mask) are precautions that are usually required. The specific barriers used to interrupt the route of transmission of pathogens will depend on the type of disease or infection and, most importantly, the mode of transmission of those pathogens associated with the disease or infection.

Three factors are involved with the use of isolation precautions: a source of the infecting microorganisms (patients, personnel, visitors), a susceptible host, and a means of transmission. The CDC guidelines for isolation precautions are designed so that the routes of transmission of the microorganisms are interrupted or blocked within the hospital. These recent guidelines eliminated the previous categories of isolation precautions (that is, strict isolation, contact isolation, respiratory isolation, tuberculosis isolation, enteric precautions, drainage and secretion precautions) and previous disease-specific precautions into three designations of precautions based on the route of transmission (that is, contact, droplet, airborne) for a smaller number of specified patients known or suspected to be infected or colonized with highly transmissible or epidemiologically important pathogens. These are known as Transmission-Based Precautions, as described previously. These precautions are to be used in addition to Standard Precautions dependent on the patient's known or suspected diagnosis (Box 2-4; Table 2-1).

There are five primary transmission routes: contact (directly with the host or indirectly with the host's linen, equipment); droplet (sneeze, cough, talking); airborne (evaporated droplet, dust particle); common vehicle (food, water, medications); and vector borne (mosquitoes, flies, rats). Diseases that can be transmitted airborne include measles, varicella, and tuberculosis. Droplet transmission conveys meningitis, influenza, streptococcal pharyngitis, and pneumonia. Infections of the skin, gastrointestinal tract, and wounds are most likely to be spread by direct or indirect contact, especially when body fluids, secretions, excretions, or blood are involved. Box 2-5 presents the activities that caregivers, other personnel, and, at times, visitors must perform to reduce the spread of infection in the hospital.

A cart containing protective garments, biohazard bags, and other materials should be located outside the patient's

Box 2-4 Transmission-Based Isolation Precautions

CONTACT PRECAUTIONS

Hands: Wash with CHG antiseptic soap upon leaving the room.
Gloves: Wear gloves upon entering the room.
Gown: Wear a gown when having direct contact with the patient, environmental surfaces, or patient items. Remove before leaving the room.
Room: Private or cohort
Dedicated Equipment: Patient care items (thermometer, stethoscope, blood pressure cuff) should remain in the room. If any item must be removed, it must be disinfected or placed in a bag labeled "biohazard."

DROPLET PRECAUTIONS

Hands: Wash thoroughly upon entering and leaving the room.
Mask: Required when working within 3 feet of the patient.
Room: Private
Patient Transport: Place a surgical mask on the patient if possible.

AIRBORNE PRECAUTIONS

Hands: Wash thoroughly upon entering and leaving the room.
Mask: An N-95 respirator (dust-mist respirator) must be worn when entering the room. It must fit snugly around the nose and face. Discard the mask upon leaving the room.
Room: Private room with negative air flow. Door must remain closed.
Patient Transport: Place surgical mask on the patient if possible.

Note: For each of these categories visitors are to report to Nurse's Station before entering the room. Permission granted to use this material by the Epidemiology Department of the Ohio State University Medical Center, Columbus, OH, April 2001.

Table 2-1 Isolation Precautions

Isolation Type	Common Clinical Syndromes	Room Assignment	Mask	Gown	Gloves	Patient Transport/ Discontinuing Isolation
Contact	MRSA VISA, VRE Aminoglycoside resistant Gram negatives Uncontrolled diarrhea *(Clostridium difficile),* lice, scabies, impetigo	Private room or cohort patient with same infection Dedicated equipment in the room	No	Yes, with direct contact with patient, environmental surfaces, or items in the patient's room	Yes CHG soap for hand washing	Minimize transport as feasible Clearing the patient from MRSA or VRE isolation should *not* be attempted if receiving antibiotics (that treat that infection) See specifics below for D/C of isolation*
Droplet	Mumps (rubella) *Neisseria meningitidis*	Private room; does *not* require negative air flow	Yes, when working within 3 feet of patient	No	No	Minimize transport of patient Mask patient when transport is necessary†
Airborne	Measles (pulmonary) Tuberculosis	Private room with negative air flow; keep door closed	Yes—Dust Mist Mask (N-95)	No	No	Minimize transport of patient Mask patient when transport is necessary‡
Airborne *plus* Contact	Chickenpox and disseminated herpes zoster in immunocompromised hosts	Private room with negative air flow; keep door closed	Yes—Dust Mist Mask (N-95)	Yes	Yes	Minimize transport of patient Mask patient when transport is necessary Continue for duration of illness

From Epidemiology Department. The Ohio State University Medical Center, Columbus, OH, 2001.

AFB, Acid-Free Bacillus; *MRSA*, Methicillin-Resistant Staphylococcus Aureus; *Mtb*, Myobacterium Tuberculosis; *VISA*, Vancomycin Intermediate Staphylococcus Aureus; *VRE*, Vancomycin-Resistant Entercoccus.

VRE, Discontinuation at the admission of initial diagnosis is discouraged; outpatient is preferred; 3 paired negative perirectal screens plus original site (if present or inguinal or axillary or umbilical areas); pairs should be obtained at least 7 days apart.

*MRSA, Three negative anterior nares screens *plus* original site (if present), obtained 24 hours apart.

†Isolation for *Neisseria meningitidis* may be discontinued after 24 hours of appropriate antibiotic therapy.

‡Isolation must be continued for Mtb until there are 3 negative AFB smears.

room so the items can be accessed before anyone enters the room. Containers for disposal of contaminated items should be located in the patient's room. The requirements for the amount and type of protection required for each category are listed on a color-coded card that is usually placed on the door or wall next to the patient's room (see Box 2-4). The medical record will indicate the isolation precautions in effect for the patient. Visitors of a patient who is in isolation will need to report to the Nurse's Station before entering the room. The caregiver must be aware of the means of transmission of various diseases or infections so that he or she will be able to protect the patient and himself or herself when working with the patient in an area other than the patient's room (that is, dialysis unit, rehabilitation unit or department, radiology unit, medical laboratory, patient's home). Consideration should be given to activities that may need to be performed before or after treatment (that is, cleansing of treatment and transportation equipment, separation of the patient from other persons, use of protective garments) when the patient is treated away from the room. In addition, it is important for the caregiver to know and understand the isolation system or precautions used in the facility so they are followed and the means of protection are used properly.

Occasionally, the term "protective isolation" may be used to designate a patient whose condition or disease causes a high risk of becoming infected through contact with another person. Patients with extensive open burns or wounds, a compromised immune system (that is, low white blood cell count), or a systemic infection (that is, *sepsis*) are examples of patients who may benefit from protective isolation. If this approach is used, it may be necessary for any person who enters the patient's room to apply protective garments to reduce or prevent the transmission of pathogens to the patient. The sequence and method for applying the garments are usually more important than the method and sequence used to remove them when the patient is in protective isolation. The sequence and method of application are described later in this chapter.

Box 2-5 Fundamentals of Infection Precautions

Proper hand-washing techniques and glove wearing
Use of masks, respiratory protection, eye protection, and eye shields (especially when fluid splashes or sprays are anticipated)
Use of gowns and protective apparel
Handling and disposal of linen and protection of laundry personnel
Cleaning or disposal of eating utensils and dishes
Patient placement (private room or with a person with the same disease)
Transportation of an infected patient
Use and care of patient care equipment and articles (disposal of sharps)
Routine and terminal cleaning of the patient's environment (use of disinfectants, consistent housekeeping activities in the patient's room and treatment areas)

APPLICATION OF PROTECTIVE GARMENTS

The caregiver may need to be protected from the patient, or the patient may have to be protected from the caregiver. In either situation, it is likely that protective clothing will be required. This section will describe a method that can be used to apply clothing before treatment of a patient who has been placed in protective isolation (Procedure 2-3) and a method that can be used to remove clothing after treatment of a patient who has been placed in isolation (Procedure 2-4). When the patient is in protective isola-tion, the garment-application sequence is extremely critical, but the garment-removal sequence is less critical. When the caregiver is to be protected from the patient, the garment-application sequence is less critical, but the garment-removal sequence is extremely critical.

Text continued on p. 41

PROCEDURE 2-3

Clothing Application for Protective Isolation

1. Wash your hands as described previously for medical asepsis.
2. Apply a cap, but avoid touching your hair as much as possible. Include all of your hair in the cap and, if possible, cover your ears (Fig. 2-3, *A* and *B*).
3. Apply a mask, handling it by its ties or edges. Position the metal or plastic band of the mask over your nose, or center the dome type of mask over your nose and mouth. Gently open the mask so that the bottom edge fits over your chin. Tie the upper ties snugly behind your head and above your ears; tie the lower ties snugly behind your neck. Avoid touching your neck or cap as you tie the mask. (*Note:* In some settings it may be preferred to apply the mask before the cap) (Fig. 2-3, *C* to *E*).
4. Open the outer package of a sterile disposable gown and the sterile gloves and place them on a table or counter in a sterile field at the approximate height of your waist. The inner cover of the gloves should remain closed (Fig. 2-3, *F* to *H*).
5. Wash your hands as described previously for surgical asepsis. (The medical asepsis technique may be acceptable for certain specific protocols.) Dry your hands thoroughly and avoid touching your clothing or other objects with the washed areas of your skin.

PROCEDURE 2-3

Clothing Application for Protective Isolation—cont'd

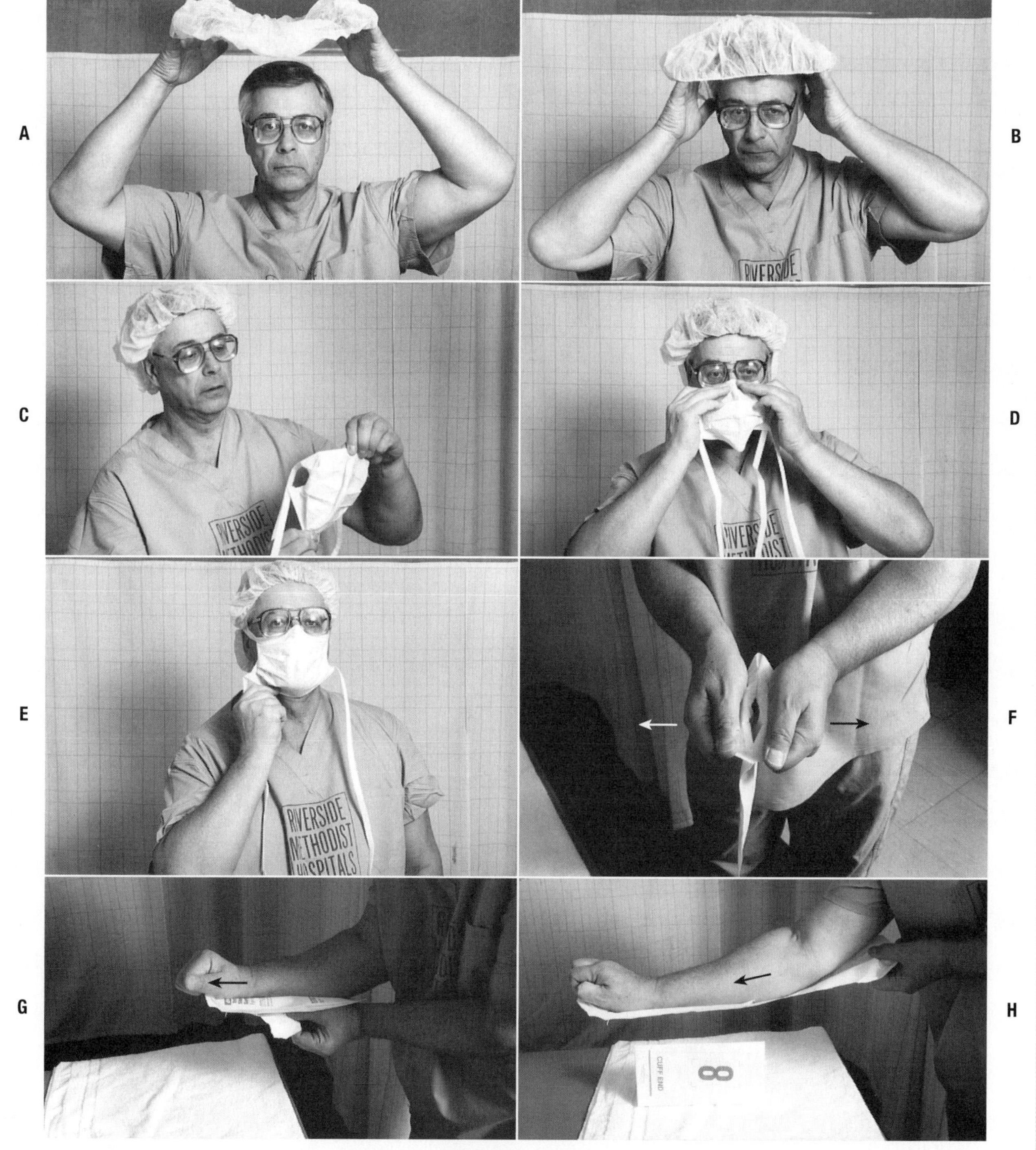

FIG. 2-3 Application of protective garments.

Continued

PROCEDURE 2-3

Clothing Application for Protective Isolation—cont'd

6. Grasp the center of the gown with one hand, pick it up, and allow it to unfold without touching your body, clothing, or any other object. The gown will be folded inside out and you should avoid touching the outside of the gown (Fig. 2-3, *I*).
7. Gently shake the gown so that it opens fully and insert your left or right hand and arm into the left or right sleeve; DO NOT ALLOW YOUR HAND TO EXTEND THROUGH THE GOWN CUFF; in this way a closed-glove technique can be used. Insert your other arm into the other sleeve and keep that hand inside the cuff (Fig. 2-3, *J* and *K*).
8. Request another person to tie the neck and waist ties snugly without touching the outside of the gown or the person's body. DO NOT ALLOW YOUR HANDS TO EXTEND THROUGH THE GOWN CUFFS when the gown is being tied (Fig. 2-3, *L* and *M*).

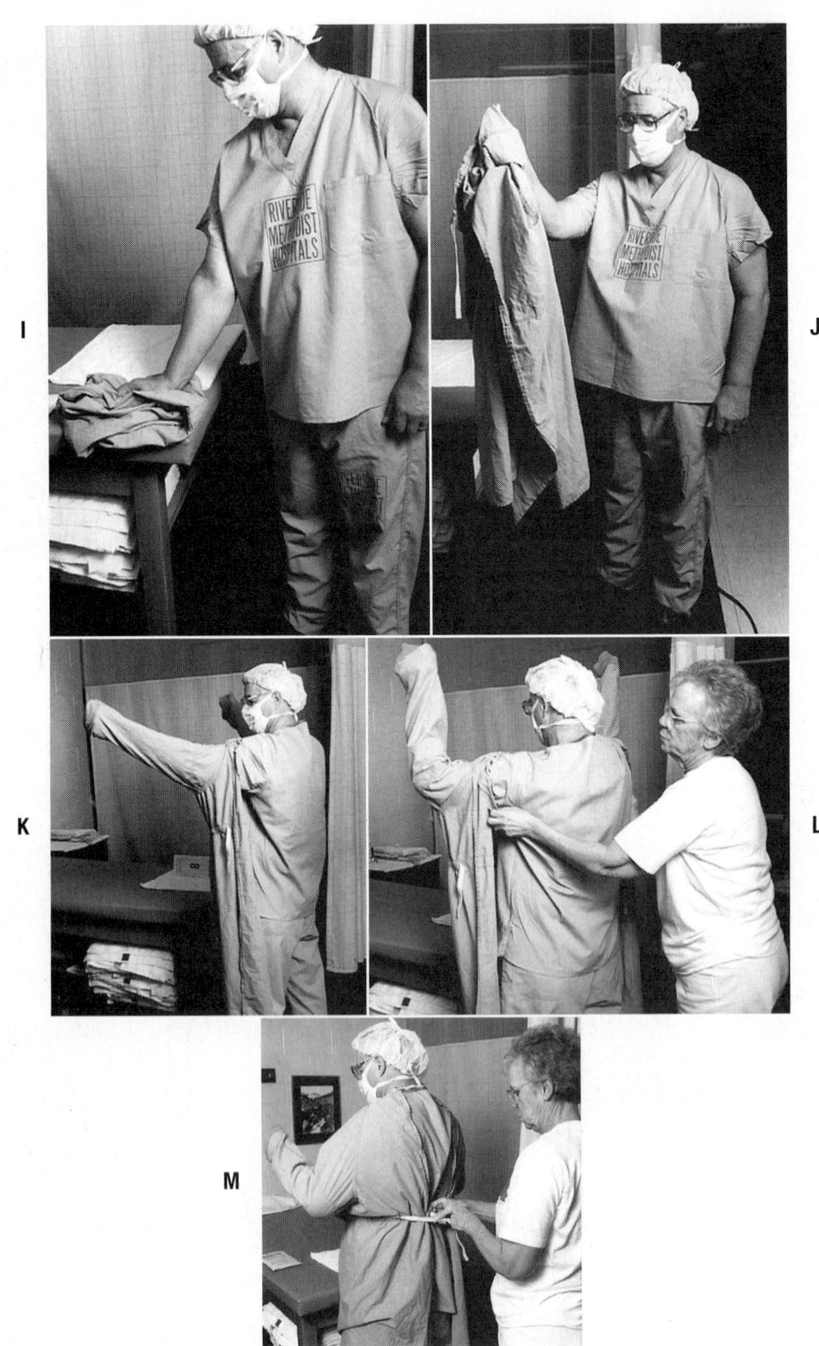

PROCEDURE 2-3

Clothing Application for Protective Isolation—cont'd

9. When a disposable gown is applied, with assistance from another person, care must be used to avoid contamination of the waist tie. Figure 2-3, *N* and *O*, shows proper handling of the tag of the tie so that the tie and gown remain sterile; the upper portion of the tag is sterile and the bottom portion is not.
10. Carefully open the inner packet containing your gloves and pick up one glove with your hand, which is still inside the gown cuff. Place the glove palm down on its proper hand, so that the thumb of the glove rests on the thumb of your hand and the fingers of the glove are directed toward your elbow (Fig. 2-3, *P* to *R*).
11. Grasp the cuff of the glove through the cuff of the gown and peel the cuff over your hand to seal or enclose your hand within the glove cuff and then gently maneuver your fingers and hand into the glove. Your other hand remains within the gown sleeve; do not extend it beyond the cuff (Fig. 2-3, *S* to *U*).

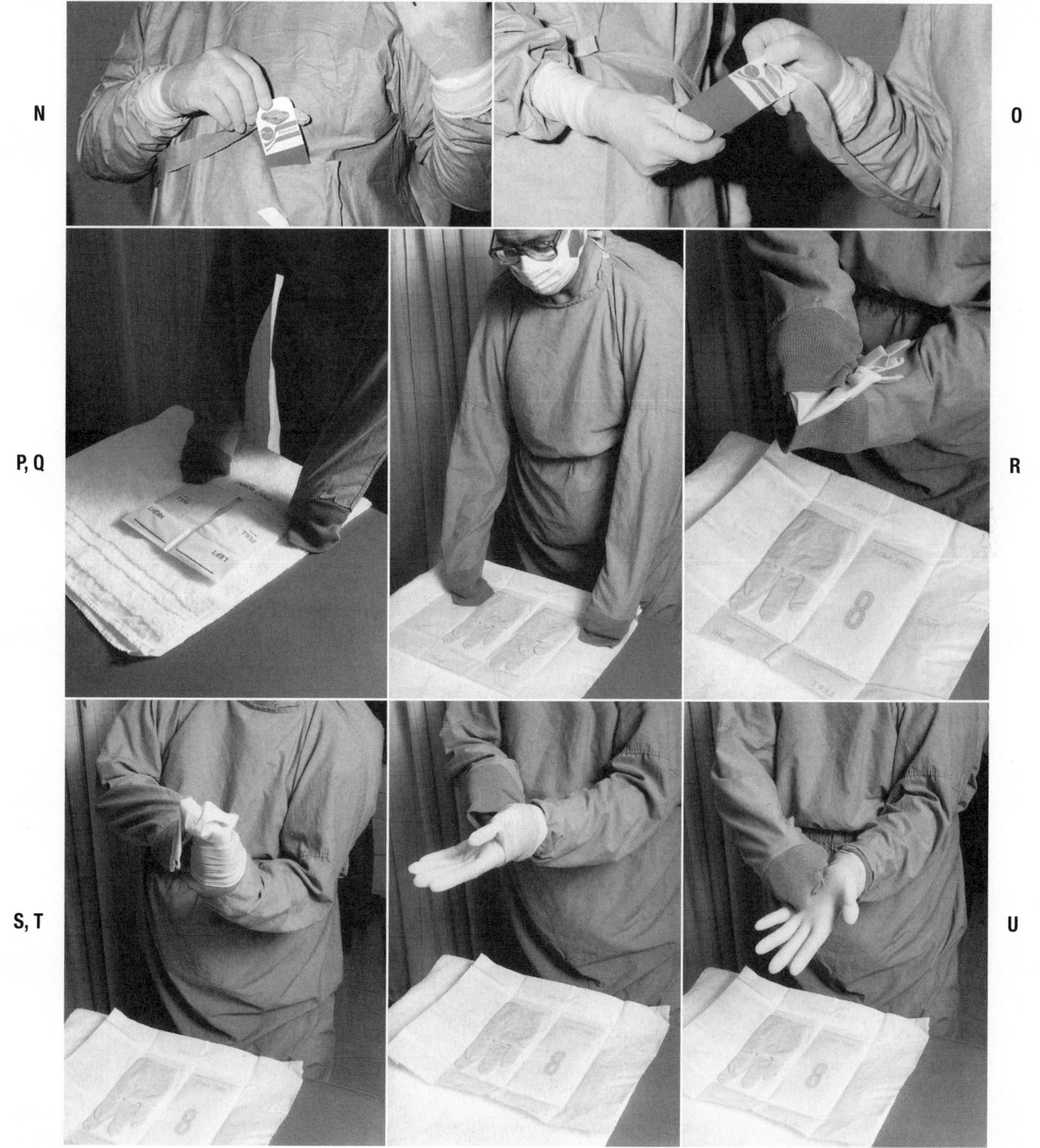

Continued

PROCEDURE 2-3

Clothing Application for Protective Isolation—cont'd

12. Repeat steps 10 and 11 to apply the other glove. Once both gloves have been applied completely, hold them above waist level and avoid touching your gown or other objects to maintain sterility. A sterile towel can be wrapped over your gloved hands to protect them until it is time to treat the patient (Fig. 2-3, *V* to *Z;* Fig. 2-4, *A* and *B*).

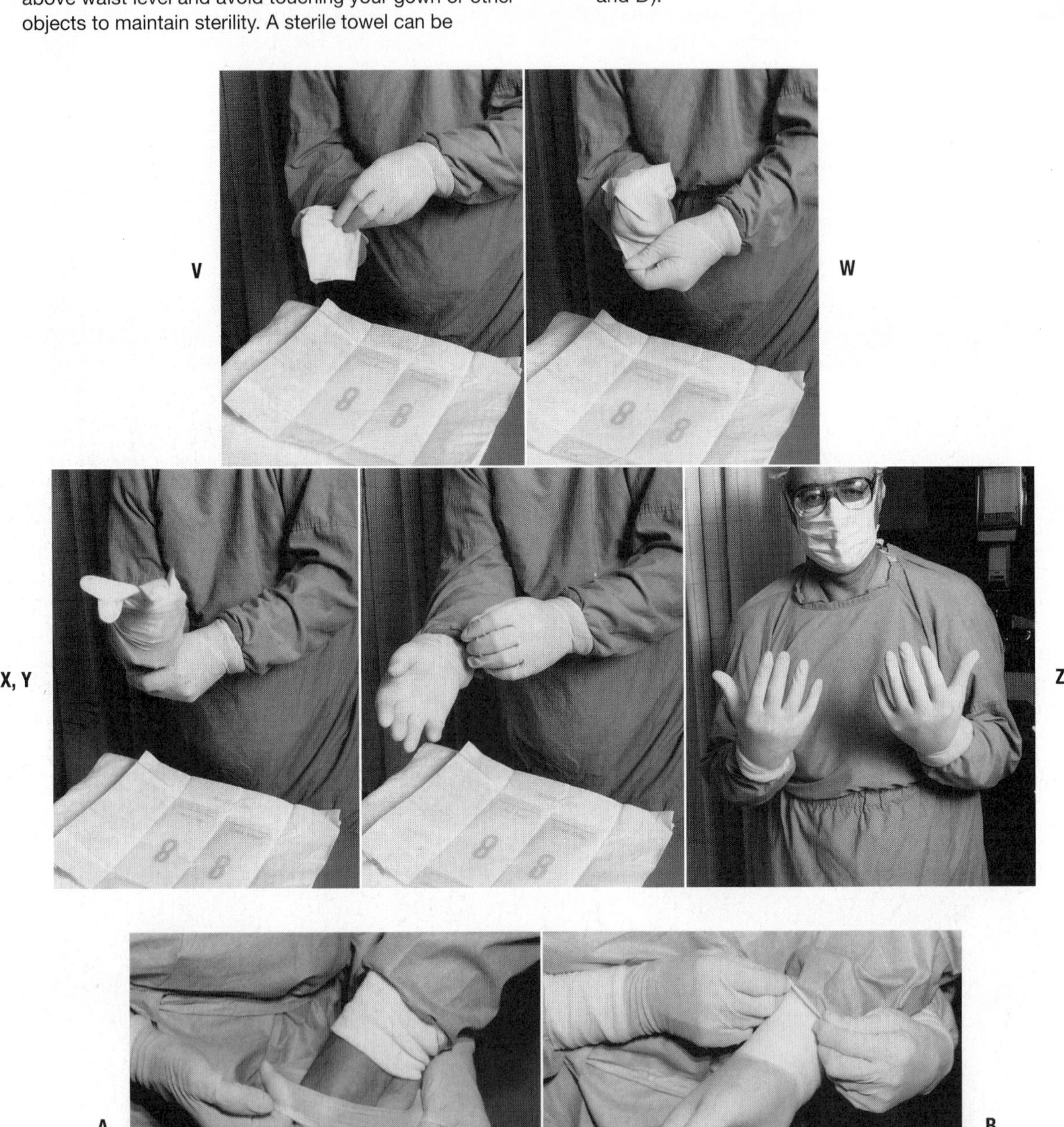

FIG. 2-4 **A,** Two-person method to apply sterile gloves; all garments and gloves are sterile at this time. **B,** Glove is applied over the gown cuff.

PROCEDURE 2-4

Clothing Removal for Isolation Precautions

1. Untie the waist tie of the gown and have another person carefully untie the neck tie. You should avoid touching your neck, cap, or the outer side of gown when untying the gown (Fig. 2-5, *A* and *B*). Refer to Procedure 2-6 for guidance when no assistant is available.
2. Grasp the outer front shoulders of the gown by crossing the arms (that is, your left hand grasps the right front shoulder and your right hand grasps the left front shoulder). Gently remove the gown by pulling it over your arms with your arms extended in front of your body. Avoid touching the outer side of the gown with your bare arms or clothing. Gently roll the gown into a ball so that it will be turned inside out and dispose of it. Avoid touching your skin or clothing with the gown or with your gloves (Fig. 2-5, *C* to *G*).
3. The glove cuffs will have been turned down as the gown sleeves are removed from your arms. To remove the right glove, grasp the *outside* of it with your left hand and gently remove the glove so that it is inside out and discard it. Use your ungloved right hand to grasp the *inside* of the left glove and gently remove that glove so that it is inside out; discard it. Avoid touching the outside of the left glove with your ungloved hand or the ungloved skin with the left glove after the right glove has been removed (Fig. 2-5, *H* to *K*).

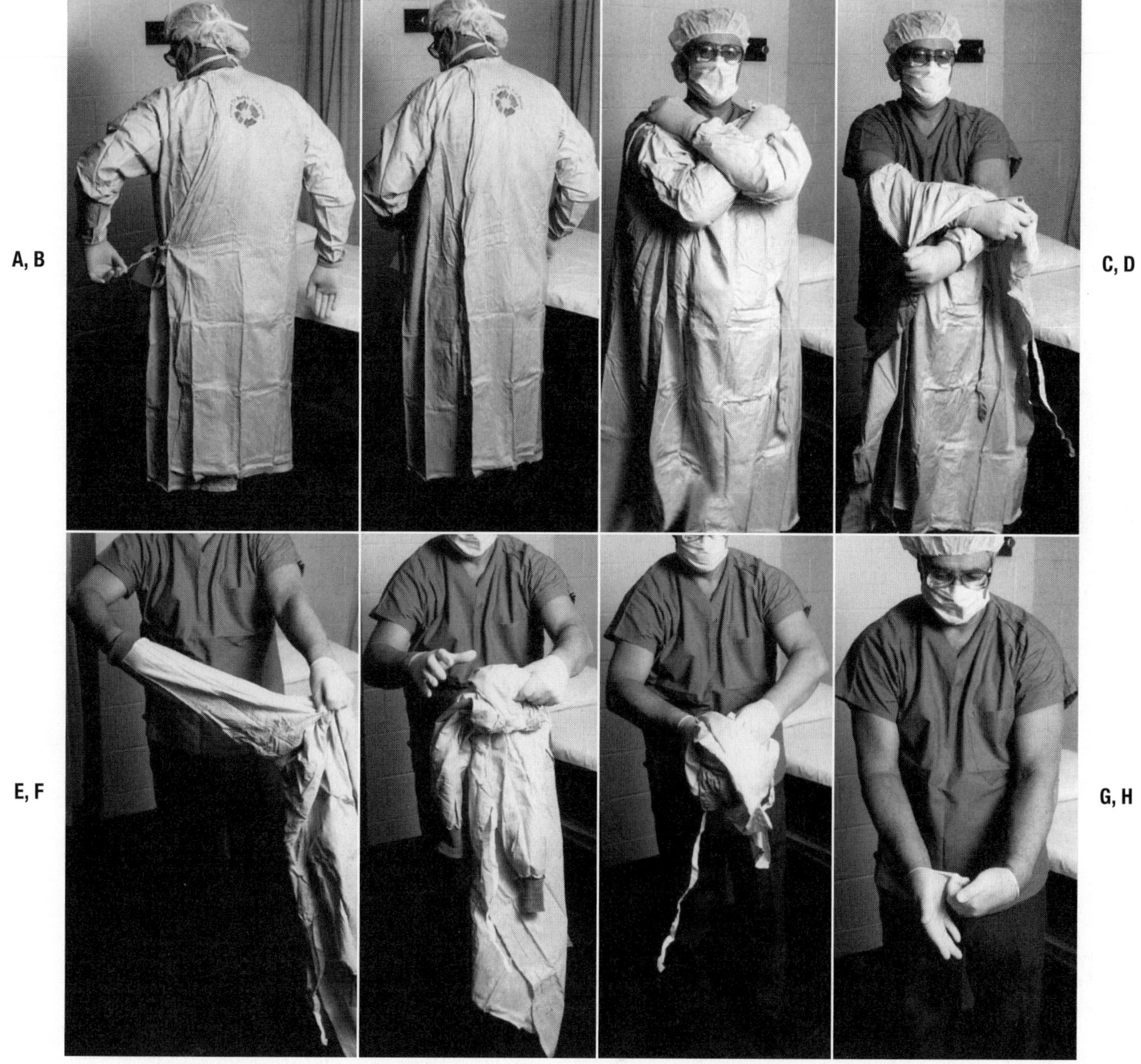

FIG. 2-5 Removal of protective clothing.

Continued

PROCEDURE 2-4

Clothing Removal for Isolation Precautions—cont'd

4. Wash your hands as described for medical asepsis.
5. Remove your mask by carefully untying each set of ties and handling it by the ties. Avoid touching the center of the mask with your hands and dispose (Fig. 2-5, *L* and *M*).
6. Remove the cap by handling it by its ties or by gently grasping the center at the top and gently lift it from your head and dispose (Fig. 2-5, *N* and *O*).
7. Wash your hands as described for medical asepsis.

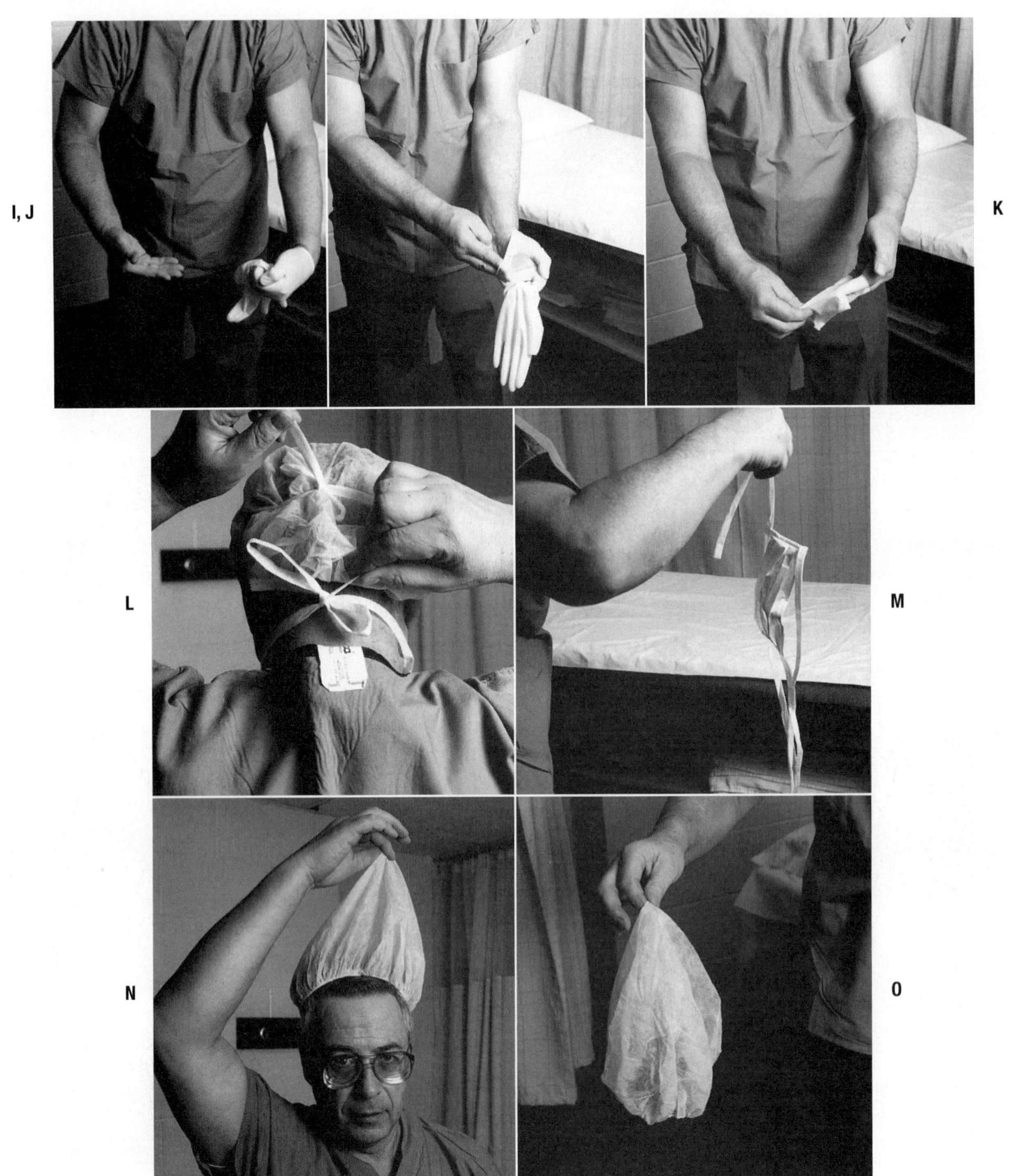

Each facility or nursing unit will have its own specific protocols related to the application and removal of protective clothing. The information in this chapter is sufficient to allow a caregiver to satisfactorily protect himself or herself or the patient, but it may not be as complete or specific as individual facility protocols. Therefore the caregiver should become familiar with the established protocols at the facility where patient care is provided.

After treating the patient in protective isolation, your gloves and clothing can be removed in any sequence because there is very little danger that you will become contaminated from a noninfectious patient. However, you should wash your hands after removing the gloves and clothing and avoid contact between your hands and your eyes, ears, nostrils, and mouth until you have washed your hands thoroughly.

Closed-Glove Technique for Asepsis

The closed-glove technique is to be used to reduce the possibility of glove contamination when the gloves are being applied. The exterior surface of the gloves is protected from contact with sources of contamination when this technique is performed properly (see Fig. 2-3; *P-U* and *V-Z*).

Open-Glove Technique for Asepsis

There are situations in which the closed-glove technique is impractical or undesirable. The open-glove technique can be used in these situations, but it has a greater potential for glove contamination than the closed-glove technique unless you use extreme caution when you apply the gloves (Procedure 2-5).

PROCEDURE 2-5

Open-Glove Technique for Asepsis

1. Perform preparatory activities of hand washing and applying the cap, mask, and gown as described in Procedure 2-3, items 1 to 3.
2. Open the package containing the sterile gloves and place the gloves in the sterile field. Open the inner packet carefully and arrange the gloves so that the cuffs are nearest you by touching only the *inside* of the folded cuffs with your hands. Avoid touching the outer surface of the gloves with your hands as you prepare to apply the first glove (Fig. 2-6, *A*).
3. To apply the first glove, grasp the inner side or surface of the folded cuff of the glove. *Caution:* Do not touch the outside of either glove with an ungloved hand. Insert your hand and fingers into the glove and apply the glove as if you were applying a dress glove, but allow the cuff to remain folded; do not attempt to adjust the cuff or the fit of the glove at this time (Fig. 2-6, *B* and *C*).
4. Using your gloved hand, lift the other glove by sliding your gloved fingers between the underside of the cuff and the outer side of the palm of the other glove. *Caution:* Do

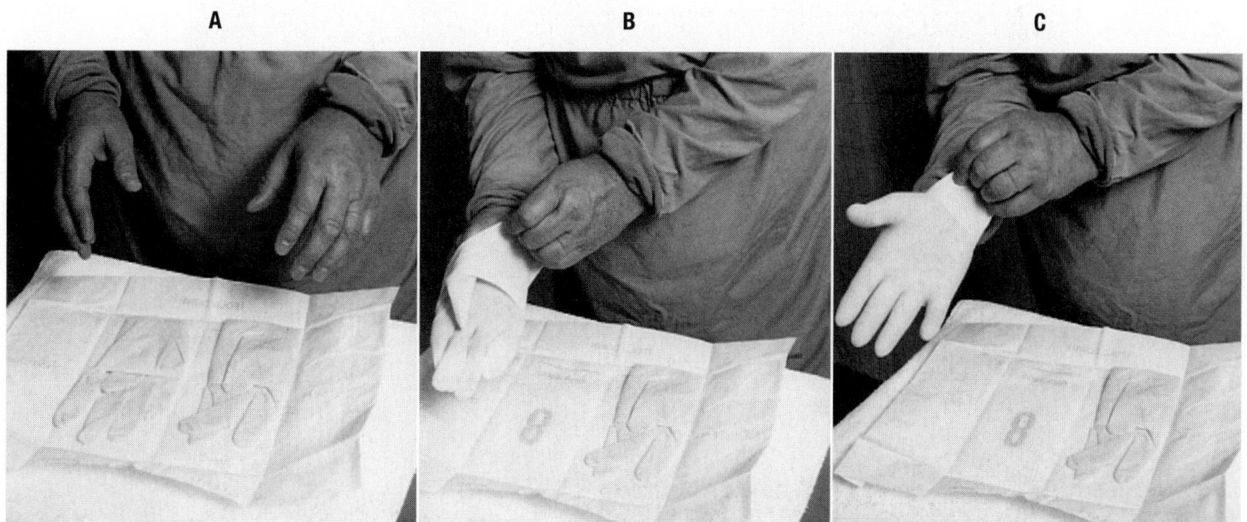

Fig. 2-6 Open-glove application technique.

Continued

PROCEDURE 2-5

Open-Glove Technique for Asepsis—cont'd

not touch the inside surface of the second glove or your ungloved hand with your gloved hand; to do so will contaminate them. Insert your hand and fingers into the glove, but do not allow the thumb of the hand you are using to apply the second glove to touch the inside of the cuff of that glove (Fig. 2-6, *D* to *F*).

5. Pull the cuff of the second glove over the cuff of the gown by holding the outer surface of the cuff; avoid touching the skin of your hand or the sleeve of the gown with the outside of the first glove that was applied.
6. Once the cuff of the second glove is in place, slide your fingers under the cuff of the first glove and pull the cuff of that glove over the cuff of the gown (Fig. 2-6, *G*).
7. Adjust the fingers of the gloves as necessary, but avoid touching any nonsterile objects. Keep your hands above waist level and slightly away from your body until you begin the patient care activity (Fig. 2-6, *H* and *I*).

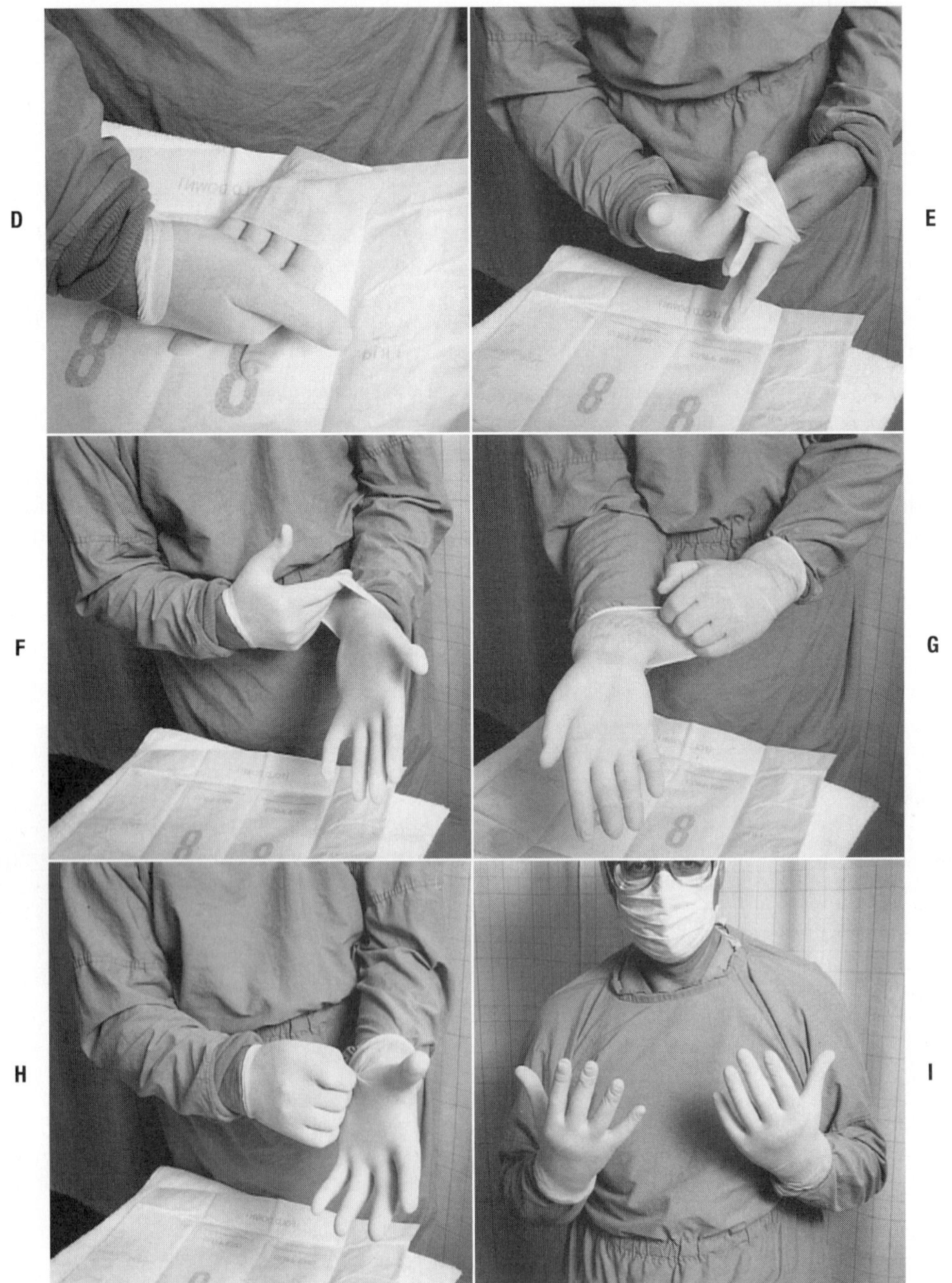

REMOVAL OF CONTAMINATED PROTECTIVE GARMENTS

Frequently you will have to remove your contaminated protective garments without assistance after treatment of a patient for whom you had to use contact isolation precautions. When this situation occurs, you must avoid contaminating yourself while removing the garments. To protect yourself, do not touch any area of your body (that is, your skin, eyes, ears, or hair) with your gloved hands. The sleeves and front of your gown will be the areas most likely to be contaminated; so do not touch those areas with your ungloved hands. You should remove your gloves without touching their outer surface with an ungloved hand. The paper type of gown can be removed similarly to the way you would remove a cloth gown, and you should not touch the gown sleeves or front with your ungloved hand. You can release the neck and waist ties by tearing them rather than untying them (Procedure 2-6).

Consider the furniture, sinks, linen, and other objects in the room may be contaminated and avoid touching them with any unprotected surfaces of your body. Remember to perform proper hand-washing techniques before you apply and after you remove your protective clothing. Finally, do not wear protective clothing outside the patient's room or remove equipment from the room for use with patients in another area of the facility.

The following are some of the precautions you should follow when you treat a patient who is in protective isolation:

- Apply your protective clothing carefully and follow the recommendations for application that have been provided.
- Avoid causing excessive air currents in the patient's room; move slowly and arrange linen or equipment carefully.
- Do not enter the patient's room with protective clothing or equipment that has been worn to treat patients in another area of the hospital because you may bring undesired microorganisms into the patient's environment.
- Remember to perform proper hand washing before applying and after removing your protective clothing. Adherence to these precautions will help to protect both you and the patient from becoming infected.

Disinfection, Decontamination, and Disposal

Careful handling is necessary to prevent injuries from needles, scalpel blades, and other sharp instruments or equipment during their use, disposal, cleaning, or handling during or after patient care. Needles should not be uncapped until they are used and should not be manipulated by hand when uncapped. They should be placed in a puncture-proof container after use, along with scalpel blades and other sharp items.

Hands and other skin surfaces should be washed immediately and thoroughly after they have been contaminated by blood, wound drainage, or other body fluids to which standard

PROCEDURE 2-6

Independent Removal of Contaminated Protective Garments

Untie the waist tie and then carefully remove one glove by turning it inside out with the opposite hand. *Caution:* Do not touch the bare skin of your hand with the glove of your other hand as the glove is being removed. Dispose the glove.

Untie the neck tie with your ungloved hand, but avoid touching the back of the gown, your neck, or your cap. Remove the gown, using your gloved hand to grasp the opposite outer anterior shoulder of the gown and your ungloved hand to grasp the opposite inner anterior shoulder of the gown. Gently turn the gown inside out and remove it from your arms. Avoid touching the outside of the sleeve or cuff with your ungloved hand; dispose the gown. The remaining glove should roll down to expose the inside of the glove at your wrist.

Remove the remaining glove by grasping the inner surface of the glove at the cuff or by inserting one or two fingers at the base of your palm; peel the glove off by turning it inside out. Avoid touching your ungloved hand to the outside of the glove. Dispose it.

Wash your hands as described previously.

Remove the mask and cap as described previously.

Wash your hands as described previously.

An alternative method is as follows:

Untie the waist tie and remove your cap, if it was applied after the mask, by grasping the top of it and lifting it from your head. Avoid touching your hair with your gloved hand. Dispose of the cap.

Grasp the outside of one glove at the cuff and fold it down to form a wide cuff; do the same to the opposite glove. Remove one glove by turning it inside out. Avoid touching your exposed hand with the outside of the other glove.

Remove the opposite glove by grasping the inside of the cuff of the glove and turning it inside out. Avoid touching the outside of the glove or the sleeve of the gown with your exposed hand. Dispose of the glove. Wash your hands, but avoid getting the cuffs of the gown wet.

Untie the mask or grasp the inside of the mask with one hand and the elastic strap with the other hand and remove the mask carefully. Avoid touching the exposed skin of your hands or face with the outer side of the mask. Dispose of the mask.

Untie the neck tie of the gown and shrug the gown forward off your shoulders, or grasp the *inside* of the gown at the shoulders and pull it inside out over your extended arms. Roll the gown into a small ball by handling the inside of the gown. Avoid touching your clothing or exposed skin with the outside of the gown. Dispose the gown.

Wash your hands as described previously.

precautions apply, even if gloves have been worn. The gloves should be removed carefully to avoid contacting your skin with the external surface of the gloves. The soiled gloves should be disposed in a nonporous container; the same pair of gloves must not be worn to treat more than one patient.

Soiled linen should be handled as little as possible and with minimal movement to prevent contamination of the air and the persons who handle the linen. It should be disposed and transported in bags that are leakproof and clearly designated as containing potentially contaminated linen. The risk of disease transmission from soiled linen contaminated with pathogenic microorganisms is negligible, but reasonable care should be taken when such linen is handled.

Protective clothing contaminated with blood or other body fluids subject to standard precautions should be disposed and transported in bags or other containers that are nonporous and leakproof. Any person who is involved with the bagging, transporting, or laundering of contaminated clothing should wear gloves.

Infective waste products such as feces, urine, bulk blood, or suctioned fluid can be disposed by carefully pouring them into a drain or toilet connected to a sanitary sewer, if this is permitted by institutional or local public health policies and procedures. In some instances, the waste product may have to be placed in a plastic bag that can be sealed so that it can be transported. Individual bedpans and urinals, if not made of a disposable material, must be cleaned thoroughly and sterilized before use by another patient. Persons who are involved with the handling of these waste products should wear gloves and a gown may be necessary if soiling of the handler's clothing is anticipated.

Protective clothing and apparel should be available to all caregivers and personnel who treat, transport, or handle items used for the patient whose condition requires the use of standard precautions. Items that should be available are gloves (either disposable or reusable), gowns, masks, and protective eyewear such as eye shields or safety glasses. The necessary items should be applied before treatment of the patient or before items associated with the patient are handled. Disposable gloves usually do not provide as much protection as individually sized, packaged gloves. Disposable gloves are usually one-size-fits-all gloves and may not conform closely to the wearer's hands and wrists. Furthermore, these gloves can slip easily and can be removed inadvertently during patient care. However, they can form an effective barrier between the caregiver's hands and the patient when applied and used properly. Regardless of the type of gloves you use, be careful when removing them to avoid any contact between the outside of the glove and your skin. Gloves should be worn routinely in situations in which it is necessary to control bleeding, perform a venipuncture, perform oral or nasal suctioning, perform endotracheal intubation, change a contaminated dressing, and handle or clean contaminated instruments or equipment. Usually it is not necessary to wear gloves to measure blood pressure or temperature. However, if there are other reasons to wear gloves when performing these two procedures, they should be worn.

A gown, mask, and protective eyewear should be worn when there is spurting blood and in any other situation in which splashing of blood or other body fluids containing blood is anticipated or expected. Again, these examples are related to the patient for whom standard precautions are in effect. There can be several other reasons or patient conditions that could necessitate the wearing of protective clothing. You should follow specific institutional or agency policies and procedures regarding the use of protective clothing.

Spills of body fluids should be cleaned as soon as possible and the surface where the spill occurred should be cleansed with a solution of one part 5.25% sodium hypochlorite (bleach) diluted in 10 parts water or with an EPA-approved hospital disinfectant. Towels or linen used to clean up the spill must be disposed properly and the person involved in cleaning the spill should wear gloves and may have to consider whether a gown should be worn. Generally it is better to be overprotected than underprotected when dealing with body fluids.

Regulations established by OSHA are in effect for health care facilities and are designed to protect their employees. The facility has the responsibility to provide its employees with information and instruction in techniques to protect themselves from infectious diseases, especially blood-borne diseases. Specifically, each health care facility must do the following:

- Educate its employees on the methods of transmission and the prevention of HBV and HIV.
- Provide safe and adequate protective equipment and teach the employees where it is located and how to use it.
- Teach the employees about work practices used to prevent occupational transmission of disease, including but not limited to standard precautions, proper handling of patient specimens and linens, proper cleaning of body fluid spills, and proper waste disposal.
- Provide proper containers for the disposal of waste and sharp items and teach the employees the color-coding system used to distinguish infectious waste.
- Offer the HBV vaccine to employees who are at substantial risk of occupational exposure to HBV.
- Provide education and follow-up care to employees who are exposed to communicable disease.

The responsibilities of health care employees have been outlined by OSHA. These include the following:

- Use protective equipment and clothing provided by the facility whenever the employee contacts, or anticipates contact, with body fluids.
- Dispose waste in proper containers, using knowledge and understanding of the handling of infectious waste and color-coded bags or containers.
- Dispose sharp instruments and needles into proper containers without attempting to recap, bend, break, or otherwise manipulate them before disposal.
- Keep the work and patient care area clean.

- Wash their hands immediately after removing gloves and at all other times required by hospital or agency policy.
- Immediately report any exposures such as needle sticks or blood splashes or any personal illnesses to a supervisor and receive instruction about any follow-up action.

Decontamination There are several methods that can be used to clean or decontaminate equipment or a surface area. By definition, *decontamination* is "to remove, inactivate, or destroy blood-borne pathogens on a surface or item to the point where they are no longer capable of transmitting infectious particles and the surface or item is rendered safe for handling, use, or disposal."*

Sterilization *Sterilization* is used to destroy all forms of microbial life, including high numbers of bacterial spores. An item can be sterilized by being subjected to steam under pressure, or autoclaved; by being subjected to ethylene oxide, a gas; by being subjected to a dry heat source; or by being immersed in an EPA-approved chemical sterilant for 6 to 10 hours or according to the manufacturer's instructions. This last method should be used only for instruments or equipment that cannot be sterilized with heat, such as instruments or items that penetrate skin (that is, needles or scalpel blades) or that contact areas of the body that are not contaminated.

Disinfection High-level *disinfection* destroys all forms of microbial life except high numbers of bacterial spores. Hot-water pasteurization, at 80°C to 100°C for 30 minutes, or exposure to an EPA-approved sterilant chemical as mentioned previously for 10 to 45 minutes or as directed by the manufacturer, are the common methods used for this type of disinfection. This method can be used for reusable instruments or items that come into contact with mucous membranes (such as endotracheal tubes).

Intermediate-level disinfection destroys most viruses, most fungi, vegetative bacteria, and the tuberculosis bacterium, but it does not kill bacterial spores. The EPA-approved hospital disinfectant chemical germicides labeled for tuberculocidal activity and commercially available hard-surface germicides or solutions that contain at least 500 ppm of free available chlorine are the solutions most commonly used to accomplish this type of disinfection. Common household bleach in a solution of approximately ¼ cup per gallon of water will produce an appropriate solution.

Low-level disinfection destroys most bacteria, some viruses, and some fungi, but it does not kill the tuberculosis bacterium or bacterial spores. The EPA-approved hospital disinfectants without a label claim for tuberculocidal activity are used for this type of disinfection. These types of agents are excellent cleaners and can be used for routine housekeeping or to remove soiling in the absence of visible blood contamination.

*Rules and regulations. *Federal Register* 56:64175, December 6, 1991.

Environmental disinfection is used to clean and disinfect surfaces that have become soiled and is done by use of any cleaner or disinfectant that is intended for environmental use. Environmental surfaces include floors, woodwork, mat or treatment table pads, countertops, sliding or transfer boards, and sinks.

When liquids are used as cleaning agents, the person who uses them should protect the skin from repeated or prolonged contact with the agent by wearing gloves and other protective clothing as necessary.

Any item that is to be disinfected or sterilized should be cleaned thoroughly first to remove residual organic matter such as blood, excrement, or tissue. Different microorganisms will require different methods and levels of disinfection. The CDC, the local health department, or a hospital infection-control department can be contacted for current information regarding the best method to use and the level necessary to destroy or control various microorganisms.

According to institutional policies and procedures, the patient's room and the treatment area should be cleaned routinely by housekeeping personnel using EPA-approved cleansing products. It is unlikely the pathogenic microorganisms that are usually present on the walls, floors, carpet, furniture, and other objects in the area will be transmitted to persons or patients. Simple actions such as disposing linen that drops onto the floor; avoiding shaking or rapidly moving linen, which could create air currents and lift microorganisms from the floor onto clothing; avoiding placing contaminated linen or protective clothing against your clothing to reduce the transfer of microorganisms; and promptly discarding dressings and soiled linen according to institutional or agency policies and procedures will assist in reducing the transmission of microorganisms.

Protective Clothing As described previously, protective clothing is recommended to safeguard the caregiver and the patient when it is necessary to reduce the transmission of pathogens from the caregiver to the patient, or vice versa. Gloves offer protection to the caregiver's hands to reduce the likelihood of becoming infected with microorganisms from an infected patient. They also reduce the likelihood that the patient will receive microorganisms from the caregiver and reduce the possibility that a colony of microorganisms will develop on the caregiver's hands that could be transmitted to patients or to other personnel. Suggestions on the application, use, removal, and disposal of gloves are presented elsewhere in this chapter.

The mask is designed to reduce the spread of microorganisms that are transmitted through the air. It protects the wearer from the inhalation of particles or droplets that may contain pathogens. It also acts as a filter to reduce the transmission of pathogens from the wearer to the patient. The proper techniques for application, positioning, removal, and disposal of the mask are presented elsewhere in this chapter.

A gown is used to protect the wearer's clothing from becoming contaminated or soiled by contact with a contaminant. It also provides a barrier to decrease the transmission of microorganisms from the caregiver's clothing to the patient or to the environment. Techniques for the proper application removal and disposal of the gown are presented elsewhere in this chapter.

Protective eyewear, such as goggles, facial shield, or eyewear with side shields, should be worn to prevent fluids from entering the eyes. It is especially important that protective eyewear be worn when blood splashes or spurts are likely to occur and when other body fluids are likely to be sprayed or splashed onto the face.

Disposal Instruments and equipment used to treat a patient should be cleaned or disposed according to institutional or agency policies and procedures. Contaminated reusable equipment should be placed carefully in a container, labeled, and returned to the appropriate department for sterilization. Contaminated disposable items should be placed carefully in a container, labeled, and disposed according to institutional or agency policies and procedures.

Anyone who handles these instruments or equipment should wear gloves and should wash the hands before and after the gloves have been applied and removed. Needles, scalpels, and other sharp instruments should be placed in puncture-proof containers. No attempt should be made to recap, bend, or break the needle before it is disposed. The ear tips of a "community" or departmental stethoscope should be wiped with alcohol before and after each use. In some instances, it may be necessary to clean the diaphragm with alcohol. If the cuff of the sphygmomanometer becomes contaminated, it should be disinfected in a manner similar to that used for clothing items. Each patient should have an own individual thermometer. If this is not possible, the thermometer must be sterilized or receive high-level disinfection before it is used for another patient.

Contaminated or soiled linen should be disposed with minimal handling, sorting, and movement. It can be bagged in an appropriate bag and labeled before transport to the laundry, or the bag can be color coded to indicate the type or condition of linen it contains.

Contaminated dressings, bandages, materials, paper items, and other disposable items should be properly placed in a nonporous container or bag, labeled, and disposed according to institutional or agency policies and procedures.

Other contaminated items such as toys, magazines, personal hygiene articles, dishes, and eating utensils should be disposed or disinfected and should not be used by others until they have been disinfected.

These precautions require greater emphasis when you are caring for patients whose susceptibility to infection is greatest. Patients with open burns or wounds, with a disease that compromises the immune system, or who are receiving chemotherapy or body irradiation are examples of patients who are more susceptible to transmitted pathogens. Protection of patients from pathogens is important for all patients, but is particularly important for patients who have a reduced capacity to resist or overcome infection.

SUMMARY

The caregiver may be required or find it necessary to treat a patient who has a transmissible pathogen or who needs to be protected from pathogens that may be in the environment. Therefore the caregiver must be aware of methods to protect the patient and himself or herself. The most effective method for the caregiver to use to reduce the transmission of pathogens is to routinely wash the hands. Other methods include maintaining a barrier between the caregiver and the patient and to dispose of dressings, sharps, and contaminated items properly. Most hospitals require all employees to adhere to the procedures established in the CDC's standard precautions for blood-borne pathogens.

The caregiver should be able to apply and remove a dressing to protect the patient and himself or herself from contamination. The method of selecting the appropriate dressing and its application should be known by the caregiver so that proper wound care will be provided.

Each institution has the responsibility to protect its employees from occupational exposure and transmission of pathogens. The institution's employees have the responsibility to follow the institution's policies and procedures regarding infection control. The desired outcome is to protect patients, visitors, and employees from contracting or transmitting pathogens. Information about the use of aseptic techniques and protective clothing, the proper handling of dressings and bandages, and methods to control the spread of disease in the hospital or a similar health care setting has been provided.

self-study ACTIVITIES

- Explain your duties or obligations when you treat a patient in isolation and when you treat a patient in protective isolation.
- Demonstrate the sequence you would use to apply and remove protective clothing when treating a patient in isolation and when treating a patient in protective isolation.
- Explain the concept and principles associated with standard precautions and describe the actions you would perform to comply with those principles when you provide patient care or treatment.

problem SOLVING

1. In your clinical setting, a patient has been referred to you who has a disease that is transmissible by air and is in isolation. How will you prepare yourself to treat him in his room? In the course of his stay, he has progressed and is able to be treated in a site away from his room. What precautions would be required to transport and treat him in this area?

Assessment of Vital Signs

objectives *After studying this chapter, the reader will be able to:*

- Provide the rationale for the need to measure, monitor, and record a patient's vital signs.
- Locate and palpate a patient's arterial pulse at various sites.
- Describe and define blood pressure.
- Accurately measure and record a patient's blood pressure, pulse and heart rates, respiration rate, and body temperature; determine the person's sense of pain.
- Describe the expected normal and abnormal changes in blood pressure, heart rate, and respiration rate resulting from exercise and other factors.
- Explain to a patient or family member the significance of measuring and monitoring vital signs.

key terms

Anoxia Absence of oxygen in the tissues.

Apical pulse The pulse that is found when a stethoscope is placed on the chest wall over the apex of the heart; may also be found by palpation.

Apnea The absence of breathing.

Arrhythmia Variation from the normal rhythm.

Auscultation Listening for sounds produced within the body using the unaided ear or the stethoscope.

Bradycardia A slow heart beat (that is, pulse rate less than 60 beats per minute); may be a normal finding in a well-conditioned person or an abnormal finding.

Cardiac output The amount of blood that is pumped from the heart during each contraction.

Diaphoresis Profuse perspiration.

Diastole The period when the least amount of pressure is exerted on the walls or the arteries during the heartbeat; usually indicates the resting phase of the heart.

Dyspnea Labored or difficult breathing.

Dysrhythmia Disturbance of rhythm.

Ectopic Arising or produced abnormally.

Expiration The passive phase of respiration when the person breathes out; also referred to as *exhalation.*

Fever Body temperature that is above the normal level; also referred to as *pyrexia.*

Hypertension Abnormally high blood pressure.

Hypotension Abnormally low blood pressure.

Inguinal Pertaining to the groin.

Inspiration The active phase of respiration when the person breathes in; also referred to as *inhalation.*

Intubation The insertion of a tube, as into the larynx to maintain an open airway.

Korotkoff's sounds Sounds heard during auscultatory determination of blood pressure; believed to be produced by vibratory motion of the arterial wall as the artery suddenly distends when compressed by a pneumatic blood pressure cuff. The origin of the sound may be within the blood passing through the vessel or within the wall itself.

Occlude To fit close together; to close tight; to obstruct or close off.

Orthopnea A condition in which breathing is easier when the person is seated or standing.

Pulse A palpable wave of blood produced in the walls of the arteries with each heartbeat or contraction.

Rale An abnormal discontinuous nonmusical sound heard on auscultation of the chest, primarily during inhalation; also called a *crackle.*

key terms—cont'd

Rectal Pertaining to the rectum, or the distal portion of the large intestine.
Respiration The act of breathing.
SOB Shortness of breath.
Sphygmomanometer An instrument used to measure blood pressure; it may use a mercury column or an enclosed air-pressure spring system.
Stethoscope An instrument used to convey sounds produced in the body of a person to the ears of the examiner; it is composed of a diaphragm, tubing, and earpieces.
Stridor A shrill, harsh sound, especially the respiratory sound heard during inspiration in laryngeal obstruction.
Syncope A temporary suspension of consciousness caused by cerebral anemia; fainting.
Systole The period when the greatest amount of pressure is exerted on the walls of the arteries during heartbeat; usually indicates the contractile phase of the heartbeat.
Tachycardia An abnormally fast heart beat (that is, pulse rate greater than 100 beats per minute).
Vital signs Measurement of a person's body temperature, heart and respiration rates, and blood pressure; also referred to as *cardinal signs*.

INTRODUCTION

The patient's *vital signs*—blood pressure (BP), heart rate, *respiration* rate, and body temperature—are important because they are indicators of general health or physiologic status. In addition, the determination of a patient's sense or level of pain is frequently included with the measurement of vital signs. Normal values or ranges have been established for vital signs and significant deviations from these norms may indicate an abnormal condition. It is important for the caregiver to know the normal values and determine the normal and abnormal changes that may occur as a result of illness, trauma, exercise, or physical condition.

For most patients, a baseline measurement of the vital signs at rest should be established so that changes in the values caused by exercise or other activity factors can be determined. It is particularly important to establish baseline values for the following types of patients:

- Elderly patients (that is, older than 65 years)
- Very young patients (younger than 2 years)
- Debilitated patients
- Patients who have performed limited aerobic activities for several weeks or months
- Patients with a previous or current history of cardiovascular problems
- Patients recovering from recent trauma or those with a condition or disease that affects the cardiopulmonary system (such as spinal cord injury, cerebrovascular injury, *hypertension*, peripheral vascular disease, or chronic obstructive pulmonary disease) or those recovering from recent major surgery

If abnormal values are found when the person is at rest, the cause of these abnormal values should be determined before the initiation of any activity that could affect the vital signs. Frequently the patient with abnormal resting values will be less able to tolerate physical activity or stress-producing events.

Measurements of the patient's vital signs can be used to establish goals of treatment, assist with the development of a treatment plan, and assess a patient's response or treatment effectiveness.

General factors that frequently cause an increase or decrease in a person's vital signs are the level or amount of physical activity, the environmental temperature, the person's age, the emotional status of the person, and the physiologic status of the person (that is, the existence of illness, disease, trauma, or use of medications).

Some possible adverse and potentially dangerous responses to activity are mental confusion; fatigue; exhaustion; lethargy; slow reactions of movement or response to commands; decreased response to verbal and tactile stimuli; complaints of nausea, *syncope*, or vertigo; *diaphoresis*; a change in appearance (such as pallor, erythema); pupil constriction or dilatation; and loss of consciousness. Many of these responses may be caused by *anoxia*. The caregiver should monitor the patient during and after treatment for any indication of these undesirable signs and symptoms. Prompt and appropriate care may need to be provided to reduce or relieve the symptoms and modifications in the treatment program may be necessary to avoid them.

BODY TEMPERATURE

Body temperature is an indication of the intensity or degree of heat within the body. It represents a balance between the heat that is produced in the body and the heat that is lost. In humans, body temperature remains relatively constant regardless of the environmental temperature. However, there are some exceptions, as when someone is exposed to extremes of heat or cold or when other factors such as humidity and physical exertion are involved.

Depending on the source, an accepted normal range for human oral core or body temperature is 96.8°F to 99.3°F (36°C to 37.3°C). The average temperature of 98.6°F

Box 3-1 Factors Affecting Body Temperature

Time of day. Body temperature is usually lower in the early morning and higher in the afternoon.
Age. Body temperature tends to decrease slightly with age and is increased slightly in the very young.
Environmental temperature. Body temperature may increase slightly in a hot environment and decrease slightly in a cold environment.
Infection. Body temperature increases when a major infectious process occurs.
Physical activity. Body temperature usually increases slightly with physical activity, but reaches a plateau as the person becomes better conditioned.
Emotional status. Body temperature increases slightly during stressful or emotional periods (such as crying or anger).
Site of measurement. Body temperature values are slightly higher if measured rectally and slightly lower if measured in the axilla when compared with oral values.
Menstrual cycle. Body temperature is slightly higher at the time of ovulation and a pregnant female's body temperature tends to be slightly higher than usual.
Oral cavity temperature. Body temperature measurement may be inaccurate if measured orally within 14 to 30 minutes of ingestion of warm or cold substances or smoking. The body core temperature probably is not affected by these factors, but a false reading is obtained as a result of the temporary changes in the temperature of the oral cavity.

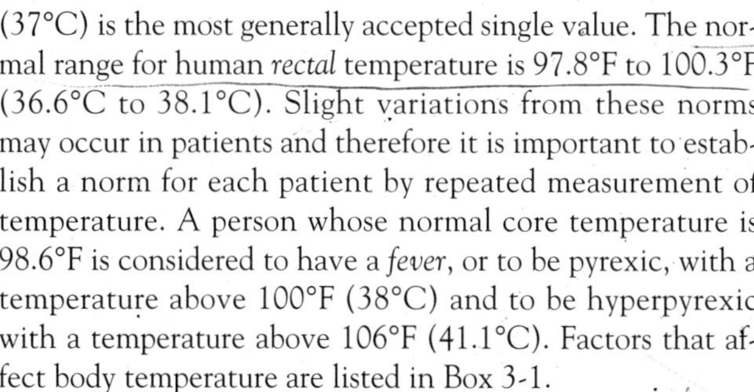

(37°C) is the most generally accepted single value. The normal range for human *rectal* temperature is 97.8°F to 100.3°F (36.6°C to 38.1°C). Slight variations from these norms may occur in patients and therefore it is important to establish a norm for each patient by repeated measurement of temperature. A person whose normal core temperature is 98.6°F is considered to have a *fever*, or to be pyrexic, with a temperature above 100°F (38°C) and to be hyperpyrexic with a temperature above 106°F (41.1°C). Factors that affect body temperature are listed in Box 3-1.

Assessment of Body Temperature

Sites used to assess a person's body temperature are the oral cavity, rectum, axilla, ear canal, and occasionally the *inguinal* fold. The most common and a convenient location to measure a person's temperature is the oral cavity, but the most accurate measurement of body temperature is obtained from the rectal cavity. Rectal or ear canal measurement can be used for infants or young (that is, preschool) children who are unable to maintain the thermometer under the tongue or to safely hold it between the lips and for unconscious patients or patients who are unable to maintain the thermometer in the mouth (such as a patient who is *intubated*). The axillary or inguinal folds are the least desirable sites because the measurement will not be accurate because air currents may reduce the accuracy of the measurement. Therefore measurement at these sites should be used only when measurement at the other sites is neither possible nor safe. If the temperature is measured by the rectal, ear, or axillary method, it should be so noted on the patient's record.

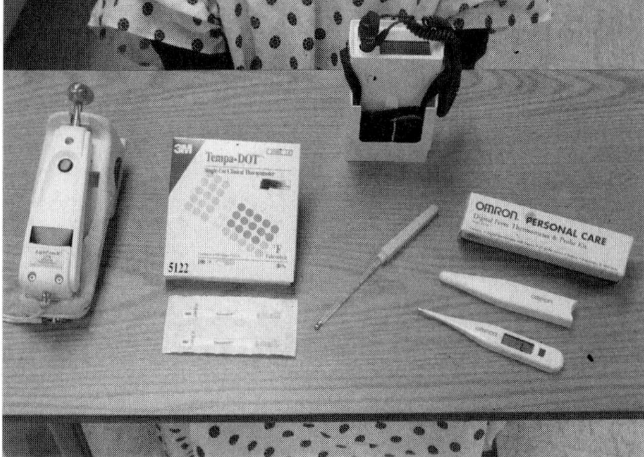

Fig. 3-1 Examples of temperature measurement devices.

Equipment available to measure body temperature includes the clinical glass thermometer or the oral electronic thermometer with a probe, both of which are reusable; the chemical thermometer, which is disposed after one use; or the ear canal electronic thermometer (Fig. 3-1). *Note:* When this text was being prepared, many stores that sell thermometers stopped selling the mercury type of oral thermometer because of the toxicity of the mercury, which becomes a public health hazard when the thermometers are destroyed. Some city and county health departments were in the process of discontinuing their use for the same reason.

Ear Thermometer A thermometer that measures body temperature on the basis of heat generated by the ear canal and its surrounding tissue is available. It is especially useful for infants, toddlers, and older persons for whom it is difficult to use an oral thermometer. Most ear thermometers require a nine-volt battery as the power source and disposable lens filters are used to protect the ear canal and lens cone. The lens filter should be cleaned thoroughly or discarded after each use to prevent cross-contamination or a false reading of the unit. The temperature value is obtained from a liquid crystal display (LCD) in a window on one side of the thermometer. The unit has two settings: rectal and oral. The rectal setting is used for infants and toddlers and the oral setting is used for other persons. These setting selections allow the unit to measure and report a temperature that is consistent with the sites for which a glass thermometer is used. Regardless of the setting selected, the lens cone is placed in the person's ear canal (Fig. 3-2). It is suggested that a normal or baseline temperature be established for an individual before the need to measure the temperature during an illness, especially when the person is an infant or a toddler. Two or three serial measurements should be taken for infants younger than 3 months and for toddlers younger than 3 years when the presence or absence of a fever is a critical finding or when the operator is unfamiliar with the unit. When the individual has been lying on the ear for a period, that ear should not be used for measurement until it has been exposed to the air for 2 to 3 minutes so the ear canal temperature can become stable. If the temperature of the ear canal is not permitted to acclimate, a falsely high reading may occur. A temperature differential may exist between the person's left and right ear, and so the same ear should be used for all measurements during each period the thermometer is used. When you document the results of the measurement, you should indicate in which ear the thermometer cone was placed.

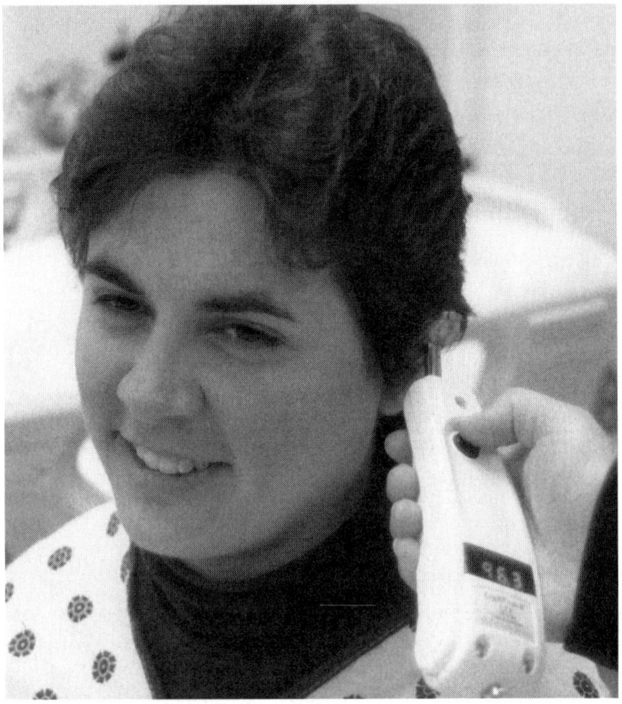

Fig. 3-2 Temperature measurement with an ear thermometer.

Oral Electric Thermometer The oral electric thermometer has a probe connected to a small rectangular unit containing a battery that measures a person's temperature and provides a digital reading. To use the equipment, a cover is placed over the probe; the probe is inserted into the mouth, positioned under the tongue and held in place by the lips. The probe remains in place for approximately 30 to 90 seconds or until the temperature reaches its final value. The probe is removed, the cover is discarded, and the temperature is recorded (Fig. 3-3).

Nursing personnel usually measure temperature, but other health care personnel should be prepared to perform this task. In addition, treatment decisions may need to be made based on the patient's body temperature or response to exercise. Exercise should not be started in a person whose body temperature is elevated before treatment. The cause of this abnormal temperature should be determined before exercise is started. The person whose body temperature is lower than normal before treatment should be monitored to be certain that treatment is tolerated and determine whether the temperature changes during or at the conclusion of the activity. The person with a normal body temperature before treatment can be monitored during or at the conclusion of

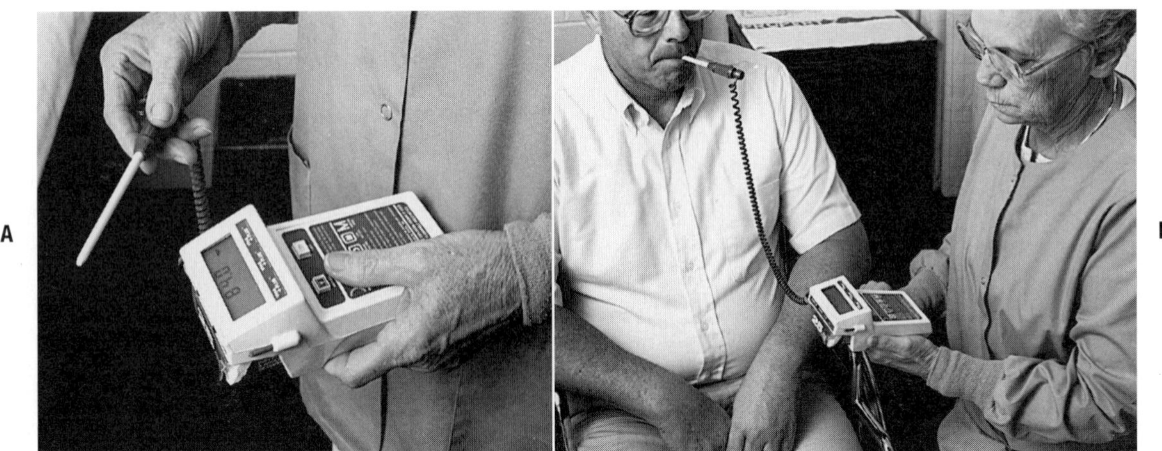

Fig. 3-3 **A** and **B,** Use of an electronic thermometer for oral body temperature.

the treatment to determine whether normal responses occur; if an excessive temperature value is measured or any signs or symptoms of excessive temperature are observed, the patient should have adequate periods of rest to allow the body temperature to become stabilized at the normal value. The patient whose body temperature becomes lower than normal during treatment may also be demonstrating an abnormal response to the treatment. In any of these abnormal situations, caution should be used if the treatment is continued and it may be prudent to have the patient examined by an appropriate medical practitioner.

Glass (Mercury) Thermometer The glass, or mercury, thermometer has a bulb containing mercury at one end of a glass tube that is calibrated in degrees that are separated into tenths. A patient should only use a thermometer that is specifically designated for him or her. When it is not in use, it should be placed upright in a solution of alcohol or wiped with alcohol before use. To obtain the patient's temperature, the bulb end is placed in the mouth under the tongue and held in place by the lips, not by the teeth. It should remain in the mouth for 3 to 5 minutes and then removed. The temperature is determined by holding the small end of the thermometer, positioned horizontally at eye level. The temperature is observed and recorded to the nearest tenth (that is, 98.3, 99.3, 100.2). Steps to measure body temperature orally using a glass thermometer are listed in Procedure 3-1. Use of an oral electronic thermometer is described in Procedure 3-2, and the use of the ear canal electronic thermometer is described in Procedure 3-3.

PROCEDURE 3-1

Measuring Body Temperature Orally with a Glass Thermometer

Wash your hands and obtain a thermometer, recording form, pen, and an alcohol wipe to clean the thermometer.

Position the patient and explain the procedure. Observe the patient and evaluate signs or symptoms related to body temperature: skin color, temperature (hot, warm, cool), and condition (moist, dry). Clean the thermometer bulb with an alcohol wipe, or wipe it dry if it has been stored in alcohol or a similar solution.

Check the level of the mercury in the thermometer to be certain it is below 96°F, or 33°C. If it is higher than those values, hold the end of the thermometer opposite to the bulb and shake the thermometer with several quick wrist movements.

Instruct the patient to open the mouth, position the thermometer bulb under the tongue, and instruct the patient to hold the thermometer in place with the lips, not with the teeth, and to breathe through the nose.

Leave the thermometer in place for approximately 3 to 5 minutes, though some sources indicate that 7 to 8 minutes may be necessary to obtain an accurate value.

Remove the thermometer using your thumb and index finger and lightly clean the thermometer by wiping from the top to the bulb end when you clean it or when you attempt to read the scale.

Read the thermometer by holding it horizontally at eye level so that the mercury column is clearly visible. Each long line on the scale is 1 degree, and each small line is two tenths of a degree. A special line usually marks 98.6°F, or 37°C.

Clean and place the thermometer into its container and wash your hands.

Record the results, using even increments to report tenths (such as 97.6°F, 98.6°F, or 99.2°F).

PROCEDURE 3-2

Measuring Body Temperature Orally with an Electronic Thermometer

Wash your hands and obtain an electronic thermometer, probe cover, recording form, and pen.

Position the patient and explain the procedure. Observe the patient and evaluate signs and symptoms related to body temperature: skin color, temperature (hot, warm, cool), and condition (moist, dry).

Turn the unit on and apply the disposable probe cover to the probe (see Fig. 3-3, *A*).

Instruct the patient to open the mouth, position the probe under the tongue, and instruct the patient to hold the probe in place with the lips, not with the teeth, and to breathe through the nose (see Fig. 3-3, *B*).

Leave the probe in place until the digital readout or alarm indicates that a normal temperature level has been reached; note the value.

Remove the probe from the patient's mouth, discard the probe cover, turn the unit off, and wash your hands.

Record the results, using even increments to report tenths of a degree.

PROCEDURE 3-3

Measuring Body Temperature with an Ear Thermometer

Wash your hands and obtain the ear thermometer, lens filter, recording form, and pen.

Position the patient to expose one ear; an infant or a toddler may be held on your lap so the head can be stabilized; other persons may lie or sit.

Apply a clean lens filter and select either the oral or rectal setting; select "rectal" for an infant or toddler and "oral" for an older child or adult. Regardless of the setting you select, the thermometer lens will be placed in the person's ear canal.

Gently, but firmly, pull and hold the ear to straighten the ear canal. Pull straight back on an infant's ear and pull up and back on the ear of a person who is older than 1 year.

Insert the thermometer lens cone, with a clean filter applied, into the ear opening. It may be necessary to gently rock the lens cone back and forth to insert it far enough to seal the ear canal from the external air.

Maintain the lens cone in the ear canal and depress and hold the activation button for 1 second. The temperature reading will appear in the LCD window; mentally record the value.

Remove the lens cone from the person's ear and discard or thoroughly wash the lens filter if it is to be used again. *Note:* In the home, it may be appropriate to wash and reuse a lens filter, but in other environments the used lens filter should be discarded. Wash your hands.

Record the results using the value from the LCD reading; indicate whether the rectal or oral setting was used and indicate the ear that was used.

Box 3-2 Factors Affecting Pulse

Age. Persons older than 65 years may exhibit a decreased pulse rate, whereas young persons (adolescents and younger) usually exhibit an increased rate.

Gender. Male pulse rates are usually slightly lower than female rates.

Environmental temperature. The pulse rate tends to increase with high temperature and decrease with low temperature.

Infection. The pulse rate tends to increase when a major infectious process occurs.

Physical activity. Normally the pulse rate should rise rapidly in response to vigorous physical activity, plateau or stabilize as the intensity or severity of the exercise plateaus, and then decline as the intensity of the exercise declines. The postexercise pulse rate should revert to the person's resting pulse rate within 3 to 5 minutes after cessation of exercise. A person with a conditioned cardiopulmonary system will probably exhibit less change in the pulse rate and the rate should return to its normal resting level in a shorter time than that required by an unconditioned or debilitated person.

Emotional status. The pulse rate increases during episodes of high stress, anxiety, or emotion (such as anger or fear) and may decrease when the person is asleep or in a state of extreme calm.

Medications. Various medications may cause the pulse rate to increase or decrease, depending on their effect on the cardiovascular system.

Cardiopulmonary disease. Both the condition of the heart and the peripheral vascular system and their ability to function normally affect the pulse rate. For example, a patient with hypertension may exhibit a slower (lower) pulse rate, whereas a patient with hypotension may exhibit a faster (higher) pulse rate to compensate for the higher or lower BP.

Physical conditioning. Persons who perform frequent, sustained, vigorous aerobic exercise will exhibit a lower-than-normal pulse rate.

PULSE

The *pulse* is an indirect measure of the contraction of the left ventricle of the heart and indicates the rate at which the heart is beating. It is defined as the movement of blood in an artery, which can be palpated at various sites of the body or measured through *auscultation* over the apex of the heart with the use of a *stethoscope*. The rate or frequency of ventricular contractions of the heart is reported in beats per minute (bpm).

Depending on the source used, the accepted normal range for the resting pulse is 60 to 100 bpm in the adult, 100 to 130 bpm in the newborn, and 80 to 120 bpm in the child 1 to 7 years old. The normal resting pulse can be established for each patient by repeated measurement of the pulse at the same site and under the same conditions. Wide variations in pulse rate are likely to be found among patients and may or may not be indicative of abnormalities. However, unusual or abnormal findings in a specific patient should be carefully evaluated to determine their potential cause and the potential effect the treatment may have on the patient.

Factors that affect the pulse are listed in Box 3-2.

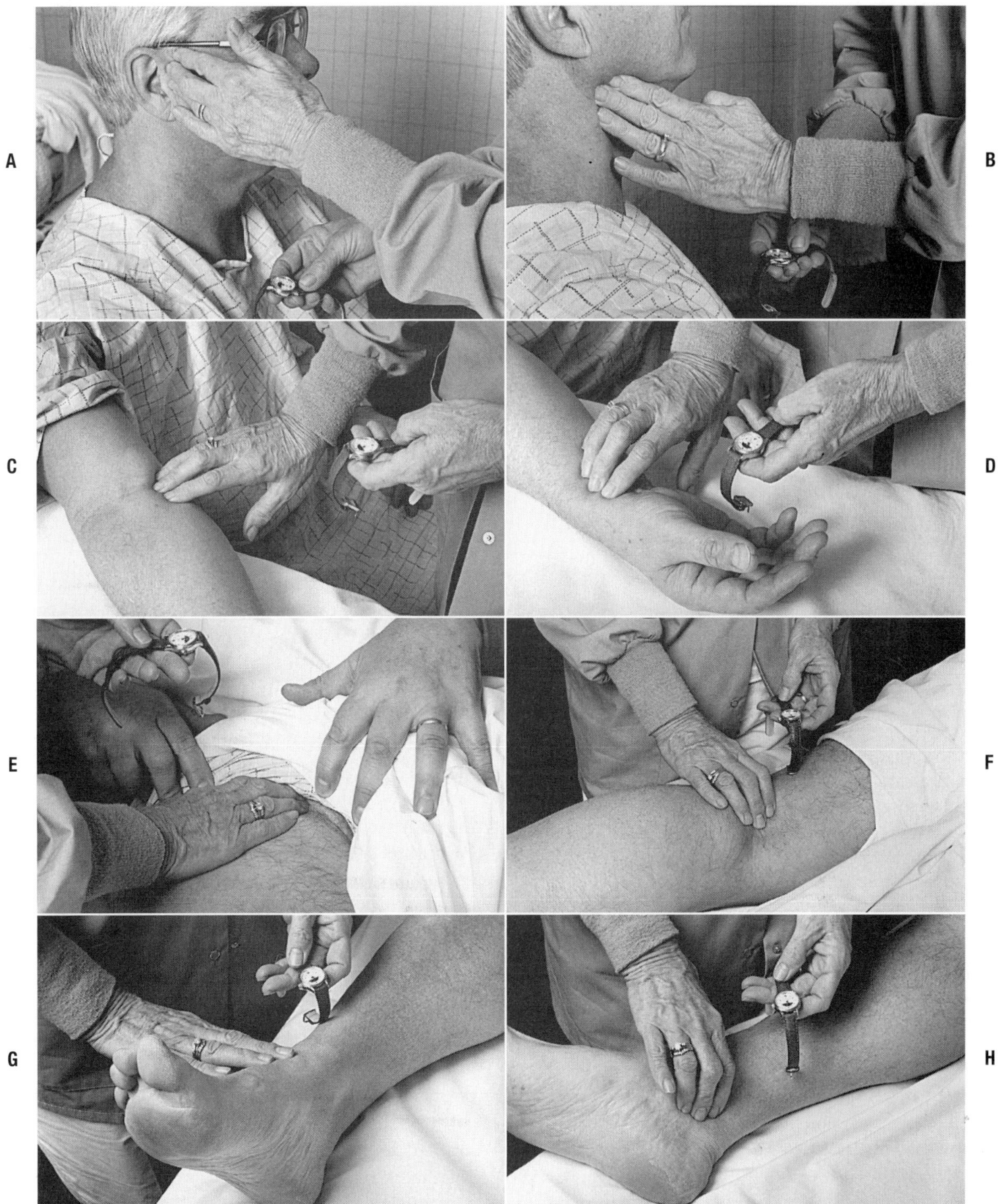

Fig. 3-4 Pulse measurement sites. **A,** Temporal; **B,** Carotid; **C,** Brachial; **D,** Radial; **E,** Femoral; **F,** Popliteal; **G,** Dorsal pedal; **H,** Posterior tibial.

Assessment of Pulse

Sites used to measure pulse are the temporal, carotid, brachial, radial, femoral, popliteal, dorsal pedal, and posterior tibial arteries (Fig. 3-4; Box 3-3) and the apex of the heart, with the use of a stethoscope. The most common sites used are the radial and carotid arteries because of their ease of access. The temporal or carotid sites can be used when access to the radial site is restricted. The carotid or radial sites are usually preferred by persons when measuring their own pulse (Fig. 3-5). The *apical pulse* site is used when the peripheral sites are inaccessible or the pulse is difficult to palpate at those sites. The inguinal, popliteal, tibial, and pedal

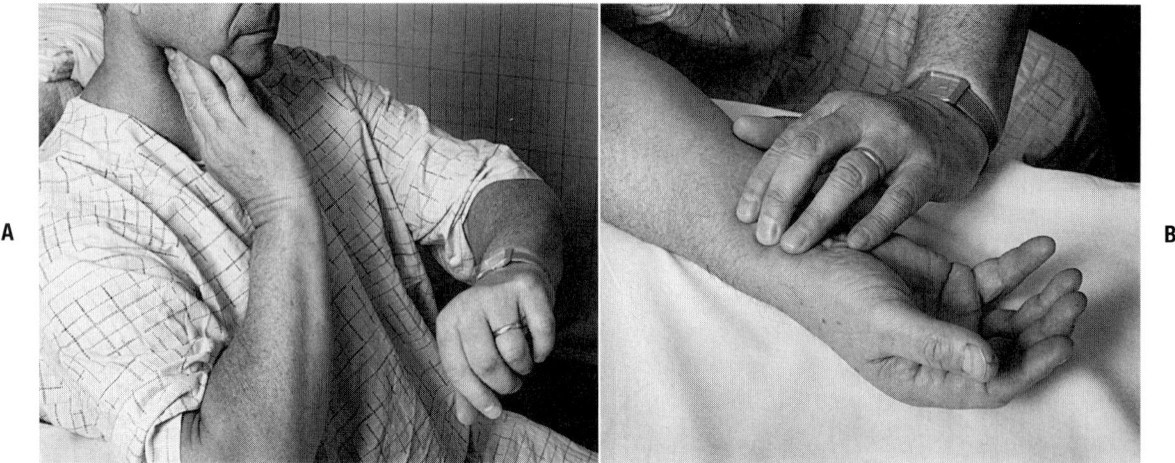

Fig. 3-5 Person measuring his own pulse at the carotid **(A)** and radial **(B)** sites.

Box 3-3 Pulse Measurement Sites

Temporal: Anterior and adjacent to the ear.
Carotid: Inferior to the angle of the mandible and anterior to the sternocleidomastoid muscle.
Brachial: Medial to the biceps in the antecubital fossa or on the medial aspect of the midshaft of the humerus.
Radial: At the wrist on the volar forearm medial to the stylus process of the radius.
Femoral: At the femoral triangle slightly lateral and anterior to the inguinal crease.
Popliteal: In the midline of the posterior knee crease between the tendons of the hamstring muscles.
Dorsal pedal: Along the midline or slightly medial on the dorsum of the foot.
Posterior tibial: On the medial aspect of the foot inferior to the medial malleolus.

Note: These sites will be accurate for most patients; however, it may be necessary to palpate the area surrounding a site to locate the pulse on some patients. (See Fig. 3-4.)

arterial sites are used to evaluate the pulse in the lower extremity. These measurements are important when patients with peripheral vascular disease or a disorder affecting peripheral blood flow are treated.

The pulse is often subjectively described according to its rate, rhythm, and volume. Examples of descriptive terms include the following:

- "Strong and regular" indicates even beats with a good force to each beat.
- "Weak and regular" indicates even beats with a poor force to each beat.
- "Irregular" indicates that both strong and weak beats occur during the period of measurement.
- "Thready" indicates a weak force to each beat and irregular beats.
- "Tachycardia" *indicates a rapid heart rate (greater than 100 bpm).*
- "Bradycardia" *indicates a slow heart rate (less than 60 bpm).*

A timepiece that will allow the evaluator to easily count the pulse for 1 minute or part of a minute (such as 10, 15, 20, or 30 seconds) is necessary to accurately measure the pulse rate. A stopwatch, clock, or wristwatch with a sweep second hand or a second digital readout is the most convenient and readily available timepiece. Materials to record the measured value and a stethoscope (if the apical pulse is to be measured) are other items that may be needed to measure the patient's pulse rate. Steps to measure pulse are listed in Procedure 3-4.

In most persons, the apical and radial pulse rates will be equal. However, in patients with cardiac disease or peripheral arterial disease, these two values may differ. Therefore the radial and apical pulse rates should be evaluated simultaneously during the initial evaluation of the patient. Two persons should monitor the two pulses simultaneously (that is, one monitors the radial pulse for 1 minute while the other monitors the apical pulse for 1 minute) and the results are compared. Any difference in the two values is referred to as the "pulse deficit." Further evaluation of the patient is necessary to determine the cause of the difference between the two pulse rates. Both the left and the right radial pulses should be compared with the apical pulse. If there is a difference between the apical and radial pulse rates, only the apical pulse should be used to evaluate the patient. Such differences should be documented in the patient's medical record.

The expected normal responses of the pulse rate to exercise have been described (refer to Box 3-2). A patient with resting tachycardia or bradycardia should be carefully evaluated by an appropriate practitioner (that is, physician, nurse, or cardiovascular exercise specialist) to determine the limitations or tolerance to exercise or treatment before treatment is initiated.

PROCEDURE 3-4

Measuring the Pulse

Wash your hands, obtain a timepiece that measures seconds, and explain the procedure to the patient. Observe the patient for signs or symptoms of stress, anxiety, or cardiovascular distress. The patient may be recumbent, sitting, or standing.

Select an arterial site and firmly, but gently, place two or three fingertips over the artery. Avoid using your thumb because you may perceive your own pulse rather than that of the patient and the thumb's pad is less sensitive than that of the other fingers. Avoid excessive pressure because it may occlude the artery. An exception to light pressure is when you attempt to palpate the popliteal artery. Very firm, deep pressure may be required to locate the artery and palpate its pulse. When determining a patient's resting heart rate for the first time, allow the person to rest supine or seated for approximately 5 minutes before the measurement. Measure the pulse rate for a full minute to reduce the potential for error and improve the accuracy of the measurement.

Mentally count each beat. If you measure the rate for 10 seconds and multiply that value by 6, the margin of error is ±6 bpm; if you measure the rate for 15 seconds and multiply that value by 4, the margin of error is ±4 bpm; if you measure the rate for 30 seconds and multiply that value by 2, the margin of error is ±2 bpm.

Record the results in bpm, indicate any variations in rhythm or volume, and identify the location you used to palpate and measure the pulse (such as 68 bpm, regular, R brachial pulse; 86 bpm, irregular [every fourth beat absent in 1 minute], L radial pulse, patient sitting).

Measurement of the apical pulse usually requires a stethoscope, but manual palpation is possible. Wash your hands and explain the procedure to the patient. The patient must be positioned so the left anterior side of the chest is accessible.

- *Manual palpation.* Place two or three fingertips on the patient's skin on the left lateral side of the base of the sternum approximately in the interspace between the fourth and fifth or the fifth and sixth ribs; then count and record the pulse rate as previously described.
- *Auscultation.* Clean the stethoscope's diaphragm and earpieces with an alcohol wipe. Position the earpieces in your ears with the earpieces directed forward. This position will be the most comfortable and the ear-pieces will be in line with the auditory canal. Warm the diaphragm with your hand or by rubbing it with a cloth. Then place the diaphragm on the patient's skin in a location similar to the one described previously. In an adolescent or adult female patient, it may be necessary to position the diaphragm slightly medially or laterally and inferior to the left breast. Count and record the pulse rate as described previously. Remove the earpieces from your ears and clean them and the diaphragm with an alcohol wipe. (*Note:* If the stetho-scope is a personal one, only the diaphragm needs to be cleaned before and after use with a patient. If the stethoscope is loaned to other persons or belongs to the department, the earpieces should be cleaned using an alcohol wipe before and after use. This action will decrease the possibility of contamination of the earpieces and diaphragm and help prevent the spread of disease or infection from one person to another.)

Box 3-4 Abnormal Responses Exhibited by the Pulse

- The pulse rate slowly increases during active exercise.
- The pulse rate does not increase during active exercise.
- The pulse rate continues to increase or decreases as the intensity of exercise or activity plateaus.
- The pulse rate slowly declines as the intensity of the exercise or activity declines and terminates.
- The pulse rate does not decline as the intensity of the exercise or activity declines.
- The pulse rate declines during the exercise before the intensity of the exercise or activity declines.
- The increased pulse rate or the amount of the increase exceeds the level expected to occur during the exercise period.
- The rhythm of the pulse becomes irregular during or after the exercise or activity (such as *dysrhythmia, arrhythmia,* or *ectopic* beats occur).

During the monitoring of the patient's pulse, the evaluator should be aware of abnormal pulse responses to exercise or other treatment activities. It may be necessary to modify or terminate treatment when these abnormalities are severe or persistent. Additional caution or a consultation with other medical personnel may be necessary before you proceed with treatment to protect the patient from harm or undue stress.

Abnormal responses of the pulse rate during or after exercise or physical activity are listed in Box 3-4.

BLOOD PRESSURE

Systemic arterial BP is a physiologic variable that reflects the effects of *cardiac output*, peripheral vascular resistance, and other hemodynamic factors. A *sphygmomanometer* (that is, a BP cuff) measures BP and is an indirect measurement of the pressure inside an artery caused by blood flow through the artery. Specifically it is the force exerted by the blood against any unit area of the vessel wall. It is composed of the systolic and diastolic pressures. The systolic pressure is the BP at the time of contraction of the left ventricle (*systole*), and the diastolic pressure is the BP at the time of the rest period of the heart (*diastole*).

Listening for *Korotkoff's sounds* with a stethoscope can identify the various phases of a person's BP. These sounds have been described as occurring in phases, as shown in Table 3-1. A great amount of practice and a quiet environment are necessary for the evaluator to differentiate these five phases. Phases I and V are the two most important phases to identify in most patients. However, in patients with a known or suspected cardiovascular condition, it may be important to identify most or all of the phases.

Depending on the source, accepted normal BP ranges in adults are systolic, 120 to 130 millimeters of mercury (mm Hg); and diastolic, 80 to 85 mm Hg. A systolic/diastolic value of 120/80 mm Hg is frequently used as the normal value (Box 3-5).

Persons whose resting systolic pressure is consistently found to measure more than 140 mm Hg or whose resting diastolic pressure consistently measures more than 90 mm Hg are usually considered to be hypertensive. A consistent reading of 180/110 is considered to be indicative of severe hypertension. Factors that are associated with or contribute to hypertension are obesity; physical inactivity; excessive use of nicotine, alcohol, or salt; arteriosclerosis; diabetes mellitus; oral contraceptives (in women); advanced age (that is, middle age or older); kidney disease; race (that is, greater incidence in blacks); and diet. In most persons, there are no signs or symptoms associated with hypertension and unless the person has the BP measured periodically, the condition often goes unrecognized and undiagnosed. Persons with hypertension are more susceptible to coronary artery disease, cerebrovascular accident, peripheral vascular disease, and congestive heart failure. Therefore it is important for all persons to have their BP evaluated several times a year.

Hypotension is defined as a systolic pressure that is consistently below 100 mm Hg. This condition is usually nonthreatening, but some hypotensive patients may experience dizziness or syncope when abruptly standing from a previous lying, sitting, or squatting position.

Factors that affect BP are listed in Box 3-6.

Assessment of Blood Pressure

The most common site used to measure BP is the brachial artery. Occasionally the femoral artery is used, particularly in patients with known or suspected lower-extremity peripheral vascular diseases.

Table 3-1 Korotkoff's Sounds

Phase	Description
I	The first faint, clear tapping sounds are detected and gradually increase in their intensity. These sounds are the initial indication of systolic pressure in an adult, according to the American Heart Association.
II	The sounds heard have a murmur or swishing quality to them.
III	The sounds become crisp and louder than those previously heard.
IV	There is a distinct and abrupt muffling of the sounds until a soft, blowing quality is heard. This phase is the initial indication of the diastolic pressure and is the best indicator of diastolic pressure in adults, according to the American Heart Association.
V	The sounds essentially disappear totally; the phase is also referred to as the "second diastolic pressure phase."

Box 3-5 Blood Pressure: Accepted Normal Values

INFANTS

Birth to 3 months: 85 to 90 mm Hg (systolic); 35 to 65 mm Hg (diastolic)

3 months to 1 year: 90 to 100 mm Hg (systolic); 60 to 67 mm Hg (diastolic)

CHILDREN

1 to 4 years: 100 to 108 mm Hg (systolic); 60 mm Hg (diastolic)

4 to 12 years: Add 2 mm Hg/year to 100 mm Hg; 60 to 70 mm Hg (diastolic)

ADOLESCENTS

100 to 120 mm Hg (systolic); 65 to 75 mm Hg (diastolic)

ADULTS

120 to 130 mm Hg (systolic); 80 to 85 mm Hg (diastolic); high normal 130 to 139 mm Hg (systolic); 85 to 89 mm Hg (diastolic)

ELDERLY (OVER 63 YEARS)

120 to 140 mm Hg (systolic); 80 to 90 mm Hg (diastolic)

HYPERTENSION RANGES

Stage 1: 140 to 159 mm Hg (systolic); 90 to 99 mm Hg (diastolic)

Stage 2: 160 to 179 mm Hg (systolic); 100 to 109 mm Hg (diastolic)

Stage 3: 180 to 209 mm Hg (systolic); 110 to 119 mm Hg (diastolic)

Stage 4: >210 mm Hg (systolic); >120 mm Hg (diastolic)

A stethoscope, sphygmomanometer, chairs, an object to support the patient's upper extremity, alcohol wipes, and recording materials are necessary to measure and record the patient's BP. The cuff must be the proper size to obtain an accurate measurement. If the bladder in the cuff is too narrow in relation to the circumference of the patient's arm, the reading will be erroneously high; if the bladder is too wide, the reading will be erroneously low. The width of the bladder should be 40% of the circumference of the midpoint of the limb. For an average-sized adult, the bladder should be 3 to 6 inches (13 cm) wide; for an infant, it should be 1 to 1½ inches (3 cm) wide; and for a large adult, it should be 6 to 8 inches (17 cm) wide. If the thigh is used for measurement, the bladder should be 8 to 9 inches (20 cm) wide. The length of the bladder is also important and should be approximately twice the width of the bladder, or 80% of the arm circumference.

Decisions regarding the size of the bladder should be based on the circumference of the patient's extremity, not on the patient's age or other personal factors. Steps to measure BP are shown in Procedures 3-5 (auscultation) and 3-6 (palpation).

If it is necessary to repeat the measurements, the cuff should be completely deflated and the patient should be allowed to sit quietly for 1 to 2 minutes before the measurements are retaken. This will allow any blood that may be trapped in the veins to be released and will allow the circulatory system to return to normal. The caregiver or practitioner should be alert to the potential sources of errors in measurement of BP so that they can be avoided or eliminated.

You will need to develop your hearing, vision, and manual dexterity so that you can accurately hear phases I and V of Korotkoff's sounds, read the value accurately, and properly operate the valve on the cuff-inflation bulb (that is, close it, open it, and control the rate of deflation) with your thumb and index finger.

You should develop the habit of reporting the values without "rounding" them to the nearest higher or lower value. For example, if you read the systolic pressure as 137 mm Hg, report it as 137 mm Hg; do not report it as 135 mm Hg.

Do not bias the findings by expecting a certain value rather than listening for it. Some patients will tell you what their usual values are before you actually take a measurement; you may have read the values determined previously by another evaluator; or you may recall the values you measured during a previous treatment session. This information may bias you into predicting or expecting similar values rather than recording the values as you hear and measure them. When you eliminate, reduce, or avoid these potential sources of errors in the measurement of a patient's BP, you will increase the accuracy and precision of your measurement.

Box 3-6 Factors Affecting Blood Pressure

Age. Younger patients (adolescents and younger) exhibit lower systolic and diastolic values. Elderly patients (65 years and older) may exhibit slightly higher systolic and slightly lower diastolic pressure.

Physical activity. Systolic pressure should gradually increase with exercise, plateau as the exercise intensity plateaus, and then gradually decline as the exercise intensity declines. It should return to its normal resting value within 3 to 5 minutes after termination of the exercise. The diastolic pressure should remain essentially unchanged throughout the exercise period, though an increase of approximately 10 to 15 mm Hg is usually not considered abnormal, but an increase of more than 10 to 15 mm Hg as a result of exercise is considered abnormal.

Emotional status. The BP will increase during episodes of high stress, anxiety, or emotion (such as anger or fear).

Medications. Various medications may cause BP to increase or decrease, depending on their effect on the cardiovascular system. Medications are frequently used to control hypertension and may result in a temporary state of hypotension in some patients.

Size and condition of arteries. Arteries that have a reduced lumen will produce an increased BP value and arteries that have decreased elasticity will produce an increased systolic value and a decreased diastolic value. These two factors tend to account for the changes that occur in the BP values of the elderly.

Arm position. The standard arm position to measure BP is as follows: the forearm is maintained at the level of the fourth intercostal space at the sternum, with the elbow extended when the person is seated or standing. No adjustment in arm position is required when the person is supine because when it is supported on the bed it is at the proper level. The BP will increase 10 to 20 mm Hg as the arm is lowered from the level previously described and will decrease 10 to 20 mm Hg as the arm is raised above that level.

Muscle contraction. The patient should not maintain arm position by contraction of his or her upper extremity musculature because this may produce an increase in the BP because of the increased resistance to blood flow caused by the muscle contraction.

Blood volume. The BP decreases when there is a loss of blood and increases with an increase in blood volume (that is, after transfusion of whole blood or plasma).

Cardiac output. Systolic BP increases with increased cardiac output and decreases with decreased cardiac output.

Site of measurement. The BP values are often higher in the left upper extremity than in the right upper extremity. If the thigh is used as the measurement site, the systolic pressure is usually higher than that found in the arm, partly because of the need to use a wider bladder in the cuff, but the diastolic pressure will be essentially the same as that found in the arm.

PROCEDURE 3-5

Measuring Blood Pressure by Auscultation

Wash your hands and obtain a stethoscope and a sphygmomanometer (Fig. 3-6, *A*). Explain the procedure and rationale for measurement to the patient. Observe the patient for signs or symptoms of stress or recent exercise. If the patient has exercised, ambulated, or experienced emotional stress, the person should rest for 15 to 30 minutes before the BP is measured. Position the patient sitting with the forearm supported on a firm object approximately at the level of the heart, with the thighs parallel to each other and the feet flat on floor. Position yourself so you are comfortable and can view the manometer gauge easily. If the patient is sitting or recumbent, you should sit facing the person. If the patient is standing, elevate the arm and support it between your arm and lateral area of the chest while you face the patient.

Expose the antecubital space of either the left or right arm; do not roll the shirt or blouse sleeve too tightly because it may partially occlude the artery. Palpate the brachial pulse so you will know where to place the diaphragm of the stethoscope.

Apply the deflated cuff to the arm with the center of the bladder over the medial aspect of the arm so it will occlude the artery when it is inflated. The cuff should be applied approximately 2½ cm above the antecubital space (about 1½ fingerbreadths) with the manometer attached to the cuff or placed so that the needle and scale can be observed easily without being held in your hand (Fig. 3-6, *B*).

After cleaning the earpieces and diaphragm with an alcohol wipe, apply the stethoscope to your ears with the earpieces directed forward. Place the diaphragm on the skin where the brachial artery was palpated, but avoid contact with the patient's clothing or with the cuff. Apply firm, but light, pressure on the diaphragm to maintain contact with the skin (Fig. 3-6, *C*).

To initially determine the amount of pressure needed in the cuff to occlude the brachial artery, palpate the radial pulse and inflate the cuff by closing the valve on the inflation bulb and squeezing the bulb until the radial pulse is no longer palpable. This value can be used as a baseline for the cuff-pressure inflation level (Fig. 3-6, D). Note this value and deflate the cuff. After waiting 30 to 60 seconds, reinflate the cuff to 15 to 20 mm Hg above the pressure that previously occluded the artery to ensure that the artery is fully occluded. (*Note:* Once the patient's systolic

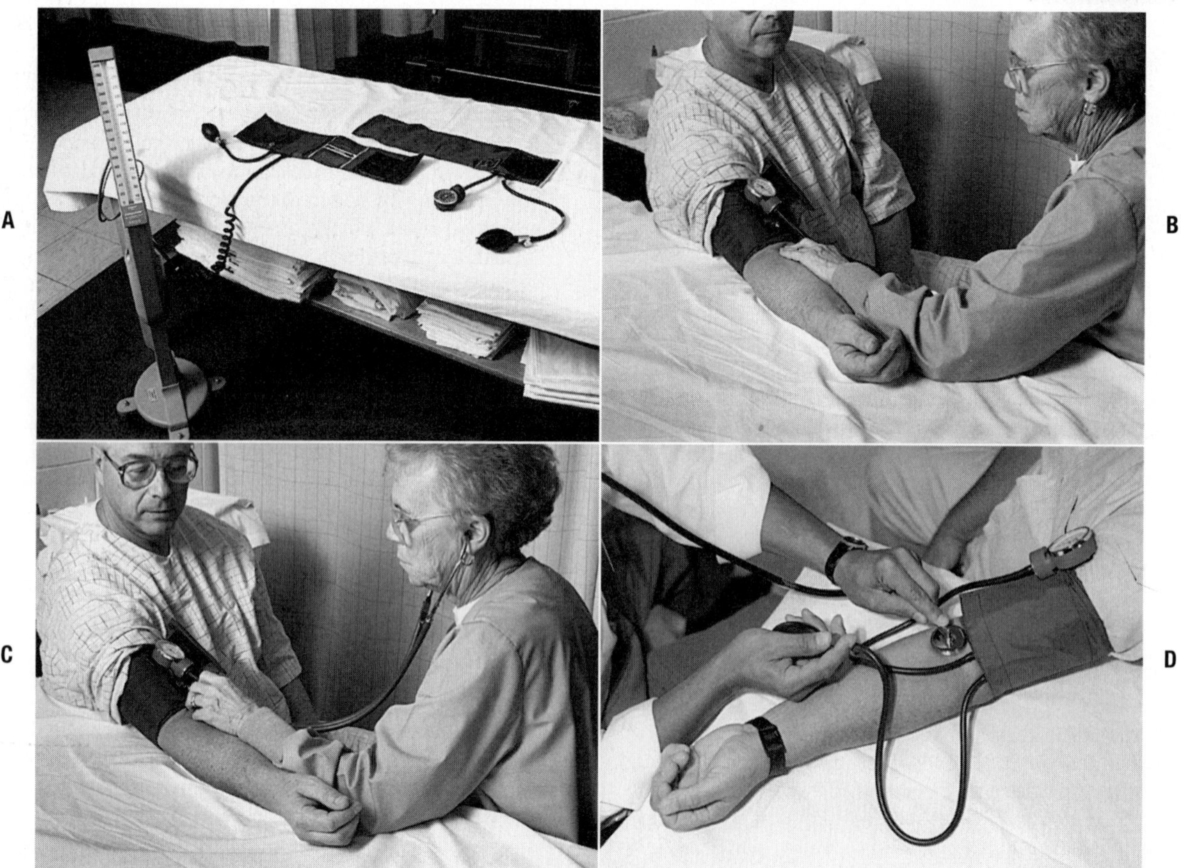

Fig. 3-6 Measurement of BP by auscultation.

PROCEDURE 3-5

Measuring Blood Pressure by Auscultation—cont'd

pressure has been determined several times and a normal systolic value has been established, the cuff can be inflated to approximately 15 to 20 mm Hg above that value each time the BP is measured.)

To deflate the cuff, release the valve on the inflation bulb so that the needle drops at the rate of 2 to 3 mm Hg per second. Listen for normal Korotkoff's sounds and mentally note the needle position (reading) when the initial sound is heard through the stethoscope. This is the systolic pressure value. Continue to deflate the cuff, listening for the absence of the sound of a pulse or beat and mentally note the needle position. This is the diastolic pressure value. Allow the cuff to deflate completely, remove it from the patient, and remove the stethoscope from your ears. Record the values, including the patient position and extremity used (such as 130/70 right upper extremity [RUE], sitting; 140/80 left upper extremity [LUE], sitting). Clean the stethoscope earpieces and diaphragm with an alcohol wipe.

PROCEDURE 3-6

Measuring Blood Pressure by Palpation

Perform steps 1 through 3 as outlined in Procedure 3-3.

Palpate the brachial artery pulse in the antecubital space with two or three fingers and maintain your fingers over the pulse.

Inflate the cuff as described previously.

Deflate the cuff as described previously and observe the manometer. Mentally note the needle position when the first pulse in the artery is palpated. This is the systolic pressure value.

Continue to deflate the cuff while observing the manometer. Mentally note the needle position when the last distinct pulse is palpated. This is the diastolic pressure.

Completely deflate the cuff and remove it from the patient.

Record the values as described previously; indicate that the palpation method was used.

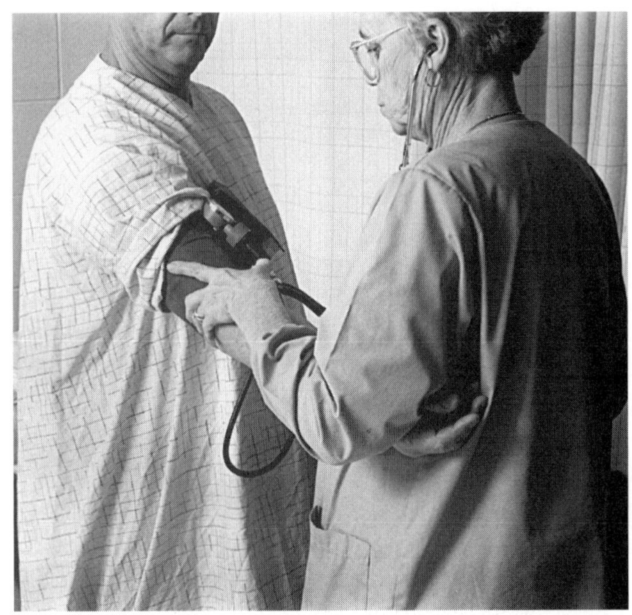

Fig. 3-7 Taking BP for a standing patient.

The patient may sit, stand, or lie for this procedure, but upper extremity must be supported with the forearm and arm at the approximate level of the heart to reduce inaccurate measurements (see Fig. 3-6; Fig. 3-7). If the extremity is positioned in a dependent (hanging) position, the hydrostatic pressure of the blood will be increased and such an increase will erroneously increase the value of the patient's BP. Do not allow the patient to position the upper extremity by contracting the muscles of the chest, shoulder, or arm. Isometric muscle contractions will partially *occlude* secondary blood vessels and the patient's true BP may be distorted. In a normal subject, no significant difference in the BP should be found, regardless of position, provided that the upper extremity is properly positioned as described. Stimuli that may influence the BP should be controlled, eliminated, avoided, or accounted for (see Box 3-6).

The measurement should be performed in a quiet, warm, comfortable environment and the cuff size must be appropriate for the size (circumference) of the patient's arm. A cuff that is proportionately too small will produce a higher value and a cuff that is proportionately too large will produce a lower value.

Unless you desire to evaluate the patient's BP in response to exercise, the patient should avoid vigorous physical activity for approximately 30 minutes before measurement. Postural position changes should be avoided in the 3 min-

Box 3-7 Abnormal Responses Exhibited by Blood Pressure

- Systolic pressure rapidly increases during active exercise.
- Systolic pressure does not increase during active exercise.
- Systolic pressure continues to increase or decreases as the intensity of the exercise or activity plateaus.
- Systolic pressure rapidly declines as the intensity of the exercise or activity declines and terminates.
- Systolic pressure does not decline as the intensity of the exercise or activity declines.
- Systolic pressure declines significantly below its resting level at the termination of exercise or activity.
- Systolic pressure declines during exercise before the intensity of the exercise declines.
- The systolic pressure rate or the amount of systolic pressure increase is excessive during the exercise or activity period.
- Diastolic pressure increases more than 10 to 15 mm Hg during the exercise or activity period.

utes before measurement. You may need to practice measuring BP to improve your accuracy and efficiency.

The expected normal responses of BP during exercise have been described (refer to Box 3-6). A patient with a resting elevated BP (hypertension) or a resting depressed BP (hypotension) should be evaluated carefully by an appropriate practitioner to determine the limitations or anticipated tolerance to exercise or treatment before treatment is initiated.

During monitoring of the patient's BP, the caregiver should be aware of abnormal BP responses to exercise or other treatment activities. It may be necessary to modify or terminate the patient's treatment if these abnormalities are serious or persistent. To ensure patient safety, additional caution or a consultation with medical personnel may be necessary before you proceed with treatment.

Abnormal responses of BP during or after exercise or physical activity are listed in Box 3-7.

RESPIRATION (PULMONARY VENTILATION)

The physical components of respiration produce an inflow (*inspiration*) and outflow (*expiration*) of air between the environment and the lungs. Air moves into and is expelled from the lungs by muscle contraction and relaxation. One respiration comprises one inhalation and one exhalation.

Depending on the source used, the accepted normal range for respiration is 12 to 18 respirations per minute for adults and 30 to 50 respirations per minute for infants. Resting values above 20 or below 10 respirations per minute are considered abnormal for adults.

Assessment of Respiration

Measurement of the rate, rhythm, depth, and character of respiration is performed by observation or tactilely. "Rate" refers to the number of breaths per minute, "rhythm" refers to the regularity of the pattern, "depth" refers to the amount of air exchanged with each respiration, and "character" refers to deviations from normal, resting, or quiet respiration. The evaluator observes or tactilely measures the rate of movement of the patient's thorax, abdomen, or both. Patients who are extremely ill and in respiratory distress may have their respiration measured by stethoscope. The amount of effort required and the sounds produced during resting respirations should be evaluated as part of the assessment.

Normal respiration requires minimal effort for inspiration and essentially no effort for expiration. A person may be classified as either an upper chest (thoracic) or abdominal breather. If an upper chest breather, the thorax elevates and expands during inspiration and the abdomen remains relatively motionless. During inspiration, the abdominal breather exhibits expansion of the abdomen and the thorax remains relatively motionless. During periods of respiratory distress, a person may exhibit both breathing patterns. Persons who have difficulty breathing while at rest experience *dyspnea*, or labored breathing. No sound should be heard during normal, resting respiration. Abnormal sounds include wheezing, *rales*, and *stridor*. Patients may also demonstrate *orthopnea*, or difficulty breathing while recumbent. This condition is relieved when the patient sits or stands. *Apnea*, or absence of breathing, and shortness of breath (*SOB*) also may be experienced by patients and may require the use of a ventilator if they persist.

A watch or clock that measures both seconds and minutes, or a stopwatch, and materials to record the results will be necessary for evaluation of a patient's respiration rate.

Steps to measure respiration rate are shown in Procedure 3-7.

The expected normal responses of the respiration rate when a person exercises have been described (Box 3-8). A patient who exhibits problems or difficulty with breathing while at rest should be evaluated carefully by a qualified practitioner to determine the person's limitations or tolerance to exercise or treatment before treatment is initiated.

During monitoring of the patient's respiration rate, the caregiver should be aware of abnormal respiration responses to exercise or other treatment activities. It may be necessary to modify or terminate treatment if these abnormalities impair function or are persistent. Additional caution or a consultation with other medical personnel may be necessary before proceeding with treatment. Frequent monitoring of the patient's respiration rate may be necessary during the initial treatment sessions to ensure the person is functioning within safe limits.

Factors that affect respiration are listed in Box 3-8. Abnormal responses to watch for while you are measuring respirations are listed in Box 3-9.

PROCEDURE 3-7

Measuring Respiration Rate

Wash your hands and obtain a timepiece that measures seconds. Observe the patient for signs or symptoms of abnormal respiration (such as gasping, panting, open-mouth breathing, use of accessory neck muscles). The patient may be sitting, lying, or standing as long as the abdomen or thorax can be observed. To avoid voluntary control of respiration by the patient, do not explain the procedure to the patient.

Simulate measurement of the radial pulse with the patient's forearm resting on the abdomen. Observe or tactilely measure the outward and inward movement of the patient's thorax or abdomen (Fig. 3-8).

Count either the inspirations or the expirations for 1 minute. (One inspiration and one expiration equals one respiration cycle.) The rate is reported in respirations per minute. Once the rate, rhythm, depth, and character of the person's respirations have been determined to be within normal parameters, the measurement period can be reduced to 30 seconds, but the number of inspirations or expirations must be multiplied by 2 to determine the rate for a full minute.

Reposition the patient's clothing or bed linen if it was removed or adjusted to expose the patient's abdomen or thorax.

Note and record the rate, depth, rhythm, and character of the person's respirations. Record the rate as respirations per minute and describe the depth, rhythm, and character of the pattern if they vary from normal.

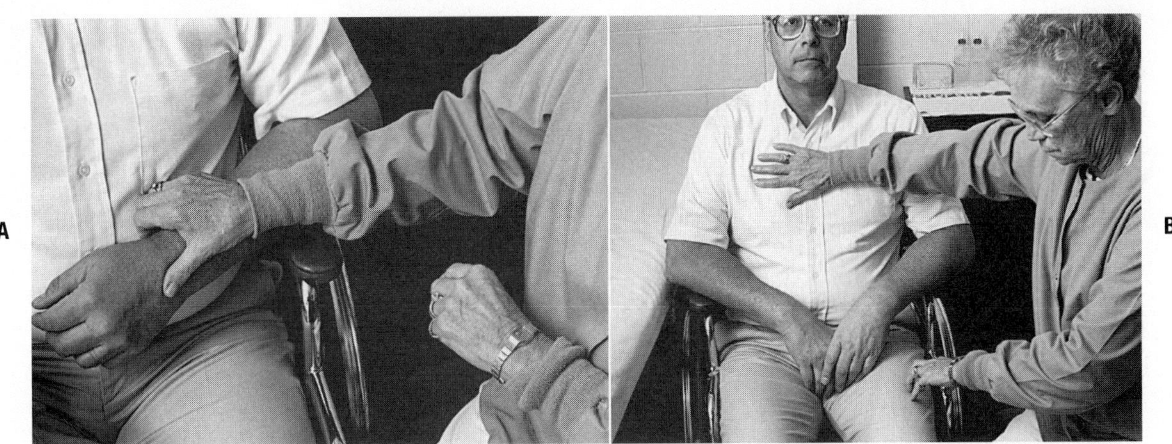

Fig. 3-8 Measuring a patient's respiration rate.

Box 3-8 Factors Affecting Respiration

Age. Both very young (infant to 3 years of age) and elderly (65 years and older) patients tend to have higher respiration rates.

Physical activity. The rate and depth of respiration increase during exercise.

Emotional status. The rate and depth of respiration increase during episodes of high stress, anxiety, or emotion (such as anger or fear).

Air quality. Impurities in the atmosphere may cause the respiration rate to increase or decrease, depending on their effects on various components of the pulmonary system.

Altitude. High altitudes cause the respiration rate to increase until a person is acclimated.

Disease. Disease that affects various components of the pulmonary system usually increases the respiratory rate and may also affect the depth of respiration.

Box 3-9 Abnormal Responses Exhibited by Respiration Rate

- The respiration rate slowly increases during exercise or activity.
- The respiration rate does not increase during exercise or activity.
- The respiration rate increases as the intensity of the exercise or activity plateaus.
- The respiration rate slowly declines as the intensity of the exercise or activity declines and terminates.
- The respiration rate does not decline as the intensity of the exercise or activity declines.
- The respiration rate declines during exercise or activity before the intensity of the exercise declines.
- The increase in the rate or the amount of increase in the patient's respiration rate is excessive during the exercise period.
- The rhythm of the respiration pattern becomes irregular during or after exercise or activity.

PAIN

Health care professionals should question or interview a patient about pain and the patient's self-report of the severity and location of pain should be the primary source of information. The initial assessment of pain should be based on a detailed history and include an assessment of the pain, its characteristics and intensity, a physical examination, a psychosocial assessment, and a diagnostic evaluation of signs and symptoms associated with the patient's cause of pain. Pain assessment should be done before or during the initial examination and evaluation. Reassessment of pain may need to be performed several times per day to determine the effect of medications or interventions designed to alleviate the pain. Written documentation of the patient's perception of pain is preferred rather than oral responses.

Many patient pain assessment tools are available for use. It is important to remember these tools are largely focused on the adult population. Special considerations should be given to the very young and very old, known or suspected substance abusers, the cognitively impaired, and those who do not speak English. When developing a pain treatment plan, clinicians should be aware of the unique needs and circumstances of patients from various ethnic and cultural backgrounds. Standards implemented by the Joint Commission on Accreditation of Healthcare Organizations (JCAHO) require pain assessment to be monitored frequently during a patient's hospitalization or admission to an extended care facility.

Assessment of Pain

In many hospital environments patient pain is considered the fifth vital sign. Some facilities have created comprehensive pain clinics or pain management teams, especially those facilities that treat cancer patients or have a large population of orthopedic or neurologic patients. Pain management teams typically include some or all of the following disciplines: an orthopedist, internist, oncologist, physiatrist, radiologist, neurologist/neurosurgeon, dentist/oral surgeon, physical therapist, occupational therapist, vocational counselor/social worker, dietitian, pharmacist, or nurse. Goals for an interdisciplinary pain team or an individual clinician are to eliminate the source of pain when feasible; teach the patient to function within pain limitations; improve pain control through conservative physical and psychologic methods; relieve drug dependency; treat underlying depression and improve psychologic well-being; address areas of secondary gain; improve family and community support systems; provide access to occupational rehabilitation; provide patient education on pain, anatomy, physiology, posture, body mechanics, and medications; improve strength, flexibility, and general physical conditioning; and maximize the patient's functional level.

In the initial assessment of pain, the clinician should document the onset and temporal pattern of pain. Ask the patient to point to the exact location of pain on the body, the clinician, or on a pain questionnaire, if available (Figs. 3-9 to 3-11; Tables 3-2 and 3-3). Determine whether the pain radiates or spreads to other parts of the body. Ask the patient to describe the pain because words can provide valuable clues as to the cause. For example, patients who describe their pain as "burning" or "tingling" are likely to have a neuropathic cause of pain, particularly if associated with subjective numbness, loss of sensation, and weakness.

An assessment of pain intensity should include an evaluation of the present pain intensity and when the pain is at its least and worst. Knowing factors that aggravate or relieve the pain helps clinicians to design a better plan of care. The patient should describe the symptoms at onset, whether they are constant or intermittent, and what activities make the symptoms worse or better (such as bending, sitting, rising, standing, walking, or lying). Ask the patient if the symptoms are worse upon awakening, as the day progresses, or in the evening. Document if the pain increases during a cough, sneeze, or strain and if the bladder function is affected. The initial pain assessment should elicit information about changes in activities of daily living, including recreational and work activities, sleep patterns, sleeping postures and sleep surfaces, mobility, appetite, and mood (Procedure 3-8).

Table 3-2 Pain Descriptions and Related Structures

Type of Pain	Structure
Cramping, dull, aching	Muscle
Sharp, shooting	Nerve root
Sharp, bright, lightninglike	Nerve
Burning, pressurelike, stinging, aching	Sympathetic nerve
Deep, nagging, dull	Bone
Sharp, severe, intolerable	Fracture
Throbbing, diffuse	Vasculature

From McGee DJ: *Orthopedic Physical Assessment*, third edition. Philadelphia: W.B. Saunders Co., 1992.

Initial Pain Assessment Tool

Date__________

Patient's name __________ Age _____ Room_____

Diagnosis__________ Physician__________

Nurse__________

I. Location: Patient or nurse marks drawing.

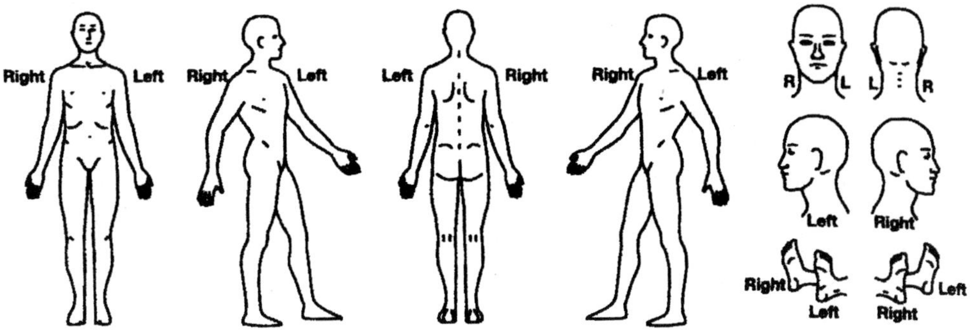

Right Left Right Left Left Right Right Left

R L L R

Left Right

Right Left Left Right

II. Intensity: Patient rates the pain. Scale used__________

Present:__________

Worst pain gets:__________

Best pain gets:__________

Acceptable level of pain:__________

III. Quality: (Use patient's own words, e.g., prick, ache, burn, throb, pull, sharp)

____

IV. Onset, duration, variations, rhythms:__________

____

V. Manner of expressing pain:__________

VI. What relieves the pain?__________

VII. What causes or increases the pain?__________

VIII. Effects of pain: (Note decreased function, decreased quality of life.)

Accompanying symptoms (e.g., nausea)__________

Sleep__________

Appetite__________

Physical activity__________

Relationship with others (e.g., irritability)__________

Emotions (e.g., anger, suicidal, crying)__________

Concentration__________

Other__________

IX. Other comments:__________

____

X. Plan:__________

____

Fig. 3-9 Initial Pain Assessment Tool. (From McCaffery M, Beebe A: *Pain: Clinical Manual for Nursing Practice.* St. Louis: Mosby, 1989.)

Simple Descriptive Pain Distress Scale[1]

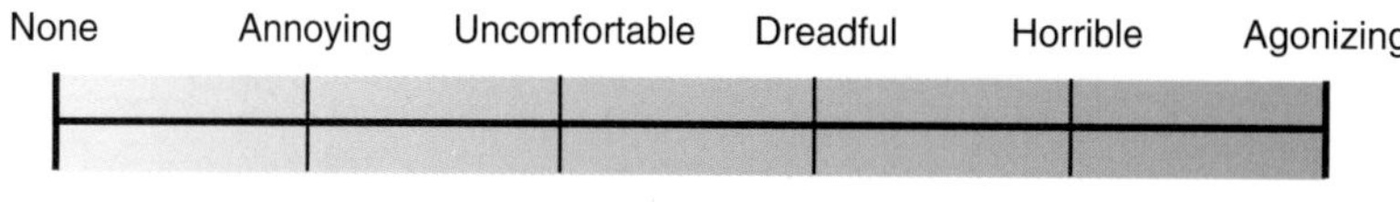

0-10 Numeric Pain Distress Scale[1]

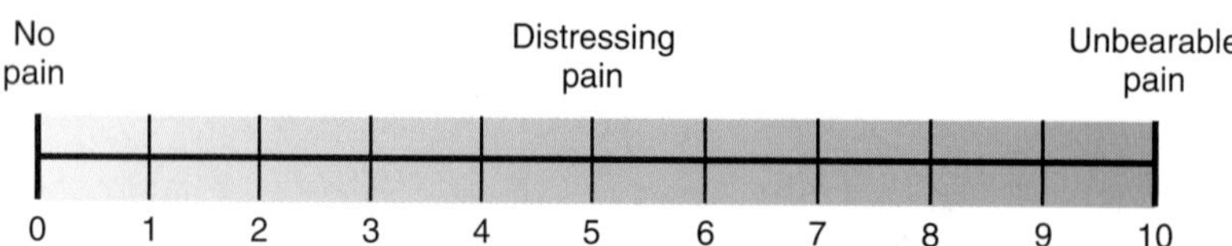

Visual Analog Scale (VAS)[2]

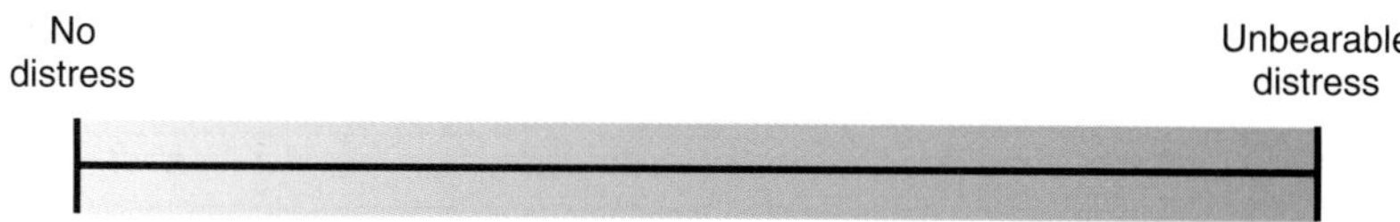

[1]If used as a graphic rating scale, a 10 cm baseline is recommended.
[2]A 10-cm baseline is recommended for VAS scales.

Fig. 3-10 Pain Distress Scale. (From Jacox A, Carr DB, Payne R, et al.: *Management of Cancer Pain. Clinical Practice Guideline.* No. 9. AHCPR Publication No. 94-0592. Rockville, MD: Agency for Health Care Policy and Research, U.S. Department of Health and Human Services, Public Health Service, March 1994.)

Instructions:
Below is a thermometer with various grades of pain on it from "No pain at all" to "The pain is almost unbearable." Put an × by the words that describe your pain best. Mark how bad your pain is AT THIS MOMENT IN TIME.

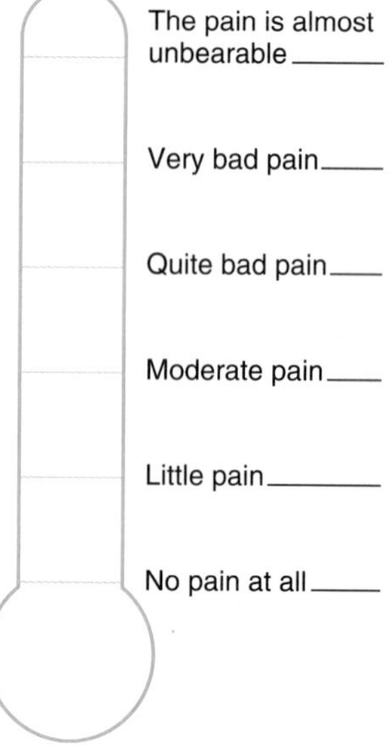

Fig. 3-11 "Thermometer" Pain Rating Scale. (From Brodie DJ, Burnett JV, Walker JM, Lydes-Reid D: Evaluation of low back pain by patient questionnaires and therapist assessment. *Journal of Orthopaedic and Sports Physical Therapy* 11:528, 1990, Orthopaedic and Sports Sections of the American Physical Therapy Association.)

Table 3-3 Pain Rating Scales for Children

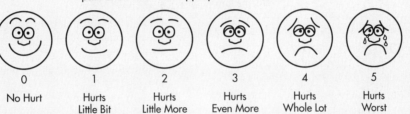

Pain Scale/Description	Instructions	Recommended Age/Comments
FACES Pain Rating Scale (Wong and Baker, 1988, 2000): Consists of six cartoon faces ranging from smiling face for "no pain" to tearful face for "worst pain"	*Original Instructions:* Explain to child that each face is for a person who feels happy because there is no pain (hurt) or sad because there is some or a lot of pain. FACE 0 is very happy because there is no hurt. FACE 1 hurts just a little bit. FACE 2 hurts a little more. FACE 3 hurts even more. FACE 4 hurts a whole lot, but FACE 5 hurts as much as you can imagine, although you don't have to be crying to feel this bad. Ask child to choose face that best describes own pain. Record the number under chosen face on pain assessment record. *Brief Word Instructions:* Point to each face using the words to describe the pain intensity. Ask child to choose face that best describes own pain and record the appropriate number.	For children as young as 3 years. Using original instructions without affect words, such as *happy* or *sad,* or brief words resulted in same pain rating, probably reflecting child's rating of pain intensity. For coding purposes, numbers 0, 2, 4, 6, 8, 10 can be substituted for 0-5 system of accomodate 0-10 system. The FACES provides three scales in one: facial expressions, numbers, and words. Use of brief word instructions is recommended.
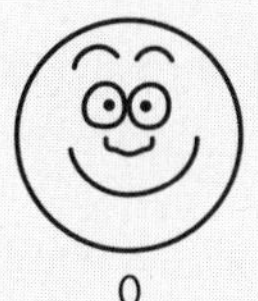 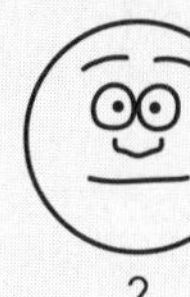 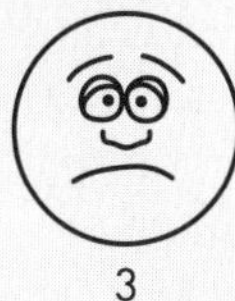 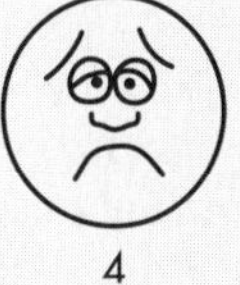  0 No Hurt; 1 Hurts Little Bit; 2 Hurts Little More; 3 Hurts Even More; 4 Hurts Whole Lot; 5 Hurts Worst		
OUCHER (Beyer, Denyes, and Villaruel, 1992): Consists of six photographs of child's face representing "no hurt" to "biggest hurt you can ever have"; includes a verticle scale with numbers from 0-100; scales for black and Hispanic children have been developed (Villaruesl and Denyes, 1991)	**NUMERIC SCALE** Point to each section of scale to explain variations in pain intensity: "0 means no hurt" "This means little hurts" (pointing to lower part of scale, 1-29). "This means middle hurts" (pointing to middle part of scale, 30-69). "This means big hurts" (pointing to upper part of scale, 70-99). "100 means the biggest hurt you could ever have." Score is actual number stated by child. **PHOTOGRAPHIC SCALE** Point to each photograph on Oucher and explain variations in pain intensity using following language: first picture from the bottom is "no hurt," second is "a little hurt," third is "a little more hurt," fourth is "even more hurt than that," fifth is "pretty much or a lot of hurt," and sixth is the "biggest hurt you could ever have." Score pictures from 0-5, with the bottom picture scored as 0. **GENERAL** Practice using Oucher by recalling and rating previous pain experiences (e.g., falling off a bike). Child points to number or photograph that describes pain intensity associated with experience. Obtain current pain score from child by asking, "How much hurt do you have right now?"	For children 3-13 years Use numeric scale if child can count to 100 by ones and identify larger of any two numbers, or by tens. Determine whether child has cognitive ability to use photographic scale; child should be able to seriate six geometric shapes from largest to smallest. Determine which ethnic version of Ouch to use. Allow child to select a version of Oucher, or use version that most closly matches physical characteristics of child. (Jordan-Marsh and others, 1994).

From Wong DL, Hockenberry-Eaton M, Wilson D, Winkelstein ML, Swartz P: Wong's Esssentials of Pediatric Nursing, 6th edition. St. Louis, 2001, p.1301. Copyrighted by Mosby, Inc. Reprinted by permission.

PROCEDURE 3-8

Assessment of Pain

In the initial assessment of pain, the clinician should document:

Pain onset

Pattern of pain

Exact location of pain

Results of a pain questionnaire, if available

Whether the pain radiates or spreads to other parts of the body

Description of the pain; that is, when is it best and worst, constant or intermittent, what activities make the pain better and worse, time of day pain is better or worse

What work or social activity is affected by the pain

SUMMARY

It is important to monitor a patient's vital signs (that is, body temperature, pulse, BP, respiration rate, and pain) because they are indicators of the patient's general health or physiologic status. The caregiver should be able to differentiate between normal and abnormal findings and should have some knowledge of the possible causes of abnormal findings. It may be necessary to measure the vital signs before, during, and after exercise or physical activity. The use of proper techniques during the measurement of vital signs will produce the most accurate findings.

In addition to measuring a patient's vital signs, a subjective determination of the response to exercise or aerobic activity can be obtained by use of a tool such as the Borg Scale of Perceived Exertion. The patient is asked to indicate the perceived level of exertion during exercise using a numeric (that is, 6 to 20 or a 0 to 10 range) or a descriptive scale. The scales progress from a minimum exertion of "none" (6) to a maximum exertion of "very, very hard" (18 to 20) or from "nothing" (0) to "very, very strong"/"maximum" (10). A printed copy of these scales can be displayed on the wall so that the patient can report the exertion level to the caregiver during physical activity. This information could be used to evaluate the patient's response to the activity, to establish patient goals, to judge progress, or to establish parameters for aerobic conditioning. Adverse responses or reactions to exercise or activity should be reported to the patient's physician or to nursing personnel and documented by the caregiver. It may be necessary to adjust or modify the exercise or activity at future sessions to reduce or eliminate undesirable reactions. If it is apparent the patient is in acute distress or the condition is life threatening, emergency procedures should be implemented immediately. Contact skilled personnel using the 911 emergency exchange or emergency number within the facility before you begin emergency care.

Pain assessment is an important part of the patient's medical history and record. Pain scales or pain questionnaires should be completed by the patient or the caregiver if the patient is unable to do so. The amount, type, location, and frequency of the pain a patient has should be reassessed throughout treatment.

self-study ACTIVITIES

- List the normal values for adult heart rate, BP, and respiration rate.
- Explain the reactions a normal adult should exhibit to aerobic exercise or activity in terms of heart rate, BP, and respiration rate.
- Discuss the factors that may affect a person's heart rate, BP, and respiration rate; indicate why it is important for the caregiver to be knowledgeable about these factors.
- Describe three factors or procedures that can adversely affect the accuracy of BP values.
- List six specific sites at which a patient's heart rate (pulse) can be accurately palpated and measured.

problem SOLVING

1. You have taken the BP on a 34-year-old female before treatment. She exercises on a bike for 20 minutes and you are to reassess her BP 5 minutes after exercise. What would you expect her BP to be now in relation to her resting BP?
2. A 35-year-old male is treated in an outpatient setting 2 weeks after a motor vehicle accident with a neck flexion-extension injury. What questions would you ask concerning his pain?
3. You are completing a clinical education experience at a children's hospital and are treating a 6-year-old child with leukemia who has frequent complaints of pain. One component of the treatment is to lessen the pain she experiences. What would you do to determine the location and severity of pain; how will you know whether your intervention is effective?

CHAPTER 4

Body Mechanics

objectives *After studying this chapter, the reader will be able to:*

- Define the term *body mechanics.*
- Describe proper body mechanics to be used for lifting, reaching, pushing, pulling, and carrying objects.
- Instruct or teach another person to use proper body mechanics.
- Explain specific precautions to be used when lifting, reaching, pushing, pulling, and carrying objects.
- Provide basic information to educate another person to care for the back.
- Use proper body mechanics for lifting, reaching, pushing, pulling, and carrying objects.

key terms

Anterior Situated at or directed toward the front of a body or object; the opposite of *posterior.*

Base of support (BOS) The area on which an object rests and provides support for the object.

Center of gravity (COG) The point at which the mass of a body or object is centered.

Dysfunction Disturbance, impairment, or abnormality of the functioning of a body part.

Friction The act of rubbing one object against another.

Gravity The force that pulls toward the center of the earth and affects all objects.

Isometric Maintaining or pertaining to the same length.

Lateral Pertaining to a side; away from the midline of the body or a structure.

Lever arm A component of a mechanical lever; it may be the force arm or the weight (resistance) arm; when the length of the force arm is increased or the length of the weight arm is decreased, a greater mechanical advantage is created for the lever system.

Lordosis An increase in one of the forward convexities of the normal vertebral columns; a lumbar or cervical lordosis can occur.

Lumbar Pertaining to the loin; lower region of the back superior to the pelvis.

Medial Pertaining to or situated toward the midline of the body or a structure.

Pelvic tilt (inclination) Movement of the pelvis so that the anterior superior iliac spines move anteriorly or posteriorly to produce an anterior or a posterior tilt or inclination of the pelvis.

Posterior Situated at or directed toward the back of a body or object; the opposite of *anterior.*

Recumbent Lying down.

Sagittal plane Anteroposterior plane or body section that is parallel to the median plane of the body.

Stoop To bend the body forward or downward by partially bending the knees.

Squat To sit on the heels with the knees fully bent.

Torque The expression of the effectiveness of a force in turning a lever system; it is the product of a force multiplied by the perpendicular distance from its line of action to the axis of motion $(T = F \times D)$.

Valsalva phenomenon or maneuver Increased intrathoracic pressure caused by forcible exhalation against a closed glottis.

Vector A quantity possessing magnitude and direction, such as a force or velocity.

Vertical gravity line (VGL) An imaginary vertical line that passes through the center of gravity of an object.

Box 4-1 Value of Proper Body Mechanics

- Conserve energy.
- Reduce stress and strain to muscles, joints, ligaments, and soft tissue.
- Promote effective, efficient, and safe movements.
- Promote and maintain proper body control and balance.
- Promote effective, efficient respiratory and cardiopulmonary function.

INTRODUCTION

Persons who are required to lift, reach, push, pull, and carry objects should be instructed to use proper body mechanics. Proper use of body mechanics will conserve energy, reduce stress and strain on body structures, reduce the possibility of personal injury, and produce movements that are safe.

Body mechanics can be described as the use of one's body to produce motion that is safe, energy conserving, and anatomically and physiologically efficient and leads to the maintenance of a person's body balance and control. Thus the person who teaches and uses proper body mechanics judiciously will better protect the patient and himself or herself from injury. Stress and strain to many anatomic structures and body systems are reduced when proper body mechanics are used so work activities and the patient can be managed with greater safety. In addition, energy expenditure can be reduced when proper habits of good body mechanics are developed to encourage comfort and efficiency of movement (Box 4-1).

Patients should be taught to breathe normally when performing active exercise to avoid the potentially adverse effects of the *Valsalva phenomenon* or *maneuver*. This phenomenon can occur when the patient holds the breath and air is trapped in the thorax, which increases intrathoracic pressure. This increased pressure can affect the circulatory system by decreasing the return of venous blood to the right side of the heart, which decreases cardiac output and increases peripheral blood pressure. These events could result in the rupture of a cerebral vessel, which could lead to death or a cerebrovascular accident. This phenomenon is most likely to occur when the patient is performing heavy resistive exercise, but could occur at any time active exercise is performed.

PRINCIPLES AND CONCEPTS OF PROPER BODY MECHANICS

Gravity and *friction* are forces that add resistance to many activities associated with lifting, reaching, pushing, pulling, and carrying an object. Therefore it is important to select and apply techniques that will, in some situations, reduce the adverse effects of gravity or friction or, in other situations, enhance the positive effects of these two forces to reduce expenditure of energy, avoid undue stress or strain to body systems, and maintain control of your body. You should review the concepts associated with mechanics as originally described by Sir Isaac Newton, especially the three laws of motion, which can be found in any basic physics or kinesiology textbook. Other forces involved with movement and body control are muscle forces and forms of external resistance.

Before lifting, reaching, pushing, pulling, or carrying an object or a patient, position yourself close to the object or adjust the position of the object so it is close to you. This will allow you to use your upper extremities in a shortened position, or as short *lever arms*. Your muscles will function more effectively and with less strain to the structures of your trunk because a lower *torque* will be required by the muscles of the upper extremity when the object is held close to your body. When the upper extremity is positioned away from the body when attempting to lift, push, pull, reach, or carry, a larger torque is required by the muscles of the extremity to perform the task. This larger torque causes more energy to be expended and increases the strain to structures of your body.

In addition to being close to the object, it is important to position your *center of gravity* (COG) as close to the object's COG as possible. The COG is where the mass of your body or an object is concentrated. Thus it is the heaviest area to move or the most difficult to adjust to a new position. Your COG is located approximately at the level of the second sacral segment in the center of your pelvis. Maintenance of the two COGs in proximity to each other will also help reduce the torque required to move or carry the object. Thus your muscles will require less energy to contract, experience less strain, and function more efficiently. You should recognize it may be easier to adjust the object's COG than adjust your own. Raising or lowering a patient's bed to adjust the COG in relation to your COG, before performing exercise, is one example of this concept.

It is important to increase your stability before lifting, reaching, pushing, pulling, or carrying. You can accomplish this by increasing your *base of support* (BOS), lowering your COG, maintaining your *vertical gravity line* (VGL) within your BOS, and positioning your feet according to the direction of movement you will use to perform the activity. When you place your feet farther apart in an *anterior-posterior* stance (that is, one foot ahead of the other foot) or in a *medial-lateral* stance (that is, with the feet farther apart in a sideward direction), you increase your BOS and these positions will help maintain your VGL within your BOS to further increase your stability.

The VGL is an imaginary line that bisects your body in the *sagittal plane* beginning at your head and continuing through your pelvis and specifically through your COG. It indicates the vertical positioning of your COG. The VGL must be within your BOS (that is, between your feet) for balance and stability. Your VGL is affected by activities that alter your COG. For example, when you attempt to stand on one foot, you must initially shift your COG over that lower extremity and foot before you can lift the other foot. Failure to shift your body weight will result in a loss of balance because your COG will not be located within your BOS. A patient's BOS can be improved when crutches, canes, or a walker are provided to aid with ambulation or stability.

Another example of a change in the position of your COG is when you reach for an object. When you reach with your arms, the relative position of your COG is changed and you will have to adjust your BOS or use more muscles to maintain your balance and stability. One way to accomplish this is to increase your BOS by widening your stance. Remember, the closer your feet are to each other, the more unstable you will be. When you *squat*, *stoop*, or *kneel*, you lower your COG, which increases your stability. Objects with a high COG tend to be unstable. Tall, columnar types of equipment (such as ultraviolet or infrared lamps, intravenous poles) frequently have a weighted BOS to lower the object's COG. In addition, the item is likely to have an enlarged or wide base so that the VGL of the object is located within its BOS.

In summary, position yourself close to an object or position the object close to you, increase your BOS, and approximate the COG of your body close to the object's COG before attempting to lift, pull, reach, or carry it.

Prepare yourself mentally and physically and plan for the series of events or movements that will be required to perform the activity. For example, before moving an object, you can estimate its approximate weight by attempting to slide, tilt or tip, or partially lift it; by looking inside its container to determine its composition; or by reading the information about the contents and its weight, which is frequently printed on the container. A patient's weight can be determined by asking him or her. The size, configuration or shape, and position of the object should be evaluated and considered to determine whether the object can be moved or controlled safely and with relative ease.

You should determine the best method to move the object before you attempt to move it. For example, will it be easier and safer to roll or slide an object rather than lift it? The move itself should be planned so all obstacles are removed and a clear path from point A to point B is established. The distance of the move and the need for and availability of assistance or use of equipment should be determined and the final location or placement of the object decided. Gravity and momentum can be useful adjuncts and should be used whenever possible. It may be helpful to rock an object back and forth to generate some momentum, or an incline or ramp may be used to lower a heavy object from one height to another. To conserve energy, you should roll, slide, push, or pull an object rather than lift it when any of those options are appropriate for the activity and the object (Procedure 4-1).

Patients and persons who assist you must be instructed about their responsibilities and tasks before they perform the activity. They must be taught or trained what to do, how to do it, and when to do it. Requesting them to repeat your instructions will help confirm their level of understanding and the level of comprehension of their roles and expected performance. In addition, you should ask them if they have any questions about their role or the expected outcome. If you are the primary caregiver, you should establish yourself as the leader or coordinator of the activity. Your instructions and directions should be brief, concise, and action oriented (such as "lift now," "push down," "stand up"). You may find it helpful to lead into the action command by using phrases such as "ready"; "one, two, three"; "first, I want you to . . ."; or "on the count of three, lift."

It is important that you give your full attention to the activity, which includes anticipating unusual or unexpected events. For example, when you assist a patient to transfer, be prepared to increase your assistance to a maximal effort at any time, even though the patient may have previously performed the transfer successfully with minimal assistance. You must guard and protect the patient until the person is able to perform the activity safely and consistently.

Your safety and that of the patient will be enhanced by prepositioning and securing the equipment required for the activity. An evaluation of the patient to determine the ability to assist or need for assistance during a transfer will also improve safety. Using mechanical devices or equipment (such as a hoist, transfer or sliding board, wheeled stretcher, or cart) and performing other previously described actions (such as raising or lowering the object, decreasing the distance of the move, or using gravity or momentum) will make the transfer safer and easier to complete. Assistance

PROCEDURE 4-1

Principles of Proper Body Mechanics

Mentally and physically plan for the activity before attempting it.

Position yourself close to the object to be moved to use short lever arms.

Maintain your VGL within your BOS to maintain stability and balance.

Position your COG close to the object's COG to improve control of the object.

Use the major muscles of the extremities and trunk to perform movements or activities and maintain your normal lumbar lordosis.

Roll, push, pull, or slide an object rather than lift it.

Avoid simultaneous trunk flexion and rotation when lifting or reaching.

Perform all activities within your physical capacity.

Do not lift an object immediately after a prolonged period of sitting, lying, or inactivity; perform some gentle stretches for the back and lower extremities first.

When performing a lift with two or more persons, instruct everyone how and when they are to assist.

should be obtained before you begin any activity that you cannot safely perform alone.

There are several precautions that you should be aware before lifting, reaching, pushing, pulling, or carrying. You must avoid simultaneous trunk flexion (bending) and rotation (twisting) when you lift or reach for an object. Prolonged trunk flexion will lead to stress and strain to muscles, ligaments, and articulations of the posterior area of the trunk and spine and perhaps the lower extremities. Therefore when an object is below the level of your waist and must be lifted, you should stoop or squat rather than flex your trunk or raise the object to avoid trunk flexion. A footstool or ladder should be used to reach an object located above the level of your head. *Caution:* Use care if you elect to use a chair or other similar object that is not designed for standing. If you do use a chair, be certain to stand on the seat within the BOS of the legs of the chair. Finally, you must be fully aware of your personal abilities and the limits of your strength, stamina, and motor control as they relate to lifting, reaching, pulling, pushing, and carrying. You must perform within the known limits of your physical abilities to avoid injury to yourself or the patient.

Your primary goal is to perform any activity safely, efficiently, and with minimal stress or strain. The use of proper body mechanics, clear and concise instructions to the patient or to the caregivers (that is, family, friends, or other personnel), and adherence to the precautions contained in this chapter will benefit you and the patient.

LIFTING PRINCIPLES AND TECHNIQUES

Through the years, several lifting methods or techniques have been described, proposed, and used. Each of the methods focuses on the posture or position of the *lumbar* spine and how it is maintained during lifting. The lumbar area is where most lifting injuries or associated activities (such as, shoveling, raking, or reaching above the head) occur.

Stress to the lumbar spine can be caused by or result from the posture or position a person uses to lift, the weight or size of the object lifted, the repetitiveness of the activity, the physical condition of the structures of the lumbar area, or the sustainment of a flexed lumbar spine. This stress can lead to discomfort, debilitating pain, or disability. Pain-sensitive structures of the lumbar area include various ligaments, lumbodorsal fascia, the anulus fibrosus of the intervertebral disk (IVD), the vertebral facets, nerve roots, muscle tissue, and the vertebral body. Therefore persons who lift and reach as part of their daily life should be advised to avoid activities, postures, and positions that may lead to injury. Precautions to follow when lifting and reaching are presented in Procedure 4-1. Injury resulting from lifting may be caused by the single act of lifting a heavy object, by lifting improperly, or by repetitive lifting. Most upper and lower back injuries are caused by cumulative episodes of microtrauma caused by repetitive lifting or overuse of the same muscles even when light objects are involved. To avoid injury and resultant *dysfunction* related to lifting, it is important that a person maintains general body strength and flexibility, proper nutrition, appropriate rest and sleeping habits, good posture, and uses proper body mechanics. Box 4-2 describes some of the common causes of back discomfort, which if avoided, may prevent future discomfort or injury.

Lumbar, or "back," belts have been advocated as a preventive measure for use by a person whose job requires frequent or repetitive lifting. It has been hypothesized that such a belt, when applied properly, increases the intradiscal pressure and serves as a reminder to the wearer to use proper body mechanics when lifting. Research has shown that there is no evidence that the proper use of a "back belt," or lumbar belt, effectively prevents injury to structures of the lumbar area. Therefore it is more important for the lifter to use proper body mechanics and follow lifting precautions than rely on an external support.

The lumbar spine should be maintained in its normal, or "neutral," position of *lordosis* when lifting is performed (Box 4-3). This position tends to reduce stress on the major struc-

Box 4-2 Common Causes of Back Problems or Discomfort

- Faulty posture
- Stressful living and work habits—inability to relax or staying in a prolonged posture
- Faulty, improper use of body mechanics
- Repetitive, sustained microtrauma to structures of the back and trunk
- Poor flexibility of muscles and ligaments of the back and trunk
- Decline in general physical fitness
- Episodes of trauma that culminate in one specific or final event ("the final straw"): Stress, strain, or tear of muscle or ligament occurs. Disk may change shape and impinge on nerve roots. Vertebral joints may become irritated.
- Improper lift, push, pull, reach, or carry motion may cause trauma to back structures.

Box 4-3 Rationale for Lumbar Lordosis Posture

- Lordosis reduces mechanical stress to the lumbar ligaments and IVD.
- Compression forces to the IVD are directed anteriorly rather than posteriorly, a direction that reduces the potential for a posterolateral rupture of the disk.
- Lumbar spine stability is increased because of the approximation of the vertebral facets.
- Function of the lumbopelvic force couple is maximized.
- Anterior and posterior lower trunk muscles and hip and thigh extensor muscles are positioned to function more effectively.

tures of the lumbar area and, when combined with partial or full flexion of the hips and knees, will reduce the tendency to bend forward at the waist during the lift. Forward bending at the waist with the hips and knees straight and the lumbar spine in a flexed position when lifting or reaching produces excessive stress to many of the structures of the lumbar area. Flexion of the hips and knees allows the lifter to lower the COG closer to the COG of the object and provides an effective position for the muscles of the lower extremities to perform the lift. *Isometric* contraction of the abdominal muscles at the beginning of the lift assists to increase the intraabdominal pressure to simulate a pneumatic cylinder that may provide additional stability and decreases the load to the lumbar spine. *Caution:* The lifter should be instructed to avoid the Valsalva maneuver when contracting the abdominal muscles.

Persons whose job or occupation requires them to perform frequent or repetitive lifting or reaching overhead may have developed faulty body mechanics or habits for these activities. If they have not sustained an injury or if they are recovering from and injury and are preparing to return to work, it will be important to teach them to lift or reach using proper body mechanics and precautions. It may be worthwhile for the caregiver to observe the person at a work environment and to understand the requirements of the job or occupation. Although it is not possible to prevent all back injuries caused by lifting, patient education and practice using proper techniques have the potential to reduce injury and prevent loss of function.

Lift Techniques

Deep Squat Lift. A full squat is performed to position the hips below the level of the knees. The lifter's feet straddle the object and the upper extremities are positioned parallel to each other. The lifter's hands grasp the opposite sides, the handles, or under the bottom of the object. The lifter's trunk is maintained in a vertical position and the lumbar spine remains in lordosis with an anterior *pelvic tilt (inclination)* (Fig. 4-1).

Power Lift. Only a half squat is performed so the hips remain above the level of the knees. The lifter's feet are positioned parallel to each other and remain behind the object, with the upper extremities positioned parallel to each other. The lifter grasps the opposite sides, the

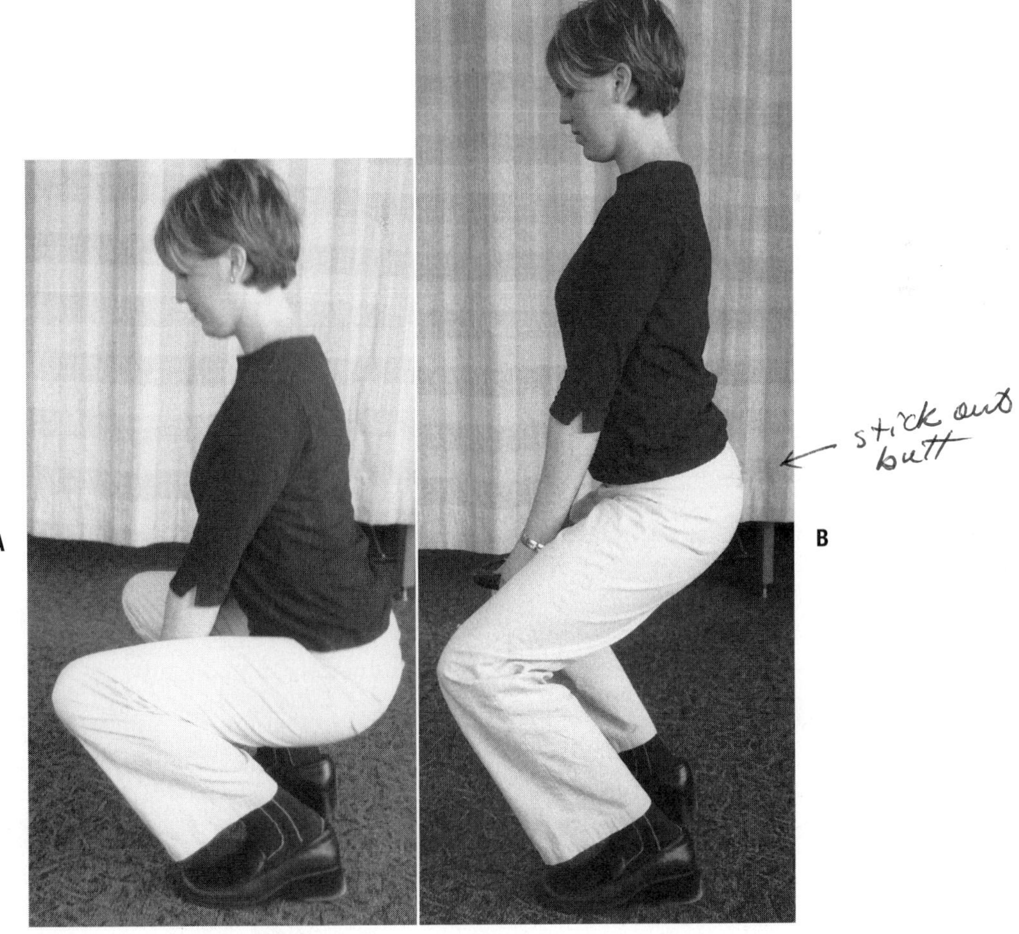

Fig. 4-1 Deep squat lift. **A,** Start position; **B,** Continuation of lift.

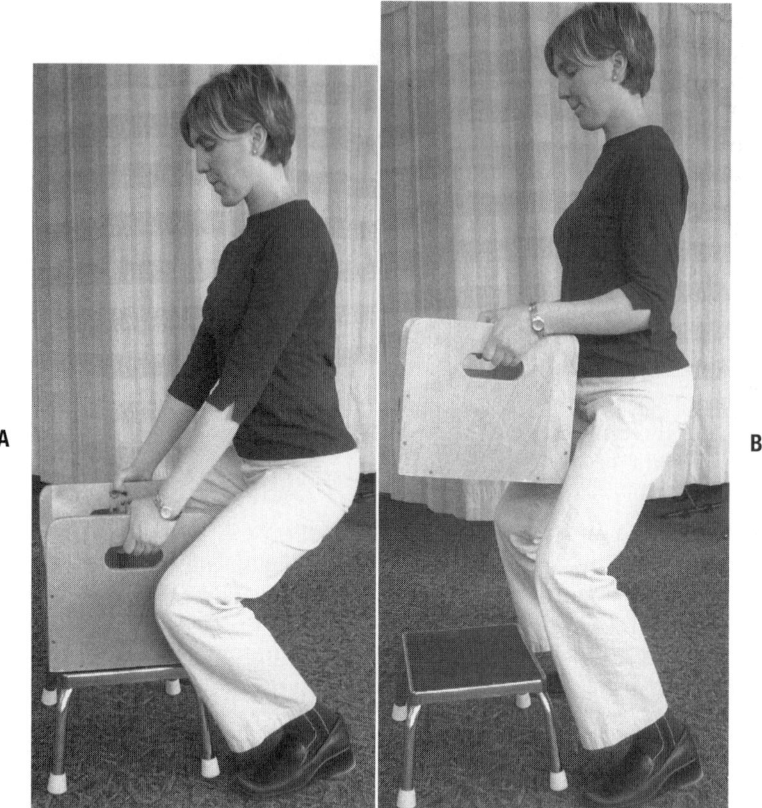

Fig. 4-2 Power lift. **A,** Start position; **B,** Midpoint of the lift.

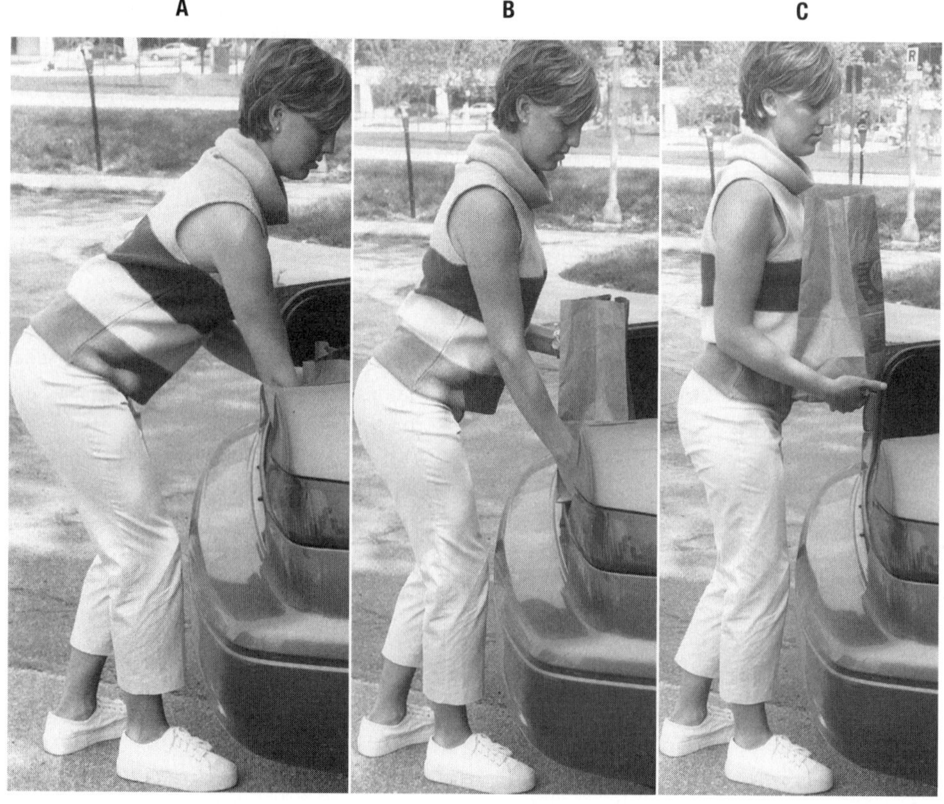

Fig. 4-3 Straight leg lift. **A,** Start position; **B,** Midposition of the lift; **C,** Completion of the lift.

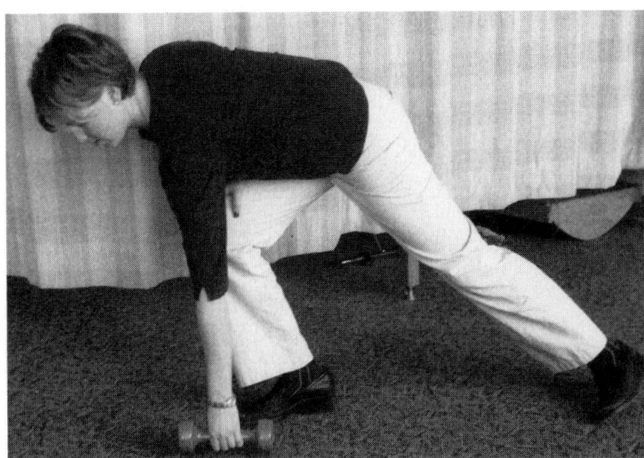

Fig. 4-4 One-leg stance lift ("golfer's lift").

handles, or under the bottom of the object. The lifter's trunk is maintained in a more vertical than horizontal position and the lumbar spine remains in lordosis with an anterior pelvic tilt (Fig. 4-2).

Straight Leg Lift. The lifter's knees are only slightly flexed or may be fully extended. The lower extremities are either parallel to each other or straddle the object and the upper extremities are either parallel to each other or grasp the opposite sides of the object. The trunk may be positioned either vertically or horizontally and the lumbar spine remains in lordosis (Fig. 4-3).

One-Leg Stance Lift ("Golfer's Lift"). The one-leg stance lift can be used for light objects that can be lifted easily with one upper extremity. The lifter faces the object, with the body weight shifted onto the forward lower extremity. To pick up the object, the weight-bearing lower extremity is partially flexed at the hip and knee while the non–weight-bearing lower extremity is lifted into extension to counterbalance the forward movement of the trunk (Fig. 4-4). The lifter picks up the object in a manner similar to the way a golfer removes a golf ball from the cup and returns to an upright position.

Half-Kneeling Lift. To perform the half-kneeling lift, the lifter aligns the body by kneeling on one knee positioned behind and on one side of the object and positions the opposite lower extremity to one side of the object with the foot flat and the hip and knee flexed approximately 90 degrees. The object is grasped and lifted by the upper extremities, placed on the thigh of the flexed lower extremity, and moved close to the body before the flexed lower extremity begins rising to standing. The opposite lower extremity assists with raising the body as the person continues to stand (Fig. 4-5). The lumbar spine is maintained in its normal lordosis throughout the lift. This lift allows the lifter to secure the object close to the body before standing. This is a useful lift for persons of small stature or whose upper extremity strength is limited and whose initial unilateral lower extremity strength and overall balance while rising to standing are exceptional. *Caution:* Persons with a knee condition that would be exacerbated by kneeling should avoid this lift and rotating or twisting the trunk to position the object on the thigh should be avoided.

Traditional Lift. To perform the traditional lift, the lifter faces the object with the feet anteroposterior on each side of the object and the lower extremities in a full squat. This position provides a low COG and a wide BOS for the lifter. The person grasps the underside of the object with the upper extremities parallel or anteroposterior to each other. The lift is begun by the flexor muscles of the upper extremities to partially lift the object and then the lower extremities are used to raise the body and object to an upright position as the hips and knees extend. The object should be held close to the body and the lumbar spine should maintain its normal lordosis throughout the lift (see Box 4-3; Fig. 4-6). The lift provides stability for the lifter and makes use of the large extensor muscles of the lower extremities to raise the body to full standing. *Caution:* This lift must be performed by the lower extremities, not by the back. To accomplish this, elevation of the hips and pelvis before the body is raised by the lower extremities must be avoided and the normal lumbar lordosis must be maintained.

Stoop Lift. When an object rests below the level of the waist, but can be reached without squatting, the lifter can stoop to lift. The person partially flexes the hips and knees and maintains the lumbar spine in its normal lordosis. The lifter grasps the object and uses the lower extremities to raise the body and the object. To improve stability and balance, the feet are positioned at shoulder width and slightly anteroposterior to each other. When the object can be lifted by one upper extremity (that is, suitcase, briefcase, tool carrier, pail, shopping bag with handles), the other upper extremity can be used for support (Fig. 4-7). This lift requires less energy expenditure than a lift that uses a deep or full squat.

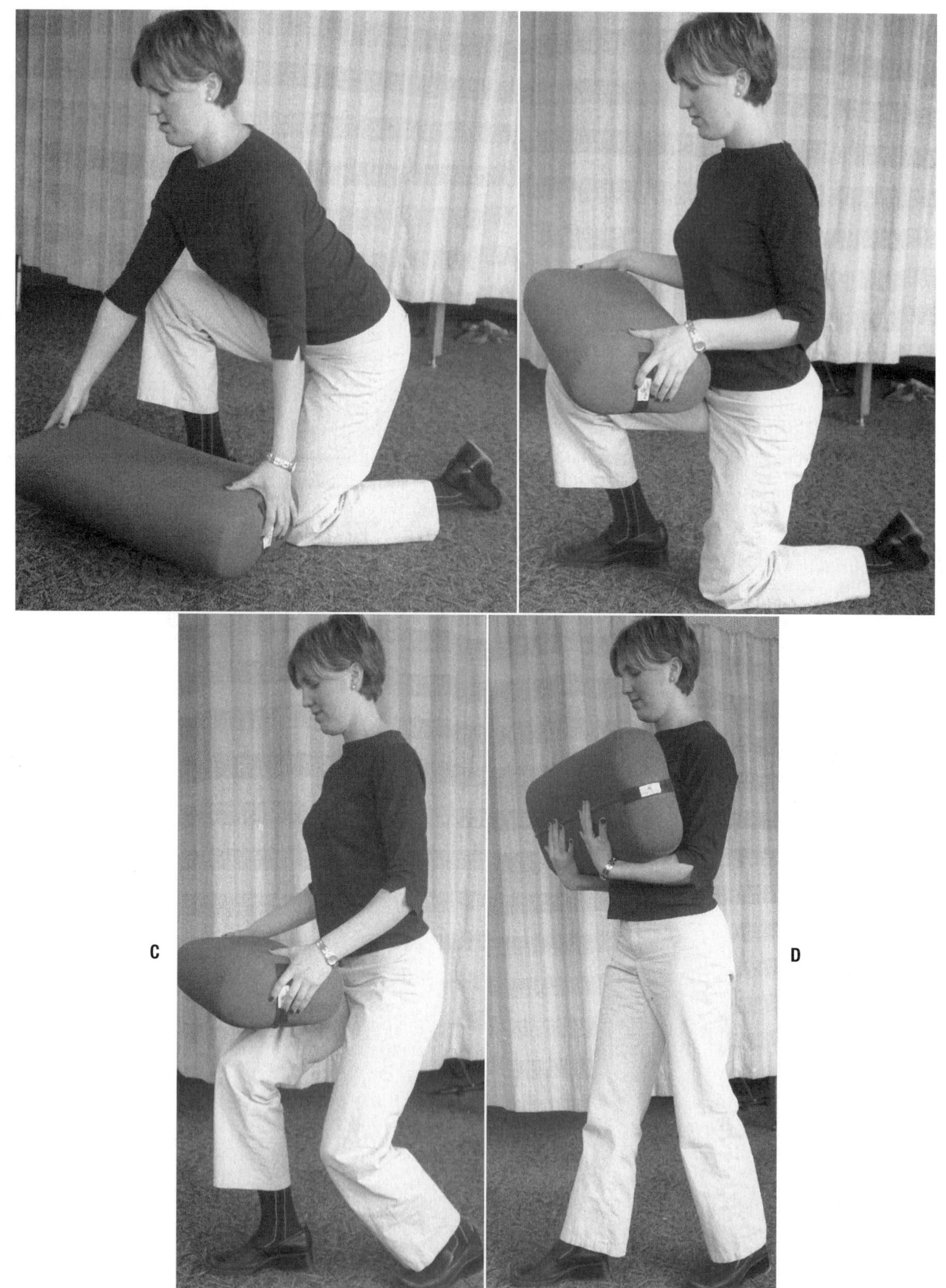

Fig. 4-5 Half-kneeling lift. **A,** Start position; **B,** Support position; **C,** Midpoint of the lift; **D,** Completion of the lift.

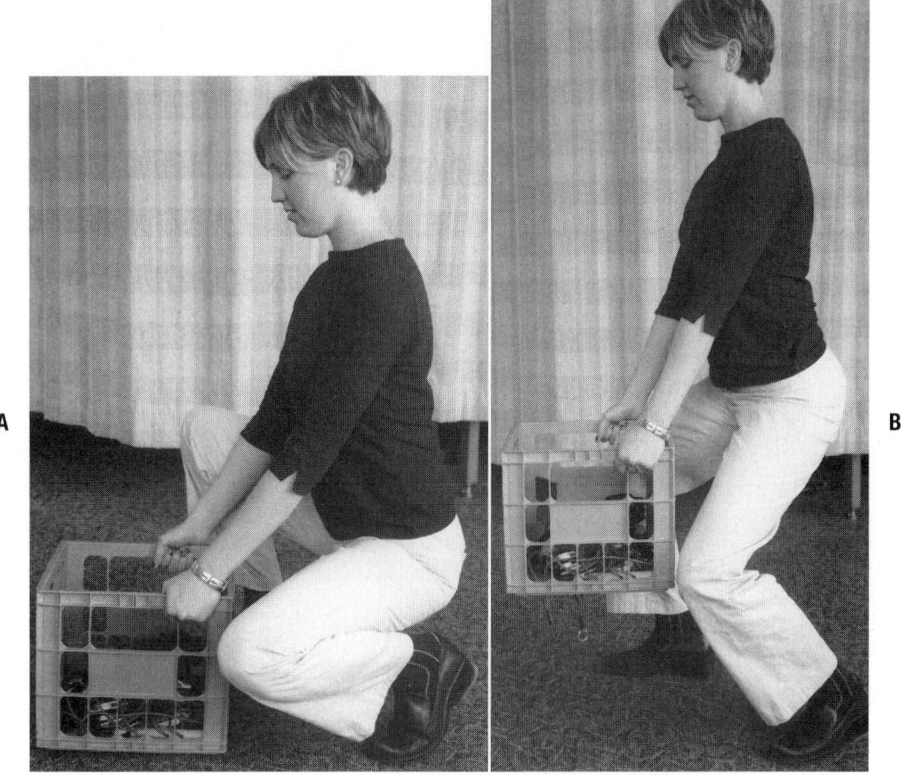

Fig. 4-6 Traditional lift. **A,** Start position; **B,** Continuation of the lift.

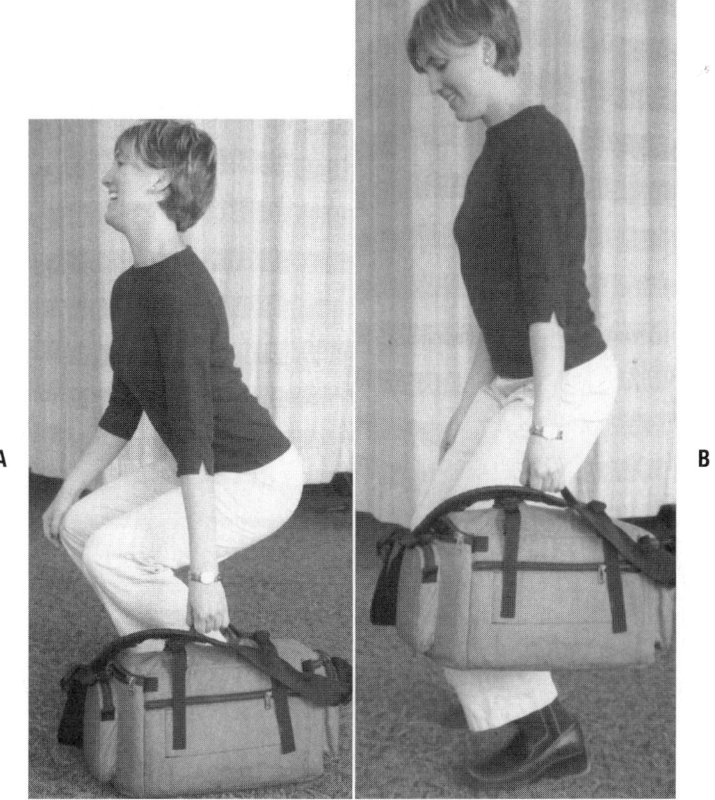

Fig. 4-7 Stoop lift. **A,** Start position; **B,** Continuation of the lift.

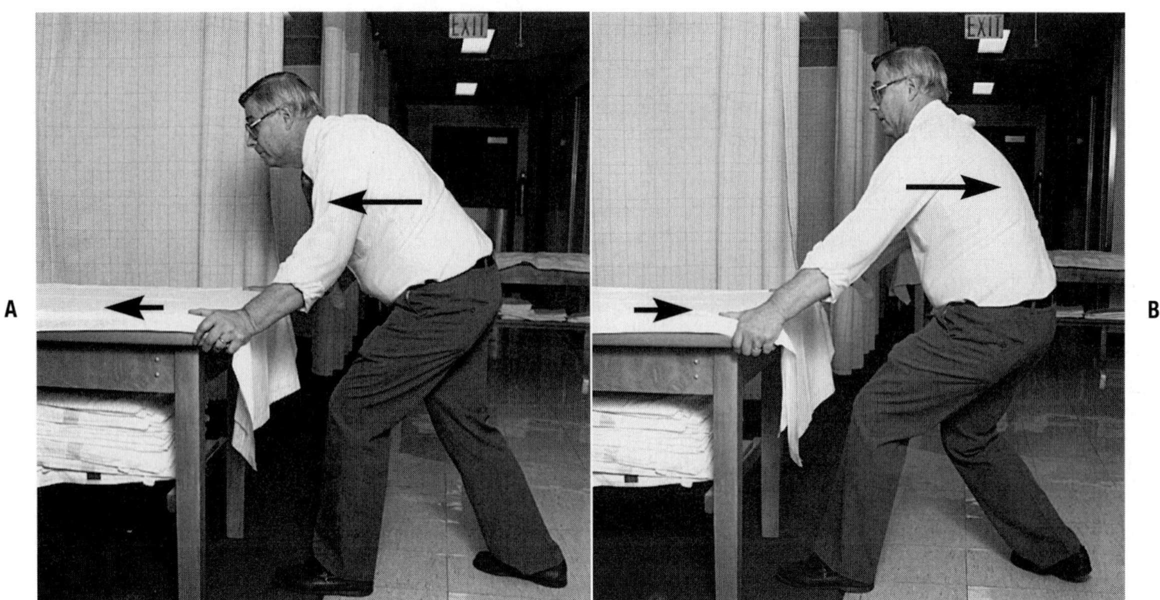

Fig. 4-8 **A,** Pushing an object; **B,** Pulling an object.

PUSHING, PULLING, REACHING, AND CARRYING

Many of the same principles described for lifting also apply to pushing and pulling activities. Use a crouched or semisquat position to push or pull (Fig. 4-8). This position lowers your COG nearer to the object's COG, which increases stability, reduces energy expenditure, and improves control of the object. The force of the push or pull should be applied parallel to the surface over which the object is to be moved and in the line of movement desired. This reduces the effects of friction and moves the object in the proper direction. Initially, consideration should be given to how to overcome the effects of inertia and friction and the influence of *vector* forces. Inertia and friction are forces that impede the movement of an object. More force is required to start the movement of a stationary object than to continue its movement; therefore you should prepare yourself to exert greater effort when beginning to push or pull an object than you will need to continue to push or pull it. You may find that rocking the object to generate some motion helps to overcome its inertia; similarly, tipping or partially lifting the object to reduce contact between the object and the surface on which it rests reduces the friction between the object and the underlying surface. You can turn or redirect the direction of movement of the object by the use of a force that alters the vectors of motion. You can accomplish this by pushing harder with one upper extremity than with the other, by pulling with one upper extremity and pushing with the other upper extremity, or by positioning your body at one corner of the object and pushing or pulling at an angle to the line of forward motion. Remember that, in most situations, energy will be conserved if an object is moved by sliding, rolling, or turning rather than by lifting or carrying.

Reaching for an object above your shoulder or head will be less strenuous if the object is lowered or if you raise your position by standing on a wide-based footstool or ladder (Fig. 4-9). These actions approximate the COG of the object and your COG, allow the use of shortened extremity lever arms, and decrease strain to back structures. An object at arm's length should be brought closer to one's body before being lifted to reduce the torque produced by long lever arms. For example, move a patient from the center of the bed or mat to one edge of the bed or mat before performing exercises or help the *recumbent* patient to move up or down or to sit up so he or she is nearer to you. When carrying an object, hold it close to your body, using your arms as short lever arms, and maintain its COG near your COG. Localize the COG of bulky objects by folding or otherwise positioning extended portions of the object toward its center. If you carry an object in a backpack or chest pack, be certain both shoulder straps are used and the weight is distributed in the pack with the weight close to your COG. You should avoid carrying the pack over one shoulder because it will affect your COG and require you to alter your posture, leading to increased strain of several structures (such as muscles, ligaments, tendons, joint surfaces).

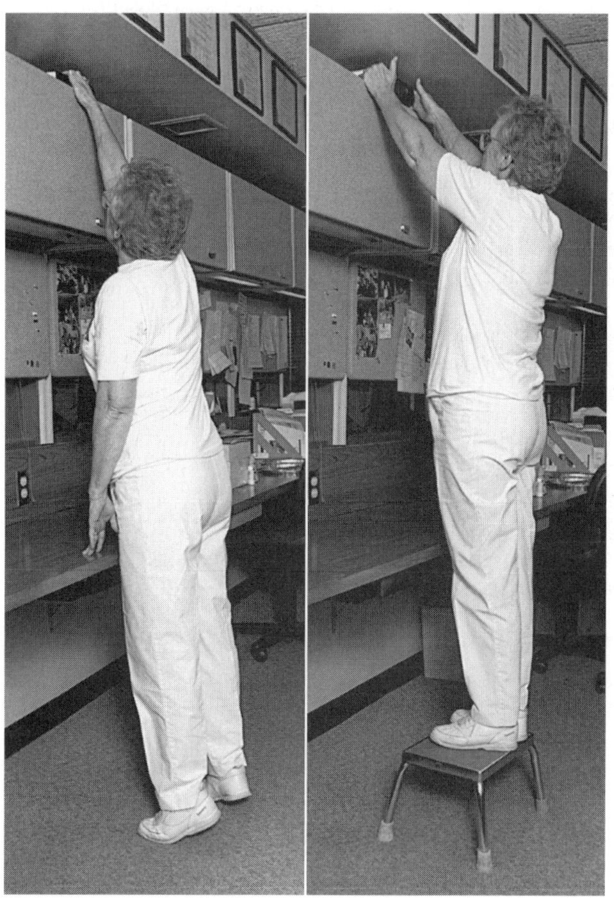

Fig. 4-9 Reaching for an object above the shoulder.

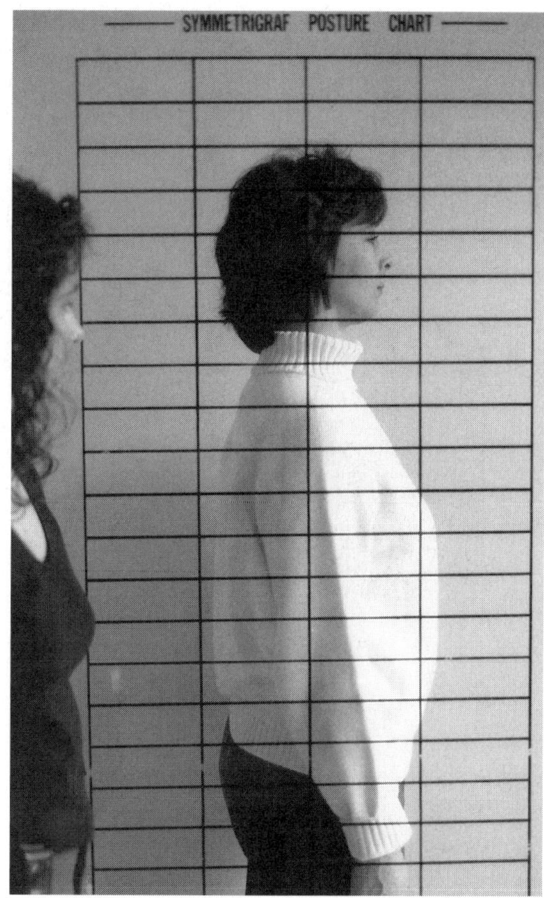

Fig. 4-10 Assessing standing posture using a posture grid.

POSTURE AND BODY CONTROL

Good posture, strength, and flexibility are important factors to prevent back and neck problems. Chronic joint sprains and muscle strains are often caused by many hours of tension placed on muscles or joints because of poor posture. Poor physical condition leads to the loss of strength and endurance necessary to perform physical tasks without strain and is a predisposition to injury. Sustained posture, even if in good alignment, can cause fatigue. Reaching with heavy loads, sitting for long periods with the back unsupported, working with objects that are too low or far away, and even sleeping on a too firm or a sagging mattress can cause back and neck pain and decreased range of motion.

As caregivers, it is our responsibility to observe a patient's posture while sitting, standing, and moving regardless of the diagnosis (Fig. 4-10). Persons with a history of low back pain or dysfunction and those whose life-style or occupation predisposes them to trauma to structures of the back (that is, repetitive lifting) should be educated in ways to prevent further back injuries. Because sitting puts more stress on the back than lying, standing, or walking, it is important to instruct those patients about proper sitting techniques when sustained sitting is necessary in their jobs (Fig. 4-11). The most important achievements in good sitting posture are a resting position for the upper extremities and correction of a forward head posture (Fig. 4-12). Sustained standing causes postural fatigue throughout the musculoskeletal system and techniques for lessening this fatigue should be provided (Boxes 4-4 and 4-5). Correcting faulty posture and guiding patients in healthy habits of good nutrition, physical fitness, stress management, rest, and exercise will assist them to attain a healthier life-style.

An initial assessment or evaluation of the individual should be performed before starting patient education. Observe the individual's posture and review any previous history related to the present condition, the mechanisms of the current injury, onset and type of symptoms, previous treatments, and current life-style and work activities, including the work environment (see Box 4-2).

Most patients, regardless of their condition or cause of injury, will benefit from basic education related to care of the structures of the back. This education is usually performed through a formal program frequently referred to as a "back

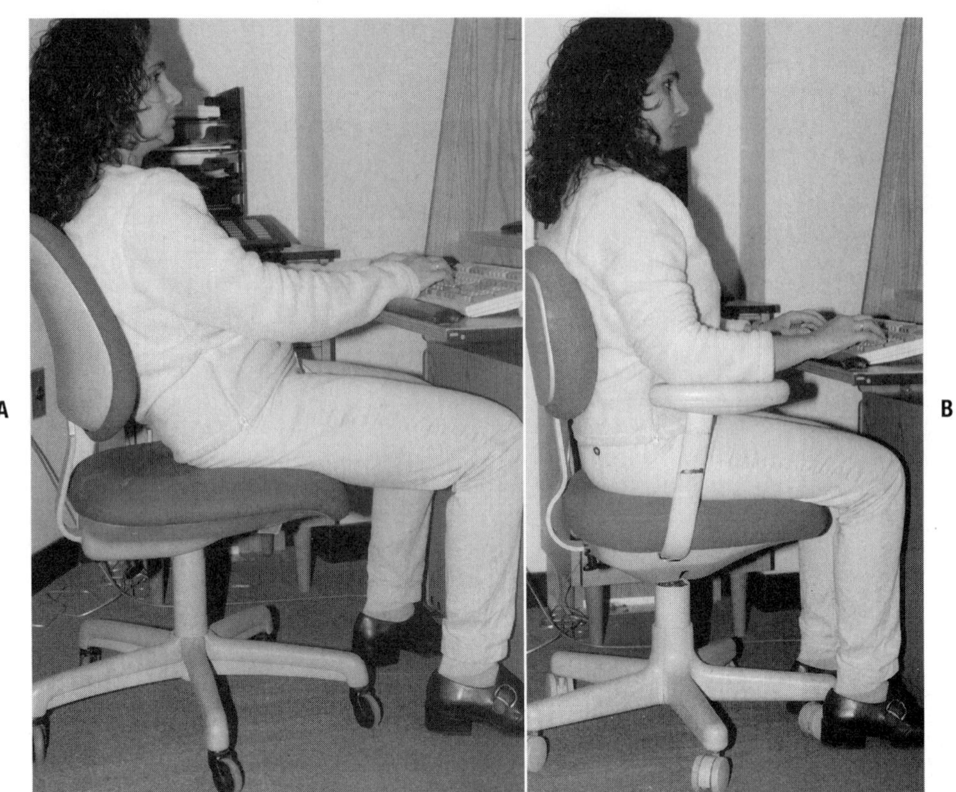

Fig. 4-11 Seated posture at a computer terminal. **A,** Improper seated posture; **B,** Proper seated posture.

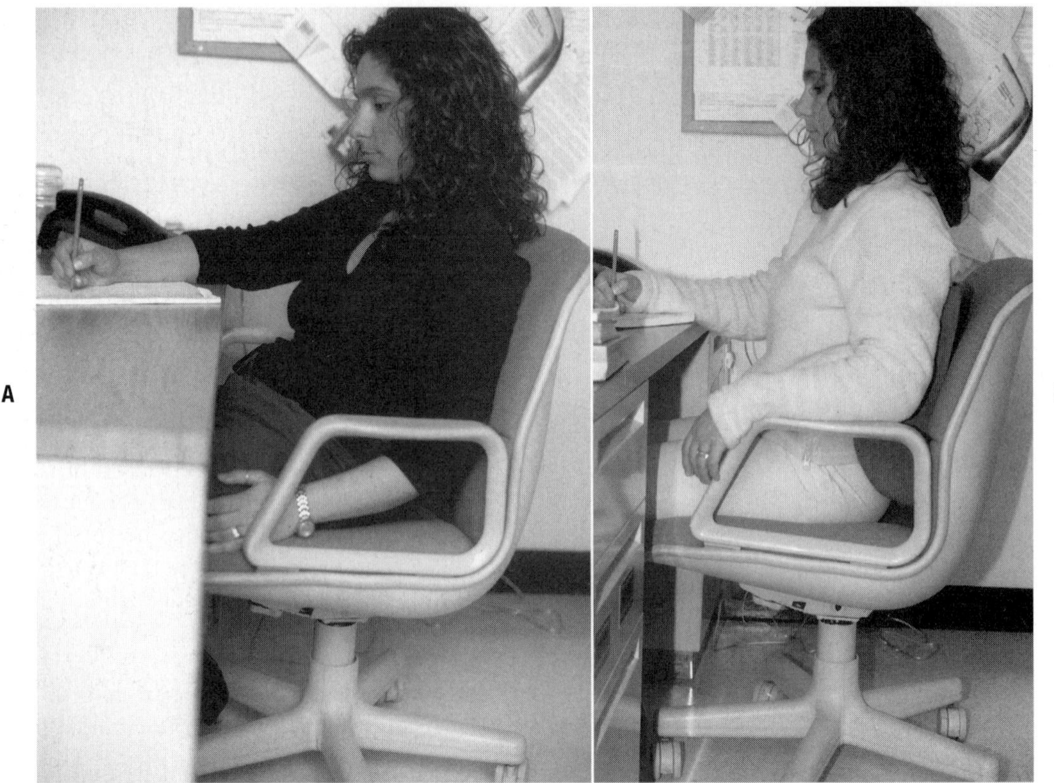

Fig. 4-12 Seated posture at a desk. **A,** Improper seated posture; **B,** Proper seated posture. Notice use of a back support.

Box 4-4 Principles for Proper Posture

Maintain the normal anterior and posterior curves of the spine for proper balance and alignment.

Stand and sit with your body erect so that your shoulders and pelvis (hips) are level; avoid slouch, or "round back" positions.

Stand with abdominal wall flat, head in neutral, shoulders level, chin parallel to the floor and slightly tucked, and your body weight evenly placed on each leg; keep your knees straight or slightly flexed; and maintain lumbar lordosis.

Sit with your head in neutral, chin tucked or parallel to the floor, and elbows, knees, and hips flexed to 90 degrees with your feet flat on the floor or supported in a slightly inclined position. Your forearms and low back curve should be supported during prolonged sitting. Avoid slouch, or "round back" posture.

Avoid standing or sitting in one position for a prolonged time; occasionally alter the position. Move your head, neck, shoulders, back, hips, knees, and ankles periodically.

Stand with your ankles, knees, hips, and shoulders aligned; keep your head over your body, not in front of the shoulders.

Lie on your back or side with your hips and knees partially flexed. Use a pillow under or between the knees for support and avoid lying prone. Use a small or medium-sized pillow to support your head, but do not position it under the shoulders. Use a bed mattress that is firm and provides support to the natural curves of the spine.

Box 4-5 Guidelines to Reduce Stress-Producing Positions or Activities

Alter your posture or position frequently; avoid prolonged standing or sitting.

Avoid bending at the waist while working, washing your face, brushing your teeth, or performing activities that are below your waist (such as bathing children in a bathtub, removing clothes from the washer or dryer); sit, stoop, or kneel instead of bending.

For activities that require prolonged standing, use a cushioned mat and wear low-heeled shoes with good arch supports. Place one foot on a footstool or railing and alternate feet occasionally for comfort (as when ironing or washing dishes). Perform a 30-second exercise routine every hour that includes low back flexion and extension, hip and knee flexion (knee to chest while standing), neck extension, lateral bending, and shoulder range of motion in all planes.

When seated at a work station for prolonged periods, keep your elbows, knees, and hips level and bent at 90 degrees; your feet should be flat on the floor or supported at a slight incline. Your forearms should be supported by armrests and your back by the chair back or a rolled pillow. A back-support cushion should support your low back curve if necessary.

When seated at a computer terminal, the vision display terminal should be directed about 10 degrees below horizontal. The chair used should encourage a supported lumbar lordosis with a seat pan that is tilted slightly forward. The keyboard should be pushed forward to permit the arms to rest in front of it, ideally, with the wrists supported on a padded surface. A 30-second exercise break every hour to include neck flexion, extension, and lateral bending stretching exercises, chin tucks, wrist flexion and extension stretches, shoulder pendulum exercises, tennis elbow stretch, and standing back bends are recommended.

Enter and leave an automobile with a sideward rather than a twisting motion of the trunk. Adjust your car seat so your knees are at the same level as your hips, use a lumbar support and stop frequently when driving long distances to walk or stretch your arms, legs, and back. Keep your chin tucked and head held erect (Fig. 4-13).

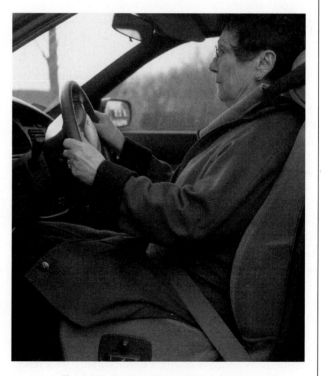

Fig. 4-13 Proper seated posture for driving.

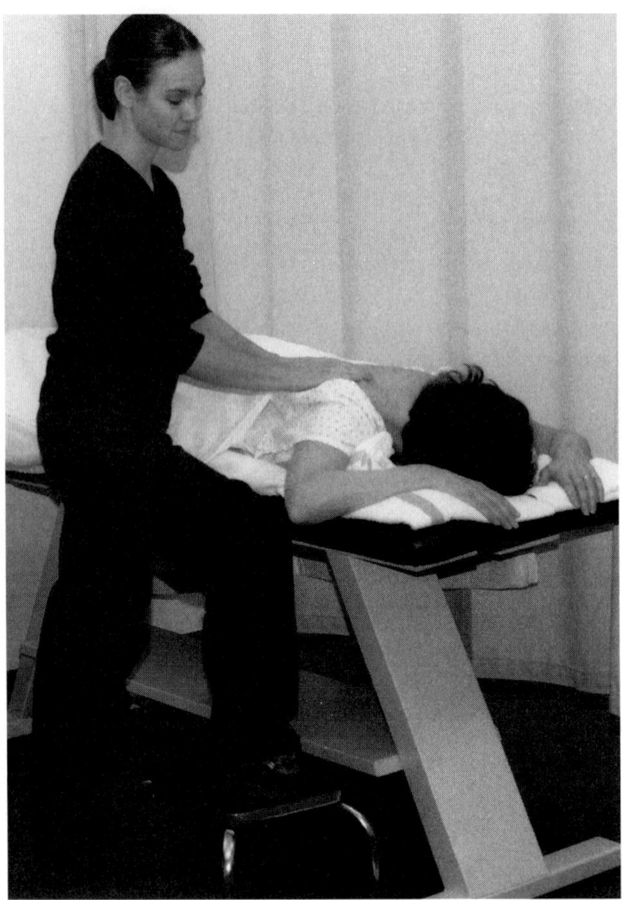

Fig. 4-14 Use of a footstool to relieve stress to the lumbar spine.

school." However, simple instructions and reminders can provide the patient or family member with information to protect the back structures. In this text, only the most basic information is presented.

Initially the patient should receive information about the basic anatomy of the body, especially the structures that affect the back. Instruction in the use of proper body mechanics and how to correct faulty standing, sitting, or recumbent postures should be presented. Suggestions on ways to identify and correct improper work, recreational, or daily life habits will be beneficial. Some simple exercises for a healthy back include the pelvic tilt, knee to chest while supine, partial sit-ups, hamstring stretches, hip stretch, press-ups, wall slides, neck glide and neck stretches. Methods that can be used to protect or relieve back stress, such as the placement of one foot on a footstool while standing (Fig. 4-14) or the use of a lumbar cushion or roll while sitting (see Fig. 4-12, *B*), should be recommended (see Box 4-5). Information about the use of body mechanics should be given to the patient. Instruction in ways to maintain the proper condition and function of muscles, ligaments, and joint structures through the use of relaxation, flexibility, strengthening activities, and aerobic exercise are important components of patient education.

The person should be cautioned to balance work, recreational activities, and rest activities to avoid chronic overuse syndromes or the development of a specific dysfunction. It may be necessary to evaluate the person's work or home environment so specific suggestions related to those settings can be given. The person should be advised to reduce, eliminate, or frequently change sustained or repetitive positions, postures, and activities that cause back stress, strain, or discomfort such as trunk flexion, prolonged sitting or standing, and combined lifting and twisting motions (see Box 4-5). The names and locations of qualified practitioners who can be contacted when professional advice or treatment is needed should be made available. There are many booklets, brochures, posters, videotapes, and other educational materials available for the patient. Most treatment units that care for patients with back dysfunction will have these materials.

The patient should be encouraged and motivated to develop a sense of individual responsibility for the proper care of the back. The patient must realize he or she is the only person who has direct control over life-style, behavior, posture, and use of the body; therefore the most appropriate person to assume responsibility for the care of the back is the individual as long as sufficient information and guidance to be independently responsible has been provided (Boxes 4-6 to 4-9).

Box 4-6 Guidelines for Lifting Activities

- Stoop or squat to lift any object that is below the level of your hips.
- Widen your feet to increase your BOS and improve your balance and stability.
- Move close to the object before you lift; keep it close to your body as you lift or carry it.
- Keep the lumbar curve in your lower back as you lift; do not flatten your lower back when you lift.
- Mentally plan the lift; be certain you can safely lift the object without assistance, that you have sufficient space to perform the lift, and that you test the weight of the object before you lift it.
- Do not lift and twist your back at the same time; pivot on your feet when you need to turn.
- Do not lift quickly or with a jerky motion.
- Move the object by pushing, pulling, sliding, or rolling rather than by lifting it when possible; pushing is better than pulling.
- Avoid repetitive, sustained lifting; use equipment or assistance to lift heavy objects.
- Use care when removing groceries, tools, or other items from the trunk of a car; do not bend at the waist and lift; bend your hips and knees slightly and move the object close to you before lifting it.

Box 4-7 Guidelines for Pushing and Pulling Activities

- Crouch and face the object squarely.
- Use your arms and legs to push or pull; push with your arms partially bent.
- Push or pull in a straight line; your force should be parallel to the floor.
- Be certain there are no objects in your path and doorways are wide enough for the object to pass through.

Box 4-8 Guidelines for Reaching Activities

- Stand on a footstool or ladder to reach an object that is above your head or to place an object above your head.
- Move the object close to you before lowering or raising it; be certain you will be able to control the object safely.
- Hold the object close to your body as you step down from or onto the footstool.
- Do not simultaneously reach and twist your body.

Box 4-9 Guidelines for Carrying Activities

- Carry all objects by holding them close to your body; the best positions are in front of your body at the level of your waist, midchest, or on your back.
- If you carry an object in one hand (such as a suitcase, briefcase), alternate carrying it in one hand and then in the other; do not twist your back when moving the object from one hand to the other; stoop to lift it from the floor.
- Balance the load whenever possible.
- Some bulky or heavy objects can be carried on your shoulders, especially if you must carry them for a substantial distance.
- Avoid carrying or balancing a small child on one hip; use an infant carrier or hold the child close to your chest.
- When a backpack is used, apply both shoulder straps.

SUMMARY

The use of proper body mechanics assists the caregiver to avoid excessive and unnecessary stress or strain to various body systems, reduces energy requirements, and enhances patient safety. For these reasons, persons, including the patient, should be instructed in the use of proper body mechanics and posture when they perform lifting, reaching, carrying, pushing, and pulling activities.

Effective body mechanics depend on the stability of your BOS, maintenance of your VGL within your BOS, your foot and body positions in relation to an object, and your use of short lever arms when you lift or reach. Information should be provided to patients about ways to reduce stress-producing posture or to improve work position and methods to provide stretching, strengthening, flexibility, and relaxation to body areas that are overused during work. Finally, a sense of personal responsibility for the proper care and use of one's body should be developed by each caregiver and patient.

self-study ACTIVITIES

- Define your concept of proper body mechanics.
- Describe at least four adverse effects that could occur if you used improper body mechanics to lift, push, pull, reach, or carry an object or to transfer a patient.
- Outline a program or the instructions you would provide to a patient to promote proper back care.
- Describe different types of lifts and explain when you would use them.
- Outline and describe five suggestions you would provide to a person who desires information about the prevention of low back stress or injury.
- Describe the use of proper body mechanics when moving a recumbent person, lifting any object from the floor, pushing or pulling a piece of equipment, reaching and removing any object from a shelf above your head, and carrying an object with both upper extremities or one upper extremity.

problem SOLVING

1. You and another student are asked to educate a group of 10 nursing students in the most effective and safest use of body mechanics for lifting, pushing, pulling, and reaching. Before you meet with them, you must review your plan and teaching methods with your clinical instructor. What plan will you prepare, what teaching methods will you use, and what equipment will you need?
2. You are treating a patient whose job requires him to transfer 5-pound boxes at a rate of 5 per minute from a waist-high conveyor belt to a pallet on the floor. The boxes contain fragile items and can be stacked only two boxes high. What suggestions or instructions would you give him or his employer to enable him to perform the task safely and effectively?

CHAPTER 5

Positioning and Draping

objectives *After studying this chapter, the reader will be able to:*

- Describe appropriate positioning of the trunk, head, and extremities with the patient supine, prone, side lying, or sitting.
- Describe appropriate draping of the patient.
- Discuss precautions related to positioning a patient who is supine, prone, side lying, or sitting.
- Present a rationale for the use and application of proper patient positioning.
- Present a rationale for the use and application of proper draping of a patient.

key terms

Abduction Movement away from an axis or from the median plane of the body; movement of a body part away from the middle of the body.

Adduction Movement toward an axis or toward the median plane of the body; movement of a body part toward the middle of the body.

Blanch To become pale.

Comatose Pertaining to or affected with coma; a state of unconsciousness.

Contracture Shortening or tightening of the skin, muscle, fascia, or joint capsule that prevents normal movement or flexibility of the involved structure.

Extension Movement that increases or straightens the angle between two adjoining body parts or bones.

Flexion Movement that decreases the angle between two adjoining body parts or bones.

Hyperextension Extension of a limb or part beyond the normal limit; overextension of a limb or part.

Ischemia Deficiency of blood in a part because of functional constriction or actual obstruction of a blood vessel.

Ischial tuberosity The protuberance of the ischium; the inferior, distal portion of the pelvis.

Maceration The softening of a solid by soaking.

Necrosis Morphologic changes indicative of cell death.

Occipital tuberosity The protuberance of the occipital bone; the posterior area of the skull.

Perineum The pelvic floor and associated structures occupying the pelvic outlet.

Prone Lying face downward on the vertical (front) surface of the body; lying on the abdomen and chest.

Recumbent Lying down.

Restraint (physical) Any manual method or physical or mechanical device, material, or equipment attached or adjacent to the patient's body that he or she cannot easily remove and restricts freedom of movement or normal access to the body.

Restraint (drug) Medication used to control behavior or to restrict the patient's freedom of movement and is not a standard treatment for the patient's medical or psychiatric condition.

Reverse T position The position of the upper extremities when they are abducted to 90 degrees and externally rotated at the shoulders and with the elbows flexed to 90 degrees.

Rotation The pivoting of a body part around its axis.

Seclusion The involuntary confinement of a person in a room or area where the person is physically prevented from leaving.

key terms—cont'd

Shear An applied force that tends to cause an opposite, but parallel, sliding motion of the planes of an object; stress is created to the object.

Spasticity Continuous resistance to stretching by a muscle because of abnormally increased tension.

Supine Lying with the face upward or on the dorsal (back) surface of the body; lying on the back.

T position The position of the upper extremities when they are abducted to 90 degrees and internally rotated at the shoulders and with the elbows flexed to 90 degrees.

INTRODUCTION

Patient positioning must be considered before, during, and at the conclusion of treatment and when a patient is to be at rest for an extended period. Although patient comfort must be considered and constitutes one reason to position a patient, the caregiver must be aware the position of comfort may be the position that could lead to the development of a soft-tissue *contracture*. Therefore frequent changes in the patient's position, approximately every 2 hours, may be necessary to prevent contractures or to relieve pressure to the skin and subcutaneous, circulatory, neural, lymphatic, or other structures. The greatest pressure occurs to the tissues that cover bony prominences. Table 5-1 provides an outline of the areas that receive the greatest pressure when the patient is in a specific position.

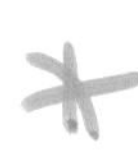

The caregiver should use caution when positioning a patient who has decreased sensation to pressure, is unable to alter position independently and safely, has minimal soft-tissue protection over bony prominences, and is unable to express or communicate discomfort. The patient's trunk, head, and extremities should be supported and stabilized and proper alignment of the axial and appendicular skeletal segments should be maintained to provide a position that will promote efficient function of the patient's body systems. The patient should be positioned to enable the caregiver to administer treatment effectively, efficiently, and safely; therefore the caregiver should determine how the patient's position may affect body mechanics and the treatment program before initiation of treatment.

Table 5-1 Bony Prominences That Often Cause Pressure Injuries

Area	Supine Position	Prone Position	Side-Lying Position (lowermost extremity)	Side-Lying Position (uppermost extremity)	Sitting Position
Head and trunk	• Occipital tuberosity • Spine of scapula • Inferior angle of scapula • Vertebral spinous processes • Posterior iliac crest • Sacrum	• Forehead • Lateral ear • Tip of acromion process • Sternum • Anterosuperior iliac spine	• Lateral ear • Lateral ribs • Lateral acromion process	—	• Ischial tuberosities • Scapular and vertebral spinous processes (if leaning against back of chair)
Upper extremity	• Medial epicondyle of humerus	• Anterior head of humerus	• Lateral head of humerus • Medial or lateral epicondyle of humerus	• Medial epicondyle of humerus (if resting on a hard surface)	• Medial epicondyle of humerus (if resting on a hard surface)
Lower extremity	• Posterior calcaneus • Greater trochanter, head of fibula, and lateral malleolus with excessive hip external rotation	• Patella • Ridge of tibia • Dorsum of foot	• Greater trochanter of femur • Medial and lateral condyles of femur • Malleolus of fibula and tibia	• Medial condyle of femur • Malleolus of tibia	—

PRINCIPLES AND CONCEPTS

The patient should be draped, with use of clean linen, to expose only the areas or body parts to be treated, with the remainder of the patient's body covered to maintain modesty and warmth. Precautions must be taken to avoid unnecessary exposure of sensitive areas of the patient's body. For example, draping of the anterior chest (breasts) of females and the *perineum* (genitalia) of both males and females must be performed carefully and may need to be adjusted periodically to ensure the drape is secure.

The linen used to drape each patient should be clean and unused before being applied to the patient. Because the drape material may become soiled with perspiration, lubricants, or wound drainage, the patient's clothing should not be used as a drape. In many instances, undergarments and outer garments may need to be removed from the patient to prevent soiling and to add to the patient's comfort. Before removal of any garments, explain to the patient the need for their removal and obtain the patient's permission. You may need to assure the patient that modesty will be maintained throughout the treatment session or activity.

Remove or reduce folds or wrinkles in the linen beneath the patient to avoid increased skin pressure. Folded or wrinkled linen creates a thickness greater than that of the other areas of the linen and may cause localized pressure. Linen that is used to protect the patient's axilla, perineum, or gluteal cleft must be discarded as soon as it is removed from the patient because it is likely to be soiled. This linen should never be reapplied to the patient or used for any other patient until it has been laundered.

Be certain to instruct or direct the patient how to position and initially drape the body. A gown or other suitable item should be given to the patient if removal of clothing or protection of sensitive areas is required. The treatment table or mat should be prepared with linen and pillows before the patient is positioned. The caregiver's instructions and directions should inform the patient exactly what to do, how to lie on the table, and how to apply the gown and drape.

Pillows, rolled towels, or commercially available devices can be used to support or stabilize body segments to relieve strain to the patient's joints, ligaments, muscles, tendons, connective tissue, and nerves. A firm mattress usually enhances proper positioning, but the patient's condition and ability to alter a position should be considered when determining the type of surface on which the person will sit or lie (Procedure 5-1).

POSITIONING

The recommendations provided for short-term positioning should be appropriate for most patients. However, there are differing opinions about the use (or nonuse) and placement of pillows, towel rolls, bolsters, and similar items. Specific patient needs and the treatment to be given will affect the position the caregiver selects. The positions described in this text should be modified based on criteria the caregiver

PROCEDURE 5-1

Guidelines for Positioning and Draping

Introduce yourself to the patient; provide your name and status (that is, physical therapist, physical therapist assistant, physical therapy student, aide, technician, occupational therapist, certified occupational therapist assistant); and confirm the patient's name and current, relevant information (that is, diagnosis, complaints, previous treatment and response, physician).

Inform the patient of the planned treatment, apply the principles of informed consent, and obtain consent for treatment.

Specifically describe how the person is to be positioned; provide assistance if required.

If the person is wearing street clothes, indicate the specific articles of clothing to be removed or request permission to remove them if assistance is necessary.

Provide temporary clothing or linen to protect modesty and provide warmth.

Have sufficient linen, pillows, and equipment needed for the treatment available in the cubicle or treatment area.

Provide safe and secure storage for the patient's valuable items.

Specifically describe how you desire the patient to use linen items, gown, robe, or exercise clothing to cover (drape) the body; provide privacy while disrobing.

Instruct the patient to inform you when he or she is positioned and draped, or confirm the person is clothed or draped so that you may enter the cubicle.

At the conclusion of the treatment:

Instruct the patient to remove drape items and temporary clothing and to reapply clothing; provide assistance if required; provide privacy while dressing.

Provide linen so the patient can remove perspiration, massage lotion, electrotherapy gels, water, or other substances.

Return valuables.

Dispose used linen in proper container.

Prepare the cubicle or treatment area for future use or assign the task to another person.

Note: Depending on the gender of the caregiver and the patient and the area or areas of the patient to be exposed for treatment, it may be necessary for the caregiver to request another person to assist the patient in undressing, positioning, draping, and redressing to protect modesty.

determines to be necessary for each patient. Specific patient conditions, such as the loss of or decreased sensory awareness, paralysis, decreased skin integrity, poor nutrition, impaired circulation, and a predisposition to contracture development, require special attention to positioning. For a patient with any of these conditions, it will be necessary to inspect the patient's skin, especially over bony prominences, before and immediately after the treatment session. Areas that are red indicate areas of pressure and pale, or *blanched*, areas may indicate severe, dangerous pressure. Complaints of numbness or tingling are indicators of excessive pressure, as is localized edema or swelling. *Caution:* Pressure to a localized area of soft tissue, especially when there is an underlying bony prominence, produces local *ischemia*, which over time can lead to tissue *necrosis*. You must be particularly aware of these possible consequences when you treat a patient whose condition involves the contributing factors described previously in this paragraph (Box 5-1).

Restraints, or safety straps, may be used to protect the patient from rolling or falling and to prevent injury. They are recommended for short-term use only and not to hinder or restrain the patient for several hours. The patient who is *comatose*, experiences *spasticity*, has extensive paralysis, or is unable to mentally or physically maintain a safe position may require some form of temporary restraint or protective positioning. These protective measures are to be differentiated from the use of prolonged restraints.

In general, unless a patient needs to be restrained for protection or to protect others from harm by the patient, physical or drug restraints are not to be used without the voluntary consent of the patient. Furthermore, a restraint should be used only when less restrictive interventions have been tried and found to be ineffective. Some examples of restraints are wrist or ankle belts or straps, a tightly wrapped bed sheet that constrains the patient's upper and lower extremities and trunk, a cloth body garment (such as Posey vest, "straight jacket"), and, at times, bed rails when they are elevated. A drug can be a restraint when it is used to control behavior or restrict a patient's freedom of movement and when the drug is not a usual form of treatment for the patient's condition. Some items that are not considered to be physical restraints are straps used for surgical or radiographic positioning, an arm board used to protect an IV infusion site, orthopedic appliances, table top chairs, postural supports, and the therapeutic holding or comforting of children.

Rules, regulations, and guidelines related to the use of restraints and *seclusion* have been developed and are enforced by various state, local, and federal agencies and by accreditation organizations. Examples of these agencies and organizations include local and state mental health agencies; the Department of Public Health (DPH); the Centers for Medicare and Medicaid Services (CMS) (formerly known as the Health Care Financing Administration [HCFA]) of the Federal Department of Health and Human Services; the Joint Commission on Accreditation of Healthcare Organizations (JCAHO); and the American Osteopathic Association (AOA). Facilities regulated or accredited by any of these agencies or organizations should have written policies and procedures for the application, use, and alternative actions associated with restraints and seclusion. Examples of alternative measures or actions include having a family member present with the patient, scheduled timing for toileting activities, use of pain management techniques, bowel and bladder function assessment and training activities, the use of cushions or pads for support, music or television for distraction, frequent changes of scenery, frequent verbal instructions or directions, and rearrangement of furniture for better access by the patient to objects or controls.

Standards and rules related to the use of restraints and seclusion are contained in the Patient Rights Standards promulgated by HCFA in July 1999. The HCFA based the standards on the concept that "patients have the right to be free from the use of seclusion or restraint, of any form, as a means of coercion, convenience, or retaliation by staff," with the term "discipline" being added to the statement later. Compliance with these standards, and the rules that accompany them, is required for any facility that treats patients who are insured by Medicare or Medicaid as a Condition of Participation (CoP). Although many questions have arisen regarding the interpretation of the HCFA standards, it is clear that the use of restraints and seclusion in the short-term and long-term care of patients will be monitored closely by various local, state, and federal agencies and accreditation organizations. Two additional documents that support the intent of the HCFA standards are the Patient Rights and Organization Ethics standards established by JACHO and the Patient's Bill of Rights contained in the Consumer Bill of Rights and Responsibilities (CBRR) developed by the Presidential Advisory Committee on Consumer Protection and Quality in the Health Care Industry. The caregiver is obligated to be knowledgeable about and comply with the rules, regulations, and policies and procedures related to the appropriate use of restraints or seclusion of a patient. Additional sources for information about the use of restraints or seclusion for patients are the *Federal Register*, Vol. 64, No. 127; the current accreditation standards from JCAHO;

Box 5-1 Rationale for Proper Positioning

- Prevent soft-tissue and joint contractures.
- Provide patient comfort.
- Provide support and stability of patient's trunk and extremities.
- Provide access and exposure to areas to be treated.
- Promote efficient function of patient's organ systems.
- Provide position changes to relieve excessive, prolonged pressure to soft tissue, bony prominences, and circulatory and neurologic structures.

publications from the American Hospital Association (AHA) and its state organization; and publications from city, county, or state mental health departments.

Supine Position

Place a small pillow or a cervical roll under the patient's head, but avoid excessive neck and upper back *flexion* or scapular *abduction* (round shoulders) (Fig. 5-1). A small pillow, rolled towels, or small bolster can be placed in the popliteal spaces (that is, behind the knees) to relieve lumbar lordosis and promote comfort. Some patients may prefer to use a small lumbar roll or pillow. *Caution:* The item behind the knees will encourage hip and knee flexion and may contribute to lower-extremity contractures of the iliopsoas (hip flexor) and hamstring (knee flexor) muscles. This position should not be maintained for a prolonged period. A small, rolled towel or small bolster can be placed under the patient's ankles to relieve pressure to the calcaneus (heel), but knee *hyperextension* should be avoided.

The patient's upper extremities may be elevated on pillows or positioned in whatever way the patient desires for comfort (as by the patient's side, in a *reverse T position*, or folded on the chest). The patient's body and extremities should be totally supported on the mat or table; no part or portion of the body or extremities should project beyond its surface. *Caution:* If the patient's hands or feet extend beyond the mat or treatment table, they could be injured if they are struck by a large piece of equipment or other object. Therefore do not position the patient so the hands or feet project off the mat or treatment table, especially if they are screened by a cubicle curtain or sheet and would extend into an area used by personnel to move equipment or walk.

Remember: The areas of greatest pressure when the patient is *supine* are the *occipital tuberosity*, spine and inferior angle of the scapula, spinous processes of the vertebrae, posterior iliac crests, sacrum, and posterior calcaneus (see Table 5-1). Other possible pressure areas, depending on how the patient is positioned, are the medial epicondyle of the humerus, head of the fibula, greater trochanter of the hip, and lateral malleolus if excessive external *rotation* of the hip occurs. A rolled towel or sandbag can be used to maintain the hip in a neutral position. The hip should be moved toward internal rotation and the towel or sandbags should be placed against the lateral aspect of the soft tissue of the thigh and lower leg.

Prone Position

Place a small pillow or towel roll under the patient's head or he or she may turn the head to the left or right (Fig. 5-2). Some *prone*-lying patients may be more comfortable if they rest their forehead on a folded towel or special headrest. A

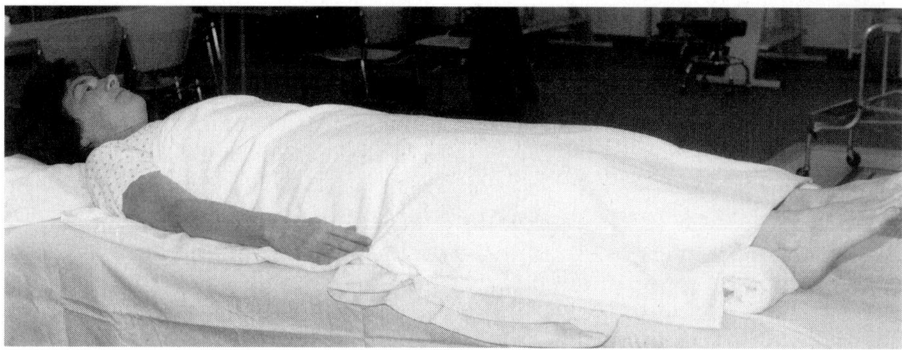

Fig. 5-1 Supine position.

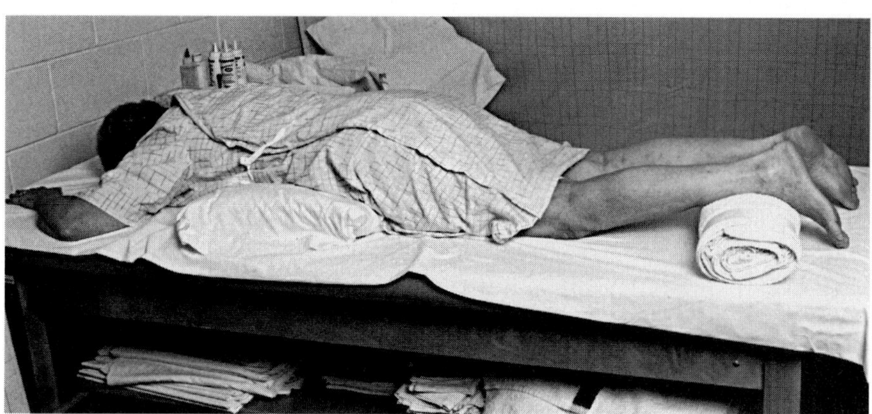

Fig. 5-2 Prone position.

treatment table that has a cut-out portion for the face and supports the head is the most comfortable for positioning the patient (Fig. 5-3). This type of table usually maintains the neck in neutral or a slightly flexed position. A pillow placed under the patient's lower abdomen will reduce the lumbar lordosis. (For some patients, maintenance of the normal lumbar lordosis may be desired and a pillow may be placed under the upper or middle chest or positioned lengthwise from the pelvis to the thorax to maintain the lordosis.) A rolled towel should be placed under each anterior shoulder area to adduct the scapulae and reduce the stress to the interscapular muscles. A treatment table with forearm rests can also be used to alleviate stress to the interscapular muscles (see Fig. 5-3). The use of a pillow, towel roll, or small bolster under the anterior portion of the patient's ankles will relieve stress on the hamstring muscles and will allow the pelvis and lower back to relax. *Caution:* The pillow placed at the ankles causes knee flexion and may contribute to a contracture of the hamstring (knee flexor) muscles. To avoid the development of a contracture, this position should not be maintained for a prolonged period.

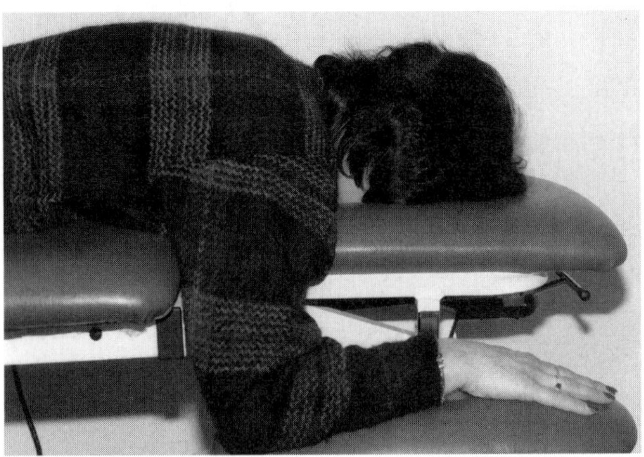

Fig. 5-3 Treatment table with a cutout for the face and adjustable armrests.

The patient's upper extremities may be positioned for comfort (as along the sides, in a *T position*, or with the hands under the head).

Remember: The areas of greatest pressure when the patient is prone are the forehead or lateral ear, tip of the acromion process, the anterior head of the humerus, sternum, anterosuperior iliac spine, patella, crest of the tibia, and dorsum of the foot (see Table 5-1).

Side-Lying Position

Initially the patient should be positioned in the center of the bed, mat, or table with the head, trunk, and pelvis aligned (Fig. 5-4). Both of the patient's lower extremities should be flexed at the hip and knee. The uppermost lower extremity should be supported on one or two pillows and positioned slightly forward of the lowermost extremity. The lowermost lower extremity provides stability to the patient's pelvis and lower trunk. One or two pillows should be used to support the patient's head. A folded pillow placed at the patient's chest is used to support the uppermost upper extremity and prevent rolling forward. It may be necessary to place a folded pillow along the posterior area of the patient's trunk to prevent rolling backward.

If you determine that the patient will not be able to maintain a side-lying position independently and safely, safety straps should be applied. The lowermost upper extremity can be positioned to promote patient comfort and stability. If the lowermost greater trochanter requires protection, place a pillow distal to the trochanter under the patient's lowermost lower extremity and a second pillow under the trunk proximal to the trochanter. *Caution:* The patient whose condition predisposes the development of a pressure ulcer should be positioned to avoid direct pressure to the downmost trochanter. You can accomplish this by placing the person in a slightly reclined position.

Remember: The areas of greatest pressure when the patient is in a side-lying position for the lowermost portion of the body are the following: the lateral ear, lateral ribs,

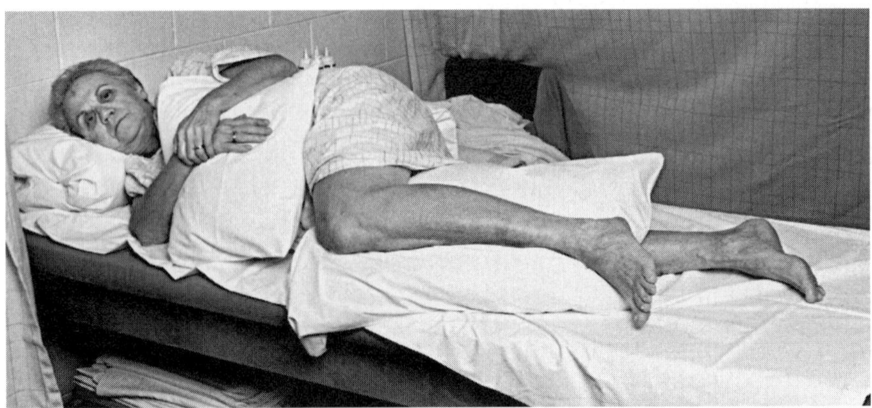

Fig. 5-4 Side-lying position.

lateral acromion process, lateral head of the humerus, medial or lateral epicondyles of the humerus, greater trochanter of the femur, lateral condyle of the femur, the malleolus of the fibula; the medial condyle of the femurs and the malleolus of the tibia if the uppermost lower extremity is positioned directly over the lowermost. The greatest areas of pressure for the uppermost portion of the body are the following: the medial epicondyle of the humerus (if resting on a hard surface) and the medial condyle of the femur and malleolus of the tibia.

Sitting Position

The patient should be seated in a chair with adequate support and stability for the trunk, which can be provided by pillows, belts, or straps or the back of the chair or by leaning forward onto a treatment table. The patient's lower extremities should be supported by placing the feet on a footstool, on the footrests of a wheelchair, or on the floor. The distal, posterior thigh tissue and deeper structures should be free of excessive pressure from the edge of the chair or wheelchair seat. When the patient receives treatment with the trunk leaning forward against the treatment table, one or more pillows can be used to support the anterior area of the trunk. Use one or more pillows behind the patient when he or she sits with the trunk leaning back against the chair. The patient's upper extremities can be supported on pillows, on the chair armrests, on the treatment table, on a lap board or by placement on a pillow in the patient's lap (Fig. 5-5). To improve access to the patient's back, he or she can sit in an armless chair with the chair back directed to the left or right.

Remember: The areas of greatest pressure when the patient is sitting are the *ischial tuberosities* and the posterior area of the thigh. Other possible areas of pressure are the sacrum and the spinous processes of the vertebrae if the patient leans against the chair back and the medial epicondyle of the humerus if the elbow rests on a hard surface such as a lap board.

In general, a patient should not be positioned for an extended period (more than 30 minutes) in any position that causes or produces the following:

- Excessive rotation or bending of the spine
- Bilateral or unilateral scapular abduction or a forward head position
- Compression of the thorax or chest
- Plantar flexion of the ankles and feet
- Hip or knee flexion; hyperextension of the knees
- *Adduction* and internal rotation of the glenohumeral joint
- Elbow, wrist, or finger flexion
- Hip adduction or internal/external rotation

These positions promote excessive stress or strain to various structures and may promote the development of a soft-tissue contracture or patient discomfort (Box 5-2). You must observe the areas of pressure in those patients who are susceptible to skin irritation or breakdown (such as the elderly, those who lack sensation, and those who are paralyzed). A reddened or blanched area that does not return to a normal appearance within an hour after the treatment session must be monitored. The use of the position that

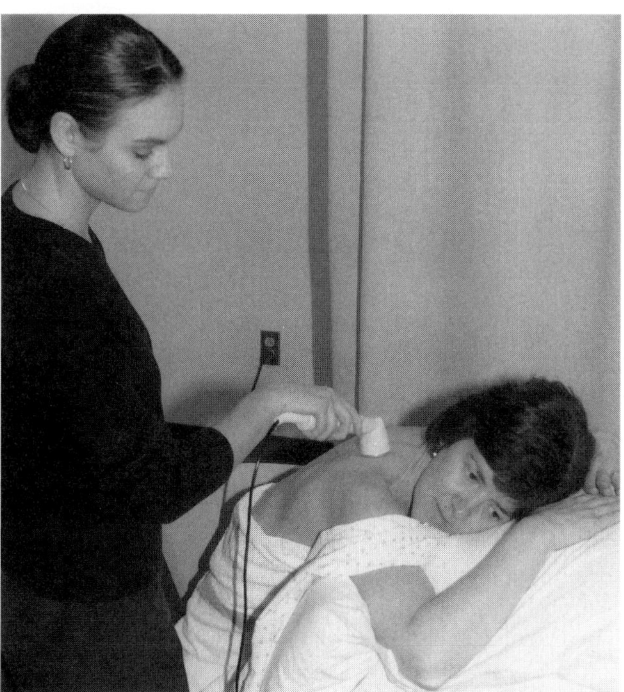

Fig. 5-5 Patient seated for treatment; notice pillows to support trunk, head, and upper extremities; only the area to be treated is exposed.

Box 5-2 Common Soft-Tissue Contracture Sites Related to Prolonged Positioning

SUPINE
Hip and knee flexors
Ankle plantar flexors
Shoulder extensors, adductors, and internal rotators
Hip external rotators

PRONE
Ankle plantar flexors
Shoulder extensors, adductors, and internal/external rotators
Neck rotators, left or right

SIDE LYING
Hip and knee flexors
Hip adductors and internal rotators
Shoulder adductors and internal rotators

SITTING
Hip and knee flexors
Hip adductors and internal rotators
Shoulder adductors, extensors, and internal rotators

Note: Forearm, elbow, wrist, and finger contractures can develop depending on the position used.

Box 5-3 Precautions for Patient Positioning

Avoid the presence of clothing or linen folds beneath patient.
Observe skin color before, during, and after treatment.
Protect bony prominences from excessive and prolonged pressure.
Avoid positioning the patient's extremities beyond the support surface.
Avoid excessive, prolonged pressure to soft tissue and circulatory and neurologic structures.
Use additional caution when positioning patients who are mentally incompetent or confused, comatose, very young or elderly, paralyzed, or lacking normal circulation or sensation.

caused the problem should be avoided in the future. Various positioning aids (such as elbow and heel protectors, footboards, seat cushions, lap boards, slings, splints, cones, or bolsters) can be helpful to reduce soft-tissue stress, support or stabilize a joint or segment, relieve pressure, or immobilize a segment. However, these items must be applied carefully and removed or adjusted periodically to avoid secondary problems. Straps on protective devices or splints may occlude peripheral circulation if applied too tightly; an unpadded lapboard may cause excessive pressure to the medial humeral epicondyle; and bolsters, cushions, or cones may create a source for the development of perspiration, which may lead to skin *maceration* if not dissipated. Therefore cautious and judicious use of these aids is recommended (Box 5-3).

Remember to be particularly careful when positioning the patient who is elderly, mentally confused, mentally incompetent, very young, comatose, paralyzed, agitated, or known to have an impaired cardiopulmonary system. These persons may not tolerate remaining in one position for more than a few minutes. Their circulation or respiration may become impaired and their skin may develop a lesion more readily as a result of pressure or *shear* forces created by the position. They may have more difficulty complying with instructions to maintain a given position, they may lack the ability to sense the need to change their position, or they may be unable to alter their position without assistance. These patients should be monitored frequently to avoid the adverse complications associated with positioning.

PREVENTIVE POSITIONING

It is recommended a patient's position be altered frequently to avoid excessive or prolonged pressure, reduce the development of contractures, avoid postural malalignment, and prevent other adverse effects. In addition, there are specific positions that should be avoided for certain patients because their diagnosis or condition predisposes them to complications related to short-term or prolonged positioning. The functional ability or capacity of the patient may be compromised because of problems caused by improper positioning techniques, which may affect the patient's independence or quality of life. Some conditions in which selected positions should be avoided are discussed in the sections that follow.

Transfemoral Amputation

For the patient with a transfemoral amputation, prolonged hip flexion should be avoided. The residual limb (RL) should not be elevated on a pillow while the patient is supine for more than a few minutes of each hour. The amount and length of time the patient is permitted to sit should be limited to no more than 40 minutes of each hour. Each of these positions promotes the development of a contracture of the patient's hip flexor muscles. If those muscles become contracted, the patient is apt to experience difficulty using a prosthesis for ambulation. In addition, it may not be possible to fit the patient with a prosthesis if contractures occur.

Hip abduction of the RL should be avoided to prevent a contracture of the hip abductor muscles. If this contracture develops, the patient will experience difficulty ambulating with a prosthesis. The patient should be encouraged to maintain the pelvis in a level position and to maintain the trunk in proper alignment while *recumbent* to avoid developing back discomfort and an abnormal posture. When the patient stands or is recumbent, the RL should be maintained in *extension*. Periodic prone lying is recommended.

Transtibial Amputation

For the patient with a transtibial amputation, prolonged hip and knee flexion should be avoided. The RL should not be elevated on a pillow while the patient is supine for more than a few minutes of each hour. If the RL is elevated, the knee should be maintained in extension. The amount and length of time the patient is permitted to sit should be limited to no more than 40 minutes of each hour. Each of these positions promotes the development of a contracture of the patient's hip flexor and knee flexor muscles. If these muscles become contracted, the patient will experience difficulty using a prosthesis for ambulation. In addition, it may not be possible to fit the patient with a prosthesis if contractures occur. When the patient sits, stands, or is recumbent, the hip and knee should be maintained in extension. Periodic prone lying is recommended.

Hemiplegia

When the patient's upper extremity is involved, prolonged shoulder adduction and internal rotation; elbow flexion; forearm supination or pronation; wrist, finger, or thumb flexion; and finger and thumb adduction should be avoided. These positions are most likely to lead to soft-tissue contractures caused by muscle spasticity, reduced function of the opposing muscles, and lack of active or passive motion. The use of a sling to support the involved extremity places the shoulder in adduction and internal rotation, the elbow in flexion, the forearm in pronation, and the wrist and fingers may be flexed. This is a position of comfort for many patients, but if contractures of the muscles of the upper extremity develop, the potential for functional use of the extremity will be reduced; therefore the upper extremity should be positioned in varying amounts of shoulder abduction and external rotation, elbow extension, slight wrist extension, thumb abduction and extension, and finger extension and slight abduction.

When a patient's lower extremity is involved, prolonged hip and knee flexion, hip external rotation, and ankle plantar flexion and inversion should be avoided. These positions are those most likely to lead to soft-tissue contractures caused by muscle spasticity, reduced function of the opposing muscle, and lack of active or passive motion. The potential for function of the lower extremity will be reduced if contractures develop; therefore the lower extremity should be positioned in varying amounts of hip and knee extension, hip abduction and internal rotation, and ankle dorsiflexion and eversion.

However, static positioning of the extremities may not be the most effective treatment technique depending on the patient's neurologic condition and response to positioning. The extremities should be exercised several times per day and should not remain in a single position for a prolonged period.

The normal alignment of the patient's head and trunk should be maintained when the person is sitting or lying. Frequent adjustments of posture or position may be necessary to ensure proper alignment.

Rheumatoid Arthritis

Rheumatoid arthritis is a systemic disease and one of the major systems involved by the disease is the musculoskeletal system, especially the joints. Prolonged immobilization of the affected extremity joints should be avoided, particularly if the joint is maintained in flexion. Bony prominences, especially the elbows and greater trochanters should be protected for the person who is immobile in bed. Gentle, careful, and frequent active or passive movement of the involved joints should be performed several times per day unless the joints are in a state of acute inflammation. The uninvolved joints should be exercised actively.

Contractures may develop even when various therapeutic measures are used. Carefully applied exercise can benefit most patients, but each patient should be given a treatment plan specifically designed for him or her. The patient will need to assume a great deal of the responsibility to maintain the body at its maximal level of function after being instructed by the appropriate caregiver or practitioner.

Split-Thickness Burns and Grafted Burn Areas

Healing or regenerating skin is apt to develop scar tissue and contractures are likely to occur. It is important to avoid prolonged positioning of the joints that have been affected by the burn or graft used to repair the wound. It is particularly important to avoid positions of comfort. A position of comfort for the patient with a burn is the position that does not produce stress or tension to the wound or graft. Prolonged flexion or adduction of most peripheral joints should be avoided when the burn is located on the flexor or adductor surface of a joint. The patient should be encouraged to perform gentle, careful, and frequent active movement of the involved joints and should exercise the uninvolved joints actively. When the patient is unable to perform active exercise, passive exercise should be performed. *Caution:* The caregiver must adhere to the physician's instructions when treating a recently grafted area.

Usually the patient should not be permitted to assume the position that provides the greatest comfort for an extended period because contractures are more likely to develop when the position of comfort is maintained. Once a contracture has developed, time, exercise, and perseverance by the patient and health care providers will be necessary to return the joint to a normal position and functional use. The patient is likely to experience a great deal of pain and discomfort during the process used to restore normal joint motion. Everyone involved with the care and management of the patient, including the patient, must understand that prevention of a contracture is far more desirable and less costly than the treatment required to overcome one.

These examples of patient conditions illustrate the need for proper positioning techniques for selected patients. Many other patient problems require thoughtfulness and planning to prevent the development of contractures or maintain function. The general rule to remember is prolonged immobilization and failure to change positions frequently are precursors to the development of contractures, pressure areas, and decreased function.

DRAPING

The primary reasons to appropriately drape or clothe a patient are to expose or free the area to be treated while the patient's modesty is protected and a comfortable body temperature is maintained. The caregiver must be aware that each patient has a concept of modesty. Some patients may be embarrassed or consider their body excessively exposed when only the upper or lower extremity is uncovered. Others may seem to have a disregard for their modesty and may expose themselves, to the embarrassment of other patients or the caregiver. A patient's cultural, religious, or personal preferences may affect the caregiver's ability to drape the patient to expose areas of skin or body parts sufficiently for treatment. For example, a woman who adheres to the Muslim religion (Islam) may not permit any area of her body to be exposed, especially to a male caregiver. Similar limitations may exist for nuns or other devout religious persons who are members of a particular group or sect. Therefore before positioning and draping of a patient, it will be important for the caregiver to determine whether the patient has specific requests or preferences that would affect the

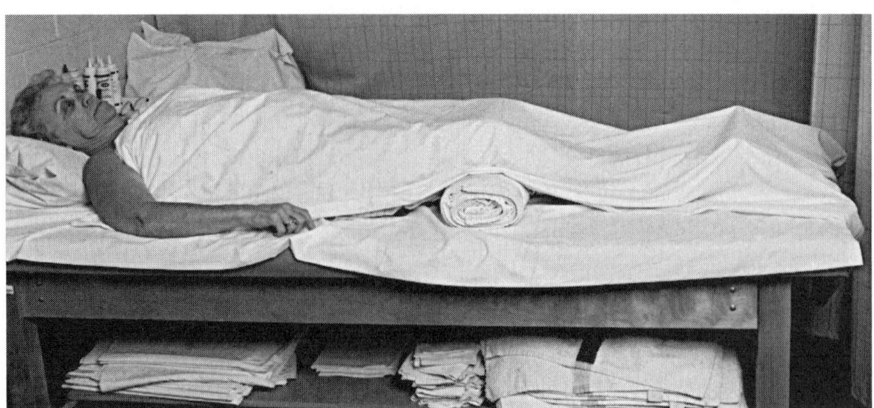

Fig. 5-6 Draping of a supine patient for treatment of the upper extremity.

Box 5-4 Rationale for Patient Draping

Provide modesty for patient.
Maintain appropriate body temperature.
Provide access and exposure to areas to be treated while protecting other areas.
Protect the patient's skin or clothing from being soiled or damaged.

draping process. Each patient should be informed of the type of clothing to be worn for the treatment session, or the facility may provide suitable clothing. Before treatment, the caregiver should inform the patient that clothing may need to be removed and why such removal is necessary. The patient should be told that the body will be protected by linen or substitute garments, except for the areas to be treated. In some instances the caregiver will need to inform the patient that clothing may become soiled even though clean linen is used as protection.

The area to be treated must be exposed and have freedom of motion so treatment can be performed effectively and observation or palpation of the area can occur. However, if the patient senses or experiences exposure of a sensitive area of the body (such as the perineum, gluteal region, or anterior chest area in female patients), it is doubtful the treatment session will be effective (Box 5-4).

Another person may have to assist the patient to apply proper clothing or drape material in preparation for treatment. If it is necessary to undress the patient, request permission to do so. To avoid or reduce the transference of disease or infection from one patient to another, only clean and previously unused linen and garments should be used for each patient. Soiled linen and garments must be properly disposed at the conclusion of each treatment session. If body fluids have soiled the items, wear gloves when you handle them and discard them in an appropriate container. If an undergarment is removed, it is imperative the patient's modesty is preserved throughout the treatment session.

Remember: Some patients may be reluctant to remove their clothing, although you have indicated their modesty will be preserved. You can help to reduce their apprehension by providing sufficient and appropriate drape materials, by instructing them how to apply or use the items, by being certain the treatment cubicle is shielded by a closed curtain or door, by asking their permission to enter the cubicle and ensuring the person is draped, and, if necessary, by having a caregiver of the same gender as the patient assist the patient to undress and dress. Access to the treatment area should be permitted only for those persons required to provide treatment. Whenever the caregiver leaves the treatment cubicle, the patient should be dressed or draped so the body is not unduly exposed in case another person enters or looks into the cubicle.

With the patient supine, the upper extremities can be exposed for treatment (Fig. 5-6). Either the caregiver or the patient should remove any restrictive clothing, splints, or other devices to expose the areas to be treated. It may be necessary to provide a gown for the patient and to be certain any clothing that was not removed does not restrict movement or access to the extremity. A towel, gown, or sheet can be used to drape the patient's anterior chest and lower extremities. The drape should not restrict joint motion or access to the area to be treated. In some instances it may be necessary to apply the drape into the axilla to shield the anterior and lateral areas of the chest.

With the patient supine, the lower extremities can also be exposed for treatment (Fig. 5-7). Either the caregiver or the patient should remove any restrictive clothing, splints, or other devices to expose the areas to be treated. Any clothing that is not removed should not restrict motion or limit access to the area to be treated. A towel or sheet can be used to drape the patient's perineum (groin); this must be applied

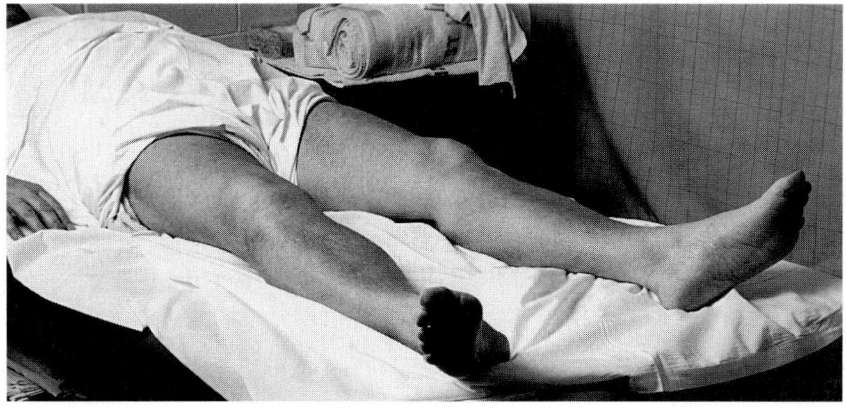

Fig. 5-7 Draping of a supine patient for treatment of the lower extremities.

high in the groin and under the thigh to shield the perineum fully. Be certain the drape remains secure throughout the treatment and that it does not restrict joint motion of the hip or knee. The patient's upper body and opposite lower extremity, if it is not to be treated, should be covered for warmth and to preserve modesty.

Draping material is frequently used to absorb perspiration, water, and various lubricants or to prevent these fluids from contacting the patient's clothing. It is also used to protect the patient's modesty and maintain body warmth. Therefore this material must not be used on another patient and must be disposed at the termination of treatment. The patient should be instructed or assisted to dress at the end of the treatment. The caregiver should evaluate the patient's response to treatment at its conclusion. Specific draping techniques necessary for massage are beyond the scope of this text and are not presented; however, they are available in other textbooks.

SUMMARY

Proper techniques to position and drape a patient are important because they protect the patient from injury, provide stabilization to an area, provide access while exposing only the specific area to be treated, maintain the person's body temperature, and protect him or her from unnecessary exposure of body areas, especially the breasts and perineum.

Prolonged use of any one position should be avoided to reduce the development of a soft-tissue contracture. Pillows, towel rolls, or similar devices can be used to promote comfort and stability, but these should be used with caution to avoid contractures. The caregiver should be aware of the body areas that will be affected most by pressure and the positions selected, so they can be protected or the pressure relieved periodically.

self-study ACTIVITIES

- List at least three possible adverse effects of improper or prolonged positioning on the musculoskeletal, neuromuscular, and cardiopulmonary systems.
- Describe why proper patient positioning and draping are important for the practitioner.
- Explain why or how the patient positions presented in the text provide comfort for the patient.
- Outline the precautions you would use if it were necessary for you to position a patient who has decreased sensation, is elderly, is mentally confused, is unable to independently change position, has impaired respiration, or has impaired peripheral circulation.
- Explain how you would position and drape a patient for treatment to the right upper and lower extremities while supine and for treatment to the left upper and lower extremities while side lying.

problem SOLVING

1. A 55-year-old female inpatient with rheumatoid arthritis and acute inflammation of her left knee is to be examined and evaluated for exercise. Explain the procedures for draping, precautions, and positioning to the patient.
2. A 65-year-old male with a left cerebral vascular accident has arrived in the department for treatment. The treatment plan includes passive, active assistive, and active exercise to the right upper and lower extremities. He wears a sling to support the right upper extremity and an ankle-foot orthosis (AFO) on the right lower leg. Describe the procedures for assisting, draping, and positioning this patient.
3. An outpatient arrives for treatment with ultrasound and deep tissue massage to the upper back and posterior neck and shoulder areas. What instructions or directions would you give her before positioning for treatment and how would you position her for maximal comfort and exposure of the area to be treated?

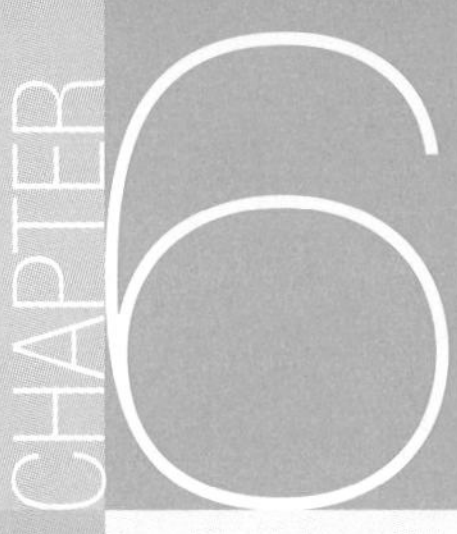

Basic Exercise: Passive and Active

objectives *After studying this chapter, the reader will be able to:*

- Differentiate among passive exercise, active assistive exercise, active exercise, and active resistive exercise.
- Provide rationale for the use or objectives of each form of exercise.
- Discuss the principles of preparation for these forms of exercise.
- Discuss the principles of application of these forms of exercise.
- Demonstrate the application of passive, active assistive, and active resistive exercise.

key terms

Active assistive exercise Exercise performed by a person with manual or mechanical assistance; can be static or dynamic.

Active exercise Exercise performed by a person without any mechanical assistance from another person.

Active resistive exercise Exercise performed by a person against manual or mechanical resistance.

Atrophy A decrease or reduction in the size of normally developed cells, tissues, organs, or body parts.

Capsular pattern A characteristic pattern for a given joint that limits joint motion and indicates that a problem exists within that joint.

Concentric contraction An overall shortening of a muscle as it develops tension and contracts; positive work is performed or movement is accelerated.

Contraction A drawing together or a shortening or shrinking (for example, a muscle contracts).

Dorsal Directed toward or situated on the back surface.

Eccentric contraction An overall lengthening of a muscle as it develops tension and contracts to control motion performed by an outside force; negative work is performed or movement is decelerated.

End feel The quality of the movement a person senses when pressure is applied passively to a joint at the end of its available range of motion.

Extrinsic Being, coming, or acting from the outside; not inherent.

Hypertrophy An increase in the cross-sectional size of a fiber or cell.

Isokinetic exercise A form of active resistive exercise; the speed of movement of the limb is controlled throughout the arc or range of motion, and the resistance offered is in direct proportion to the force offered by the patient throughout the range of motion of the exercise.

Isometric contraction A muscle contraction that develops tension, but does not perform any mechanical work; there is no appreciable joint motion and the overall length of the muscle remains constant.

Isotonic contraction A muscle contraction whereby tension is developed and movement of a joint or body part occurs; an eccentric or concentric contraction may be used and the muscle may lengthen or shorten.

Joint play The laxity or elasticity of a joint capsule that allows movement of the joint surfaces within the capsule.

Length-tension curve The curve that accounts for the active and passive elements of muscle tension and dictates that optimal tension is developed at one point known as *rest length,* the point in its range where peak torque is developed.

Passive exercise Exercise performed on a person by manual or mechanical means; no voluntary muscle contraction occurs.

Phlebitis Inflammation of a vein.

key terms—cont'd

Pronation The position of the forearm that places the hand palm downward; medial rotation of the forearm. The motion occurs in the forearm.

Proprioceptive neuromuscular facilitation (PNF) A treatment technique that uses various stimuli to affect the muscle or joint proprioceptors to facilitate or alter movement responses.

Range of motion (ROM) The normal extent of movement in a joint; the amount of motion allowed between two bony levers.

Resistance A force external to the body that creates additional work for a muscle when it contracts.

Soft tissues Tissues that lack bony or skeletal components; these include muscle, ligament, joint capsule, tendon, skin, and fascia.

Stretching Any therapeutic technique or procedure designed to lengthen or elongate shortened soft-tissue structures and to increase the range of motion.

Supination The position of the forearm that places the hand palm upward; lateral rotation of the forearm. The motion occurs in the forearm.

Thrombophlebitis Inflammation of a vein associated with the formation of a thrombus.

Thrombus An aggregation of blood factors, primarily platelets and fibrin, with entrapment of cellular elements that frequently leads to a clot and obstruction of a blood vessel.

Volar Pertaining to the palm; indicating the flexor surface of the forearm, wrist, or hand.

INTRODUCTION

Exercise is an important therapeutic intervention that is used to improve the functional capacity of many patients. Some general goals of exercise are to enhance the metabolic and physiologic function or capacity of muscle, maintain or improve joint motion and range, and enhance efficiency of the cardiopulmonary system and independent function of the body. Exercise can affect strength, endurance, joint flexibility, coordination, and one's general sense of well-being.

There are two basic types of exercise: active and passive. Each type has several benefits and limitations. In general terms, *active exercise* requires the patient to assist with or independently perform the exercise with the use of active, voluntary *contraction* of muscle. In contrast, *passive exercise* is used for the patient who is unable or not permitted to contract the muscles or to avoid undesired muscle contraction, pain, or adverse effects to the cardiopulmonary, musculoskeletal, or neuromuscular systems that may be associated with muscle contractions. When exercise is performed, the caregiver should consider the effect of gravity, the amount and type of stability and support necessary for the patient during the exercise, the purpose of the exercise, the ability of the patient to perform or participate in the activity, and the safety measures or protection required to avoid injury or an increase in the patient's symptoms or condition.

Support should be provided to relieve stress to a joint or body area, control the weight of an extremity or a body part, or compensate for the loss of muscle strength. The caregiver may need to use one or both hands to provide support to the segment or area. Support is used to promote motion or movement, whereas stabilization is used to avoid, limit, or prohibit movement. Stabilization is appropriate to protect the site of a recent, healing fracture; extensive soft-tissue trauma or damage; recently injured, healing musculotendinous structure; and where movement of an uninvolved joint or body part is to be avoided. The caregiver will need to use both hands to stabilize the area by grasping above and below the site of the problem or securing one structure (such as the scapula) while moving or mobilizing another structure. In some instances, an external splint or bandage can be used as the stabilizing force provided that it does not restrict or prevent movement that is desired. The hand positions used by the caregiver may need to be revised as the exercise is performed to maintain proper control, support, or stability. Reference to the photographs in this chapter will assist in identifying where to apply your hands to provide support and stabilization. Future decisions about hand placements should be based on the caregiver's knowledge, skill, experience, and competence.

The caregiver must integrate knowledge of the musculoskeletal, neuromuscular, and cardiopulmonary systems to properly determine and apply an exercise program. In addition, concepts and principles such as torque, force, force couples, levers, axis of motion, joint structures and components, muscle contractility and elasticity, stresses to skeletal and soft tissue, joint biomechanics, ligamentous and muscular attachments, sensation, neural innervation patterns, and muscle tone should be considered and applied by the caregiver. An explanation of these terms, concepts, and principles is beyond the scope of this textbook; see the Bibliography for appropriate resources. The desired outcome of exercise must be determined and measured throughout the treatment program. Patient progression toward preestablished objectives or goals is the key determinant of the effectiveness of the treatment program and its procedures, techniques, or activities. This progression should be measured frequently and recorded in the patient's medical record.

TYPES OF EXERCISE FOR RANGE OF MOTION

Passive exercise is the movement of a joint or body segment by a force external to the body, within an unrestricted and normal *range of motion (ROM)* and without an active, voluntary muscle contraction by the patient. The external force may be applied manually by the patient or by another person, mechanically by use of weights or pulleys or a continuous passive motion (CPM) unit, the passive mode on an isokinetic unit, or by gravity. Passive exercise or passive range of motion (PROM) differs from passive *stretching*. When PROM is used, no increase in joint range should be expected; the goal or objective is to maintain the unrestricted joint range. When passive stretching is used, the goal or objective is to increase the restricted joint range to the full joint range. Only PROM techniques will be described in this text.

Active exercise is the movement of a joint or body segment produced by active, voluntary muscle contraction by the patient within the unrestricted, normal ROM. No increase in joint range should be expected, but strength and endurance can be increased.

Active assistive exercise is a form of active exercise whereby an external force is used to assist the patient to perform the exercise. The assistance may be applied manually, mechanically, or by gravity. The patient must still perform active, voluntary muscle contractions to the extent that he or she is able. This technique may be used when muscular weakness, fatigue, or pain limit the patient's performance and when active, voluntary muscle contractions are desired.

These forms of exercise are used to preserve or maintain the normal ROM of a joint or segment, to maintain or improve strength and endurance, and to prepare the patient for future activities.

Indications for Passive Exercise

In general, passive exercise is used when a patient is unable to perform any form of active exercise. Examples of indications for PROM are when there is paralysis, when the patient is comatose, when pain occurs if an active muscle contraction is attempted, when recovery from trauma or a surgical procedure prohibits active muscle contraction, or to avoid exercise of an unhealed fracture whose healing would be disrupted with active muscle contraction. Passive range of motion is also used to counteract the negative aspects of immobilization, to evaluate joint range and flexibility, to provide sensory stimulation and awareness, and to reduce stress on the cardiopulmonary system.

Passive exercise is usually contraindicated when passive movement increases the patient's symptoms or intensifies the condition and when the person is capable of and would benefit from some type of active exercise.

Several benefits can result from passive exercise: it can assist in preserving and maintaining existing ROM; it can minimize the development of muscle shortening or the development of capsular, ligamentous, or tendinous adhesions resulting from immobilization; and it can assist in maintaining the mechanical elasticity of muscle. Passive exercise also assists in maintaining local circulation and maintaining or developing a patient's awareness of joint motion by enhancing kinesthesia, proprioception, mental imaging, and sensory awareness. Passive exercise can be used to evaluate joint ROM, stability, flexibility, and muscle tone. Cartilage nutrition and movement of the synovial fluid in the joint capsule are enhanced by passive exercise. The movement the patient is expected to perform with active exercise can be demonstrated passively to assist in learning the desired movement. Finally, passive exercise may reduce or inhibit pain when proper support is given to a specific joint or body segment (Box 6-1).

Box 6-1 Benefits of Passive Exercise

Preserve and maintain ROM.
Minimize contracture formation.
Minimize adhesion formation.
Maintain mechanical elasticity of muscle.
Promote and maintain local circulation.
Promote awareness of joint motion (that is, sensory awareness).
Evaluate joint integrity and motion.
Enhance cartilage nutrition.
Inhibit or reduce pain.

Passive exercise has some limitations of which the caregiver should be aware. It cannot prevent muscle *atrophy*; maintain or increase muscle tone, strength, or contractile endurance; or reduce adipose tissue. Although passive exercise can assist in maintaining local circulation, it is not as effective as active exercise. The caregiver will usually find that it is difficult to apply passive exercise when the patient's muscles are fully innervated and the patient is conscious or when pain occurs with motion.

At times, passive exercise may appear to the caregiver to be of little value and it may become a boring task. The best results can be expected when passive exercise is performed by a conscientious individual who integrates what is palpated, sensed, and observed during treatment. The progression to active assistive exercise, observation of changes in the joint range, and being alert to additional patient responses to the exercise program are the responsibilities of the primary caregiver, particularly if the exercise activities are assigned to supportive persons (such as family members, aides, assistants).

Indications for Active Exercise

In general, active exercise is used when a patient is able to voluntarily contract, control, and coordinate muscular movements with or without assistance, when there are no contraindications to its use, and when its established benefits are desirable to fulfill the goals of the patient's treatment.

Active exercise may be contraindicated in patients with cardiopulmonary dysfunction, an unhealed and unprotected fracture site, an unhealed and unprotected recent surgical site, or severe soft-tissue trauma. Caution in the use of active exercise is recommended when soft-tissue or joint pain or joint swelling is apparent as occurs with acute osteoarthritis, acute rheumatoid arthritis, or hemophilia. If active exercise increases the patient's symptoms or the condition intensifies when improper or substitutive movement patterns are used, active exercise may be contraindicated.

Benefits associated with active exercise include maintaining the physiologic elasticity, strength, and contractile endurance of muscle and increasing the local circulation. Active exercise also provides increased sensory awareness of joint motion, which is associated with proprioception, kinesthesia, and coordination. The cardiopulmonary functions of cardiac output, capillary efficiency, stroke volume, oxygen uptake, gas exchange in the lungs, and overall cardiac efficiency can be maintained or improved when multiple muscles perform simultaneously and the patient is in a deconditioned physiologic state. Active exercise such as repetitive ankle dorsiflexion-plantar flexion ("ankle pumping") can be used to assist in preventing the development of a *thrombus*, *thrombophlebitis*, or *phlebitis* in the peripheral veins of the lower legs. The stimulus of stress, produced by muscle contraction, will assist the tendon-bone interface to maintain its structural integrity. Finally, active exercise can improve muscle strength in a patient whose strength is measured at a grade of "fair" (50% or less of normal) on a manual muscle test. Muscles that are initially stronger than fair need to contract against external *resistance*, in addition to the weight of the segment, to increase the strength of the muscle (Box 6-2).

Active exercise will not develop strength in muscles when the initial strength was measured at a grade of "good" (75% or more) on a manual muscle test. Furthermore, cardiopulmonary efficiency in the normally conditioned or well-conditioned individual may be maintained, but will not be increased unless vigorous aerobic exercise is performed.

Active exercise is usually more beneficial for a patient than passive exercise, but the caregiver must determine which type of exercise should be used. A treatment program may begin with passive exercise, progress to active assistive exercise, then to active free exercise, and eventually lead to *active resistive exercise* depending on the goals of treatment and the patient's physical abilities. This progression requires the skill and knowledge of the caregiver to determine when the exercise progression can or should occur. The patient should be encouraged to perform within his or her ability, but at maximal effort levels whenever possible. *Caution:* Patients should be reminded to breathe normally while performing active exercise to avoid the potential adverse effects of the Valsalva phenomenon described in Chapter 4.

Passive ROM and active ROM can be performed in the traditional anatomic planes or in diagonal planes of motion using the patterns of *proprioceptive neuromuscular facilitation (PNF)*. Motion may also be performed in specific arcs or planes of motion of any joint to better affect a given muscle or portion of the joint range. The caregiver will need to decide which motions to perform and whether to perform them through the full range or through a portion of the range. The decisions should be based on evaluation and observation of the patient's responses to the exercise and the patient's condition.

Box 6-2 Benefits of Active Exercise

- Maintain physiologic elasticity, strength, and contractile endurance of muscle.
- Increase local circulation.
- Increase awareness of joint motion and sensory awareness.
- Maintain and improve cardiopulmonary functions, especially with aerobic exercise.
- May prevent thrombus formation in lower extremities using ankle flexion-extension movements (that is, "ankle pumping").
- Maintain and promote structural integrity of tendon-bone interface.
- Improve muscle strength with the use of external resistance.

PREPARATION FOR APPLICATION OF PASSIVE AND ACTIVE RANGE OF MOTION

Initially you should examine and evaluate the patient and obtain information from the medical record or other reliable sources to assist you in determining the goals of treatment and the type of exercise to be used. Introduce yourself, and explain the rationale, or purpose, and the desired outcome of treatment. Obtain the consent of the patient to perform treatment before you begin. You should be prepared to respond to questions regarding the treatment before you start the exercise program.

Position the patient to have access to the extremities, align and support the trunk and extremities, enhance your body mechanics, and provide patient comfort to the extent that it is compatible with the treatment. Restrictive clothing, orthoses, and linen should be removed or loosened. Be certain there is sufficient space to perform the treatment and drape the patient to protect modesty, maintain warmth, and expose the area or segment to be treated. Remember to use proper body mechanics when performing the exercises. This can be done by adjusting the height of the bed, the position of the patient on the bed or treatment table, or in a chair and by positioning yourself close to the person. Obtain assistance to move or position the patient when necessary (Procedure 6-1 and Box 6-3).

PROCEDURE 6-1

Procedures for Basic Exercise Activities

Examine and evaluate the patient to determine the exercise needs and establish appropriate outcome goals; inform the patient of the purpose or purposes of the exercise program.

Develop a treatment plan designed to meet the patient's needs and outcome goals (that is, frequency, duration, sequence); obtain consent from the patient.

Select the treatment activities, techniques, and procedures that will be most likely to fulfill the predetermined needs and outcome goals effectively and within an acceptable period.

Be prepared to protect structures that are unstable or vulnerable to injury when the exercise program is performed (such as hypermobile joints, healing fracture and surgical sites, muscle and ligamentous strains or sprains).

Instruct the patient about performance responsibilities and maintaining a breathing pattern during active exercise so that the Valsalva maneuver will be avoided.

Perform movements smoothly and slowly throughout the unrestricted ROM; resistive exercises should be performed within the patient's physical limits.

Proper precautions should be used during the exercise program, equipment must be secure and free from damage, and the patient and caregiver should use proper body mechanics.

The caregiver should monitor the effects of the exercise with all patients, especially those with known cardiopulmonary dysfunction.

The exercise plan, activities, techniques, or procedures should be revised or modified depending on the patient's response and progress toward the outcome goals; the program should be discontinued if adverse effects occur and persist for 24 hours or longer.

Box 6-3 Principles of Exercise Activities

The patient should not be challenged to exceed maximal physical capabilities.

Instruct the patient to maintain a breathing pattern to avoid the Valsalva maneuver.

Avoid applying excessive stress to the patient's skin, soft tissues, joints, and bones when manual or mechanical resistance is used.

Protect structures that are unstable or vulnerable to injury, such as hypermobile joints, healing fracture sites, healing surgical sites, and muscle or ligamentous strains or sprains.

Monitor the effect of exercise closely for the patient who has a known history of cardiopulmonary dysfunction.

Evaluate the equipment used to be certain that it is secure and stable and functions properly.

Use proper body mechanics as you participate in the exercise program.

PRINCIPLES OF PASSIVE EXERCISE

Passive exercise can be a beneficial treatment approach when a patient is unable to actively move a body segment; to avoid pain, undesired movements or patterns of motion, development of undesired muscle tone, and stress to a localized site of poor integrity; and to reduce cardiopulmonary stress. The patient does not assist with the movements; instead, an external manual, mechanical, or gravitational force is used to provide motion of the segment. Examples of mechanical forces are free weights, a pulley system, an isokinetic exercise unit in the passive mode, and a CPM unit. A gravitational force, or the effect of gravity on a joint or muscle, can be used with specific positioning of the segment to permit gravity to affect the structure. None of these forces is described or depicted in this text, but sources of such information can be found in the Bibliography.

Manual PROM can be performed by the patient (self-performed ROM), family member, or trained professional. Gentle, firm support and stabilization, through proper hand placement and control, should be provided to avoid stress to the structures or segment being moved. Practice will assist the caregiver to determine the best hand placements (areas of grasp) to use to provide smooth, controlled, and complete motion with minimal adjustments. All planes of motion of the joint should be exercised, which may require moving the joint through a variety or combination of motions. Although it is possible to exercise, or passively move several joints simultaneously, you should initially evaluate the range of each joint individually. This will assist in determining whether there is a limitation in the range of one or more of the joints. If all joint ranges of the segment or extremity are similar, time can be saved by performing PROM to multiple joints simultaneously. However, one must be cautious to avoid applying too little or too much motion to one or more of the joints of the extremity.

Passive range of motion should be performed through the entire unrestricted, normal range of the joint and soft tissue. The caregiver must be aware of normal joint range parameters and must perceive or sense the resistance, or lack of it, from the soft tissue or joint capsule and other joint structures as the exercise is being performed. This is the concept of *end feel*, or the "feel" of the resistance of the tissue at the end or completion of the range. To determine that feel, an excess pressure known as "overpressure" is applied at the end of the range. End feels are described as "soft" when *soft tissues* are compressed or stretched (as in elbow or knee flexion), "firm" when joint capsules or ligaments are stretched (as in hip rotation), "hard" when a bony block or resistance is reached (as in elbow extension), or "empty" when no end feel is elicited because the patient does not permit full motion to occur, usually because of acute pain. An abnormal end feel may result from muscle guarding, muscle spasm, muscle spasticity, or an intraarticular block such as a torn meniscus or articular cartilage or a loose body in the joint. The caregiver should evaluate the ROM in relation to these normal and abnormal end feels, or *capsular patterns*, and adjust the treatment as necessary.

Muscles that cross more than one joint (that is, multijoint muscles) must be identified and given special consideration when PROM is performed. Some examples of multijoint muscles are the biceps and triceps, *extrinsic* finger flexors and extensors, the quadriceps, the hamstrings, and the gastrocnemius. It is important to differentiate between the available or normal joint range and the muscle range when multijoint muscles are involved. To allow full joint motion to occur, multijoint muscles must be relaxed and must not be lengthened simultaneously over the joints they cross. Joint motion is important because it assists in maintaining proper capsular and ligamentous flexibility. Motion over the full muscle range is performed to assist in maintaining the length or flexibility of the muscles and tendons that cross a given joint. Multijoint muscles must be lengthened simultaneously over each joint they cross to maintain their functional length. This concept is particularly important when you are applying PROM to the extrinsic flexors and extensors of the fingers. For example, to maintain the length of the extrinsic finger extensors, wrist flexion should be combined with finger flexion. Conversely, to maintain the length of the extrinsic finger flexors, wrist extension should be combined with finger extension. However, there is at least one patient condition for which full lengthening of the extrinsic finger flexors usually is contraindicated: the patient with a spinal cord injury that has spared the C6 nerve root may benefit from tightness or limited range of the extrinsic finger flexors. Limited range of the finger flexors, when combined with active wrist extension, can provide the person with a passive grasp. As the wrist is extended, the finger flexors, already limited in length, are elongated or stretched over the *volar* area of the wrist, which further shortens them. When this occurs, a gross, passive grasp develops, known as a "tenodesis" (tendon fixation or suturing) grasp or movement. Relaxation of the wrist extensors allows the hand to lower and releases the passive tension on the finger flexors. This is the opening phase of the grasp-and-release action.

Other persons with a spinal cord injury may benefit if their erector spinae muscles are not elongated by passive exercise because their trunk stability when they sit may be improved by the limited length or range of those muscles. Stability of a hypermobile joint may be enhanced if the muscles that cross or support the joint are not elongated fully, but a contracture of the joint should be avoided.

Although most of the photographs in this text show the patient to be supine or prone when PROM is performed, other positions can also be used depending on the patient's condition. Many PROM activities can be performed with the patient sitting in a wheelchair (or other type of chair), side lying, or standing. Mechanical devices such as pulleys or CPM units can be used as replacements or adjuncts to manual PROM techniques.

Research studies have not specifically determined the frequency or number of repetitions necessary for PROM to be effective. Many factors affect joint or muscle range and there is no assurance that PROM will, in and of itself, maintain the free, unrestricted range of a given joint or muscles. The use of protective equipment, positioning regimens, general medical and nursing care, and the type of illness or trauma affect the results of PROM activities. The skill, knowledge, and judgment of the caregiver are required to reach decisions regarding the actual protocol that is applicable for each patient. Therefore the caregiver must evaluate the patient's response to treatment frequently and consistently.

The caregiver must also understand and recognize which muscles or soft tissues are affected by the application of PROM. In general, a passive movement should be performed in the direction *opposite* to the movement the muscle would produce if it were to contract actively. For example, passive elbow extension is performed to lengthen the biceps, passive knee flexion is performed to lengthen the quadriceps, and passive ankle dorsiflexion is performed to lengthen the gastrocnemius-soleus muscle complex. This concept can be applied to movement of other muscles, soft tissues, and joints. A muscle or soft tissue that is limited in its ability to relax or lengthen will produce a contracture in the *same* direction as the movement the muscle would produce if it were to contract actively. Some muscles that can and often do produce contractures are the biceps, hamstrings, and gastrocnemius.

Before starting PROM, determine the purpose or goal of each exercise and explain this goal to the patient. It is helpful to establish a sequence for the exercise program so you will be more likely to perform each motion and less likely to omit a motion. For example, perform all shoulder movements and then move to the elbow and to the forearm, wrist, and fingers. For the lower extremity, perform all hip, then all knee, and then all ankle and foot movements. In some situations, it may be desirable or beneficial to perform two or more movements simultaneously; in other situations, it may be undesirable to combine movements. These situations will be explained as they arise in the progression of the exercise program.

You must be alert during the application of PROM so you will perceive and determine the patient's response to the exercises. These exercises are passive for the patient, but the caregiver must be physically and mentally involved. Position yourself so you are able to observe the patient's face as you perform each exercise; you should also be positioned so you can exercise the extremity nearest to you. Avoid reaching across one extremity or the patient's trunk to exercise the more distant extremity, to reduce strain to your body, decrease the expenditure of energy, and assure safety for the patient.

All motions should be performed slowly, with a brief pause or hold at the point of greatest joint range or elongation of a muscle. You should sense or perceive when the terminal, unrestricted joint range or muscle elongation has occurred and stop the exercise at that point. *Remember:* Passive exercise is different from stretching and no increase in joint range or muscle length should be anticipated with PROM.

Proper support and stabilization of segments and joints must be incorporated into the exercise. The patient must develop trust and confidence that the caregiver will not cause further injury or pain during the performance of the exercises. This trust and confidence can be established by the manner the caregiver physically handles the patient and by explaining the intent or purpose of each exercise. After several exercise sessions have been completed, it should not be necessary to explain the intent or purpose of each exercise unless new exercises are initiated (Procedure 6-2).

PROCEDURE 6-2

Application of Passive Exercise

Position the patient for support, stability, and access to the area or segment to be exercised; drape as necessary.

Explain the purpose and goals of exercise; obtain consent for treatment.

Position the patient to promote use of proper body mechanics by the patient and caregiver.

Grasp the part to be treated to provide support, stability, and control during exercises. Refer to the photographs and instructions in this chapter for specific information.

Perform exercises through the complete, unrestricted ROM.

Perform the predetermined number of repetitions and frequency of exercises based on patient needs and goals.

Perform the exercises smoothly and slowly; pause at the start and end positions of the exercise.

At the conclusion of treatment, position the patient for proper alignment, support, and safety; drape or replace clothing for modesty and body temperature control.

Evaluate the patient's response to treatment; document important findings.

TRADITIONAL PROM MOVEMENTS

Cardinal or Anatomic Planes of Motion

The cardinal planes of motion are associated with and described according to the anatomic position. A person who is standing upright is considered to be in the anatomic position with the upper extremities relaxed along the sides of the trunk, shoulders externally rotated, forearms supinated, and fingers extended and adducted; lower extremities parallel and in neutral rotation, heels approximately 4 inches apart, and toes directed forward; and the face directed forward with the head in neutral flexion-extension, rotation, and lateral bending.

The three cardinal planes are the sagittal, frontal or coronal, and transverse. The sagittal plane is a vertical plane that divides the body into left and right components; flexion and extension occur in this plane. The frontal plane is a vertical plane that divides the body into front (anterior) and back (posterior) components; abduction and adduction occur in this plane, with the exception of the thumb. The transverse plane is a horizontal plane that divides the body into upper and lower components; rotation occurs in this plane.

Upper Extremity Movements

Traditional Anatomic Planes Position the patient supine on a firm surface; properly draped; and close to the near edge of the treatment table, mat table, or bed. Other positions can be used depending on the patient's condition and the caregiver's preference.

ARTICULATION: Scapulothoracic

Movement: Scapular elevation and depression (Fig. 6-1)

Hand placement and motion: Cup the inferior angle with one hand while resting the other hand on the superior border of the scapula; move the scapula upward and downward.

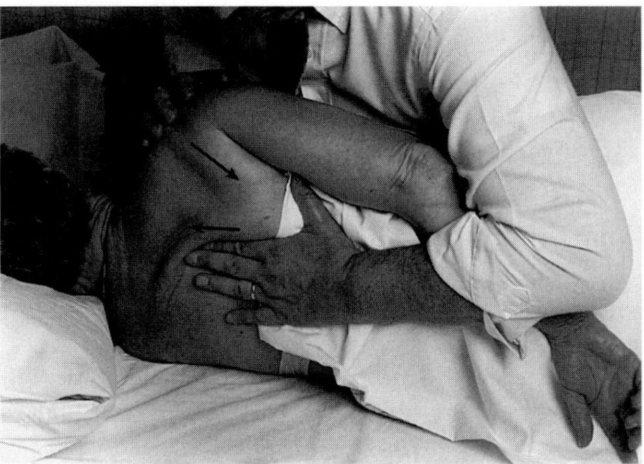

Fig. 6-1 Scapular elevation and depression.

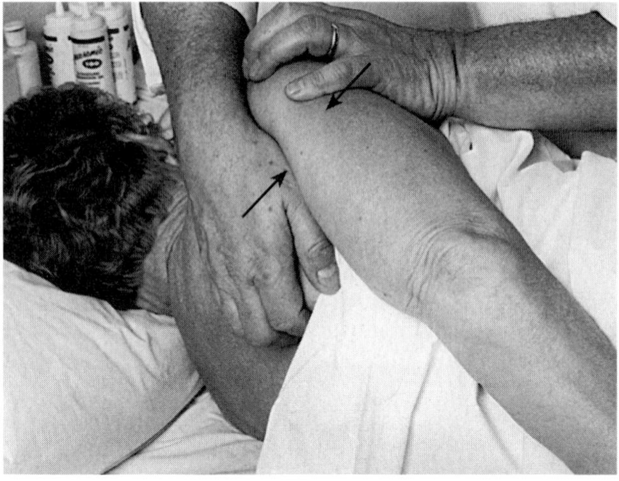

Fig. 6-2 Scapular protraction.

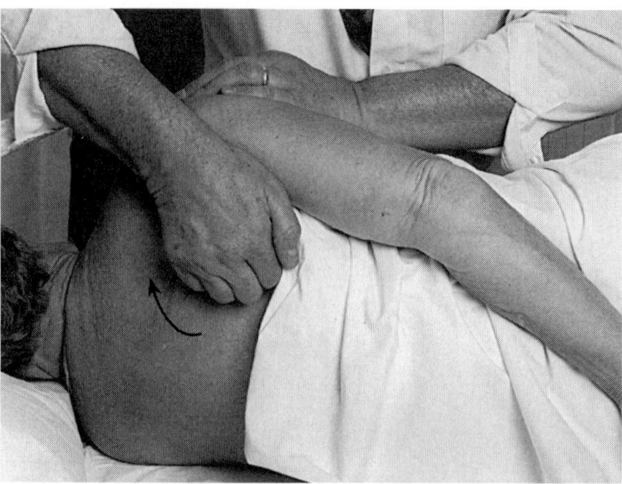

Fig. 6-3 Scapular vertebral border lift.

ARTICULATION: Scapulothoracic
Movement: Scapular protraction (abduction) and retraction (adduction) (Fig. 6-2)
Hand placement and motion: Rest one hand over the medial (vertebral) border while resting the other hand over the acromion process of the scapula; move the scapula toward and away from the spinous processes.

ARTICULATION: Scapulothoracic
Movement: Scapular vertebral border lift ("winging") (Fig. 6-3)
Hand placement and motion: Slide the fingertips of one hand under the medial (vertebral) border of the scapula; gently lift the scapula from the ribs. It will be easier to grasp the vertebral border if the patient's upper extremity is relaxed behind the trunk while in a side-lying position.

ARTICULATION: Glenohumeral
Movement: Shoulder flexion and extension (Fig. 6-4)
Hand placement and motion: For the right upper extremity, grasp the right wrist and hand with your left hand and grasp the right elbow with your right hand; lift the extremity through the available range and return. Extension of the arm beyond the midline of the body produces hyperextension. You can accomplish this with the patient supine with the shoulder at the edge of the support surface or with the patient in a side-lying or prone position.

ARTICULATION: Glenohumeral
Movement: Shoulder abduction and adduction (Fig. 6-5)
Hand placement and motion: Grasp the wrist and elbow; move the extremity away from the trunk and return. The elbow may be extended or flexed, but avoid shoulder flexion and maintain the arm horizontal to the floor. It may be necessary to externally rotate the humerus to reduce impingement of the humeral head on the acromion process. In some instances it may be helpful to prevent excessive elevation of the scapula by placing one hand over its superior border. When the exercise is performed with the elbow extended, you will have to adjust your position by moving toward the patient's head.

ARTICULATION: Glenohumeral
Movement: Shoulder horizontal adduction and abduction (Fig. 6-6)
Hand placement and motion: Grasp the wrist and elbow; begin with the patient's shoulder abducted to 90 degrees and parallel to the floor. Lift the arm up and across the upper chest and return. To attain full abduction, the patient's shoulder must be at the edge of the supporting surface to allow the humerus to clear the edge of the table. The elbow may be flexed or extended.

ARTICULATION: Glenohumeral
Movement: Shoulder internal (medial) rotation (Fig. 6-7)
Hand placement and motion: Abduct the shoulder to 90 degrees; flex the elbow to 90 degrees. Position yourself opposite the patient's elbow and face the person. Grasp the patient's wrist with one hand and support the hand; rest the other hand on the acromion process or use it to support the distal end of the humerus. Move the forearm forward toward the floor, causing the humerus to rotate. Stop the motion when the acromion process tips forward, indicating that the head of the humerus has been blocked by the acromion.

ARTICULATION: Glenohumeral
Movement: Shoulder external (lateral) rotation (Fig. 6-8)
Hand placement and motion: Use the same hand placement described for internal rotation. Move the forearm backward toward the floor, causing the humerus to rotate. Stop the motion when the forearm is horizontal to the floor. (*Note:* Shoulder internal/external rotation can be performed with the elbow extended and the extremity positioned along the patient's side. Grasp the humerus

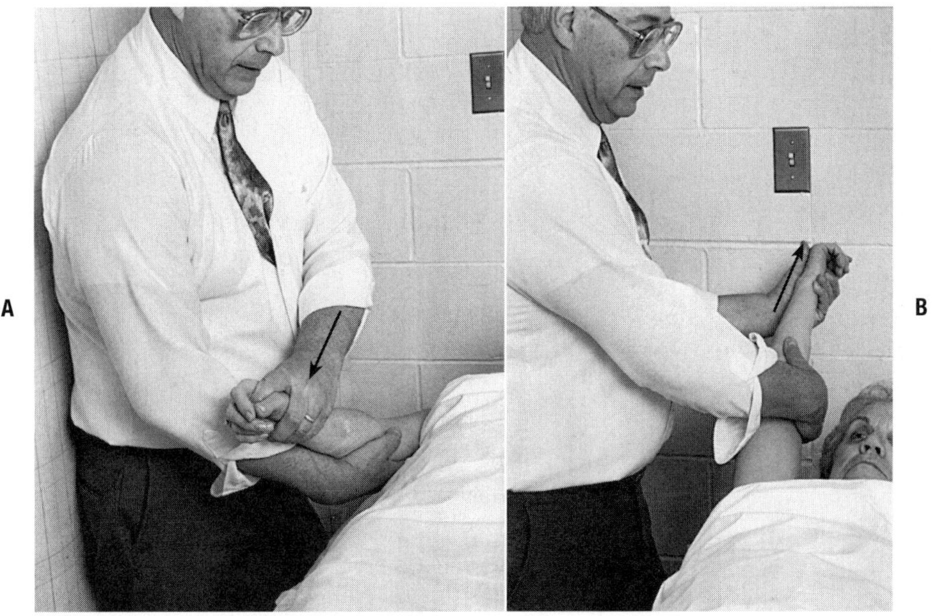

Fig. 6-4 **A,** Hand position for shoulder extension. **B,** Shoulder flexion.

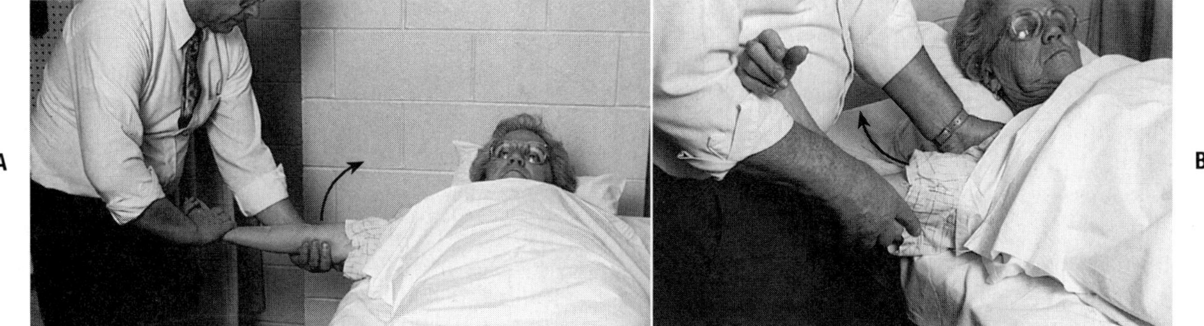

Fig. 6-5 **A,** Shoulder abduction, elbow extended. **B,** Shoulder abduction, elbow flexed.

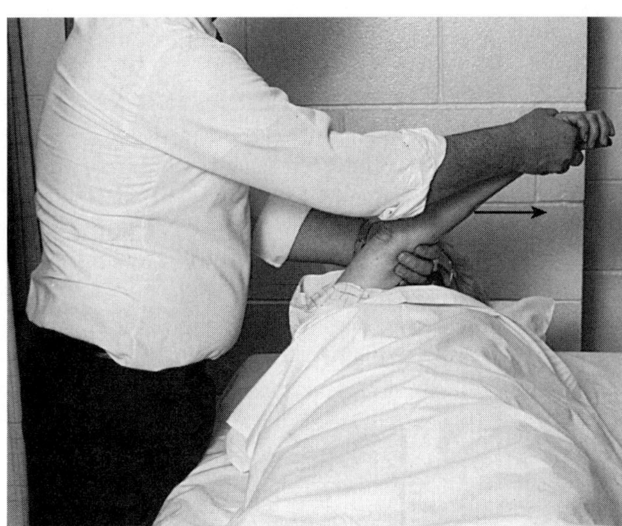

Fig. 6-6 Shoulder horizontal adduction.

A

B

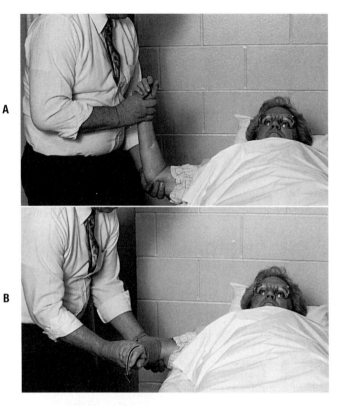

Fig. 6-7 **A,** Hand positions for shoulder rotation. **B,** Internal (medial) shoulder rotation.

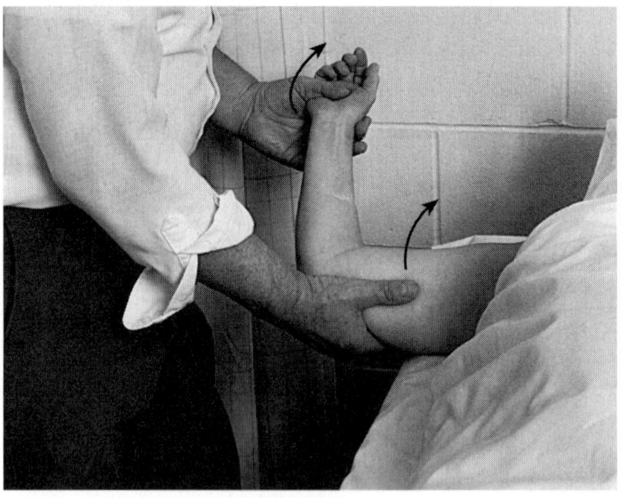

Fig. 6-8 External (lateral) shoulder rotation.

just above the epicondyles and grasp the forearm at the wrist; turn or roll the entire extremity inward and outward. As an alternative method, start with the humerus next to the trunk and the elbow flexed to 90 degrees. Grasp the distal end of the forearm, support the patient's hand, and move the forearm toward and away from the

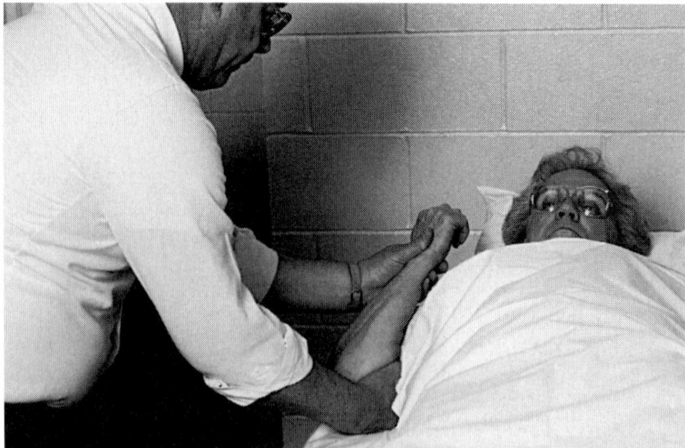

Fig. 6-9 Elbow flexion.

chest without abducting or adducting the shoulder. When this technique is used, internal rotation will be incomplete because the forearm will strike the chest before the complete range is attained.)

ARTICULATION: Humeral-ulnar

Movement: Elbow flexion and extension (Fig. 6-9)

Hand placement and motion: For the right upper extremity, grasp the patient's distal forearm and support the hand with your left hand; use your right hand to support and stabilize the distal end of the humerus. Flex and extend the elbow with the forearm neutral, pronated, and supinated, but avoid any shoulder motion.

ARTICULATION: Radial-ulnar

Movement: Forearm *supination* and *pronation* (Fig. 6-10)

Hand placement and motion: For the right forearm, grasp the distal end of the forearm and support the patient's hand with either your left or your right hand; use your other hand to support and stabilize the humerus. Supinate and pronate the forearm. This exercise can be performed with the elbow flexed or extended, but the motion must occur in the forearm. Avoid shoulder rotation and reduce stress to the wrist by grasping the distal end of the forearm. This motion can be combined with elbow flexion and extension.

ARTICULATION: Carpal-radial-ulnar

Movement: Wrist flexion and extension (Fig. 6-11)

Hand placement and motion: Grasp the patient's hand over its palmar and *dorsal* surfaces with one hand; use the other hand to support and stabilize the forearm. Move the palm toward the forearm and move the dorsum toward the forearm. Allow the patient's fingers to relax and do not stress the carpals. This motion can be performed with the elbow flexed or extended. After the range of the extrinsic finger flexors and extensors has been evaluated, you may desire to combine wrist and finger flexion and wrist and finger extension. Review the information on multijoint muscles before combining wrist and finger motions.

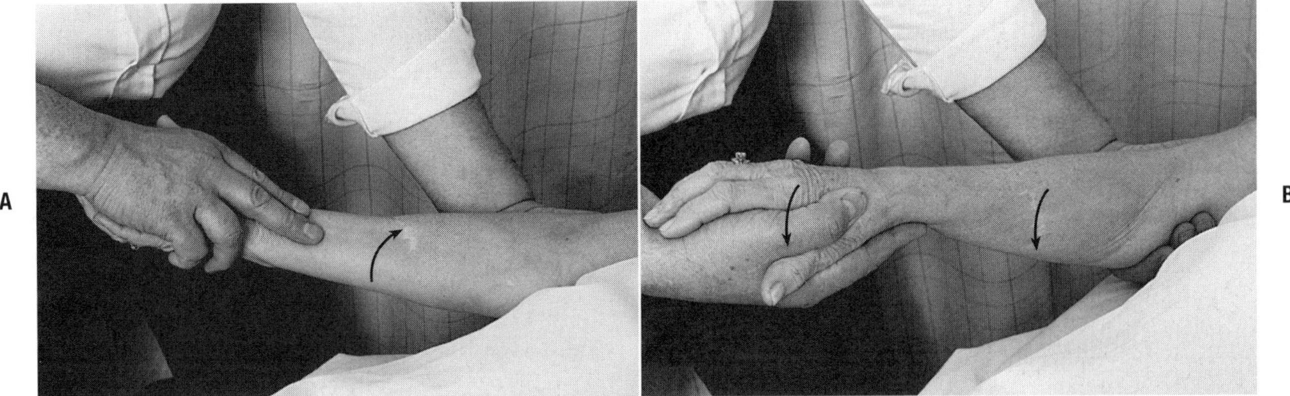

Fig. 6-10 **A,** Elbow extension with forearm supination. **B,** Forearm pronation.

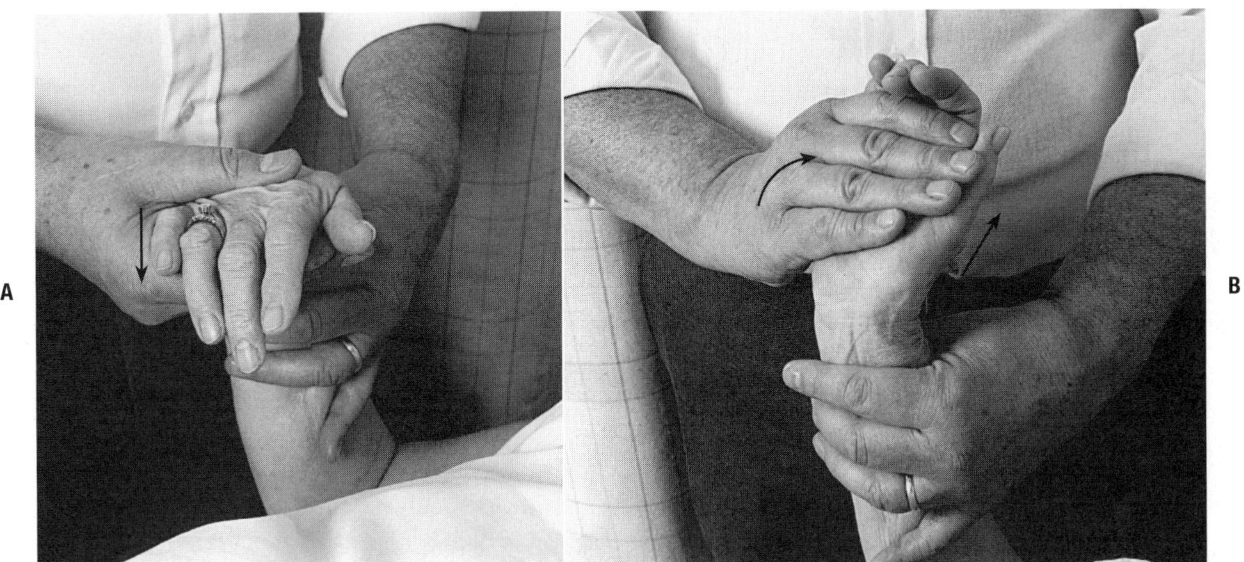

Fig. 6-11 **A,** Wrist flexion. **B,** Wrist extension.

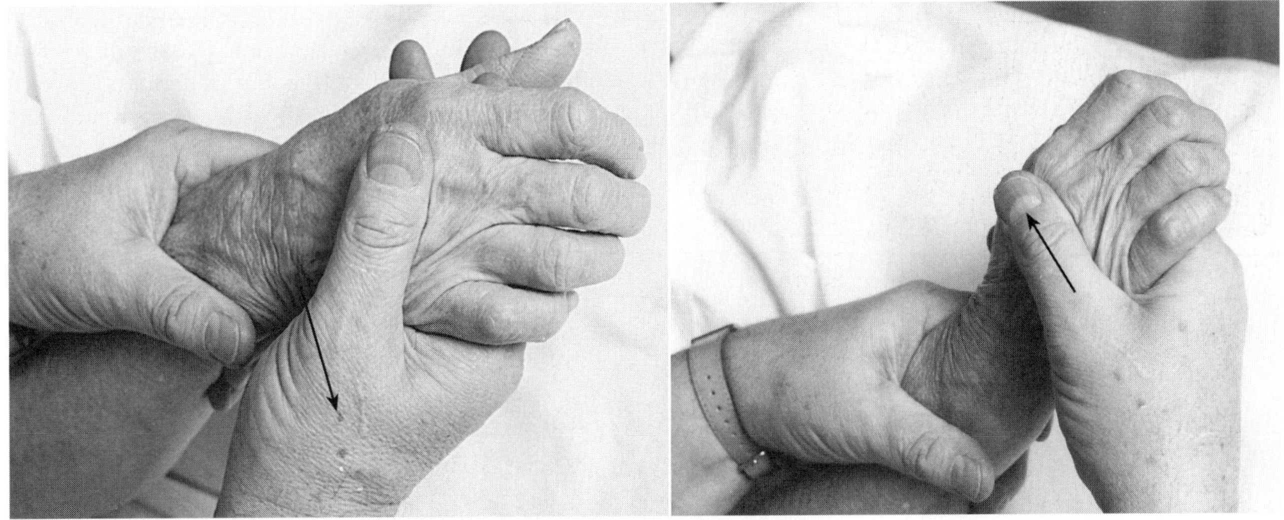

Fig. 6-12 **A,** Ulnar deviation of the wrist. **B,** Radial deviation of the wrist.

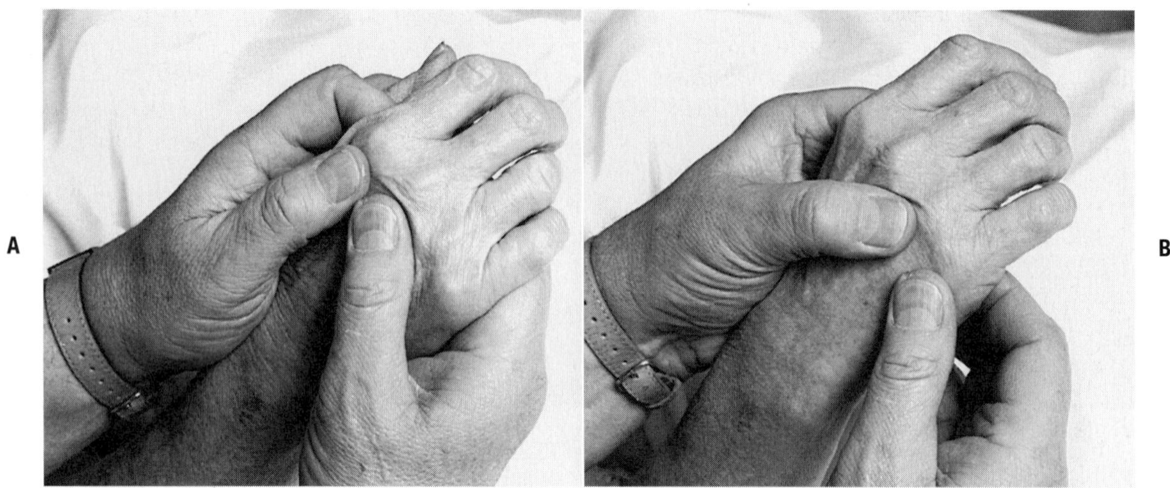

Fig. 6-13 Elevation, **A,** and depression, **B,** of individual metacarpal heads.

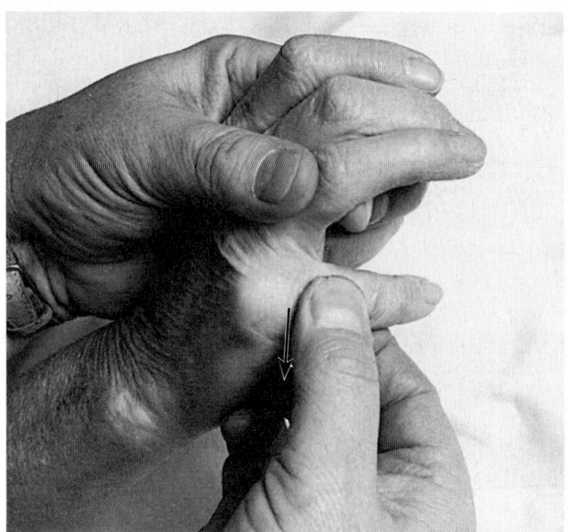

Fig. 6-14 Flexion of the MCP joint.

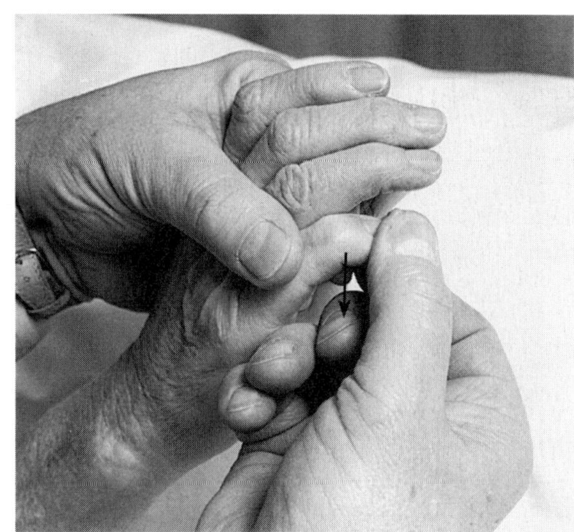

Fig. 6-15 Flexion of the distal interphalangeal (DIP) joint.

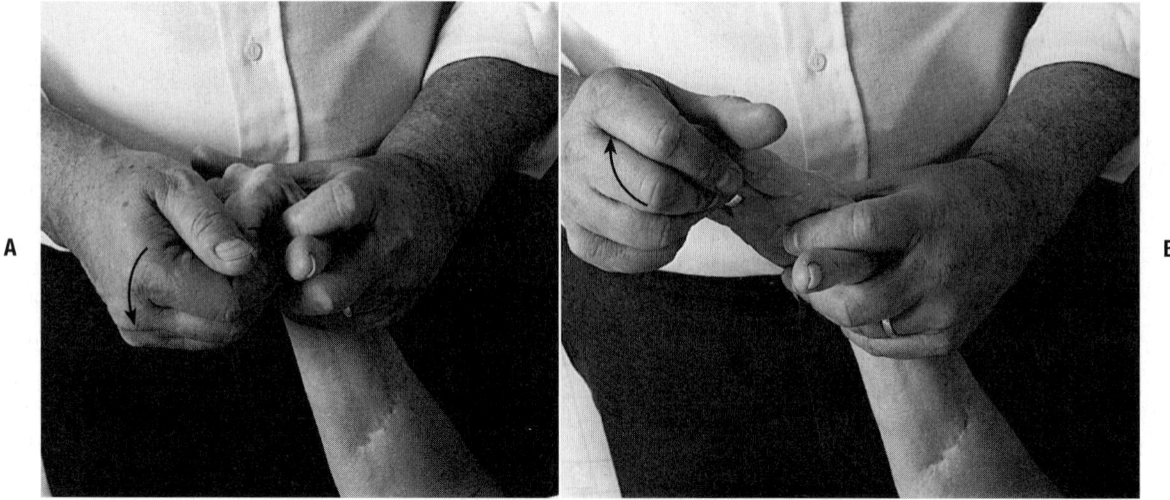

Fig. 6-16 **A,** Finger flexion. **B,** Finger extension.

ARTICULATION: Carpal-radial-ulnar
Movement: Wrist radial and ulnar deviation (Fig. 6-12)
Hand placement and motion: Grasp the patient's hand as described for wrist flexion and extension; maintain the hand in neutral flexion-extension. Move the hand in a radial and ulnar direction, but avoid wrist flexion and extension.

ARTICULATION: Metacarpal head *joint play*
Movement: Elevation and depression of individual metacarpal heads (Fig. 6-13)
Hand placement and motion: Grasp the dorsal and palmar surfaces of the metacarpal of a finger just proximal to its head with the thumb and index finger of one hand; use your other hand to stabilize the adjacent metacarpal with a similar grasp. Using the first hand, move the head of one metacarpal upward and downward, but do not allow the adjacent metacarpal to move. Progress to the next metacarpal until all four distal metacarpals have been moved. This technique should not be applied to the thumb.

ARTICULATION: Metacarpophalangeal (MCP)
Movement: Flexion and extension (Fig. 6-14)
Hand placement and motion: Grasp the dorsal and palmar surfaces of a metacarpal just proximal to the metacarpal head with the thumb and index finger of one hand and use the thumb and finger of your other hand to grasp the dorsal and palmar surfaces of a proximal phalanx. Stabilize the metacarpal while you move the phalanx upward and downward. Perform the motion for each articulation on each hand; use the same techniques for the thumb.

ARTICULATION: Distal and proximal interphalangeal (DIP and PIP, respectively)
Movement: Flexion and extension (Fig. 6-15)
Hand placement and motion: Use the grasp described for MCP flexion and extension. Stabilize the more proximal phalanx and move the more distal phalanx upward and downward. Perform the motion for each articulation on each hand and use the same technique for the thumb.

ARTICULATION: The MCP and interphalangeal (IP) (combined motions)
Movement: Finger flexion and extension (Fig. 6-16)
Hand placement and motion: Place one hand over the patient's extended fingers; use your other hand to support and stabilize the forearm. Fold the fingers into a fist gently and return them to an extended position; use the same technique for the thumb by flexing the thumb into the palm and returning it to an extended position. Maintain the wrist in a neutral position. This motion can be performed with the elbow flexed or extended.

ARTICULATION: MCP
Movement: Abduction (Fig. 6-17)
Hand placement and motion: Use one hand to grasp and stabilize the DIP joints of the first, second, and third fingers; use your other hand to grasp the fourth finger. Keeping the MCP and IP joints extended, gently move the fourth finger away from the third finger. Then stabilize the first and second fingers and move the third finger away from the second finger. Next, stabilize the second, third, and fourth fingers and move the first finger away from the second finger. The second finger can be moved to the left and to the right independently and without stabilization of any of the other fingers. (*Note:* These motions are performed independently of the thumb and are used to maintain the web spaces between the four fingers.)

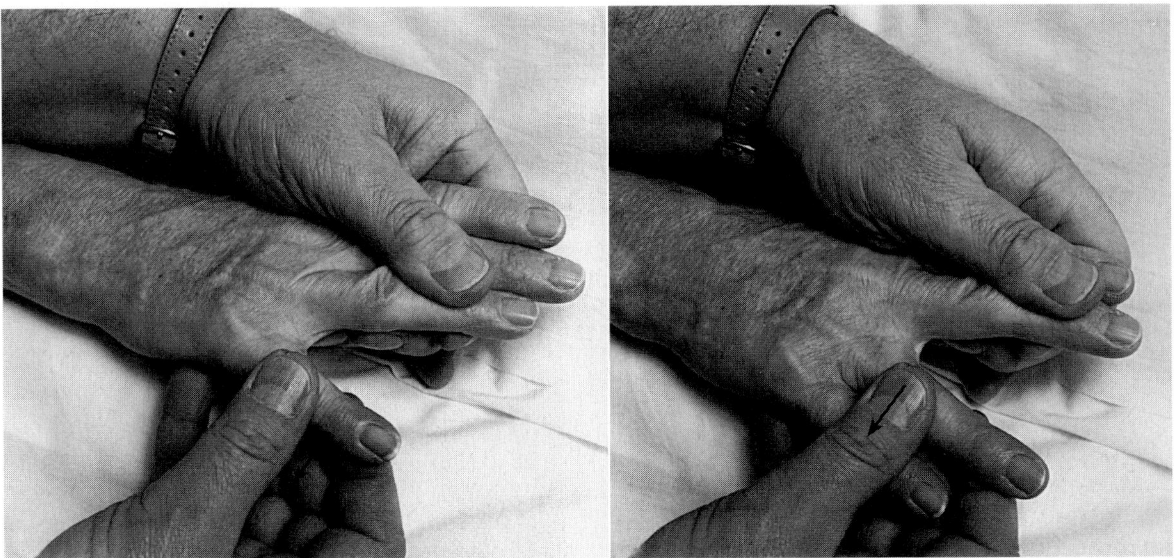

Fig. 6-17 Abduction of the MCP joints.

ARTICULATION: Thumb metacarpal-carpal and MCP
Movement: Thumb opposition (Fig. 6-18)
Hand placement and motion: Grasp the patient's thumb with the thumb and fingers of one hand; use your other hand to grasp the fifth metacarpal and finger. Roll the thumb toward the fifth finger, maintaining the MCP and IP joints in extension. Return the thumb to a position of full extension to maintain its web space.

ARTICULATION: Metacarpal-carpal of the thumb
Movement: Thumb abduction and adduction (Fig. 6-19)
Hand placement and motion: Grasp the patient's thumb with the fingers and thumb of one hand; use the other hand to stabilize the second metacarpal. Lift the thumb away from the palm so that it is perpendicular to the palm, but maintain the MCP and IP joints in extension. Return the thumb to the palm parallel to the second metacarpal.

ARTICULATION: Metacarpal-carpal of the thumb
Movement: Thumb extension and flexion (Fig. 6-20)
Hand placement and motion: Grasp the patient's thumb with the fingers and thumb of one hand; use the other hand to stabilize the second metacarpal. Move the thumb away from the index finger and horizontal to the palm; widen the web space to its maximum. Return the thumb so that it rests next to the side of the second metacarpal.

ARTICULATION: Thumb MCP and IP
Movement: Thumb flexion and extension (Fig. 6-21)
Hand placement and motion: Grasp the patient's metacarpal with the thumb and fingers of one hand; use the thumb and index finger of the other hand to flex the

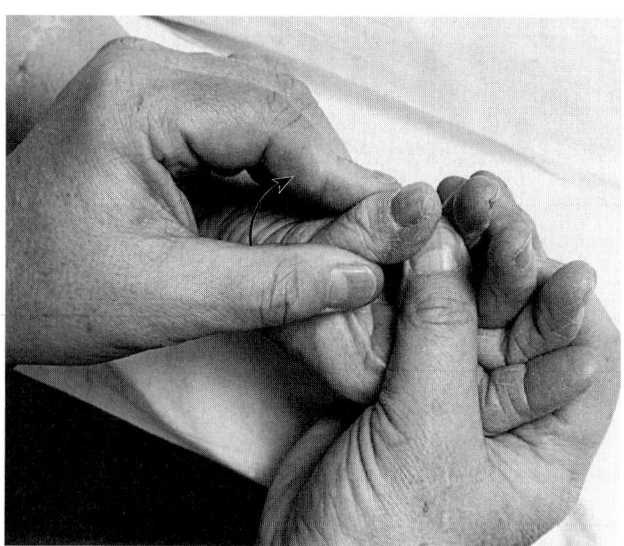
Fig. 6-18 Thumb opposition.

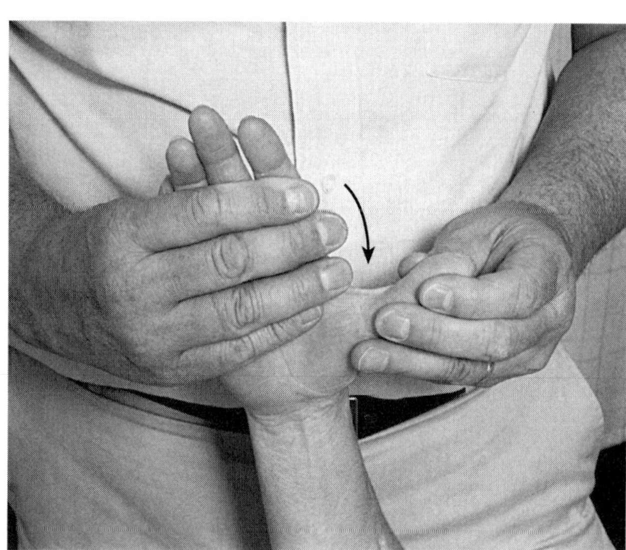
Fig. 6-20 Thumb extension.

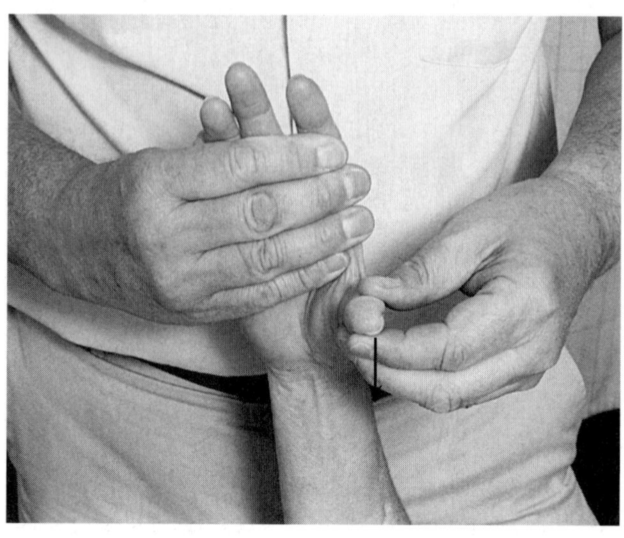
Fig. 6-19 Thumb abduction.

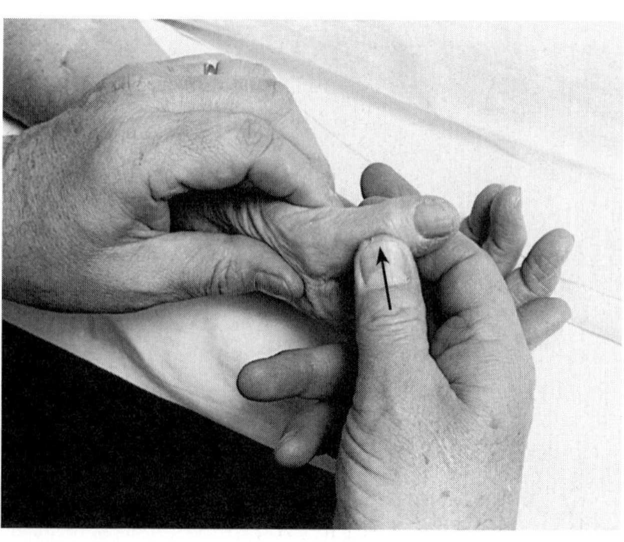
Fig. 6-21 Thumb flexion.

distal joints of the thumb. Return the distal joints to extension.

Elongation of Multijoint Muscles. Review the information presented earlier in this chapter on the concepts related to joint range and the range of multijoint muscles. All motions should be performed individually initially so that the multijoint muscle is elongated over only one joint. This will assist in determining the muscle's free unrestricted range and will prevent excessive elongation of the muscle or excessive stress to the joint and its capsule.

Biceps brachii: Start with the patient supine and the shoulder at the edge of the support surface, with the elbow extended and the forearm pronated. Grasp the elbow with one hand; use the other hand to grasp the wrist. Lower the arm below the level of the support surface (that is, hyperextend the shoulder) until you sense maximal tension in the muscle or the patient complains of discomfort along the anterior (upper) aspect of the extremity.

Triceps brachii (long head): Start with the patient supine, side lying, or sitting. Grasp the wrist with one hand; use the other hand to support the distal end of the humerus. Flex the elbow maximally and simultaneously flex the shoulder. The patient will have to be side lying, sitting, or standing for maximal elongation to occur. Terminate the motion when you sense maximal tension in the muscle or when the patient complains of discomfort along the posterior aspect of the arm (Fig. 6-22).

Extensor digitorum: Place one hand over the dorsum of all the fingers of the patient's hand; use your other hand to support and stabilize the forearm. Gently and sequentially flex the DIP, PIP, and MCP joints and carefully flex the wrist. Terminate the motion when you sense maximal tension in the muscle or when the patient complains of discomfort along the dorsal surface of the wrist, hand, or fingers. This motion can be performed with the elbow flexed or extended (Fig. 6-23).

Flexor digitorum superficialis and profundus: Place one hand over the palmar surface of all the fingers of the patient's hand; use your other hand to support and stabilize the forearm. Gently and sequentially extend the DIP, PIP, and MCP joints and then carefully extend the wrist. Terminate the motion when you sense maximal tension in the muscles or when the patient complains of discomfort along the palmar surface of the wrist, hand, or fingers. Avoid hyperextension of the MCP joints. This motion can be performed with the elbow flexed or extended (Fig. 6-24).

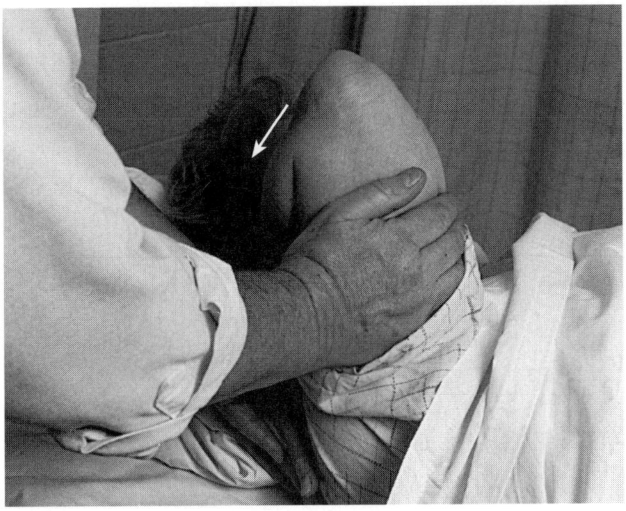

Fig. 6-22 Elongation of the triceps brachii.

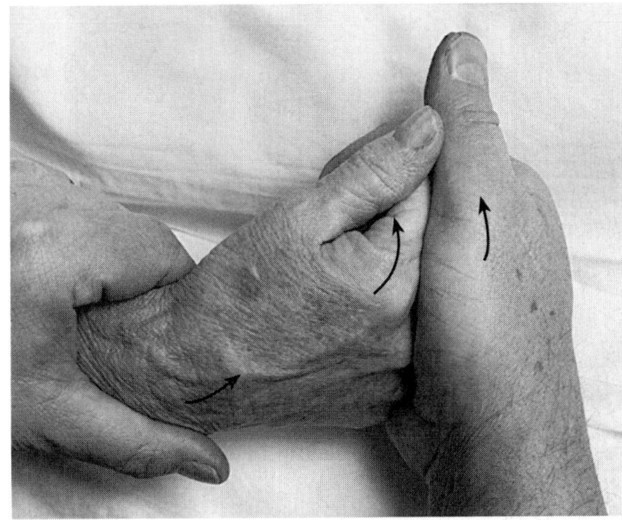

Fig. 6-23 Elongation of the extensor digitorum.

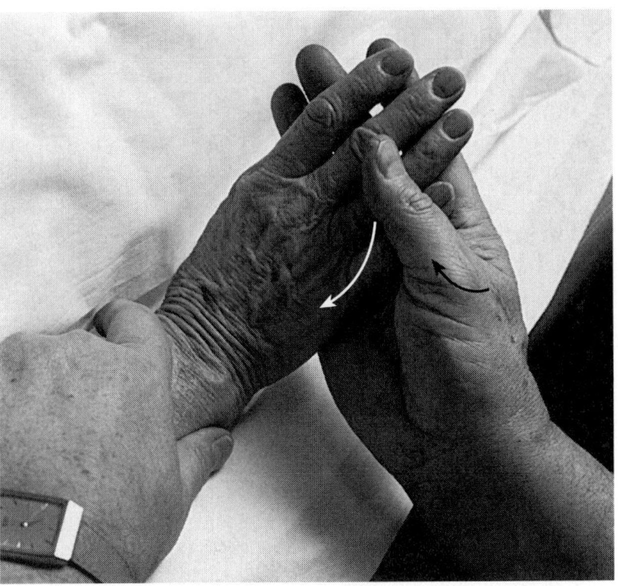

Fig. 6-24 Elongation of the flexor digitorum superficialis and profundus.

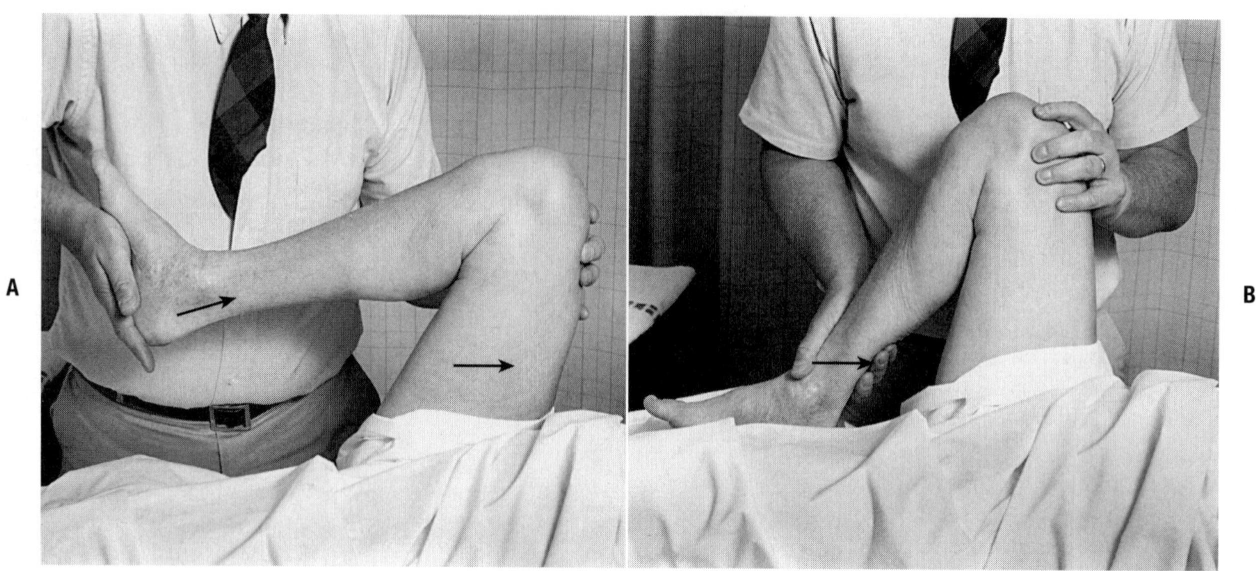

Fig. 6-25 Hip and knee flexion, **A,** and knee flexion, **B.**

Lower Extremity Movements

Traditional Anatomic Planes The primary patient position is supine on a firm surface; properly draped; and positioned close to the near edge of the treatment table. Other positions can be used depending on the patient's condition and the caregiver's preference.

ARTICULATION: Acetabular-femoral and tibial-femoral
Movement: Hip and knee flexion and extension (Fig. 6-25)
Hand placement and motion: Use one hand to cradle the patient's heel; place your other hand in the popliteal space. Lift the lower extremity, allowing the hip and knee to flex. Slide your hand from under the knee to the lateral area of the thigh to prevent hip abduction as the hip and knee flex. Approximate the thigh to the chest and the leg to the posterior area of the thigh; return to the starting position. The patient will need to have the hip at the edge of the support surface to perform hip hyperextension by lowering the extremity toward the floor. Terminate the movement when the pelvis rotates anteriorly or when lumbar lordosis is increased. (*Note:* Hip hyperextension can be performed more easily when the patient is in a side-lying or prone position.)

ARTICULATION: Acetabular-femoral
Movement: Hip flexion and extension with the knee extended (straight leg raising) (Fig. 6-26)
Hand placement and motion: Use one hand to support the distal end of the patient's leg; use your other hand to initially provide support in the popliteal space. Shift your hand from the popliteal space to the anterior area of the knee as the hip is flexed to maintain knee extension and to lift the entire lower extremity to flex the hip. Terminate the motion when you sense maximal tension in the hamstring muscles or when the patient complains of discomfort along the posterior area of the thigh or knee. Do not attempt to increase the range of the hamstrings by forceably flexing the hip with the knee extended. It may be necessary to stabilize the knee of the opposite lower extremity as you perform this motion. Some caregivers prefer to place the ankle of the exercised extremity on one shoulder and to lift the lower extremity by moving the body forward.

ARTICULATION: Acetabular-femoral
Movement: Hip abduction and adduction (Fig. 6-27)
Hand placement and motion: Use one hand to support the patient's distal leg; use your other hand to provide support in the popliteal space and to maintain the knee extended. Move the extremity away from the opposite lower extremity, keeping it parallel to the floor and in neutral internal-external rotation. Return it to a position of adduction. To attain complete adduction of the exercised extremity, the opposite lower extremity must be adducted. Some individuals adduct the extremity by lifting it above the opposite extremity so that more adduction is attained.

ARTICULATION: Acetabular-femoral
Movement: Hip adduction-side lying (Fig. 6-28)
Hand placement and motion: With the patient in a side-lying position and the uppermost hip and knee extended and the lowermost extremity flexed, use one hand to support the knee or distal area of the thigh. With the other hand, grasp the ankle and lower the extremity toward the floor and keep the knee extended.

ARTICULATION: Acetabular-femoral
Movement: Hip internal and external rotation (Fig. 6-29)
Hand placement and motion: With the patient's hip and knee extended and resting on the treatment table, use one hand to grasp the distal area of the thigh proximal to the knee; use your other hand to grasp proximally to

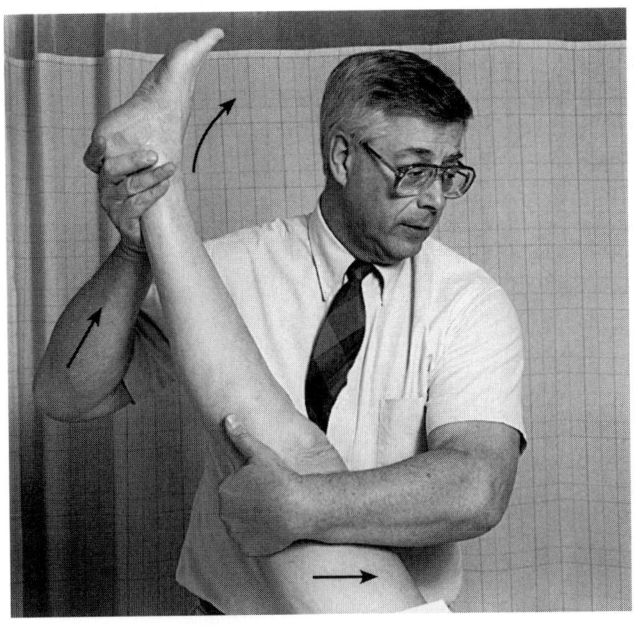

Fig. 6-26 Hip and knee extension (straight leg raise).

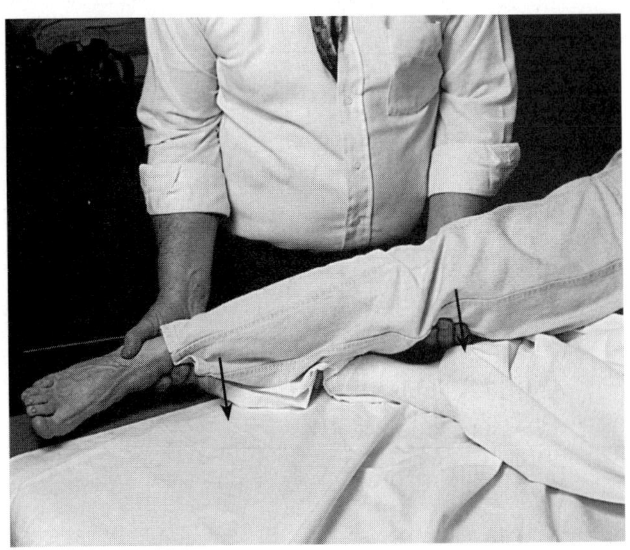

Fig. 6-28 Hip adduction in the side-lying position.

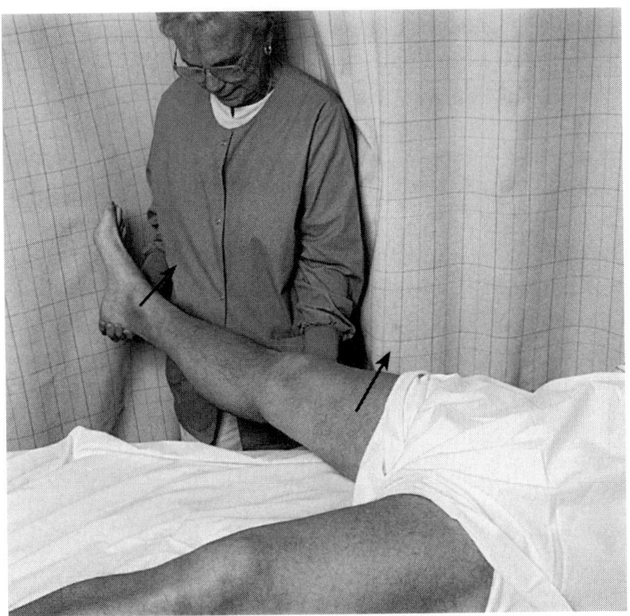

Fig. 6-27 Hip abduction.

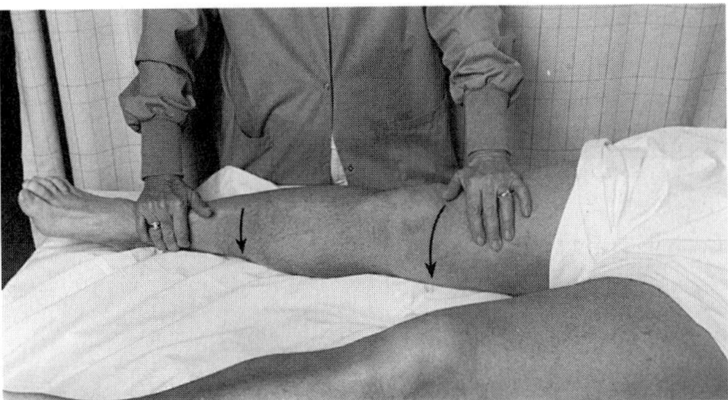

Fig. 6-29 Internal (medial) hip rotation.

the ankle. Roll the extremity inward and outward, but do not abduct or adduct the hip. Be certain motion occurs in the hip.

For an alternative technique, flex the hip and knee to 90 degrees. Use one hand to support under the patient's knee; use your other hand to grasp the ankle or cradle the leg. Move the leg inward and outward to cause the femur to rotate, but do not abduct or adduct the hip. Be cautious; avoid excessive stress to the medial or lateral aspects of the structures of the knee. Terminate the motion when you sense maximal tension in the muscle or joint or when the patient complains of discomfort in the groin or lateral area of the hip (Fig. 6-30).

ARTICULATION: Tibial-femoral

Movement: Knee flexion with the hip extended (Fig. 6-31)

Hand placement and motion: With the patient supine and the thigh supported with the knee and leg at the edge of the support surface, use one hand to support the patient's ankle; use your other hand or towel roll to protect the posterior area of the thigh. Lower the leg to flex the knee over the edge of the table. You will need to stoop to attain full range and to avoid unnecessary strain to the structures of your back.

You may also perform this motion with the patient prone. Use one hand to grasp the ankle; use your other hand to rest on the buttock. (*Note:* Place a folded towel between your hand and the patient's buttock to preserve modesty.) Bend the knee by moving the heel toward the

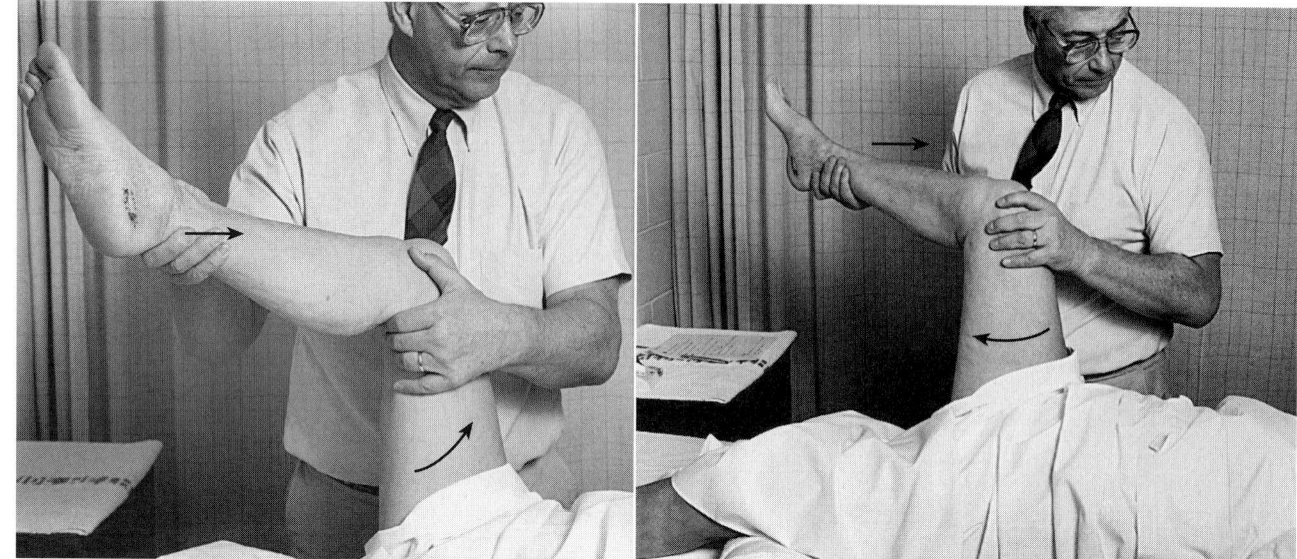

Fig. 6-30 **A,** External (lateral) hip rotation (alternative method). **B,** Internal (medial) hip rotation (alternative method).

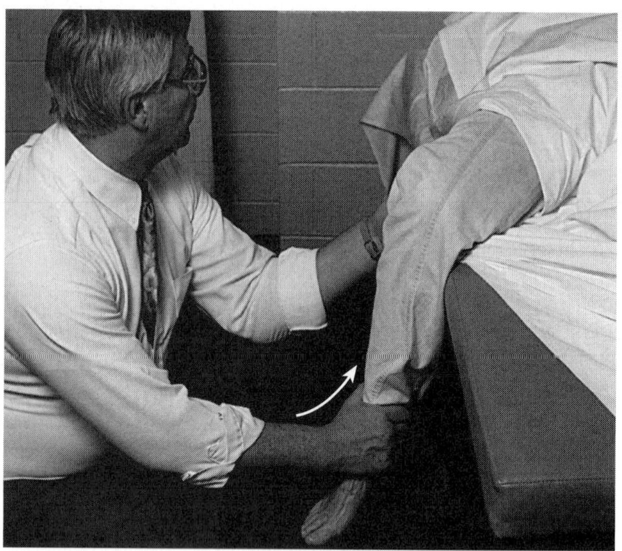

Fig. 6-31 Knee flexion with the hip extended.

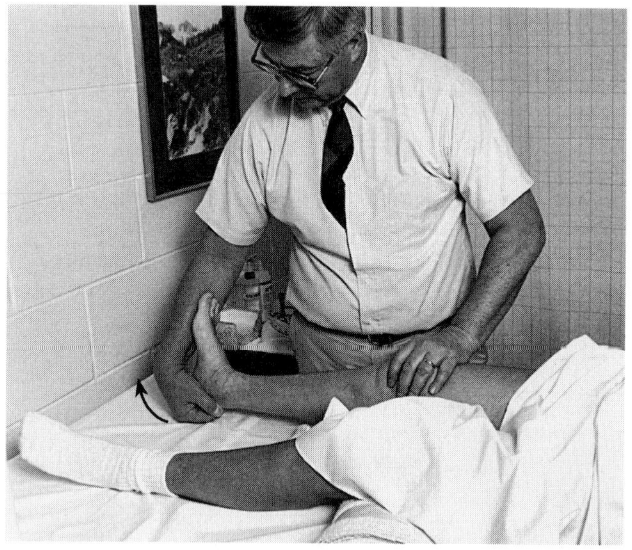

Fig. 6-32 Ankle dorsiflexion.

buttock. Terminate the motion when you sense maximal tension in the quadriceps muscle or when the patient complains of discomfort along the anterior area of the thigh or hip flexion occurs. Hip flexion indicates that the rectus femoris has reached its fullest elongation and causes anterior pelvic rotation resulting in hip flexion. To elongate the rectus femoris, the hip is extended simultaneously with knee flexion.

ARTICULATION: Crural-tibial

Movement: Ankle dorsiflexion and plantar flexion (Fig. 6-32)

Hand placement and motion: *Dorsiflexion:* Use one hand to grasp both sides of the calcaneus; place your forearm along the plantar surface of the foot; use your other hand to stabilize the distal end of the tibia. Pull downward on the calcaneus while pushing upward with the forearm against the metatarsal heads. It is important that the calcaneus move and you should avoid pushing only against the metatarsal heads or the forefoot. The knee can be extended or flexed slightly. When it is flexed, a more complete range of ankle motion will be possible because the gastrocnemius, a multijoint muscle,

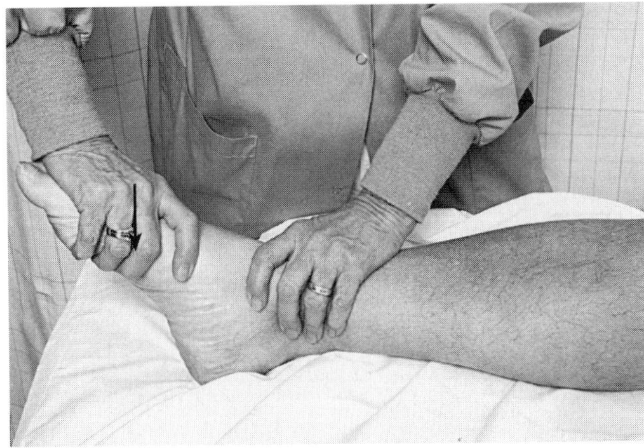

Fig. 6-33 Plantar flexion.

is partially relaxed. When the knee is extended, the gastrocnemius will be elongated more and will limit the range of ankle dorsiflexion.

Plantar flexion: Use one hand to grasp the dorsum of the foot; use your other hand to stabilize the distal end of the tibia. Press down on the foot to produce plantar flexion (Fig. 6-33), but avoid pressure over the toes.

ARTICULATION: Talar-crural

Movement: Ankle inversion and eversion (Fig. 6-34)

Hand placement and motion: Use one hand to grasp the dorsum of the foot; use your other hand to stabilize the distal end of the tibia. Turn the foot inward and outward, avoiding hip rotation. All motion should occur at the lower ankle joint.

ARTICULATION: Metatarsophalangeal (MTP) and IP

Movement: Toe flexion and extension (Fig. 6-35)

Hand placement and motion: Use one hand to grasp and stabilize the foot or to stabilize each proximal area of the bone, similar to the technique described for the fingers. Use the thumb and index finger of your other hand to grasp the phalanx immediately distal to the metatarsal being stabilized; flex and extend the phalanx. All the MTP and IP joints may be moved simultaneously after the range of each joint has been evaluated. Avoid ankle dorsiflexion or plantar flexion by stabilizing the foot. The toes can be abducted using a technique similar to that described for the fingers.

ARTICULATION: Metatarsal head joint play.

Movement: Elevation and depression of the metatarsal heads.

Hand placement and motion: Use the thumb and index finger of one hand to stabilize one metatarsal; use the thumb and index finger of your other hand to grasp the adjacent metatarsal. The metatarsal that is not being stabilized is moved upward and downward; avoid simultaneous movement of two metatarsals.

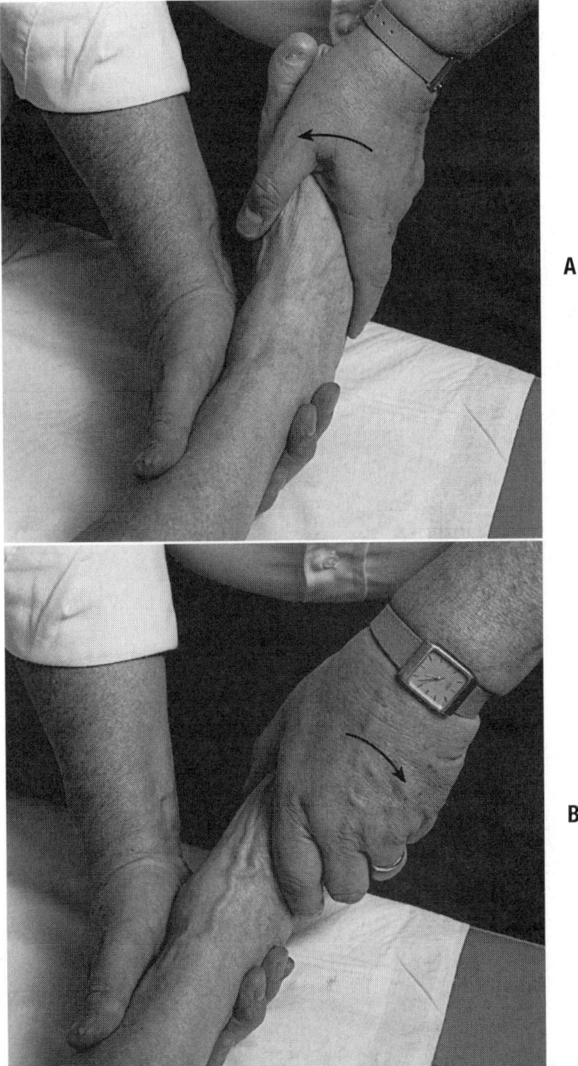

Fig. 6-34 Inversion, **A,** and eversion, **B,** of the foot.

Elongation of Multijoint Muscles

Hamstrings: Start with the patient supine and the knee extended; perform hip flexion while maintaining the knee in extension. Terminate the motion when you sense maximal tension in the hamstring muscles or when the patient complains of discomfort (see Fig. 6-26).

Rectus femoris: Start with the patient prone, and perform simultaneous knee flexion and hip extension. This motion can also be performed with the patient in a side-lying position, provided he or she is secure and you can stabilize the pelvis to prevent an anterior pelvic tilt. Terminate the motion when you sense maximum tension in the quadriceps muscle, when lumbar lordosis increases, or when the patient complains of discomfort (Fig. 6-36).

Tensor fasciae latae (iliotibial band): Start with the patient in a side-lying position and with the hip and knee

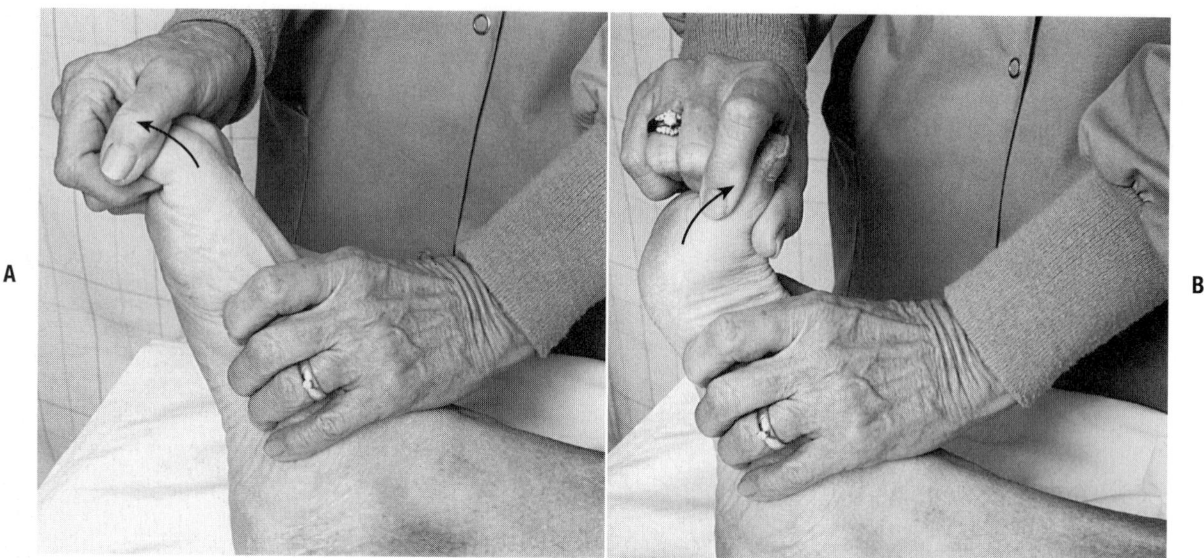

Fig. 6-35 Flexion, **A,** and extension, **B,** of the toes.

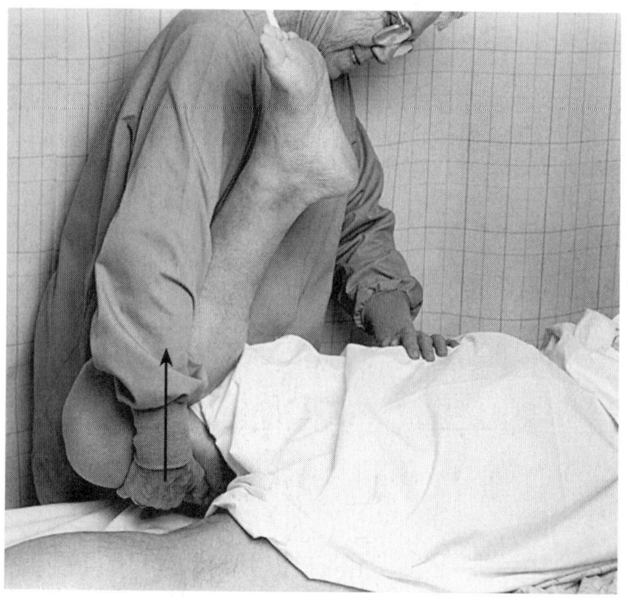

Fig. 6-36 Elongation of the rectus femoris.

PROCEDURE 6-3

Vertebral Artery Occlusion Test

Position the person supine and passively perform:

1. Full head and neck extension.
2. Full head and neck rotation to left and right with head and neck in neutral position.
3. Full head and neck rotation to left and right with head and neck in extension.
4. Simulated mobilization movements* and unilateral posteroanterior oscillation of C1-C2 facet joints with head rotated left and right (prone lying).

Maintain each position for 10 to 15 seconds or until symptoms occur; wait 10 seconds between each test after returning the head and neck to a neutral position. Positive findings include complaint of dizziness, diplopia, lightheadedness, or visual disturbances.

Adopted from Magee DJ: Orthopedic Physical Assessment. 3rd edition. Philadelphia: WB Saunders, 1997.

*Simulated mobilization movement: Passively position the cervical spine for each mobilization or manipulation without actually performing the mobilization.

of the uppermost extremity extended. Perform the motion described for hip adduction by lowering the uppermost extremity toward the floor or surface of the table. Terminate the motion when you sense maximum tension in the tensor fasciae latae or when the extremity ceases to move downward (see Fig. 6-28).

Gastrocnemius: Start with the patient supine and with the hip and knee extended. Perform the motion described for ankle dorsiflexion by moving the dorsum of the foot toward the shin; be certain the calcaneus moves. This motion can also be combined with straight leg raising. Terminate the motion when maximal tension is sensed in the gastrocnemius or when the patient complains of discomfort (see Fig. 6-32).

Trunk Movements

Traditional Anatomic Planes Proper body mechanics must be used when you attempt some of these motions to prevent unnecessary strain to the structures of your back and to protect the patient from discomfort and injury. *Caution:* Before beginning PROM to the cervical spine, the caregiver should evaluate the ability of the vertebral artery to maintain adequate blood flow to the brain using the vertebral artery occlusion test (Procedure 6-3). Patient complaints of dizziness,

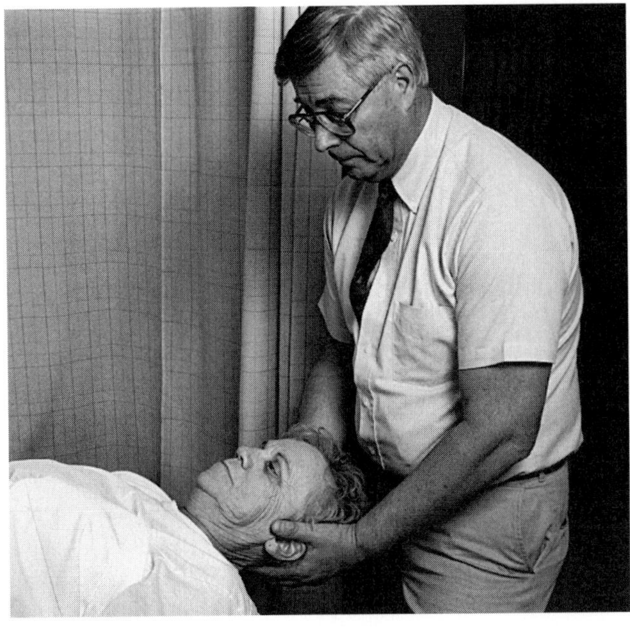

Fig. 6-37 Hand positions for midposition of the cervical spine.

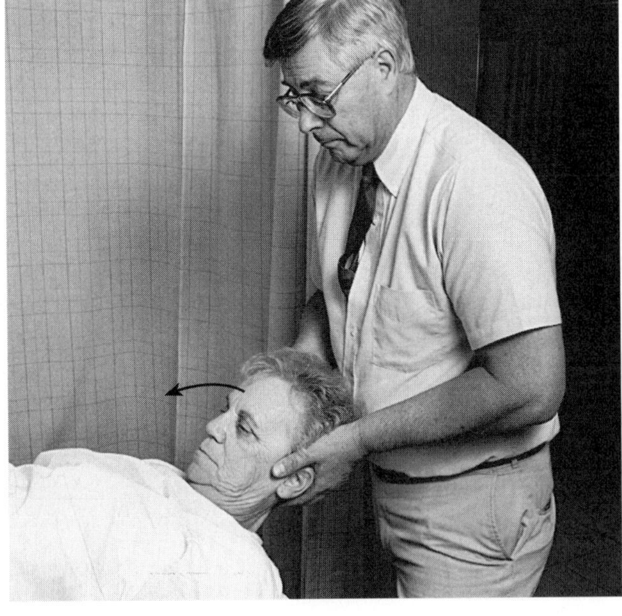

Fig. 6-38 Forward bending (flexion) of the cervical spine.

light-headedness, or visual problems (that is, diplopia) indicate a compromise of the arterial blood flow. Further treatment should be withheld or performed cautiously until the results of additional tests are available.

Cervical spine: Stand at the head and face the patient. With the patient's shoulders at the edge of the support surface, support the patient's head in your hands. Perform the motions slowly and cautiously (see Fig. 6-37).

Forward bending (flexion): Support the patient's head with your hands placed firmly at the occiput. Lift the head so the chin moves toward the chest. Encourage the patient to relax the posterior neck muscles (Fig. 6-38).

Backward bending (extension or hyperextension): Support the patient's head with your hands at the occiput. Lower the head so the occiput moves toward the floor. Encourage the patient to relax the anterior neck muscles (Fig. 6-39).

Side bending (lateral flexion): Support the patient's head at the occiput and move the head so one ear moves toward the acromion. Maintain the cervical spine in neutral flexion-extension and do not allow the scapula to elevate toward the ear. Encourage the patient to relax the lateral neck muscles on the side of the neck opposite to the direction in which you move the head (Fig. 6-40).

Rotation: Support the patient's head at the occiput and turn the head to the left and to the right. Maintain the cervical spine in neutral flexion-extension. Perform this motion slowly to avoid vertigo. Encourage the patient to relax the muscles of the neck (Fig. 6-41).

Lumbar spine: Stand on one side of the patient at the level of the pelvis with the body close to the near edge of the support surface.

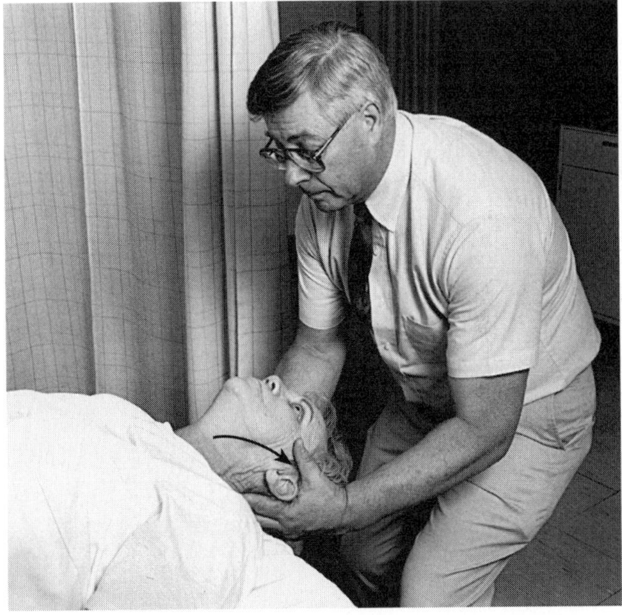

Fig. 6-39 Backward bending (extension or hyperextension) of the cervical spine.

Lumbar flexion: With the patient supine, lift both of the thighs toward the chest by performing hip and knee flexion (that is, a bilateral knee-to-chest maneuver). Elevate the distal portion of the sacrum from the support surface to produce full posterior pelvic rotation (Fig. 6-42). *Caution:* Do not attempt this maneuver when the patient's lower extremities are too heavy or too large for you to control and lift safely; be alert for indications of patient discomfort.

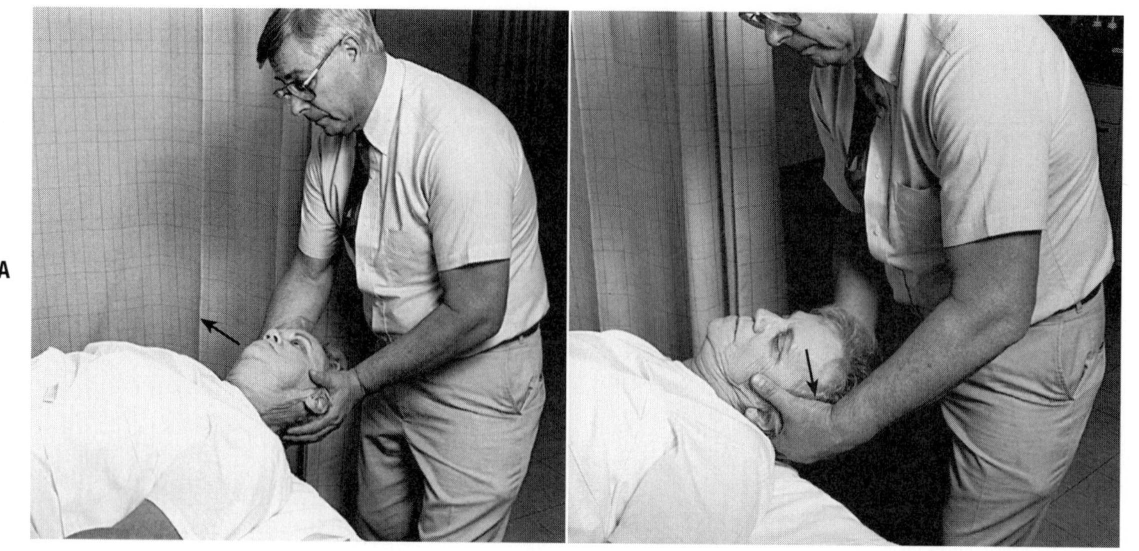

Fig. 6-40 Side bending (lateral flexion) of the cervical spine.

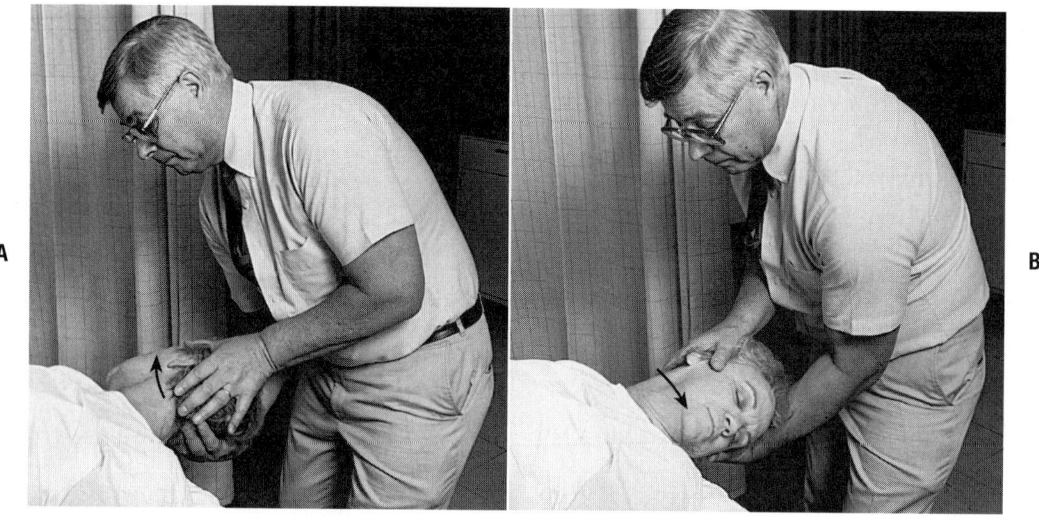

Fig. 6-41 Rotation of the cervical spine.

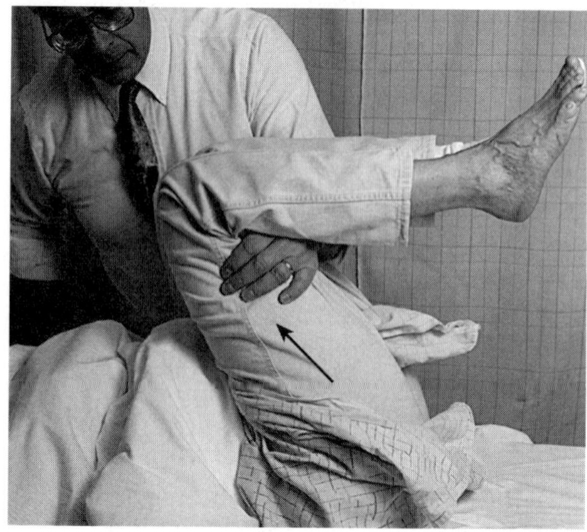

Fig. 6-42 Lumbar flexion.

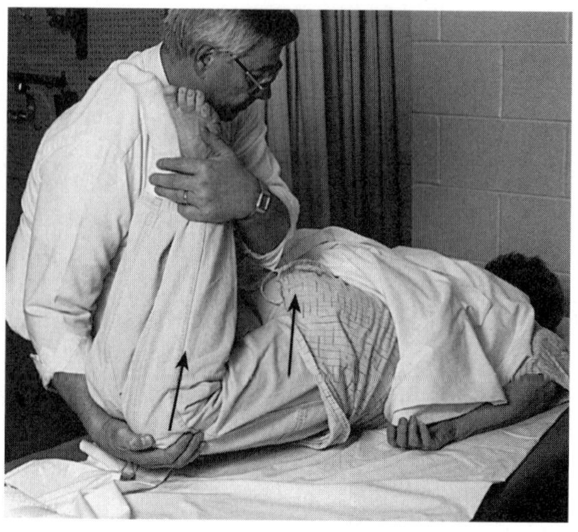

Fig. 6-43 Lumbar extension.

Lumbar extension: With the patient prone, flex both knees and lift both thighs to cause an anterior pelvic tilt and lumbar spine extension (Fig. 6-43). *Caution:* Do not attempt this maneuver when the patient's lower extremities are too heavy or too large for you to control and lift safely; be alert for indications of patient discomfort. For small patients, the patient's chest can be lifted from the support surface by grasping the anterior surface of both shoulders or the patient can perform a partial push-up to elevate the chest while maintaining the pelvis on the support surface.

Lumbar rotation: Position the patient supine with the hips and knees flexed and the feet on the support surface in a hook-lying position. Move the thighs to the left and to the right with one hand by applying a rotational force to the pelvis on the side opposite to the movement of the thighs, using your other hand to stabilize the chest. The right side of the pelvis should become elevated when the thighs are moved to the left and vice versa (Fig. 6-44). *Caution:* This activity should be performed carefully for the patient with a known hip abnormality or lumbar spine dysfunction; it is contraindicated for a patient with a recent total hip replacement or other similar surgery.

Thoracic spine: Stand at the side of the patient at the level of the upper thorax. The patient's upper extremities should be folded over the chest, and the body should be close to the near edge of the support surface.

Thoracic rotation: With the patient supine and with the hips and knees extended, grasp under the right scapula with one hand; use your other hand to stabilize over the right anterosuperior iliac spine (ASIS). Lift and rotate the upper trunk to the left, and then perform the motion in the opposite direction with your hands positioned under the left scapula and over the left ASIS. Request the patient to lift and control the head while this motion is performed (Fig. 6-45).

Diagonal Patterns for PROM Movements

Instead of using the traditional anatomic planes of motion, diagonal patterns can be used. Four of the stated and reported advantages of these patterns are as follows:

- They incorporate rotation with all movements.
- The midline of the body is crossed with many of the movements.
- The movements tend to be more functional than traditional movements.
- A combination of motions occurs within each pattern.

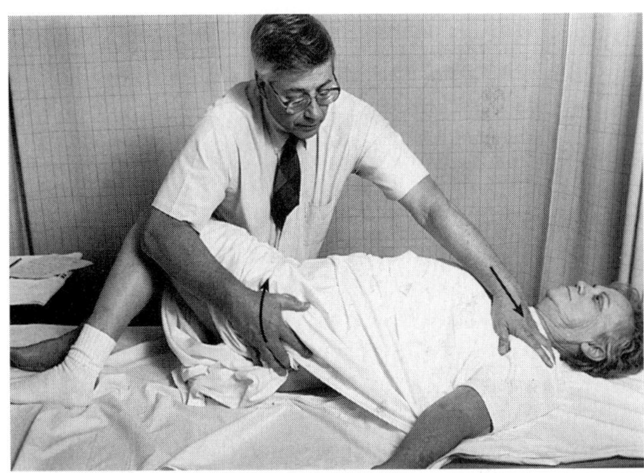

Fig. 6-44 Lumbar rotation.

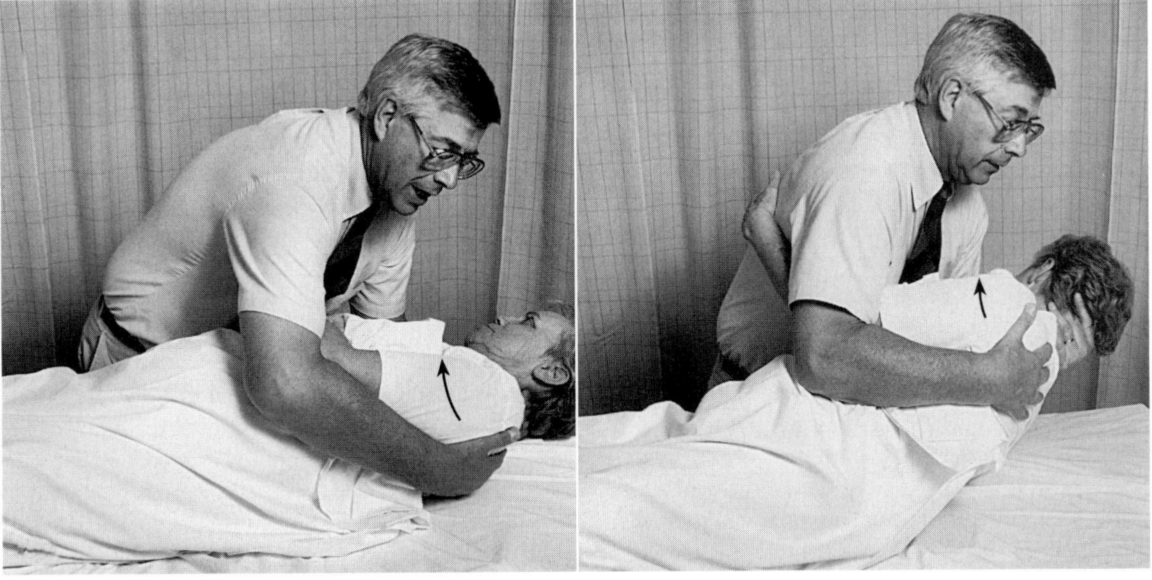

Fig. 6-45 Thoracic rotation.

Table 6-1 **Diagonal Patterns: Component Positions**

	Diagonal 1		Diagonal 2	
	Flexion	Extension	Flexion	Extension
UPPER EXTREMITY				
Scapula	Elevation, abduction, upward rotation	Depression, adduction, downward rotation	Elevation, adduction, upward rotation	Depression, abduction, downward rotation
Shoulder	Flexion, adduction, external rotation	Extension, abduction, internal rotation	Flexion, abduction, external rotation	Extension, adduction, internal rotation
Elbow	Flexion, extension	Flexion, extension	Flexion, extension	Flexion, extension
Forearm	Supination	Pronation	Supination	Pronation
Wrist	Flexion, radial deviation	Extension, ulnar deviation	Extension, radial deviation	Flexion, ulnar deviation
Fingers	Flexion, adduction	Extension, abduction	Extension, abduction	Flexion, adduction
LOWER EXTREMITY				
Hip	Flexion, adduction, external rotation	Extension, abduction, internal rotation	Flexion, abduction, internal rotation	Extension, adduction, external rotation
Knee	Flexion, extension	Flexion, extension	Flexion, extension	Flexion, extension
Ankle	Dorsiflexion, inversion	Plantar flexion, eversion	Dorsiflexion, eversion	Plantar flexion, inversion
Toes	Extension	Flexion	Extension	Flexion

The patterns were developed as components of the therapeutic approach known as PNF. The patterns can be performed actively by the patient, passively by a caregiver, or resistively against an external force. This text is not meant to be a complete resource for PNF patterning; refer to the Bibliography for *Proprioceptive Neuromuscular Facilitation* by Voss, Ionta, and Myers.

There are two basic diagonal patterns for the upper and lower extremity—diagonal 1 and diagonal 2—and each of them can be performed in flexion and extension, resulting in a total of four different movements. Thus the patterns are identified as "diagonal 1 flexion," "diagonal 2 flexion," "diagonal 1 extension," and "diagonal 2 extension." Furthermore, each pattern can be performed by the upper and lower extremity and so are termed "diagonal 1 flexion upper extremity" or "diagonal 1 flexion lower extremity," and so on. Common abbreviations of the patterns are D1 Fl UE, D2 Fl UE, D1 Ex UE, D2 Ex UE, D1 Fl LE, D2 Fl LE, D1 Ex LE, and D2 Ex LE.

The patterns are named according to the position of the proximal joint of the pattern (that is, the shoulder or the hip) at the conclusion of the pattern. Thus the pattern is initiated with the proximal joint positioned opposite to its position at the conclusion of the pattern. Each pattern contains a flexion or extension component, an abduction or adduction component, and an internal or external rotation component for the proximal joint. All three motions must be performed, especially the rotation component. Other extremity joints or components will also have a final position, but the patterns are described according to the final position of the proximal joint. Refer to Table 6-1 for a description of each pattern.

The caregiver should be positioned to be able to move in a diagonal direction as the patterns are performed. It will be necessary to pivot on your feet to avoid improper and stress-producing body mechanics. Proper positioning and movement must be used consistently by the caregiver when diagonal patterns are performed passively to reduce stress and strain and to complete each pattern.

Remember: These patterns describe the positions of the proximal components at the *completion* of the pattern. To start a pattern, the proximal joint of the extremity is placed in the position that is the reciprocal of the completed pattern. For example, to initiate D1 Fl UE, the shoulder is positioned in D1 Ex UE. How would you position the extremity to initiate D1 Fl LE or D2 Fl UE? *Note:* When PNF patterns are used for any form of active exercise, the hand placement by the caregiver should provide a tactile contact and stimulus to the major muscles involved in producing the desired extremity movement. For those situations, the caregiver's grasp must contact the skin surface overlying the muscle or muscles that are to contract and avoid contact with the muscle or muscles that are to relax during the exercise. However, when diagonal patterns are used for PMOR, hand placement is not so critical and it may be altered to provide better support and stability to an extremity. Therefore the caregiver's hand placement in the photographs depicting the use of diagonal patterns for PROM may vary from the hand positions that would be used to tactilely stimulate the contracting muscles.

Upper Extremity

Diagonal 1, Flexion with the Elbow Extended

Movement: Shoulder flexion, adduction, and external rotation. Start with the shoulder of the upper extremity slightly abducted, internally rotated, and extended. The elbow is extended and the forearm is pronated with the wrist and fingers extended (Fig. 6-46).

Hand placement and motion: For the right upper extremity, use your left hand to support the patient's hand and wrist; use your right hand to support the distal aspect of

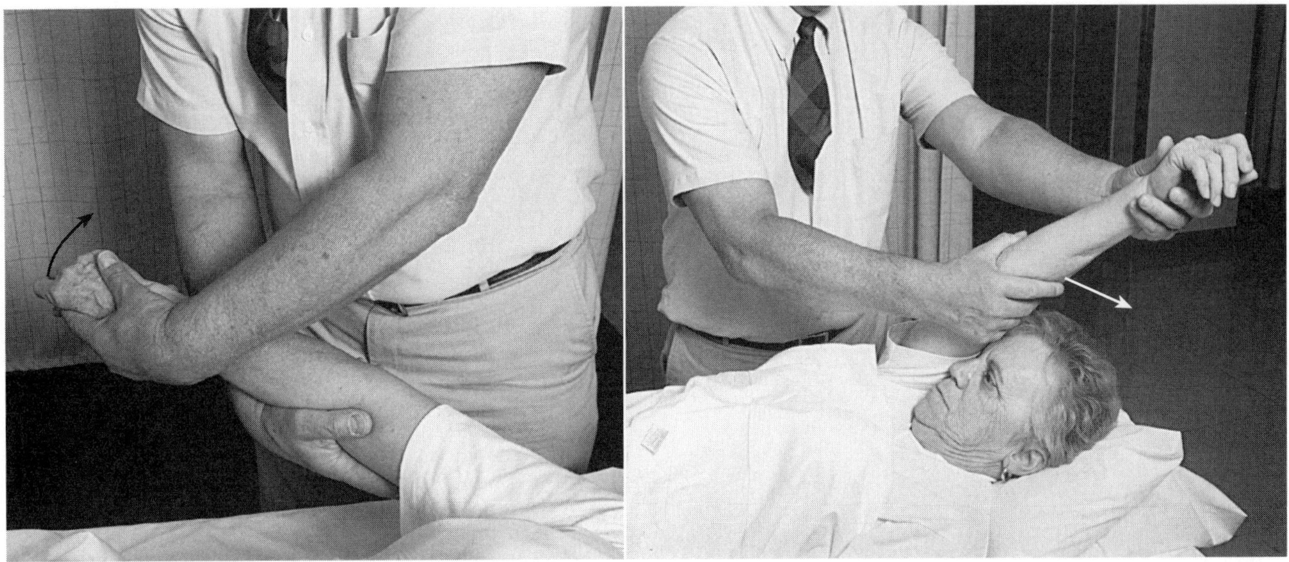

Fig. 6-46 Diagonal 1, flexion with the elbow extended.

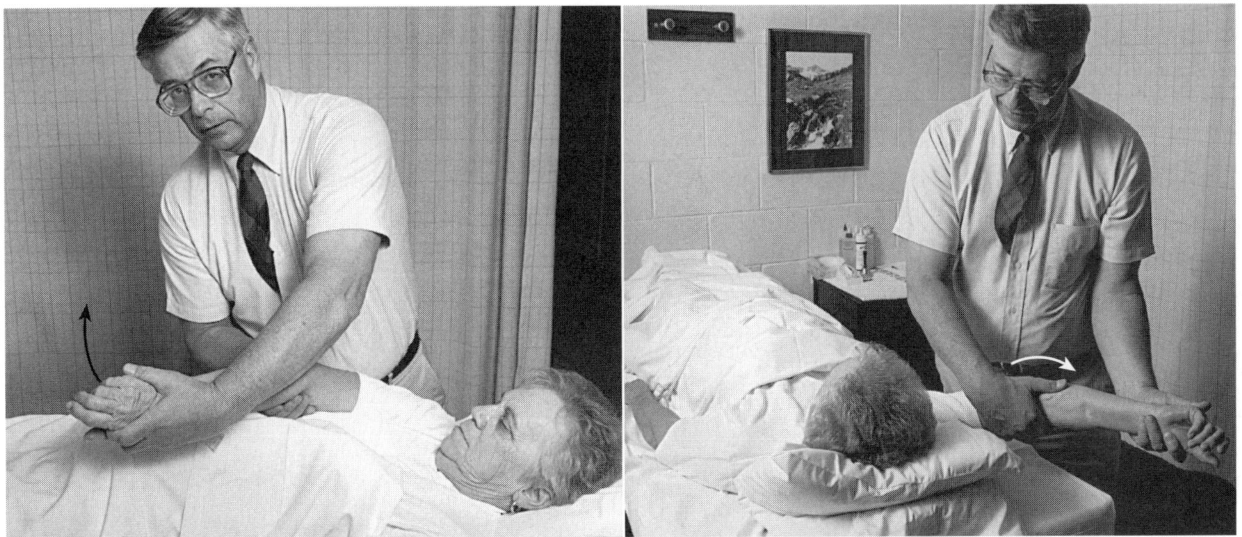

Fig. 6-47 Diagonal 2, flexion with the elbow extended.

the upper arm. Lift the extremity diagonally across the chest and over the face; simultaneously, externally rotate the shoulder, supinate the forearm, and flex the wrist and fingers. Perform diagonal flexion within the width of the shoulder. Reverse your hand placement and grip for the left extremity.

Diagonal 1, Extension with the Elbow Extended

Movement: Shoulder extension, abduction, and internal rotation. Start with the shoulder of the upper extremity adducted, flexed, and externally rotated. The elbow is extended, the forearm is supinated, and the wrist and fingers are flexed (see Fig. 6-46).

Hand placement and motion: For the right upper extremity, use your left hand to grasp the patient's hand and wrist; use your right hand to grasp the posterior distal aspect of the upper arm. Move the extremity diagonally away from the face; simultaneously, internally rotate the shoulder, pronate the forearm, and extend the wrist and fingers. Perform the diagonal extension within the width of the shoulder. Reverse your hand placement and grip for the left extremity.

Diagonal 2, Flexion with the Elbow Extended

Movement: Shoulder flexion, abduction, and external rotation. Start with the shoulder of the upper extremity positioned diagonally across the patient's body and internally rotated. The elbow is extended, the forearm is pronated, and the wrist and fingers are flexed (Fig. 6-47).

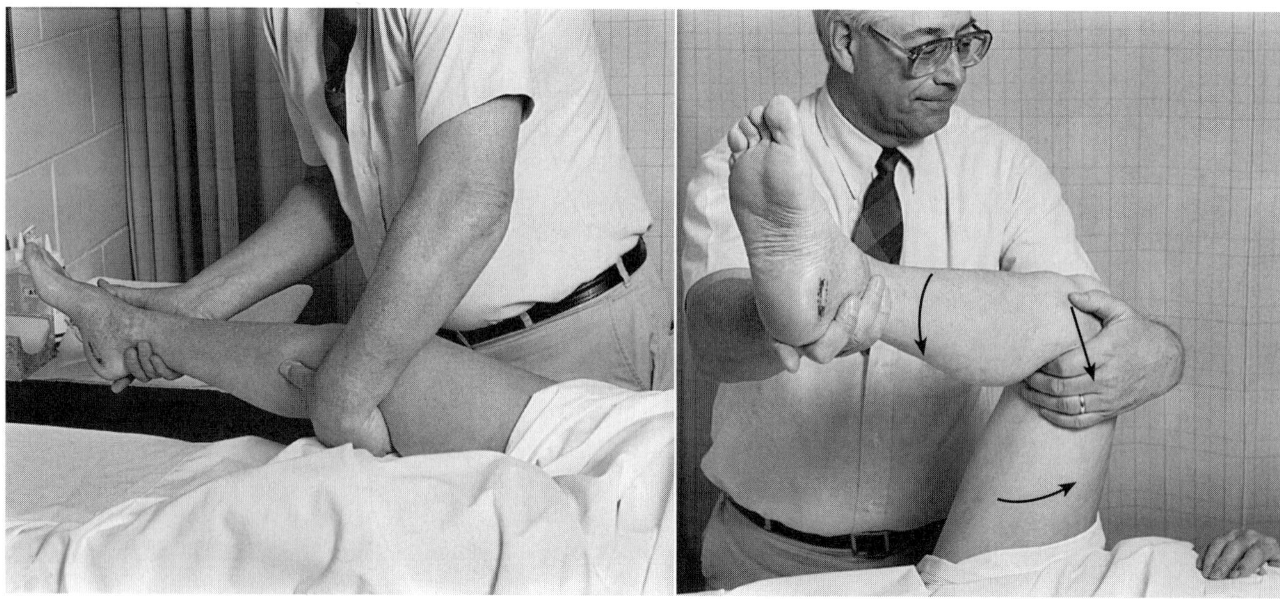

Fig. 6-48 Diagonal 1, flexion with the knee flexed.

Hand placement and motion: For the right upper extremity, use your left hand to grasp the dorsum of the patient's hand; use your right hand to grasp the dorsal surface of the forearm or the lateral surface of the upper arm. Lift the extremity diagonally up from the body into flexion, abduction, and external rotation. Perform diagonal flexion within the width of the shoulder. Reverse your hand placement and grip for the left extremity.

Diagonal 2, Extension with the Elbow Extended

Movement: Shoulder extension, adduction, and internal rotation. Start with the shoulder of the upper extremity flexed, abducted, and externally rotated. The elbow is extended, the forearm is supinated, and the wrist and fingers are extended (see Fig. 6-47).

Hand placement and motion: Retain your grasp as described for the D2 Fl pattern and move the upper extremity diagonally toward the body into extension, adduction, and internal rotation. Perform diagonal extension within the width of the shoulder.

These four patterns can be performed with the elbow flexed. Your hand placement will be similar to those described previously and the motions will be the same as those described for the upper extremity patterns with the elbow extended.

Lower Extremity

Diagonal 1, Flexion with the Knee Flexed

Movement: Hip flexion, adduction, and external rotation. Start with the hip of the lower extremity slightly abducted, extended, and internally rotated and the knee extended (Fig. 6-48).

Hand placement and motion: Use one hand to grasp and support the patient's heel; use your other hand to grasp and support the posterior distal aspect of the thigh by reaching over the thigh. Lift the extremity diagonally toward the abdomen and the opposite shoulder; simultaneously, externally rotate the hip and dorsiflex the foot. Perform diagonal flexion within the width of the hip. When this motion is performed with the knee extended, the full range of hip flexion will not be available.

Diagonal 1, Extension with the Knee Extended

Movement: Hip extension, abduction, and internal rotation. Start with the hip of the lower extremity flexed, adducted, and externally rotated and the knee extended (see Fig. 6-48).

Hand placement and motion: Maintain your hand placement as used for the D1 Fl pattern and return the extremity diagonally so the hip is extended, abducted, and internally rotated. Perform diagonal extension within the width of the hip.

Diagonal 2, Flexion with the Knee Extended

Movement: Hip flexion, abduction, and internal rotation. Start with the hip of the lower extremity slightly adducted, externally rotated, and extended and the knee extended (Fig. 6-49).

Hand placement and motion: Use one hand to grasp the lateral dorsal surface of the foot; use your other hand to grasp the posterior distal aspect of the thigh. Lift the extremity diagonally up and away from the body; simultaneously, internally rotate the hip. Perform diagonal flexion within the width of the hip.

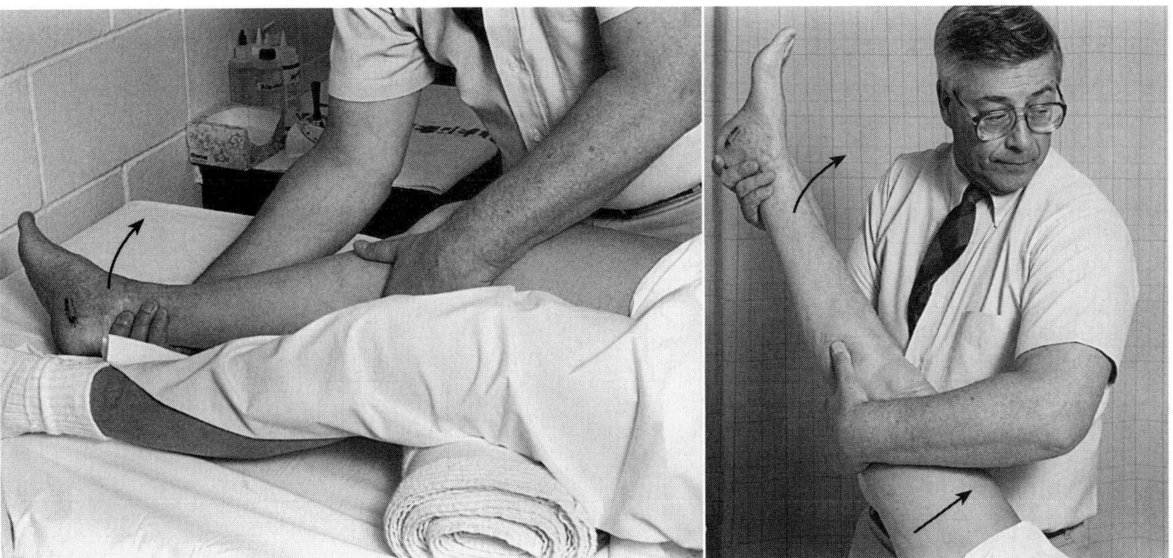

Fig. 6-49 Diagonal 2, flexion with the knee extended.

Diagonal 2, Extension with the Knee Extended

Movement: Hip extension, adduction, and external rotation. Start with the hip of the lower extremity flexed, abducted, and internally rotated and the knee extended.

Hand placement and motion: Maintain the hand placement used for the D2 Fl pattern and return the extremity diagonally toward the opposite lower extremity; simultaneously, externally rotate the hip. Perform diagonal extension within the width of the hip (see Fig. 6-49).

These four patterns can be performed with the knee flexed. Your hand placement will be similar to those described previously and the motions will be the same as those described for the lower extremity patterns with the knee extended.

ACTIVE EXERCISE

Some of the advantages, uses, and goals associated with active exercise have been described previously in this chapter. For patients who are capable, it is important for the exercise program to progress from passive to active because normal function requires muscle strength and endurance. Numerous resources that provide detailed explanations of the effects of active exercise are available; therefore such explanations are not provided in this text.

Active exercise has been described previously as any exercise in which the movement of the body or body segment is accomplished by or with an active, voluntary muscle contraction, with or without externally applied assistance or resistance. Many combinations or types of muscle contractions and assistance or resistance can be used in an active exercise program. The ingenuity and experience of the caregiver, the ability of the patient, and the goal of the exercise or program affect the selection and application of techniques. This text does not describe or present information related to resistive exercise using mechanical equipment; sources of such information can be found in the Bibliography.

Types of Muscle Contraction and Exercise

There are three basic types or forms of muscle contraction: (1) isotonic, (2) isometric, and (3) isokinetic. Isotonic contractions can be subdivided into *eccentric contractions* and *concentric contractions*. There is visible joint motion when the muscle contracts isotonically and the load, or resistance, against which the muscle contracts can remain constant or can vary. When the muscle contracts concentrically, its fibers produce a relative shortening of the muscle. When the muscle contracts eccentrically, its fibers allow a relative lengthening of the muscle. An example of a concentric contraction is contraction of the biceps to produce elbow flexion when the person is sitting or standing. An example of an eccentric contraction is contraction of the biceps to control elbow extension when one is returning the forearm from 90 degrees of elbow flexion to a completely extended position when the person is sitting or standing.

The position of the patient, especially in relationship to gravity, will affect the type of contraction produced and the muscles that produce the contraction. For example, when a person is supine and performs active shoulder flexion through the shoulder's full normal range, the shoulder flexors function concentrically from 0 to 90 degrees of flexion, whereas the shoulder extensors function eccentrically from 90 to 180 degrees of flexion. When the extremity is returned to the patient's side, the shoulder extensors function concentrically from 180 to 90 degrees of extension and the shoulder flexors function eccentrically from 90 to 0 degrees of extension. The concepts of concentric and eccentric muscle contractions can be applied to different muscles or muscle groups as you vary the position of the patient.

Isotonic exercise can be used to maintain or increase strength, power, and endurance, to promote local circulation, to enhance cardiovascular efficiency, to create *hypertrophy* of muscle fibers, to maintain the physiologic elasticity of a muscle, to maintain joint motion, and to maintain or enhance coordination. An eccentric muscle contraction develops more tension in the muscle than a concentric contraction and thus may develop strength more rapidly. External resistance or assistance can be applied manually or mechanically to either the eccentric or the concentric contraction.

In an isometric muscle contraction, there is little or no observable joint motion and no significant change in the length of the muscle. An *isometric contraction* can be performed with or without external resistance. When no resistance is applied, the contraction is frequently termed "muscle setting" (such as "quad" set, "glut" set).

Isometric exercise can be used to maintain muscle tone or, when resistance is applied, to increase strength, to focus the muscle contraction at one or several specific portions of the total joint range, and to avoid the pain associated with joint motion. It may also economize the time spent to perform the exercise. This type of exercise does little to contribute to cardiovascular fitness or joint or muscle flexibility or to maintain coordinated movement. Resistance can be applied manually or mechanically; when resistance is applied, increased tension occurs in the muscle fibers, resulting in increased strength.

A third form of exercise, termed *isokinetic exercise*, is possible when specific equipment is used. Isokinetic exercise equipment controls the speed of the patient's contractions and produces a variable resistance to the muscle as it contracts through its arc or ROM. Some equipment provides resistance to only the concentric contractions, whereas other equipment resists both concentric and eccentric contractions. Published studies indicate that isokinetic exercise strengthens muscle more efficiently than other forms of resistive isotonic exercise.

Refer to the information presented previously in this chapter to review the possible benefits and uses of passive and active exercise. Several criteria or factors must be considered when you are performing passive or active exercise to obtain the greatest benefit from the exercise and to protect the patient from injury.

Maintain the exercise activities within the physiologic capabilities of the patient, keep in mind the goals of therapy, and encourage the patient to perform at maximally tolerated levels. The Valsalva maneuver should be avoided during exercise to prevent the possibility of serious complications that could lead to a cerebrovascular accident or even death. Therefore instruct and remind the patient to breathe normally during the exercise program, particularly when performing resisted isometric exercise. Use caution to avoid causing unnecessary or excessive trauma to a skeletal or soft-tissue structure when resistance is applied and protect unstable or vulnerable structures (such as the site of a recent fracture, a hypermobile joint, a recent muscle strain, or a recent surgical site) during exercise. Finally, carefully evaluate the severity and monitor the effects of exercise for the patient who has experienced a recent myocardial infarction or has a history of cardiac dysfunction.

During exercise with a patient who has an unprotected healing fracture, avoid applying resistance to the distal segment of the fracture. Isometric and eccentric exercise may be contraindicated for those persons who are in the immediate or subacute phase of recovery from a myocardial infarction, especially if resistance is applied. Exercise that produces pain during or after exercise for a period of 24 to 36 hours may be contraindicated and this reaction should be considered a precaution for its future application. Exercise that produces abnormal results, such as an undesired or adverse change in the patient's symptoms or intensification of his or her condition, should be terminated and the program reevaluated before it is continued. Finally, certain exercise movements may be contraindicated after selected surgical procedures; an example is excessive hip movement, especially hip adduction, flexion beyond 90 degrees, and excessive external or internal rotation during the first several days after total hip replacement surgery (Box 6-4).

Box 6-4 Precautions Related to Active Exercise

Revision or cessation of an exercise program should be considered when:
Pain occurs during or persists after exercise.
Undesired cardiopulmonary stress occurs.
The breathing pattern of the patient becomes abnormal.
The patient exhibits an undesired, adverse response to exercise.
Stress occurs to an unstable area or segment.
Undesired movements or movement patterns occur.
Undesired tone of muscle develops or increases.
The patient's condition or functional ability regresses.

Types of Active Exercise

There are three common forms of active exercise: active assistive, active or active free, and active resistive. Before performing any form of exercise, introduce yourself, explain the activity, inform the patient of the desired outcome or purpose of the activity, obtain consent to participate in the program, and provide specific instructions. Once the exercise has been started the caregiver should observe the patient and correct improper performance or posture (Procedure 6-4).

PROCEDURE 6-4

Application of Active Exercise

Position the patient for support, stability, and type of active exercise to be performed; provide access to the area or segment to be exercised; and drape as necessary.

Explain the purpose and goals of the exercise, obtain consent for treatment, and select equipment if necessary.

Position the patient to promote the use of proper body mechanics by patient and caregiver.

Grasp the part to be treated to provide support, stability, control, or resistance as necessary, or orally instruct and guide the patient to perform the exercise. Refer to the photographs and instructions in this chapter for specific information.

The patient performs the exercises smoothly and slowly through the complete, unrestricted ROM with a pause at the start and end positions of the exercise.

The patient performs the predetermined number of repetitions and frequency of exercises based on predetermined abilities, needs, and goals.

At the conclusion of the treatment, the patient assumes or is assisted to assume proper alignment, support, and safety; drape or replace clothing for modesty and body temperature control.

Evaluate the patient's response to treatment; document important findings.

Isotonic Exercise Application

Active Assistive Exercise Active assistive exercise requires the patient to actively contract the muscles involved in the exercise to the maximum extent while receiving assistance from another source to perform the exercise. The assistance may be provided manually or by a mechanical or gravitational force. It is important the patient contract the muscles maximally during the exercise and the caregiver alters the assistance according to the patient's performance. The greatest amount of assistance should be provided when the patient has the greatest difficulty performing the activity. Conversely, assistance should be reduced when the patient has the least difficulty performing the activity. An eventual goal for most patients is to progress from active assistive to active exercise.

Assistance or resistance to motion can be affected by the patient's position and the relationship of the effects of gravity. The effect of gravity as a resistance force can be eliminated by the use of external assistance or patient positioning. For example, although the patient may not be able to perform full hip flexion when supine, the person may be able to perform the activity when assistance is provided manually or mechanically or when side lying and the lower extremity is supported on an elevated smooth surface. The resistance of gravity to the movement of hip flexion or extension or knee flexion or extension will be eliminated when the side-lying position is used. However, friction between the lower extremity and the surface will be created when the lower extremity is moved actively over the surface.

Before initiating the exercise, position the patient to provide stability and comfort. When you initiate the exercise, be certain to support, protect, stabilize, and control the segment being exercised, using the same hand placements described for passive exercise. Instruct the patient to actively contract the appropriate muscles through the available ROM and establish an appropriate exercise speed or rate. Your instructions may include touching, tapping, or stroking the muscle to be contracted; having the person initially perform the contraction with the opposite uninvolved muscle; demonstrating the contraction yourself; and using terms such as "bend," "lift," or "straighten." Provide assistance only to the extent necessary to allow the patient to smoothly complete the movement through the available ROM and to avoid substitute motions. The external assistance you provide can be decreased gradually as the patient demonstrates an increase in strength. The patient should progress to active free exercise when able to complete the desired movement smoothly through the available ROM without substitute motions and without assistance. The exercises may be performed in traditional anatomic planes or in the diagonal patterns described previously.

Active Free Exercise Active free exercise is performed by the patient without any assistance or resistance other than gravity and the weight of the extremity or segment involved in the exercise. The patient must have sufficient strength to perform the activity against the resistance provided by gravity. The position of the patient will affect the resistance provided by gravity. You can demonstrate to yourself how the effect of gravity is altered by attempting the same exercise while supine, sitting, standing, or prone. The more exercises you attempt and the more positions you use, the better you will be able to determine how to position a patient to obtain maximal effort while avoiding substitutive or undesired motions.

Before initiating the exercise, position the patient depending on how you desire gravity to affect the exercise and the movement to be performed. For example, do you desire gravity to resist, assist, or be neutral during the exercise? Instruct the patient to perform the desired movement through the available ROM smoothly and without any substitute motions (such as elevating the shoulders when performing shoulder flexion). If necessary, encourage or guide the patient as the activity is performed.

Establish an appropriate exercise speed to produce a smooth, controlled movement, and require that speed to be maintained. The patient should be encouraged to briefly pause (hold) at the end and start positions during each repetition. A brief rest between each bout or series of repetitions will usually be necessary to reduce the effects of fatigue (that is, two sets of 10 repetitions with a rest between the two sets).

The exercises may be performed in traditional anatomic planes or in the diagonal patterns described previously.

Active Resistive Exercise Active resistive exercise requires the addition of a resistive force other than gravity; this can be done manually or mechanically. The resistance should require the patient to use a maximal contraction to perform the activity, but the movement should be able to be completed slowly, smoothly, and through the entire available ROM. Gravity will have a resistive effect, as described previously, so the position of the patient should be considered. Furthermore, the length of the lever arm and the amount of torque the patient can develop will affect the location of the resistance. For example, greater resistance to the shoulder flexors will be required or need to be applied if the resistance is positioned above the elbow, whereas less resistance will be required if the resistance is located in the patient's hand. The shorter the lever arm, the greater the torque the patient can develop and the more the resistance the muscles will be able to overcome. The longer the lever arm the patient is required to use, the less force you will need to provide resistance. To illustrate this concept, apply resistance at various locations on a seated person's upper extremity as the person performs shoulder flexion with the elbow straight. Apply the resistance at the wrist, then at the elbow, and then at the proximal humerus, and sense the difference in the force you must develop to provide resistance as the other person performs shoulder flexion. This concept can be applied to other body segments. A goal for many patients is to progress from active free exercise to active resistive exercise, especially when a gain in muscle strength is desired.

When the patient performs an isotonic contraction, the maximal resistance able to be used is the resistance that can be overcome through the part of the range where the muscle has the weakest contractile capacity. Most muscles have the weakest contractile capacity at the beginning and the end of the ROM and most muscles tend to develop their greatest tension during the midportion of the range. (These last two statements are general statements and may not be accurate for all body positions or exercise activities. However, they do explain the general concept of the *length-tension curve* of a muscle.) Although the load (resistance) remains constant, the effect of the resistance on the muscle will vary at different points within the range as the muscle lengthens and shortens as a result of a change in the lever arm relationships of the body segments involved.

Before initiating the exercise, position the patient depending on how you desire gravity to affect the exercise, the movement required, and the amount or type of support or stabilization the patient requires. Instruct the patient to perform the desired movement through the available ROM smoothly and without any substitute motion as resistance is applied perpendicularly to the extremity or segment. You will need to determine the most appropriate site or location for the resistance to be applied based on the patient's condition, ability, exercise goals, and your awareness of the concept of lever arm length.

The body segment to which the proximal component or origin of the muscle being exercised is attached should be stabilized. The patient's body weight or position may accomplish this, or an external strap or firm surface may be required. It may be necessary to vary or adjust the resistance during the exercise to allow the patient to complete the available ROM smoothly and without substitute motions.

If manual resistance is used, the site of the application of the resistance and the amount of resistance applied can be revised during the exercise to provide maximal resistance while allowing the patient to complete the movement through the available ROM smoothly and without substitute motions. That is, the resistance lever arm can be lengthened or shortened, a new location can be used to avoid discomfort or to avoid an unstable area, or the applied resistance can be increased or decreased depending on the point in the range where the muscle is contracting.

The exercises may be performed in traditional anatomic planes or in the diagonal patterns described previously.

Isometric Exercise Application

Isometric Exercise Isometric exercise may be used when a muscle is immobilized, when a joint or soft tissue is painful when moved through its range, or when inflammation is present in the area. No observable joint motion should occur when an isometric muscle contraction is performed. Gravity has less effect on the muscle contraction when this type of exercise is used and the patient's position is not as important as it usually is for isometric exercise. The segment may be positioned at any point within the ROM depending on the patient's condition and the goal of the exercise. Manual or mechanical resistance can be applied or a patient can isometrically contract the muscles using a stationary object, such as a wall, because resistance and the length of the lever arm can be varied. The benefits of resisted isometric exercise and the reasons to select it have already been presented.

Muscle setting is a form of isometric exercise that can be beneficial to maintain some muscle tone; to maintain contractile awareness; and to allow exercise to an immobilized, innervated muscle. Before initiating the exercise, position the patient to provide a stable, comfortable position and have access to the muscle that will contract. Instruct the patient to contract or tighten (set) a specific muscle or muscle group without producing joint motion or changing the length of the muscle.

By describing the motion, you may assist the patient to use mental imaging to initiate the contraction. The use of tactile or verbal cueing to initiate the contraction by touching the muscle or telling the patient what movement the muscle will perform is another teaching method. For example, you can instruct a supine or prone patient to squeeze or pinch the buttocks together to set (contract) the gluteus maximus. If the patient squeezes the arms close to the side of the chest as if trying to hold a newspaper or small purse, the pectoral muscles will contract. When a patient has a full-length cast on one lower extremity, you can instruct the person to try to pull the kneecap of that extremity toward the hip by tightening the muscle on top of the thigh to isometrically contract the quadriceps. To facilitate this motion, have the patient perform it with the opposite, nonimmobilized quadriceps while you tactilely stroke upward on the quadriceps or gently push up on the patella. These are a few techniques that can be used to initiate an isometric contraction; you may need to consider other methods to teach a patient to contract the muscles isometrically.

Instruct the patient to maintain and hold the contraction for approximately 5 to 8 seconds and then relax. The person should be instructed to breathe normally to avoid the Valsalva phenomenon.

Isometric Resistive Exercise Isometric resistive exercise can be used to increase muscle strength through the addition of manual or mechanical resistance. The segment can be positioned at any point in the range depending on the patient's condition and the goal of the exercise. The amount of resistance and the length of the lever arm can be varied. It is particularly important to instruct the patient to breathe normally and to avoid the Valsalva phenomenon when performing isometric resistive exercise.

Before initiating the exercise, position the patient to provide stability, comfort, and access to the muscle that will contract. Determine where you desire to apply the resistance on the segment and position the segment within the available joint ROM. Be certain resistance is applied perpendicularly to the segment and instruct the patient to maintain and hold the position selected. Joint motion should not occur or be permitted. Instruct the patient to maintain the contraction for approximately 5 to 8 seconds while breathing normally and then to relax for 5 to 8 seconds before repeating the contraction. Additional information about the concept, use, and application of active exercise is contained in many of the references listed in the Bibliography.

SUMMARY

Exercise is used in the management of a variety of conditions or problems. There are several forms or types of exercise, including passive, active assistive, active, and active resistive. The caregiver must be knowledgeable and competent to be able to select the exercise type that will most benefit the patient.

There are three primary types of muscle contraction: (1) isotonic (which can be subdivided into concentric and eccentric), (2) isometric, and (3) isokinetic. Exercise can affect the person's strength, endurance, joint flexibility, coordination, and cardiopulmonary system.

Exercises can be performed with the patient positioned supine, sitting, prone, side-lying, or standing. The position selected should be based on the purpose of the exercise, the condition of the patient, the patient's ability to assume and maintain a specific position, and the equipment to be used.

The patient's response to exercise during and after each treatment session should be monitored and should include the observation of changes in the appearance of the segment exercised, evaluation of vital signs, and assessment of any changes in ROM or movement (coordination, strength, quality, or control), complaint, or indication of pain. You should provide specific support and stabilization to any unstable or pain-producing segments, such as a recent fracture site, areas of hypermobility or paralysis, or a wound or incision site. The extremity or segment should be moved through the entire unrestricted, pain-free, normal range of the associated joint or joints. Forceful movement into a restricted component of the range constitutes stretching and should be avoided when you are performing PROM exercise. A description of stretching techniques is beyond the scope of this textbook and has not been presented.

All exercises should be performed smoothly and slowly through the unrestricted range. A brief rest at the end and start position of the exercise should also be incorporated into the exercise.

The number of repetitions required to accomplish the goals of treatment will vary, just as the frequency of the exercises will vary. Some patients may benefit from or require the exercises to be performed two or more times per day for 10 or more repetitions. Other patients may benefit from or require one exercise session per day and fewer than 10 repetitions per joint or area. The patient's response to treatment, any change in the patient's condition, and the judgment of the caregiver are the factors used to determine the parameters of the exercise program.

You may apply the exercises using traditional anatomic planes, diagonal planes, or a combination of planes by using functional movement patterns or by combining two or more of these techniques. At the termination of the treatment, the patient should be repositioned with proper support, security, and alignment. Any equipment or assistive devices that were used should be stored and the treatment area prepared for other patients. Information about the patient's response to treatment or any change in condition should be documented.

self-study ACTIVITIES

- Describe some factors you would consider when determining the type of active exercise to select for a patient.
- How would you determine whether a patient had performed active exercise maximally?

- Describe how you would determine whether a patient performs active exercise properly.
- Describe the actions you would use to enhance proper active exercise motions.
- Explain what happens when you lengthen or shorten the lever arm used to apply manual resistance.
- List at least one body position you would use to place each of the following muscles in a maximal gravity-resisted position, in a maximal gravity-assisted position, and in a gravity-neutral position: middle deltoid, biceps, triceps, pectoralis major, upper trapezius, quadriceps, hamstrings, gluteus maximus, erector spinae, and abdominals.
- Explain how you would decide that a patient is ready to progress from passive to active exercise.
- What are some reasons or patient conditions for which you would perform passive exercise?
- Demonstrate the positions and motions you would use to perform concentric and eccentric contractions of the quadriceps, hamstrings, anterior deltoid, triceps, and abdominal muscles.

problem SOLVING

1. A 28-year-old patient with a C5 quadriplegia is being seen for exercises as an inpatient. What PROM exercises for this patient should be avoided and for what reason?
2. A 47-year-old patient with a left cerebral vascular accident is coming in for outpatient treatment. What possible substitute motions would you look for while performing active exercises to the right extremities?

CHAPTER 7

Transfer Activities

objectives After studying this chapter, the reader will be able to:

- Instruct and assist another person to perform various transfer techniques.
- Instruct one or more assistants to perform a safe lift transfer.
- Adjust the position of a person who is recumbent with or without the assistance of another person in preparation for the transfer.
- Teach a person independent bed mobility and functional activities preparatory to performing a transfer.
- Properly guard and protect a person during the performance of a transfer.

key terms

Dependent Requiring some level or type of assistance, which may be human or mechanical.
Exacerbation An increase in the severity of disease or any of its symptoms.
Graft Any tissue or organ for transplantation or implantation.
Hemiplegia Paralysis of one side of the body.
Ipsilateral Homolateral; on the same side.
Lateral Indicates a position away from the median plane or midline of a body or structure.
Medial Related or located toward the midline of a body or structure.
Mobility The ability to move in an environment with ease and without restriction.
Osteoporosis A decreased mass per unit volume of normally mineralized bone when compared with that in age- and sex-matched controls; loss of bone mass.
Paralysis Loss of power of voluntary movement in a muscle through injury or disease of its nerve supply.
Paresis Partial or incomplete paralysis.
Plinth A padded table for a patient to sit or lie on while performing exercises, receiving a massage, or undergoing other physical therapy treatment.
Safety belt An adjustable belt or strap that is secured around a person's waist and used to protect and control the person; also referred to as a guard, transfer, ambulation, or gait belt.
Syncope A temporary suspension of consciousness as a result of cerebral anemia; fainting.
Transfer The moving of a patient from one surface to another surface.
Vertigo A sensation of rotation or movement of one's self or of one's surroundings.

INTRODUCTION

A *transfer* is the safe movement of a person from one surface or location to another or from one position to another. Depending on the mental and physical ability of the patient, a transfer may be performed independently, with assistance (minimal, moderate, maximal, standby/supervision) or *dependently* (Box 7-1). When documenting information about the transfer, report the amount or type of assistance a patient requires to perform the transfer, the amount of time to complete it, the level of safety demonstrated, the level of consistency of the performance, and the equipment or devices used. Adjusting the patient's position or bed *mobility* activities are included in the broad definition of a transfer. The ability to move upward, downward, or from side to side; to roll; to turn over; and to move to sitting from a recumbent position are important activities for a patient to accomplish for independence. Often these movements are preliminary to the actual transfer from a bed or mat table to a wheelchair or to stand to use ambulation aids. They are also necessary to permit the patient to alter position for comfort and avoid the development of contractures or skin breakdown. The caregiver should not overlook teaching the

Box 7-1 Terminology for Transfer or Ambulation Assistance

Independent: Patient does not require any physical supervision or assistance from another person to consistently perform the activity safely and in an acceptable time. (*Note:* In some situations, specific equipment or devices may be used.)
Assisted: Patient requires assistance from another person to perform the activity safely in an acceptable time; oral or tactile cues, directions, or instructions may be used.
Minimal assistance: Patient performs 75% or more of the activity; assistance is required to complete the activity.
Moderate assistance: Patient performs 50% to 75% of the activity; assistance is required to complete the activity.
Maximal assistance: Patient performs 25% to 50% of the activity; assistance is required to complete the activity.
Standby (supervision) assistance: Patient requires verbal or tactile cues, directions or instructions from another person positioned close to, but not touching, the person to perform the activity safely and in an acceptable time. The assistant may provide protection should the patient's safety be threatened.
Dependent assistance: Patient requires total physical assistance from one or more persons to accomplish the activity safely and in an acceptable time; special equipment or devices may be used.
Guarding (close, contact): Patient requires guarding during the performance of the activity for safety; cues or directions may be used.
Close guarding: Caregiver is positioned close to, but not touching, the patient; similar to standby assistance; the likelihood the patient will require protection during the performance of the activity is minimal.
Contact guarding: Caregiver is positioned close to the patient with the hands on the patient or safety belt; it is very likely the patient will require protection during the performance of the activity.

patient to perform these movements and should emphasize their importance to the patient and the family. Preparatory activities may be needed, such as muscle strengthening, development of joint and muscle flexibility (range of motion), and development of endurance.

ORGANIZATION OF PATIENT TRANSFERS

A transfer requires planning and organization before the patient attempts to perform the transfer. The patient should be informed about the transfer and instructed how to assist with or perform it before attempting it. A demonstration of the activity by another patient or by the caregiver may assist the patient to learn how to perform the transfer. Careful attention to the safety precautions associated with each transfer will enhance the patient's confidence and lead to a more effective transfer.

Be certain to obtain and use sufficient assistance or equipment to ensure a safe procedure. When the patient is able to assist more fully with the procedure, the external assistance can be reduced or eliminated, leading to increased patient independence. Although patient independence is a frequent goal associated with transfer activities, your primary responsibility is to guard and protect the patient to avoid injury.

PREPARATION

You will have to prepare the patient, the environment, yourself, and possibly other persons before performing the transfer activity. Initially you should review the medical record and interview the patient for information to assist you in planning the activity. For example, what has the patient accomplished previously? How does the patient transfer now? What are the limitations and abilities? How much assistance is required to move in bed or to transfer? Are there specific precautions that must be used to protect the patient or to avoid further injury? Your assessment or evaluation of the patient will help to determine the person's abilities and limitations. Physical abilities that should be considered are muscle strength, joint and soft-tissue flexibility, sitting and standing balance, endurance, tolerance to sitting and standing positions, and motor control. Regarding the appropriate transfer or activity to be performed, a decision will have to be made based on your evaluation, the written information available, information from the patient, and the goals of treatment. As you mentally plan and organize the activity, you can consider whether mechanical or human assistance will be needed. Equipment such as a sliding board, a hydraulic or pneumatic lift, an electric hoist, a rope, a bed rail, and an over-the-bed frame or bar (trapeze) may be required to assist with a transfer. These devices can perpetuate dependence in a patient. Therefore they are recommended only for those patients who are unable to perform a safe transfer or when the caregiver is unable to safely assist the patient without using equipment. If equipment will be needed, obtain, position, and stabilize it and be certain it functions properly before beginning the transfer.

Introduce yourself to the patient and prepare for the transfer by explaining the activity and, in many instances, by demonstrating it. You should inform and instruct the patient about his or her role and how to assist with or perform the activity. The patient should be properly dressed for the transfer. Excessively loose clothing; excessively long trousers, slacks, or pajamas; and slippery, loose, or ill-fitting footwear should be avoided. A *safety belt* should be applied if the patient will move from one surface to another, especially during the early treatment sessions. Even though you may expect that the patient has consented to the proposed treatment, you should obtain consent after you have explained the activity and the possible risks, if any, associated with it.

PRINCIPLES

After these planning activities have been completed, you will have to apply certain concepts or principles to better ensure a safe and successful outcome. You must analyze the transfer into its component parts, such as the position of the equipment, operation of the equipment by the patient or caregiver, the position of the patient's body, and the movements the patient will have to perform. It may be necessary for the patient to practice and accomplish the component activities before the total transfer is attempted. After you have instructed the patient, ask the person to describe your instructions in his or her own words. Avoid asking the patient, "Do you understand the instructions?" Most patients will answer yes when asked such a question, even when they may not have comprehended everything you have explained. Instead, require them to explain the procedure to you to verify what they understand.

Once the transfer has begun, remain close to the patient to guard properly. Use the safety belt and the patient's knees, pelvis, or upper thorax for stabilization or control. Do not use the patient's upper extremity or clothing for guidance or stability because you will not be able to control the patient adequately and you may injure the extremity. Your instructions to the patient and to any persons who assist you should be brief, concise, and action oriented. You might instruct the patient like this: "First, lock your chair; now lift the footrests; move your hips forward; place your right foot closer to the chair and your left foot farther from the chair," and so on. Try to avoid: "Now the first thing I want you to do is . . ." Many patients will still be processing these nondirective words when you are beginning to state the actual instructions. Persons who are to assist must be informed of and understand their roles and must be instructed how to assist with the transfer. Instructions and guidance to the patient and to those who are assisting may be necessary as the transfer is performed. It may be possible to incorporate some patient teaching while the activity is performed. Encourage the patient to participate mentally and physically in the transfer maximally and within the limits of safety. The more the patient assists, the easier it will be to become independent. Present all instructions and directions slowly and allow time for the patient to process and apply them. Be certain to use proper body mechanics as you assist the patient for protection to control movements and to avoid self-injury.

PRECAUTIONS

There are several precautions you should consider when assisting a patient with a transfer, especially a standing transfer, regardless of the patient's condition. The patient should wear proper shoes to perform a standing transfer. Slippers, sandals, shoes with smooth leather soles, or socks without shoes are likely to decrease safety and should be avoided. A safety belt provides a secure object to grasp and decreases the need to use the patient's clothing. You should anticipate and be alert for unusual patient actions or equipment that may create unexpected risks. Any bandages or equipment attached to or used by the patient should be protected, including casts, drainage tubes, intravenous tubes, and dressing sites (Box 7-2).

Box 7-2 General Precautions During Transfers

Predetermine the patient's mental and physical capabilities to perform the transfer, including weight-bearing status.
The patient's clothing and footwear should be suitable for the transfer.
Mentally preplan the activities and sequence associated with the transfer.
Instruct the patient slowly and concisely; allow time to process and apply the information.
Select, position, and secure equipment before the transfer; put a safety belt on the patient.
Be alert for unusual events that may occur.
Do not guard the patient by using clothing or grasping the arm.
Position yourself to guard and protect the patient throughout the transfer.

You must determine the best position to use to protect the patient. To prevent injury to the patient as the result of a fall, it is usually best to be in front of and slightly to one side of the patient when he or she stands. Your body mechanics may be compromised when you are in this protective position, but it will enable you to provide maximal protection for the patient. At the conclusion of the transfer, you may protect the patient by applying a lap belt, engaging the bed rails, positioning the person in the center of the bed, or using other similar methods. Do not leave the patient unattended unless there is adequate support, stabilization, and protection to prevent injury.

Whenever a patient performs a transfer, it is important that the environment be free of unneeded equipment and other hazards and the area needed for the transfer is clearly visible to the caregivers and assistants. When transfers are performed in an area protected by curtains or drapes, you should know what is on the other side of the curtain when it is closed.

Precautions for Special Patient Conditions

When assisting patients with certain conditions to alter their positions in bed or on a mat or to transfer, special care and precautions must be used to avoid additional trauma or *exacerbation* of their condition. Examples of some of these patient conditions are shown in Box 7-3.

Box 7-3 Conditions Requiring Special Precautions During Transfers

1. **Total hip replacement, especially within the initial 2 weeks after surgery:** The surgically replaced hip should not be adducted or rotated, flexed more than 90 degrees, or extended beyond neutral flexion-extension. This means you must not cross the ankle of the surgically affected extremity over the opposite extremity, pull on the surgically affected extremity, or allow the patient to lie on the surgically replaced hip. You must maintain the surgical extremity in abduction when moving to and during side lying; require the patient to sit in a semi-reclining position; and require the patient to maintain the surgically affected extremity in abduction when moving from side to side.

   These precautions can also be used for the patient with a recent hip fracture or dislocation to decrease the possibility of dislocation or trauma to the fracture site.
2. **Low back trauma or discomfort:** These patients should avoid excessive lumbar rotation, trunk side bending, and trunk flexion. When turning, they may experience less discomfort if they "logroll" (that is, rolling the entire body simultaneously) rather than roll segmentally (that is, rolling the shoulders and upper trunk first, then the pelvis, and then the lower extremities). They may be more comfortable with the hips and knees partially flexed when they are in a supine or side-lying position.
3. **Spinal cord injury:** For the patient with a recent spinal cord injury, the injury site may be protected by some type of external appliance (such as a brace, a plaster or plastic body jacket, or a halo device), internal fixation (such as bone *graft*, metal rods, or wires), or a combination of the two methods. Distracting and rotational forces should be avoided, so you should not pull downward on the lower extremities and the person should be logrolled. Protective positioning or restraints will be required when this patient is in a side-lying position or sits without a back support. For the person with an injury that occurred several months or years earlier, you should be aware that osteoporosis, especially in the long bones of the lower extremities and the vertebral bodies, may be present. Even mild to moderate stress or strain to these bones may lead to a fracture. Some patients could experience a fracture when turning over or transferring from a wheelchair to the floor or to other objects. Caution should be used when you are transferring this patient from a supine to a sitting position because the blood pressure may not be stabilized.
4. **Burns:** The primary precaution is to avoid creating a shear force across the surface of the burn wound, graft site, or area from which the graft was taken. Sliding creates a shear force, which causes friction, which in turn disrupts the healing process. The patient should be instructed to elevate the body when moving to avoid the effect of shear forces.
5. **Hemiplegia:** Pulling on the involved or weakened extremities should not be used to control or move the patient. This is particularly important for the affected shoulder because the muscles will not provide adequate support to the joint because of the effects of paralysis. Many patients will experience pain or discomfort when they lie on or roll over the involved shoulder.

PROCEDURE 7-1

General Transfer Principles

Evaluate the patient to determine the mental and physical capacities to perform the transfer.
Select, position, and secure needed equipment; apply a safety belt on the patient.
Instruct the patient how to perform the transfer; demonstrate the transfer as necessary.
Practice components of the transfer as necessary before attempting the entire transfer.
Position yourself to guard and protect the patient throughout the transfer.
Request the patient initiate and perform the transfer; assist as necessary.
Guide and direct the patient throughout the transfer and guard closely.
At the conclusion of the transfer, position the patient for comfort, stability, and safety; document changes in the patient's ability or performance.

TYPES OF TRANSFERS

Transfers are designated by a variety of terms. Some transfers may be described according to the number of persons required to assist the patient (such as Plus 1, Plus 2); however, most descriptions indicate whether the patient requires assistance or can function independently. The designation of the transfer is important because it is part of the documentation to which other caregivers will refer. All persons involved with the care and management of the patient should use the same terminology when describing the transfer and there must be a consensus regarding the terminology that will be used by all caregivers (refer to Box 7-1). Once the transfer method or type has been selected, it is important for all caregivers to perform each transfer the same way with a particular patient to enhance learning and competence by the patient. If modifications are made to the transfer, each caregiver should be aware of them. The patient's family should observe the transfer and practice providing assistance while being guided by the appropriate caregiver before the patient's release (Procedure 7-1).

Standing, Dependent Pivot

The standing, dependent pivot requires at least one person to transfer the patient. The patient is elevated to a standing position, usually from a bed, *plinth*, toilet seat, or wheelchair, and pivoted so that the back is toward the object to which the person is lowered. You may be required to lift the patient to a standing position, to stabilize the knees and hips for the pivot, and to assist to sit.

Standing, Assisted Pivot

The caregiver provides assistance for the patient to stand, pivot, and transfer to another object such as a bed, wheelchair, plinth, or toilet seat. The patient must be able to provide minimal (up to 25%) to maximal (75% or more) physical effort during the transfer. Safety is often an issue with this transfer, so the caregiver must be alert at all times.

Standing, Standby Pivot

The standing, standby pivot requires the standby presence of another person. Patients using this transfer may be able to stand, pivot, and sit as they move from one object to another. The assistance required may vary from verbal cueing to close or casual guarding. Safety is still a concern with this type of transfer and you must be alert to provide protection when needed.

Standing, Independent Pivot

The patient is able to perform the entire transfer safely and consistently without any physical or verbal assistance from another person.

Sitting, Assisted Transfer

The patient is able to move from one surface to a second surface while in a sitting position with the assistance of at least one person. This transfer may require the use of a transfer or sliding board, an overhead bar or frame, overhead straps, or other equipment. These items are used to bridge the space between the two objects or to permit the patient to use the upper extremities for assistance. The patient may be able to physically assist with the transfer, but requires physical assistance, and he or she must be guarded and protected throughout the transfer.

Sitting, Independent Transfer

The patient is able to move safely and efficiently from one surface to a second surface while in a sitting position, without assistance from another person. It still may be necessary for the patient to use a transfer or sliding board, an overhead bar or frame, overhead straps, or other equipment.

Sitting, Dependent Lift

One, two, or three persons may be required to lift the patient and move the person from one surface to a second surface. A mechanical lift may be used instead of multiple persons. If a mechanical lift is used, only one caregiver is usually needed to perform the transfer. This transfer is used when the patient is totally unable to physically assist with the transfer and other persons or equipment are required.

Recumbent, Dependent Lift

The recumbent, dependent transfer is used when the patient is physically unable to assist with the transfer and is unable to be placed in a sitting position. One, two, or three persons or special equipment are required to lift and move the patient from one surface to a second surface. The equipment may be a mechanical lift, mechanical transfer stretcher, mattress pad, bed liner (such as a draw sheet), or plastic transfer board.

PRINCIPLES OF MOBILITY ACTIVITIES FOR A BED OR MAT

Mobility activities are used to adjust the recumbent patient's body position. They may be performed independently by the patient, with assistance from another person, or by use of various types of equipment. The most common movements are turning from a supine to a side-lying position and returning; from a supine to a prone position and returning; moving upward, downward, or from side to side and returning to the center; and moving from a lying to a sitting position and returning. The equipment may include bed rails; an overhead bar or frame; loops attached to the bed, mat, or mattress; or linen items such as a draw sheet.

These activities should be taught to a patient to improve independence and assist in preventing the development of skin problems or contractures as a result of lying in one position too long. The patient must become independent in all phases of bed or mat mobility to become independent in sitting or standing transfers. Remember to use proper body mechanics as you assist and guard the patient to provide safety.

The patient should mentally and physically participate in these activities even when being assisted. You can begin to initiate patient involvement by asking the patient to control the head, position the upper or lower extremities, or use the upper and lower extremities to help with the activity within the functional capacity. The patient should perform these assistive movements to promote independent movement as the condition improves. You and the patient may need to problem solve together to determine the most effective way to use the person's abilities to lead to independent movement and decrease the amount of assistance required.

To perform mobility activities with greater ease, you should attempt to reduce friction between the patient's body and the surface of the bed or mat, centralize the weight of the patient, reduce the effects of gravity, and use gravity as an assistive force. Each of these techniques will reduce the patient's and your energy expenditure and will enhance the patient's ability to move. There are many "tricks of the trade" that you can discover and apply by using your problem-solving skills and ability; some are presented later in this chapter.

Knowledge of many of the basic principles of physics and body mechanics will assist you in developing innovative and safe methods to adjust a patient's position or to perform a transfer. Role playing with a friend, classmate, or coworker and simulating specific patient conditions or limitations are excellent methods to start the problem-solving process. The better you mimic a patient's condition, the better you will be able to devise techniques to alter your position on the bed or mat.

Techniques of Dependent or Assisted Mobility Activities

To move a supine or prone patient, you should move individual body segments to reduce the effort required and to provide greater control. Begin by positioning yourself close to the side of the patient or the bed or mat table. This will allow you to use your upper extremities with short lever arms to reduce strain and increase the mechanical advantage of your muscles. By kneeling on the mat or flexing your hips and knees as you treat the patient who is in bed, you will minimize strain to your back. If it is possible to adjust the height of the bed, position it at the most comfortable and most beneficial level for you to function. Remember to apply the principles of body mechanics to reduce stress and strain to your muscles, joints, and ligaments.

Be certain to explain the activity to the patient and encourage the person to assist with each of the movements. You should continue to guide and encourage the patient throughout the activity to promote motivation and independence.

Side-to-Side Movement, Patient Supine Position one forearm under the patient's neck or upper back and one forearm under the middle of the back and gently slide the upper body and head toward you (Fig. 7-1). Do not lift the upper body, slide it on your forearms, or use a draw sheet to move the patient. It may be necessary to support the patient's head with your upper arm as you move the person. Next, position your forearms under the patient's lower trunk and just distal to the pelvis and gently slide that body segment toward you. Finally, position your forearms under the thighs and legs and

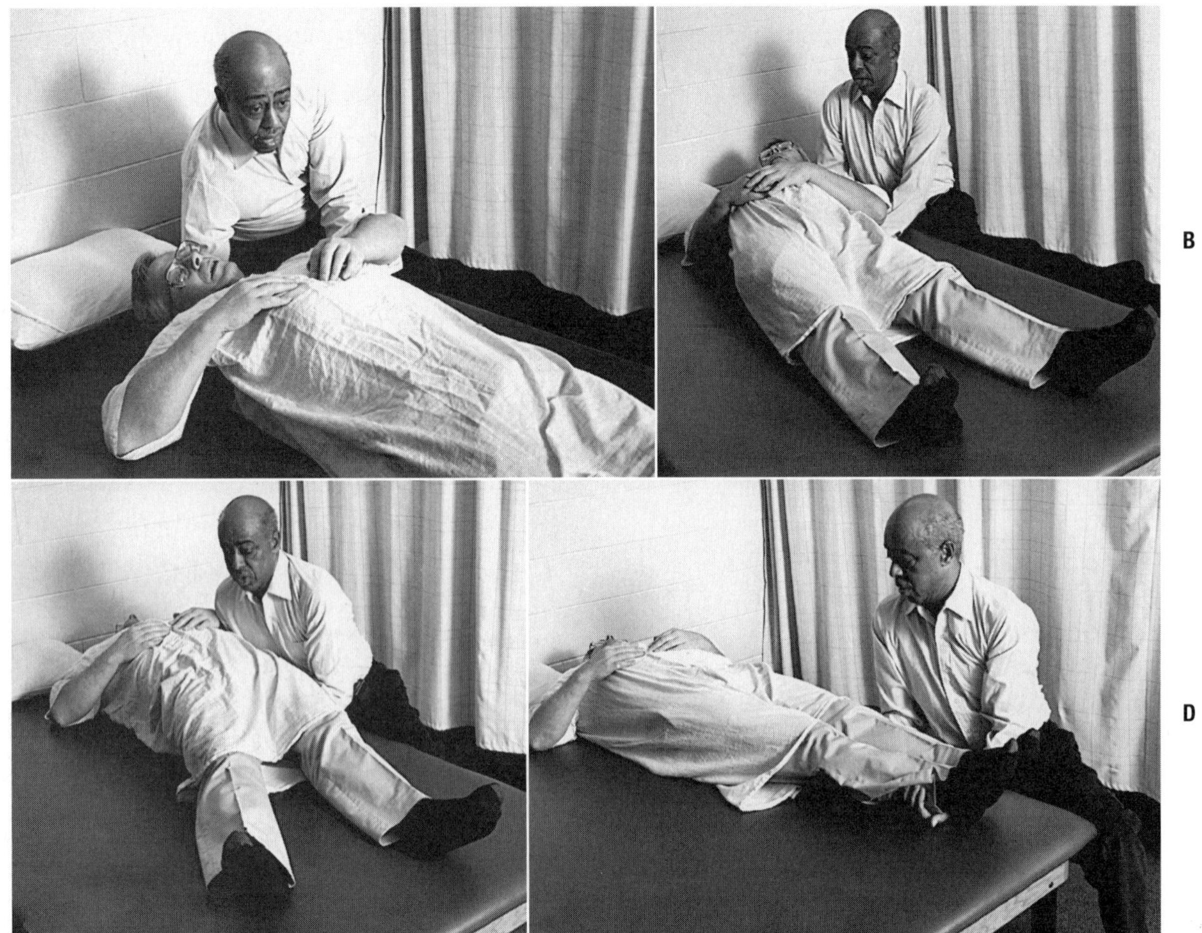

Fig. 7-1 Moving a supine patient sideward.

gently slide them toward you. When you slide rather than lift the patient toward you, the amount of energy required and the stress to your upper extremity and back muscles will be reduced. The force you use to pull and slide the patient should be applied parallel to the surface of the bed or mat to further reduce the energy required. Remember to lower your trunk by flexing your hips and knees or raise the bed before moving the patient. This will position your center of gravity (COG) as close to the patient's COG as possible. Position your feet to widen your base of support (BOS) by placing one foot in front of the other. These actions allow you to control the patient better, to reduce stress and strain to your arms and back, and to reduce the energy required to move the patient. When it is necessary to move the patient sideward over a large distance, it will be easier if each body segment is moved several times. Moving the patient closer to one side of the bed or mat is important before you perform exercise or a transfer. Having the patient close to you allows you to take advantage of the use of proper body mechanics.

Upward Movement, Patient Supine Before attempting to move the patient upward, bring the person closer to the near edge of the bed or mat, especially if the patient is lying in the center of the bed or mat. If the patient is on an adjustable bed, be certain the portion that raises the head and trunk is flat; remove any pillows from under the head and shoulders. This position will allow you to use the muscles of your upper extremities more effectively by using short lever arms. Short lever arms can develop greater force than long lever arms, with less energy expenditure and better patient control.

To initiate the move, flex the patient's hips and knees so the feet rest flat on the bed or mat. This will reduce friction between the extremities and the bed or mat surface and will position the patient so the person can assist by lifting the pelvis or pushing with the extremities. It may be necessary to support the thighs with one or more pillows if the patient is unable to maintain the position. You should face toward the patient's head and stand approximately opposite the patient's midchest level with the foot that is farthest from the bed in front of your other foot (that is, in stride in an anteroposterior position). Support the patient's head and upper trunk with your arms and lift until the inferior angles of the scapulae clear the bed or mat; your chest should be close to the patient's chest so that you will use short lever arms with your arms. This position will reduce the friction of the patient's trunk on the bed or mat, but should not place excessive strain or stress on the structures of your back. If you are unable to lift the patient's trunk or if the lift creates excessive strain or stress to your back, it may be necessary to ask another person for assistance using a draw sheet (Fig. 7-2).

Slide the lower trunk and pelvis upward approximately 6 to 10 inches; do not attempt to move the patient over a long distance unless the patient is able to assist. To move the patient farther, reposition yourself and the patient's lower extremities and repeat the process. Some patients may be able to grasp your trunk to help elevate their trunk. However, this may increase stress or strain to your back and you must determine whether it is a safe technique. If an over-the-bed frame, bar, or trapeze is available, the patient can grasp it and elevate the upper body. After you have moved the patient upward to the final position, reposition the person in the center of the bed or mat to reduce the possibility of rolling off the bed or mat.

Downward Movement, Patient Supine Initially, move the patient closer to the near edge of the bed or mat and partially flex the hips and knees. If necessary, use a pillow to support the thighs. Position yourself approximately opposite to the patient's waist or hips or at the patient's feet (Fig. 7-3). Cradle and lift the pelvis slightly before you slide the patient's upper body and head downward. Move the patient approximately 6 to 10 inches and then reposition yourself and the patient's lower extremities if further movement is required. Reposition the patient in the center of the bed or mat.

Note: Movement of a recumbent patient upward, downward, or sideward can be accomplished more easily if a small sheet or linen pad is placed beneath the patient. This item is frequently called a draw sheet or pad; it usually extends from the upper back to the buttocks or midthigh area. Two persons, one on each side of the bed or mat, grasp the sheet or pad and, on command by the leader, simultaneously move the patient by sliding. Some lifting may be required, but the primary force used is sliding (Fig. 7-4). The patient should be encouraged to assist by using the upper or lower extremities to partially elevate the trunk or pelvis. When the patient is moved upward or sideward, the upper portion of the bed should be lowered; when moved downward, the upper portion of the bed can be raised.

Note: A commercially available fabric tube sheet, which creates a low coefficient of friction between it and the surface on which the patient lies, can be used instead of a draw sheet to reduce the effort necessary to move the patient.

Move to a Side-Lying Position, Patient Supine To have sufficient space on the bed or mat, it may be necessary

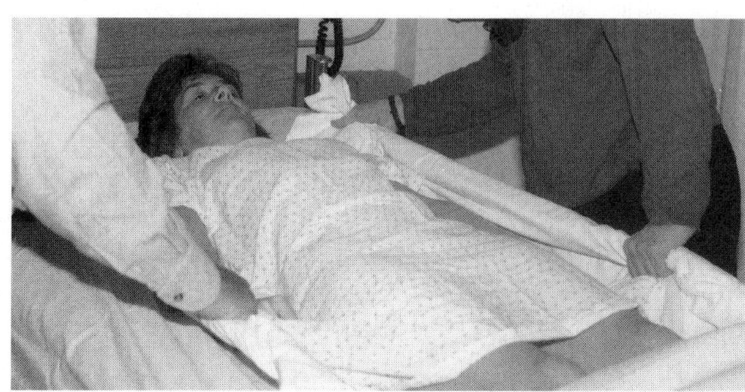

Fig. 7-2 Moving a supine patient upward using a draw sheet.

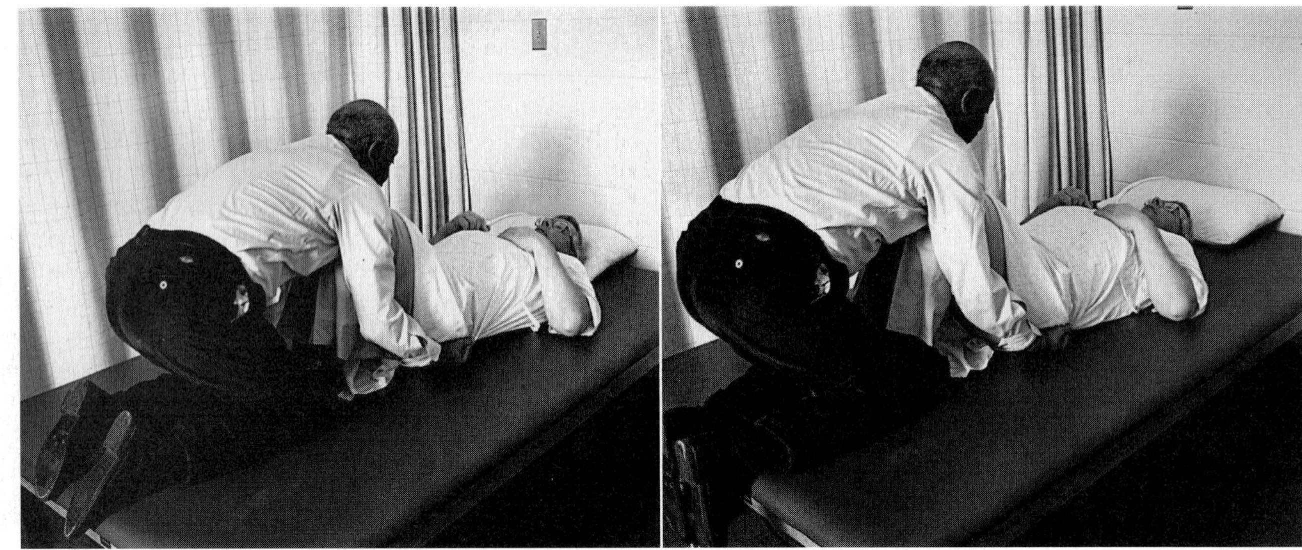

Fig. 7-3 Moving a supine patient downward.

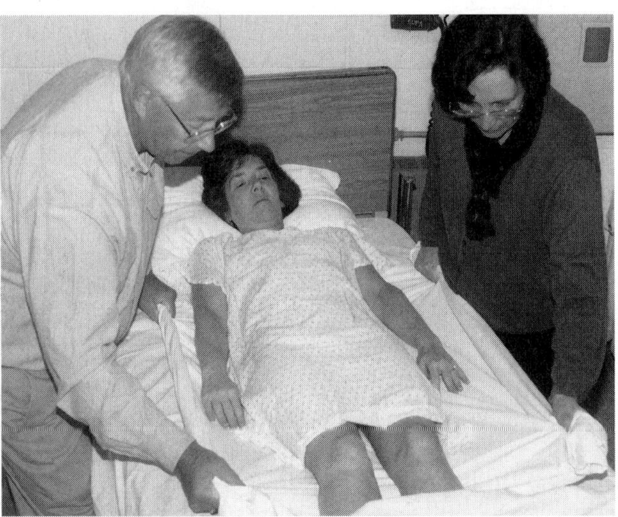
Fig. 7-4 Moving a patient downward using a draw sheet

to initially position the patient close to the far edge of the bed or mat. This is a potentially dangerous position and you, another person, a bed rail, or a wall must protect the patient from rolling off the bed or mat. Be certain the bed wheels are locked or blocked to prevent the bed from moving.

Stand facing the patient so you can roll (or turn) the person toward you to a side-lying position. When it is absolutely necessary to roll the patient away from you, be certain there is protection from rolling off the bed or mat table (that is, elevate the bed rail, block the edge with pillows, position another person at the opposite side of the bed). If you plan to roll the patient toward the right extremities, place the left lower extremity over the right lower extremity, place the left upper extremity on the chest, and place the right upper extremity in straight abduction. Roll the patient toward you by pulling gently on the left posterior scapula (shoulder) and the left posterior pelvis. Do not use the upper or lower extremity to initiate the roll because you will not be able to properly control or initiate movement of the trunk and the extremity may be injured. When the patient is in a side-lying position, flex the hips and knees and place a pillow under the head, between the knees and ankles, and along the front and back of the trunk. The downmost upper and lower extremities should be positioned for comfort. Refer to the description of the side-lying position in Chapter 5 for more complete information about this position. If the patient is to remain in this position unattended, it may be necessary to apply trunk restraints or engage the bed rails. *Caution:* Be careful when readjusting the patient's position when side lying. This is an unstable position and the patient can easily roll forward or backward. Inform the patient when you move from one side of the bed or mat to the other side. It is recommended that you maintain manual contact with the patient as you move. You should roll the patient toward you and guard the edge of the bed or mat to prevent the person from rolling too far. This will require you to stand close to the side of the bed or mat toward which you roll the patient, with at least one thigh against the edge of the bed or mat. These precautions must be followed when you are moving the patient from a supine to a prone position or from a prone to a supine position to protect and maintain control.

Move to a Prone Position, Patient Supine Move the patient closer to one side of the bed or mat and prepare to roll him or her to a side-lying position as described previously, with one modification. The arm over which the patient will roll should be positioned either close along the side with the shoulder externally rotated, elbow straight, palm up, and the hand tucked under the pelvis; or with the

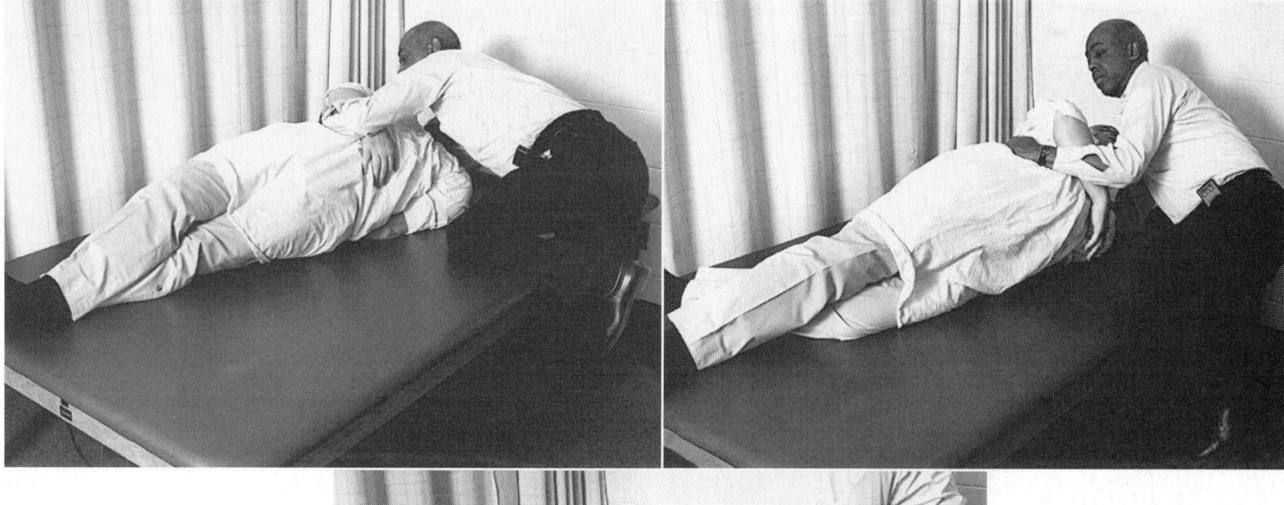

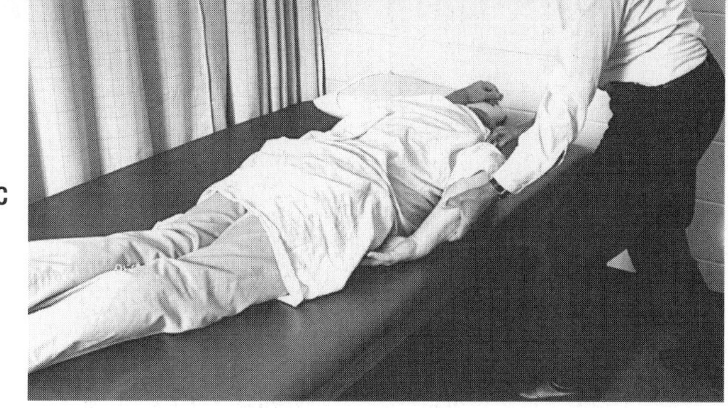

Fig. 7-5 Moving a supine patient to a prone position.

shoulder flexed so that the arm rests next to the ear with the elbow straight. The other upper extremity remains by the side (Fig. 7-5).

Stand facing the patient and roll the person to a side-lying position. Determine whether there is sufficient space to allow the roll to a prone position to be completed. If the space is insufficient, move the patient backward, while side lying, until there is sufficient space to complete the roll to prone. *Caution:* The patient is very insecure while in a side-lying position, so you must guard closely.

With the bed wheels locked, roll the patient toward you, and protect the near edge of the bed or mat by placing one of your thighs against it. This will prevent the patient from rolling off the bed or mat.

Move to a Supine Position, Patient Prone Move the patient close to one edge of the bed or mat. If the person is going to roll toward the right side, cross the left leg over the right leg. Position the right upper extremity close to the side with the elbow straight, palm up, and hand tucked under the pelvis, or the right shoulder can be flexed and the arm positioned close to the patient's ear; place the other upper extremity next to the side. Stand on the far side of the table and roll the patient toward you to a side-lying position. Determine whether there is sufficient space to allow the roll to a supine position to be completed. If the space is insufficient, move the patient forward, while side lying, until there is sufficient space to complete the roll to a supine position.

Guide the patient from a side-lying to a supine position by resisting against the posterior left shoulder and pelvis to retard the movement to a supine position. Reposition the person in the center of the bed or mat.

With the bed wheels locked, roll the patient toward you and, to protect the near edge of the bed or mat, place one of your thighs against it.

Move to a Sitting Position, Patient Supine Move the patient close to one edge of the bed or mat, and roll to a side-lying position with the lower extremities partially flexed. Elevate the trunk by lifting under the shoulders or by instructing the patient to push up using either or both upper extremities (Fig. 7-6).

Pivot the lower extremities over the side of the bed or mat as the trunk is raised. Do not allow the patient to sit unattended or unsupported.

This method is recommended for the patient who has a lower back condition that might be aggravated by trunk

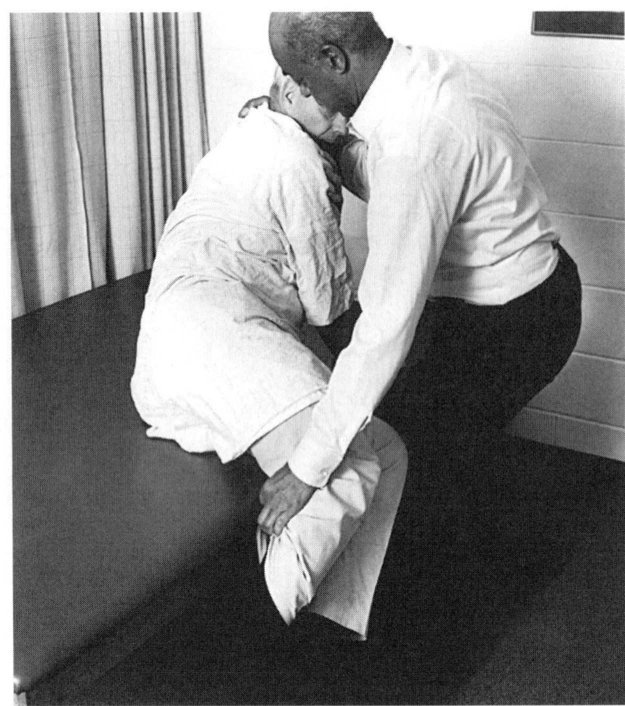

Fig. 7-6 Assisting a supine patient to a sitting position.

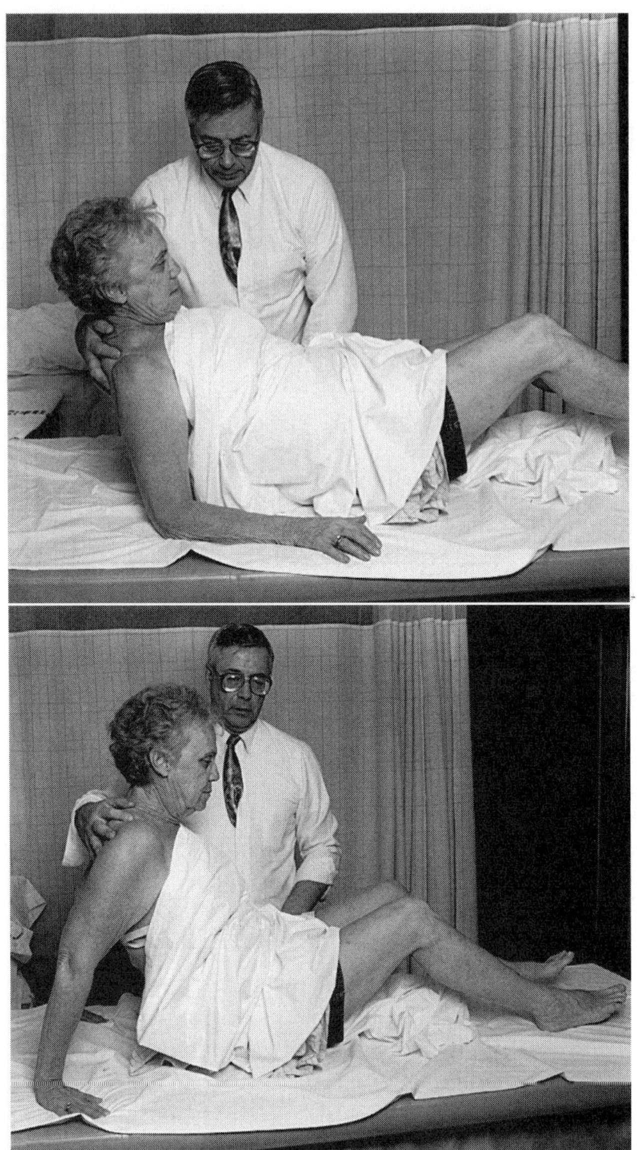

Fig. 7-7 Alternative method. Assisting a supine patient to a sitting position.

flexion or for the patient who has functional use of only one upper and lower extremity. This method concentrates the patient's body weight closer to the COG, which will make it easier for you to lift the trunk. Position your feet in an anteroposterior position to widen your BOS and to avoid twisting your back as you lift the patient.

Alternative Method Move the patient close to one edge of the bed or mat and flex the hips and knees with the feet flat on the bed or mat (Fig. 7-7). Fold the arms across the chest unless they will be used to elevate the trunk by using an over-the-bed frame, bar, or trapeze. Place one or both of your arms under the patient's upper back and head or have the patient pull or push with the upper extremities to elevate the trunk until a sitting position is attained.

Pivot the patient by supporting under the thighs and behind the back to a short sitting or dangling position. *Caution:* Do not allow the patient to sit unattended or without support, even briefly. Some patients may experience *vertigo* or *syncope* (that is, become faint) when they are moved quickly from a supine to a sitting position. Other patients may lack sufficient strength or balance to remain sitting without some form of support.

Move to Supine Position, Patient Sitting Reverse the sequence of activities described in the preceding section to move from a supine to a sitting position. Reposition the patient in the center of the bed or mat when supine.

Independent Mobility Activities

Each patient should be taught and encouraged to independently perform or assist with all bed or mat mobility activities within his or her abilities. Initially, these activities can be used while dependent or assisted bed or mat mobility activities are practiced. Instruct and guide the patient in the activities to be performed. Assistive equipment such as bed rails or overhead bars should not be used unless the patient is unable to safely perform the activity without equipment. *Remember:* These activities are necessary for the patient to be able to perform transfers and avoid soft-tissue pressure and the development of contractures as a result of prolonged immobilization.

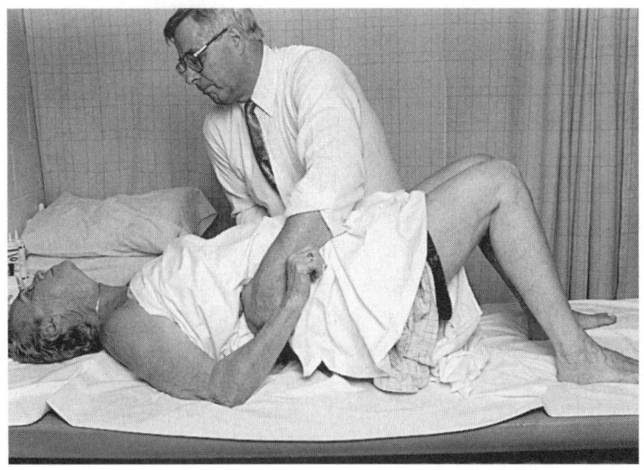

Fig. 7-8 Assisting a supine patient to move upward.

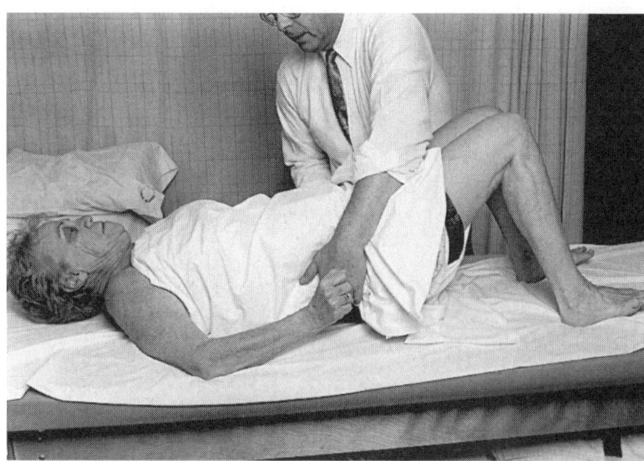

Fig. 7-9 Assisting a supine patient to move downward.

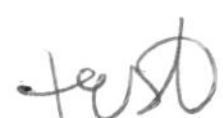

Side-to-Side Movement, Patient Supine Instruct the patient to flex the hips and knees and place the feet flat on the bed or mat, position one upper extremity next to the trunk, and abduct the other upper extremity approximately 4 inches from the trunk.

Instruct the patient to push down with the lower extremities to lift the pelvis and move it toward the abducted upper extremity and elevate the upper trunk by pushing into the mat with the elbows and the back of the head to move toward the abducted elbow. Then reposition the lower and upper extremities to move again or for comfort.

An alternative method for some patients is to elevate the pelvis and upper trunk by simultaneously pushing down with the legs and the back of the head and shift the body toward the abducted upper extremity. The patient should be taught to move to the left and to the right.

Upward Movement, Patient Supine Instruct the patient to fully flex the hips and knees, position the feet flat on the bed or mat with the heels close to the buttocks, and position the upper extremities with the elbows flexed, next to the trunk with the shoulders (scapulae) pulled up toward the ears (Fig. 7-8).

The patient elevates the pelvis using the lower extremities and elevates the upper trunk by simultaneously pushing into the bed or mat with the elbows and the back of the head, then moves upward by pushing with the lower extremities and depressing the shoulders (scapulae). The person then repositions the lower and upper extremities for successive movements. If the bed is adjustable, the upper portion should be flat and the wheels should be locked.

Downward Movement, Patient Supine Instruct the patient to partially flex the hips and knees to position the feet flat on the bed or mat; the heels should be 8 to 12 inches distal to the buttocks. The upper extremities should be positioned next to the trunk with the elbows flexed and the shoulders (scapulae) depressed (Fig. 7-9). If the bed is adjustable, the upper portion should be elevated slightly and the wheels should be locked.

The patient elevates the pelvis using the lower extremities and elevates the upper trunk by simultaneously pushing into the bed or mat with the elbows and the back of the head; moves downward by pulling with the lower extremities, simultaneously pushing up with the shoulders (scapulae) and pulling downward with the elbows or forearms. The lower and upper extremities are repositioned for successive movements.

Move to a Side-Lying Position, Patient Supine Instruct the patient to move to the far side of the bed or mat. To roll toward the right, the person simultaneously reaches across the chest with the left upper extremity and lifts the left lower extremity diagonally over the right lower extremity; then uses head flexion and the abdominal muscles to roll onto the side or uses the left hand to grasp the edge of the mattress, draw sheet, or bed rail to pull to aside-lying position.

Instruct the patient to maintain the side-lying position by using the left hand on the bed or mat and by flexing the lower extremities. A pillow will be needed for the head.

To roll to the left, the patient performs the same process with the opposite extremities.

Alternative Method Instruct the patient to move to the far side of the bed or mat. To roll to the right, the person pushes with the left upper extremity and the left lower extremity before reaching across the body. Some patients may prefer to reach with their upper extremity and push with their lower extremity to initiate the roll. To roll to the left, the patient performs the same process with the opposite extremities.

Caution: You must inform the patient about the relative insecurity of the side-lying position. Be certain you instruct

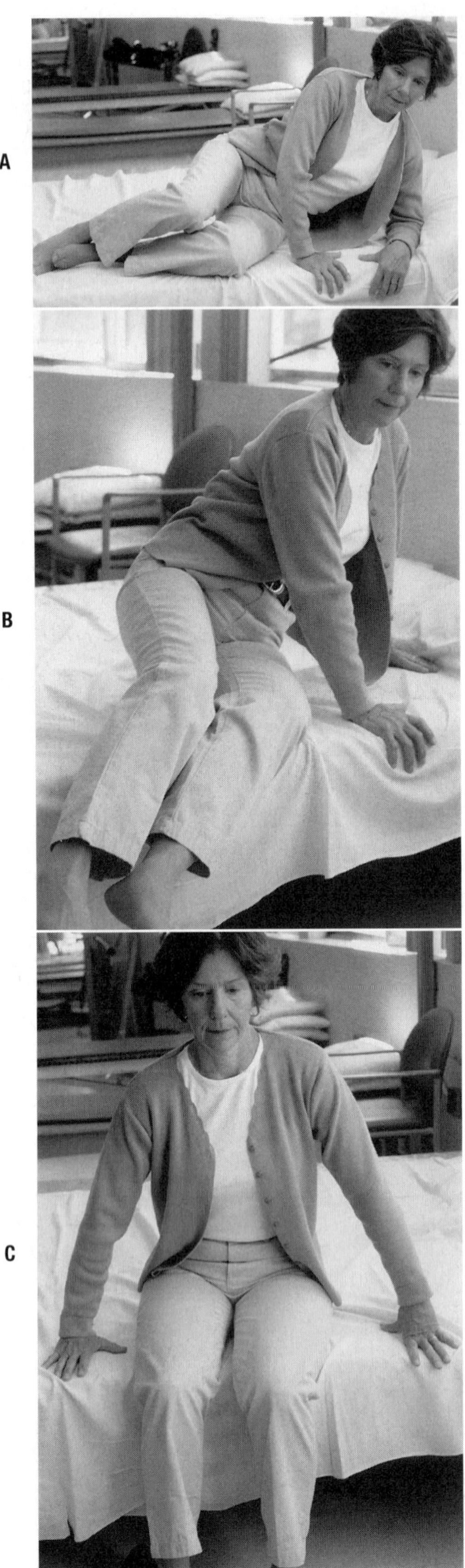
Fig. 7-10 Independent movement rising from supine.

the patient to flex the hips and knees and to place the uppermost hand in front of the chest on the bed or mat to increase stability. In addition, you may need to teach the patient to reposition the body in the center of the bed or mat to provide as much bed area in front and behind the body.

Move to a Prone Position, Patient Supine Instruct the patient to move to one side of the bed or mat. To roll to the right, the person positions the right upper extremity under the right side of the body or flexes the shoulder so it is positioned next to the right ear and then moves to a side-lying position. If the space is insufficient to roll to prone, the person repositions the body away from the near edge of the bed or mat. As the patient rolls to prone, the left upper extremity is used for protection and then adjusts the position as desired for comfort.

Move to a Supine Position, Patient Prone Instruct the patient to move to one side of the bed or mat. To roll to the right, the person positions the right upper extremity under the right side or flexes the right shoulder so that it is positioned next to the right ear. The left hand is placed flat on the bed or mat near the anterior left shoulder; the left hip and knee can be partially flexed or extended.

The patient pushes with the left upper extremity, lifts the left lower extremity over the right lower extremity, and moves to a side-lying position. If space on the bed or mat is insufficient to roll to a supine position, the person repositions the body away from the near edge of the bed or mat and then rolls to a supine position and adjusts the position as desired for comfort.

Caution: You must instruct the patient to determine his or her position on the bed or mat before any rolling activities are attempted. Depending on the width of the bed or mat, it may be necessary for the patient to adjust the position by moving forward or backward while in a side-lying position.

Move to a Sitting Position, Patient Supine Instruct the patient to move toward one edge of the bed or mat, but leave sufficient space to roll to a side-lying position. The person rolls to a side-lying position and flexes the hips and knees to maintain the side-lying position briefly, then positions the hand of the uppermost upper extremity on the bed or mat opposite to the midchest level (Fig. 7-10, *A*).

The patient pushes with the upper extremity to raise the trunk and maintains this position by resting on the elbow and forearm of the lowermost upper extremity; then elevates the trunk fully by pushing with both upper extremities to a side-sitting position (Fig. 7-10, *B*). The lower extremities can be pivoted simultaneously over the edge of the bed or mat in preparation for standing (Fig. 7-10, *C*). This technique is beneficial for the patient with low back dysfunction or pain because less stress is directed to the lumbar spine through the avoidance of rotation and flexion. The patient can return to a supine position by performing the movements in reverse sequence. Occasionally a patient with low back dysfunction

PROCEDURE 7-2

Protective Transfer to and from the Floor for a Person With Low Back Dysfunction

The patient should be encouraged to use a firm, stable object for support and to reduce stress to the back as these activities are performed.

MOVEMENT TO THE FLOOR

The patient places one hand on a firm object and moves to a single knee (half-kneeling) position, keeping the trunk erect.

The person kneels on both knees (high kneeling); then moves to all fours (hands and knees).

The patient moves the hands forward until prone or gently side sits, if not painful, then lowers onto one elbow to a side-lying position.

The patient can adjust the body position as desired.

FROM THE FLOOR TO STANDING

The patient starts from a prone position and pushes to a hands-and-knees position, or logrolls to side lying.

If on all fours, the person pushes to a high kneeling position; then moves to a half-kneeling position; then to standing; a firm object may be used for assistance.

If side lying, the person pushes to side sitting; then moves to a hands and knees position; then performs the movements listed in the previous step.

may desire to move to the floor and return to standing. Procedure 7-2 presents techniques designed to accomplish the movements safely and with reduced stress and discomfort.

Alternative Method Instruct the patient to move to the near edge of the bed or mat. If the bed is adjustable, raise the upper portion to approximately 45 degrees. Start with the hips and knees flexed and the feet flat on the bed or mat; the upper extremities are slightly abducted, with the shoulders internally rotated and the forearms resting on the bed or mat (Fig. 7-11, *A*).

The patient lifts the head and pushes with the upper extremities to elevate the trunk using a tripod support, with the hands placed on the bed or mat behind the hips with the elbows extended. By alternately moving the hands forward, the patient attains a sitting position (Fig. 7-11, *B*). The person can pivot the lower extremities over the edge of the bed or mat in preparation for standing (Fig. 7-11, *C*).

It may be necessary to alter or modify these activities for the patient who has reduced strength or reduced function of one or more of the extremities. For example, the *paralysis* or *paresis* of the *ipsilateral* upper and lower extremity that results from a cerebrovascular accident (that is, stroke) will require the patient to use the remaining functional extremities to adjust position and to be mobile in bed or on a mat. The patient who has limited function as a result of joint

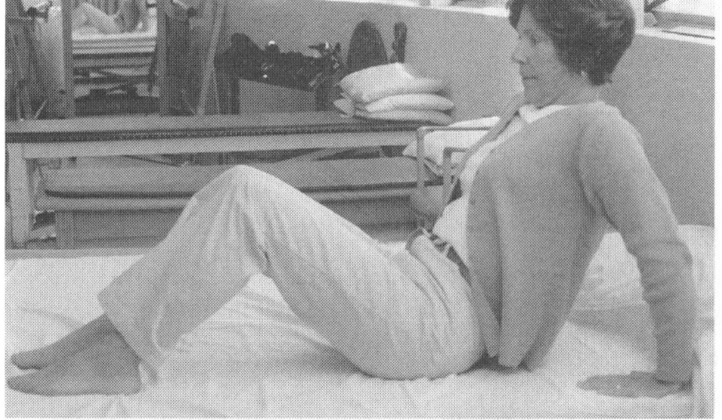

A

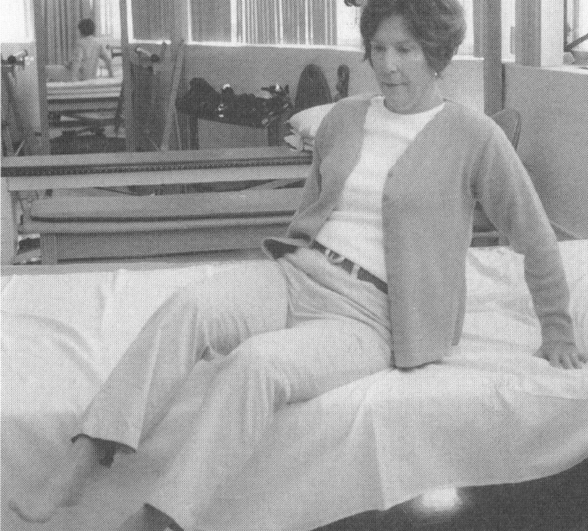

B

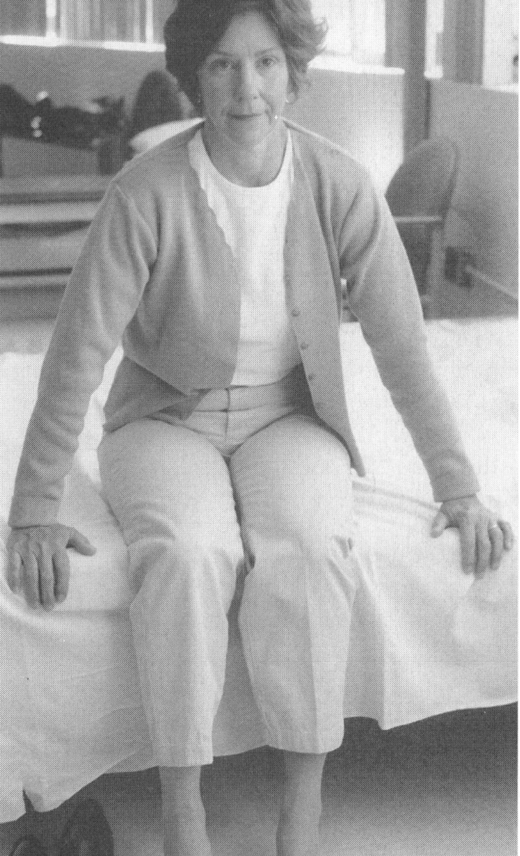

C

Fig. 7-11 Alternative method. Independent rising to sitting from supine.

disease or trauma will need to rely on the noninvolved or least involved joints to adjust position. Finally, the patient with paralysis of the lower extremities and lower trunk (that is, a paraplegic) or with paralysis of all four extremities and trunk (that is, a quadriplegic) will require a longer period of training and practice to learn how to safely and efficiently adjust position. The quadriplegic patient may require aids such as loops attached to the mattress or to an overhead bed frame, bed rails, an overhead trapeze, or loops of cloth sewn to clothing to assist to alter position. The techniques or procedures that must be learned and practiced by the patient with multiple or severe paralyzing injuries are beyond the scope of this text. Refer to the Bibliography for sources of information about these types of patient conditions.

STANDING, SITTING, LIFTING TRANSFERS

Movement to or from a Wheelchair to a Bed, Mat, Floor, or Low Plinth

Standing Transfer, Dependent Pivot A safety belt should be applied before you attempt any sitting or standing transfer, particularly during the early treatment sessions. The patient should be instructed in the procedures required to maneuver, position, and operate the wheelchair and its components. These procedures are described in Chapter 8.

Position the wheelchair parallel or at a 45- to 60-degree angle to the bed midway between the head and foot of the bed, mat, or plinth (Fig. 7-12, *A*). Apply a safety belt and lock the wheelchair with the caster wheels positioned forward to increase the BOS of the wheelchair. *Note:* The caster wheels may pivot or turn to one side when the patient performs the transfer. That movement does not cause a safety problem and the patient can continue to perform the transfer. However, the caster wheels should not be permitted to be directed backward because that position reduces the stability of the chair, particularly when the patient moves to the front portion of the seat. Remove the patient's feet from the footrests and elevate the footrests; remove or swing away the front rigging and place the patient's feet flat on the floor. Remove the armrest nearest to the bed, mat, or low plinth if the top surface of the bed, mat, or low plinth is lower than the armrest. Move the patient forward in the chair by grasping the posterior area of the pelvis and pulling on it so that the buttocks slide forward (Fig. 7-12, *B*), position the feet parallel to each other, and position the trunk over the pelvis. A patient can be taught to move the hips forward by using the upper trunk to push back against the upper portion of the seatback and sliding the pelvis forward. The trunk will need to be repositioned over the pelvis before you begin the transfer. Partially stoop and position your knees and feet outside and touching the patient's knees and feet. If able, the person can hold your middle or upper back with the upper extremities. *Caution:* Do not allow the patient to hold around your neck. You must use proper body mechanics to prevent undue strain to your back.

Grasp the safety belt at the sides of the patient's waist and inform the person when and how the move to standing is performed. If necessary, you may rock the patient to develop momentum before standing (Fig. 7-12, *C*).

Instruct the patient using terms such as "Ready, stand" or "One, two, three, stand." Instruct the patient to move the head forward to begin the transfer. As you lift on the safety belt, simultaneously straighten your lower extremities and stabilize the patient's knees by pushing in and forward with your knees to stand. Elevate the body high enough to clear the wheelchair wheel and stand the patient to the height necessary to elevate the pelvis above the level of the surface of the bed, mat, or plinth. Pivot yourself by sliding your feet and the patient toward the bed, mat, or plinth and lower onto the surface when the buttocks (pelvis) are turned so that they are directed toward the bed, mat, or plinth. *Note:* A commercially available rigid or flexible fabric disk, which allows the patient to be pivoted without moving the feet, can be placed under the feet before standing, reducing the effort required by the caregiver to perform the transfer. Set the patient on the edge of the bed, mat, or plinth and then assist to a supine position (Fig. 7-12, *D* to *G*). *Caution:* Do not leave the patient sitting unattended or without sufficient support to prevent a fall.

The return to the wheelchair is performed using the same procedures in reverse. The patient should be transferred toward the left and right side and requested to assist with the transfer. As the patient gains strength, the assisted standing transfer should be attempted.

If a safety belt or strap is not used, the assistant may lift the patient by grasping under the buttocks. However, this procedure may be difficult to perform on large patients and some patients may prefer that you not use this method. Your hands may slip or slide over the patient's clothing and it may not be as easy to control the person as it would be with a safety belt. *Caution:* You should not use the patient's clothing, including the belt, to lift or protect the patient. You could soil and tear the clothing or unbuckle the belt or cause patient discomfort if you use them as a means of control.

Standing Transfer, Assisted Pivot; Stronger Knee Stabilized When performing this transfer with a patient who has greater strength in one upper and lower extremity than in the other extremities, you should decide which direction the patient will transfer. Initially it will be easier and safer for most patients to transfer by leading with the stronger extremities. However, there are reasons to have the patient learn to lead with the weaker extremities. When the patient leads with the weaker extremity and uses the weaker upper extremity to assist with the transfer, proprioception and kinesthesia in those extremities may be improved and the patient is more likely to sense or feel them in a functional way. In addition, if the patient learns to transfer using both the left and the right extremities, the person will be better prepared to move in either direction at home or in the community depending on the location of objects such as

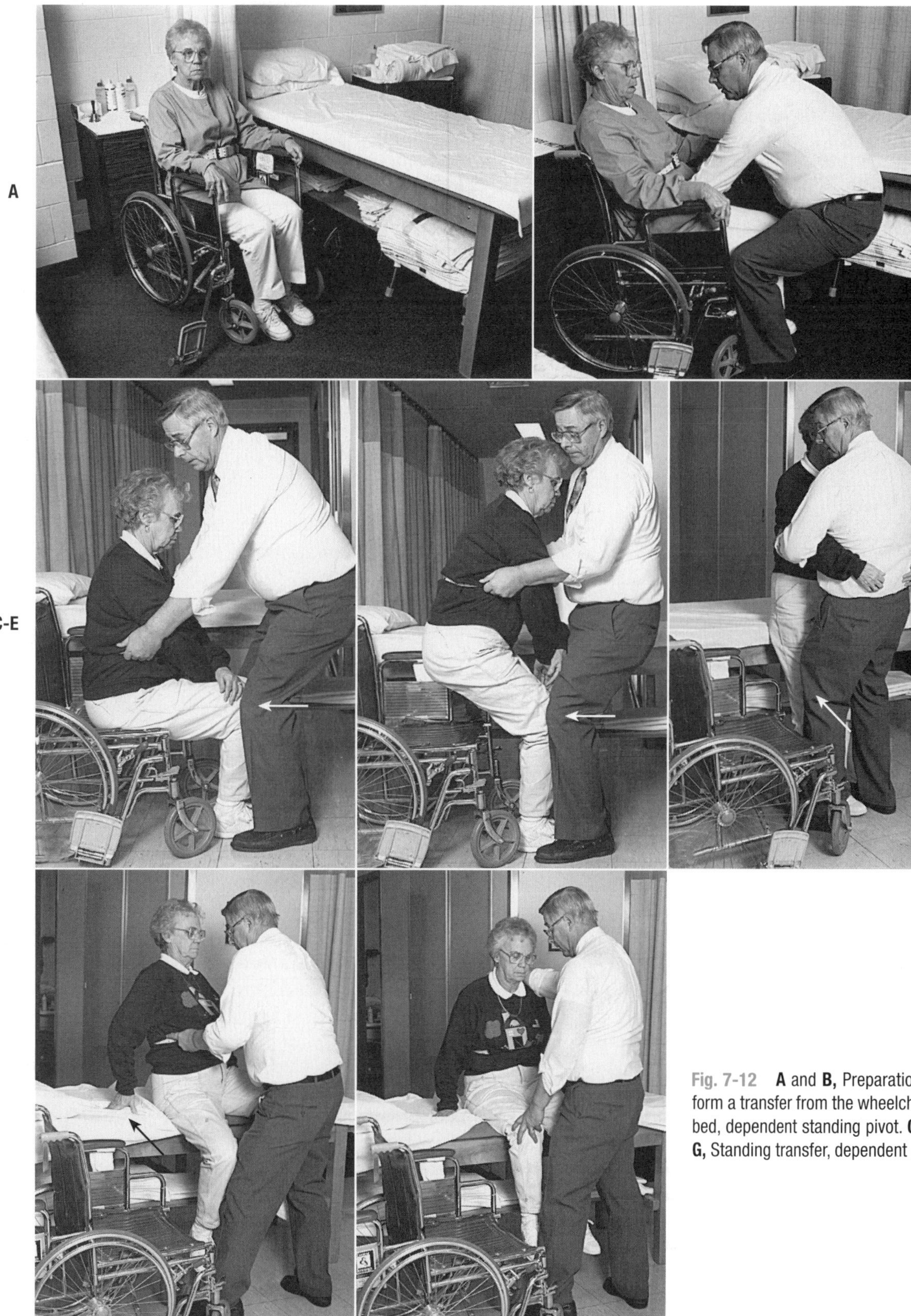

Fig. 7-12 **A** and **B,** Preparation to perform a transfer from the wheelchair to the bed, dependent standing pivot. **C** through **G,** Standing transfer, dependent pivot.

PROCEDURE 7-3

Procedures Associated With a Standing Transfer

Examine and evaluate the patient to determine whether the person has the mental and physical capacities to perform or assist with the transfer.

Position, secure, and stabilize the wheelchair and other items involved with the transfer, swing away front rigging or elevate foot plates, and apply safety belt on the patient.

Instruct the patient in the steps of the transfer, indicate the activities expected to be performed, and demonstrate the transfer as necessary. Instruct the patient to move forward in the chair, or provide assistance; position the patient's feet flat on the floor parallel or anteroposterior to each other.

The patient initiates standing with trunk momentum or by inclining the trunk forward ("nose over toes"); the caregiver is positioned in front and slightly to one side of the patient to protect and guard.

The patient uses the upper and lower extremity, or extremities, to rise to stand; assistance is provided by the caregiver as needed by use of the knees and the safety belt.

The patient stands briefly to establish balance and to acclimate to the upright position before turning or pivoting toward the object to which he or she is transferring.

As the patient turns or pivots or after the turn or pivot has been completed, the patient reaches for the object (that is, armrest, grab bar, edge of bed mattress, automobile seat) and uses the upper and lower extremity or extremities to lower onto the object; assistance is provided by the caregiver as needed.

The patient's position is adjusted for proper support, stability, and safety; any reaction and physiologic response to the activity are evaluated by the caregiver.

Remove the safety belt; document the patient's performance.

the bed, toilet, or bathtub. The patient should learn to transfer by leading with both the weaker and the stronger extremities to increase independence and to encourage use of the weaker extremities (Procedure 7-3).

Initially the patient may feel more secure if the stronger knee is blocked, a position that ensures that one lower extremity will be stable throughout the transfer. When the patient transfers by leading with the left (stronger) extremities, you should stabilize the left knee by placing your left foot next to the *medial* side of the left foot and placing your left knee on the *lateral* area of the knee. Grasp the safety belt with your right hand and place your left hand on the right shoulder or on the posterolateral area of the thorax by reaching under the right upper extremity. *Caution:* Do not use the right upper extremity or clothing as a point of control because both are insecure and you will not be able to guard the patient satisfactorily (Fig. 7-13).

Standing Transfer, Assisted Pivot; Weaker Knee Stabilized When you determine the patient is able to support weight on the stronger lower extremity safely and independently, you may choose to stabilize the weaker extremity. This stabilization will allow the patient to increase the use of the lower extremities and improve independence. When the patient transfers leading with the left (stronger) extremities, you should stabilize the weaker (right) knee by placing your left foot next to the lateral area of the right foot and placing your left knee on the medial side of the right knee. You can control the patient's trunk by grasping the safety belt with your left hand and by placing your right hand on the left shoulder or on the posterolateral area of the thorax by reaching under the left upper extremity (Fig. 7-14).

Instruct the patient to position the wheelchair parallel or at a 45- to 60-degree angle to the bed, with the stronger extremities nearest the bed. The chair should be at the midpoint between the head and foot of the bed or mat (see Fig. 7-14).

Instruct the patient to lock the wheelchair with the caster wheels directed forward, remove the feet from the footrests, and remove or swing away the front rigging. Armrests of the desk type should be reversed so the highest part is forward. Instruct the patient to move forward to the center or forward part of the seat by shifting weight off one buttock and elevating the pelvis on that side and moving it forward to the desired position in the chair or by leaning against the chair back and pushing the pelvis forward to the desired position in the chair and then moving the trunk to an erect or forward-inclined position to place the COG over the feet.

The patient positions the feet with the stronger or least affected foot posterior to the weaker or most affected foot. This position allows a stronger lower extremity to raise the body most effectively. However, that extremity will need to be advanced so it is anterior to the opposite lower extremity before the patient pivots. (*Note:* An elderly patient may perform better with the feet positioned parallel rather than anteroposterior to each other.) The person places the hands forward on the armrests and simultaneously pushes down with the upper and lower extremities while inclining the trunk forward slightly ("nose over toes") to stand. Some trunk motion can be initiated by rocking the trunk forward and back to develop momentum before attempting to stand. You may need to stabilize one or both of the knees as described previously when the patient begins the stand while you maintain control using the safety belt and the shoulder or the posterior neck. *Caution:* Do not use the patient's upper extremity or clothing for control for the reasons stated previously.

Allow the patient to stand briefly to establish balance and to determine whether light headedness or a dizzy sensation occurs. The patient pivots toward the bed so the back is nearest to the bed, reaches with the nearest upper extremity

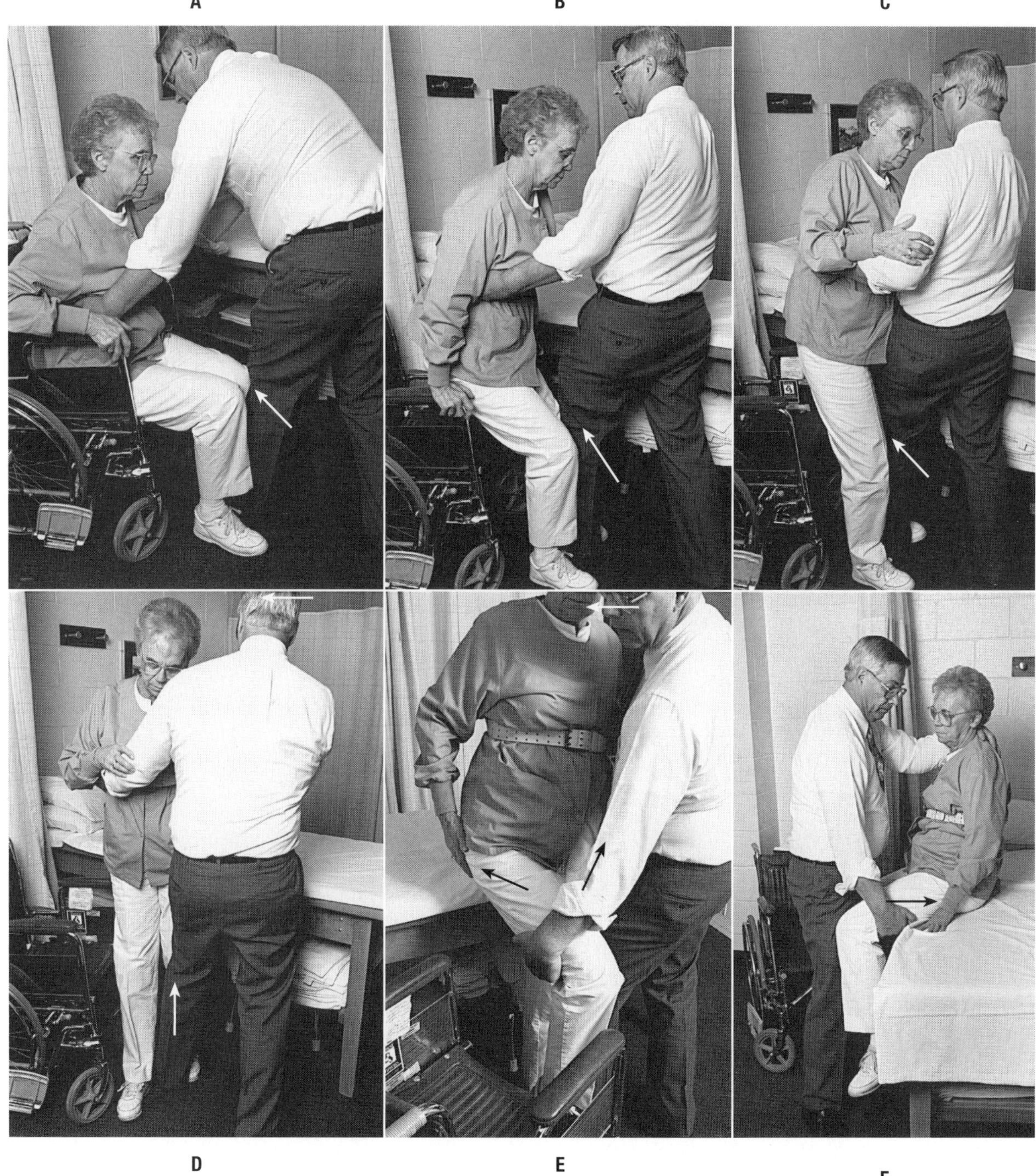

Fig. 7-13 Standing transfer, assisted pivot, with the patient leading with the stronger (left) extremities.

to the surface of the bed, and lowers to sitting on the bed. The patient places the lower extremities onto the bed and then lies down; if necessary, you may need to lift the lower extremities onto the bed and assist to recline.

Independent Standing Transfer The wheelchair should be positioned and locked as previously described. The patient should position it before lying down, or it will have to be positioned after the person sits on the edge of the bed or by another person before the transfer. Instruct the patient to rise to a sitting position using one of the methods described previously. Assistance should be provided as necessary for safety and to complete the change in position. Instruct the patient to move the hips to the edge of the bed and place the feet on the floor with the lead foot more anterior to position it for the pivot into the wheelchair. Again, an elderly patient may perform best with the feet parallel to each other. You may need to guard one or both knees as the person stands.

Instruct the patient to push to a standing position and to reach for the near armrest of the wheelchair; start to pivot, reach to the far armrest, and continue to pivot so the back is toward the chair. Next, have the person grasp the other armrest and then lower into the chair, reposition the front rigging and the footrests, place the feet on the footrests, and move the hips (pelvis) back into the chair seat.

Caution: For patients with a recent total hip replacement, care must be taken to avoid adduction of the surgically replaced hip beyond a midline position, excessive internal or external hip rotation, and excessive hip flexion, which is usually restricted to 60 to 90 degrees. The patient *must not* pivot on that extremity when standing, flex the surgically replaced hip or the trunk excessively, or adduct the hip at any time during the transfer.

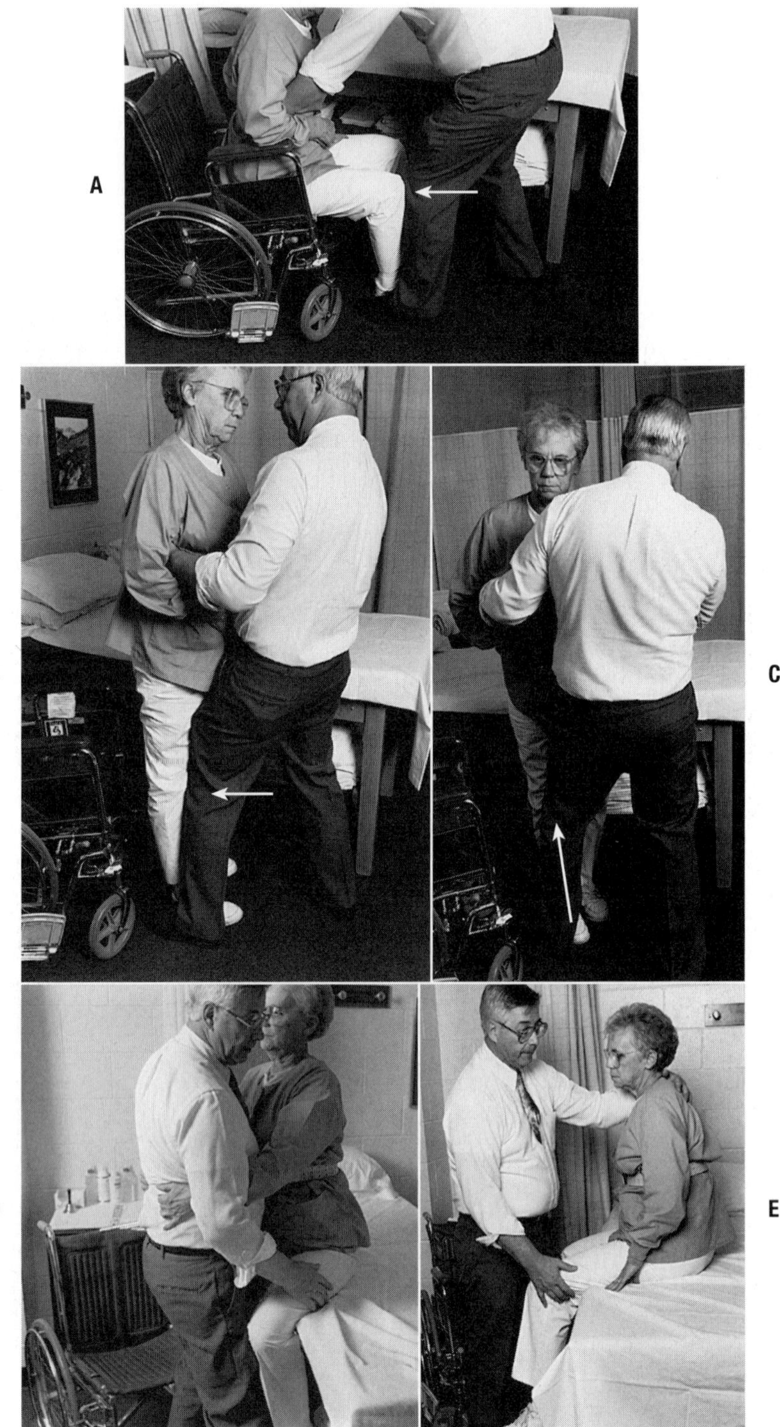

Fig. 7-14 Standing transfer, assisted pivot, with the weaker (right) knee stabilized.

Standing Transfer, Assisted Pivot with Use of a Footstool Occasionally it may be necessary for the person with short stature to use a footstool to elevate the hips to the height of a nonadjustable bed or plinth. The important principle to remember is the person should step onto the stool with the stronger lower extremity and it may be necessary to guard the opposite. The footstool should have four legs and the feet of the legs should be located beyond the edges of the top. For maximal stability, the feet should have rubber tips and the top should have a nonslip surface. The footstool should be between 8 and 12 inches high.

As with other transfers, the chair must be positioned properly and the patient should initiate the transfer with the stronger extremities nearest to the bed or plinth. The preliminary steps are the same as those listed for a standing transfer, assisted pivot. The caregiver guards the weaker knee as the patient steps onto the footstool with the stronger lower extremity. That extremity is used to lift the body high enough to position the buttocks slightly above the surface of the bed or plinth. The caregiver assists the patient to pivot so the buttocks are turned toward the bed or plinth. The person sits on the edge of the bed or plinth and establishes balance (Fig. 7-15). The caregiver can assist the patient to lie down by controlling the trunk and the lower extremities.

Another method is to instruct the patient to place the stronger foot on the footstool and to stand with assistance (Fig. 7-15, *E* to G). When this method is used, the weak lower extremity is not stabilized. *Caution:* The patient must be instructed to push down onto the footstool and to not push forward to avoid sliding or tipping the footstool.

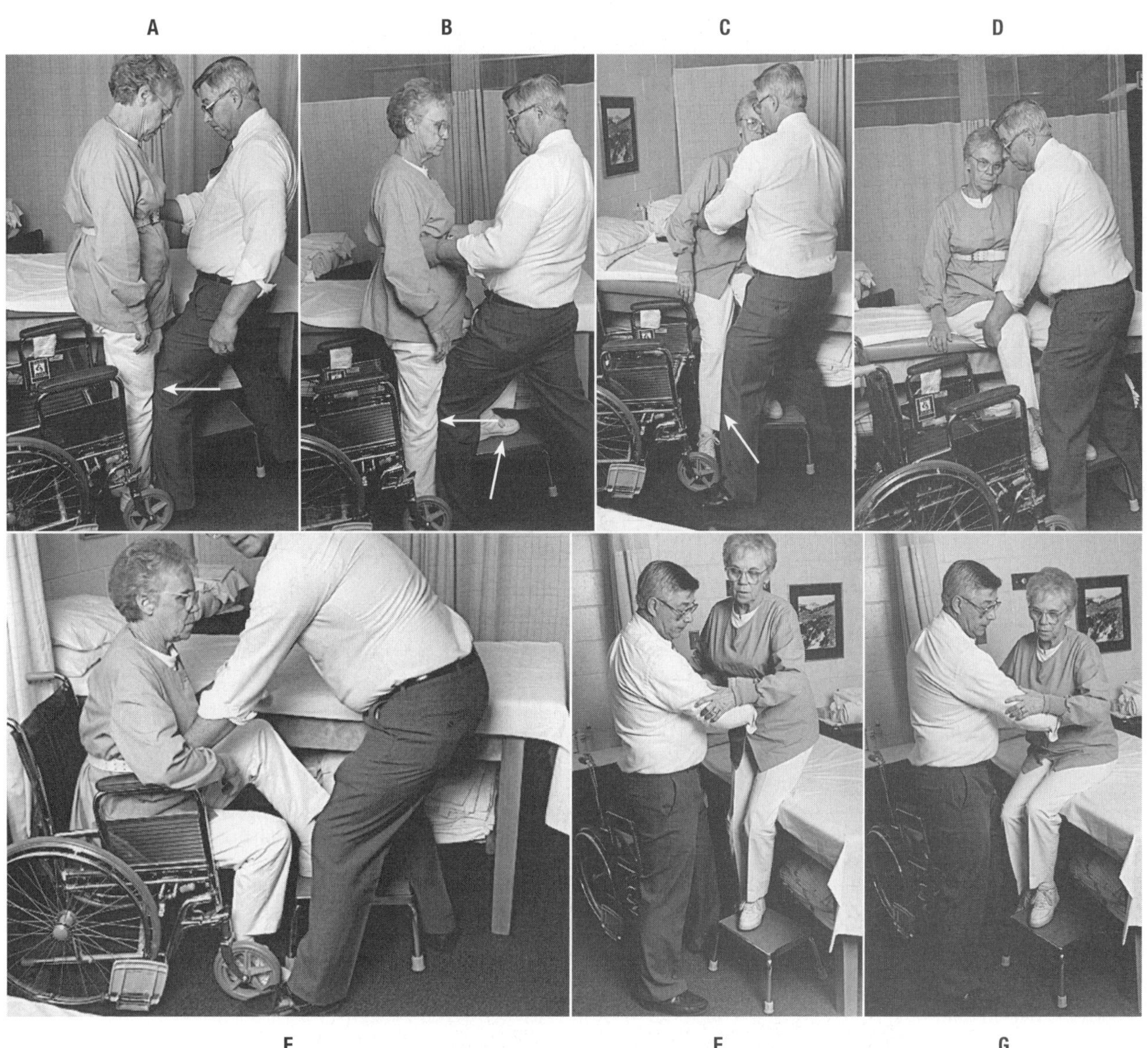

Fig. 7-15 **A** through **D,** Standing transfer, assisted pivot, using a footstool. **E** through **G,** Standing transfer, assisted pivot, using a footstool (alternative method).

Usually it is not necessary to use a footstool to transfer from the bed or plinth to a wheelchair, particularly if the bed or treatment table can be lowered. The caregiver assists the patient to sit with the legs over the edge of the bed or plinth and the stronger lower extremity slightly forward of the opposite extremity. The wheelchair is positioned at a 45-degree angle and nearest to the stronger lower extremity. Guard and assist the person to move forward leading with the stronger lower extremity so that it contacts the floor before the opposite lower extremity. When the leading foot is secure on the floor, the weaker foot is placed onto the floor. The person grasps the far armrest of the wheelchair, partially pivots on the stronger lower extremity so the back is toward the chair seat, completes the pivot, and is assisted to sit. If necessary, the knee of the weaker lower extremity may be stabilized by the caregiver.

Remember to apply and use a safety belt for these transfers. If it becomes apparent you will not be able to control or protect the patient throughout the transfer, return the person to the object from which the transfer was initiated. Transferring a patient from a wheelchair to a motor vehicle will also require a safety belt (Fig. 7-16).

Sitting Lateral Transfer Assisted with a Sliding Board

Instruct the patient to position the wheelchair at an angle to the bed and midway between the head and foot of the bed, mat, or low plinth. With the caster wheels forward and the bed wheels locked, apply a safety belt to the patient. Instruct the person to lock the wheelchair, remove the feet from the footrests, swing away or remove the front rigging, and place the feet on the floor. Instruct or assist the person to move forward in the chair and to remove the armrest nearest to the bed. The sliding board is positioned under the patient's thigh, in front of the drivewheel, so it extends from the wheelchair seat to the bed, mat, or low plinth (Fig. 7-17).

If the patient is going to move to the right, the right hand is placed on the board 4 to 6 inches from the right thigh and the left hand is placed next to the left thigh. The person performs a push-up with the upper extremities to elevate the body and begins to move toward the bed by quickly moving the head to the left and pushing toward the right with the left arm simultaneously. This procedure is repeated until the hips are on the bed. To move to the left, the position of the patient's hands is reversed. (*Note:* Some patients will be able to totally elevate the pelvis and move across the board without assistance. However, some patients will not be able to totally elevate the pelvis and must slide their buttocks, using a series of small movements, to progress across the board.) You should guard the patient's knees and use the safety belt to assist in elevating the body or moving the buttocks across the board. You can protect the patient's loss of balance by placing your hand on the upper trunk. The sliding board is removed when the person is seated securely on the bed, mat, or low plinth. The patient then lies down independently or is assisted to a lying position. *Caution:* Do not leave the patient sitting unattended.

The return to the wheelchair is performed using the same techniques in reverse order. The patient should learn to transfer to the left and right to maximize independence.

PROCEDURE 7-4

Sliding Board Transfer

If the bed height can be adjusted, it should be positioned as near the height of the wheelchair seat as possible before the transfer is attempted; the bed wheels should be locked.

BED TO WHEELCHAIR

Position the wheelchair at an angle next to the bed, facing the foot of the bed with the caster wheels forward and opposite the patient's hips. Lock the chair, remove the armrest nearest the bed, and swing away the front rigging.

Assist the patient to long sit, apply a safety belt, and assist to move to the edge of the mattress. The lower extremities may be positioned over the edge of the mattress or remain parallel to the edge of the mattress.

Position one end of the sliding board under the patient's upper thighs and buttocks; the other end should rest on the chair seat. Position yourself slightly in front and to the near side of the patient to guard and protect throughout the transfer.

Assist the patient to moving across the board and onto the chair seat. Guard and protect the trunk if the lower extremities need to be lowered from the mattress and when the board is removed.

Place the feet on the footrests, position the body for safety and comfort, and remove the safety belt.

WHEELCHAIR TO BED

Position the chair at an angle next to the bed, facing the foot of the bed and midway between the head and foot of the bed. Lock the chair and remove the armrest nearest the bed. Swing away the front rigging with the caster wheels forward.

Assist the patient to move forward in the chair. Place one end of the board under the thighs and buttocks; the other end should rest on the mattress. Position yourself slightly in front of and to one side of the patient to guard and protect.

Assist the patient to move across the board onto the mattress; the legs may dangle over the edge of the mattress, or they may be lifted onto the mattress. Guard and protect as the lower extremities are placed onto the mattress.

Remove the board; assist the patient to move toward the center of the mattress and lie down.

Position the body for safety and comfort; remove the safety belt.

This transfer is most commonly used for the patient who is unable to stand, but has functional upper extremities. A similar transfer can be performed by a patient with weakness in one upper and lower extremity and normal strength in the other extremities, but who is unable to stand safely. Some patients will require the use of a sliding board at all times, whereas other patients will develop the balance, strength, and skill to permit them to perform the transfer without the board (Procedure 7-4).

Sitting Transfer, Independent Lateral/Swinging Instruct the patient to position the wheelchair at an angle to the bed and midway between the head and the foot of the bed, mat, or low plinth. The caster wheels should be positioned forward to expand the BOS of the chair. Instruct the person to remove the feet from the footrests, remove or swing away the front rigging, and place the feet on the floor.

Instruct the patient to move forward in the chair to clear the buttocks past the drivewheel and to remove the armrest

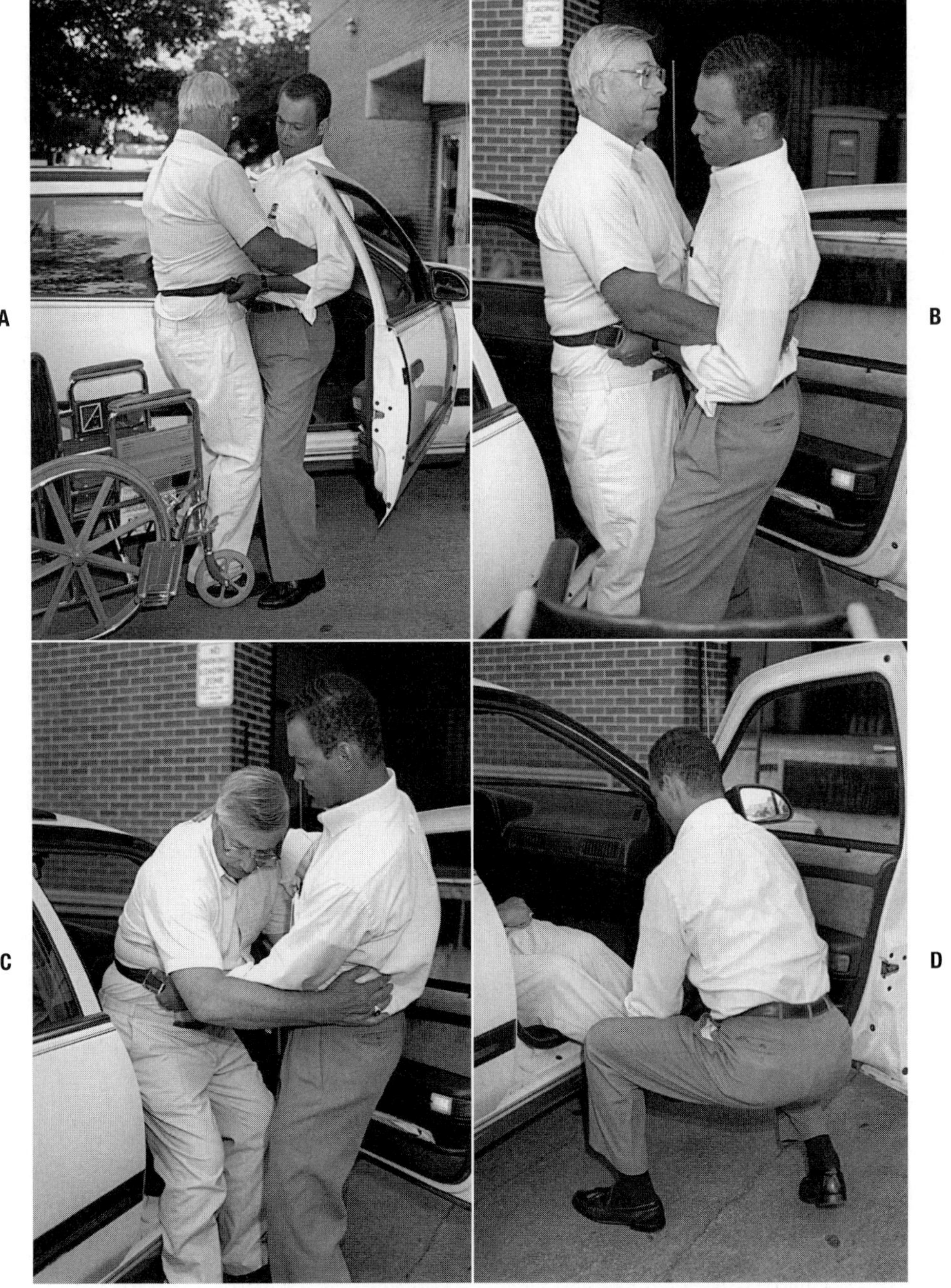

Fig. 7-16 Assisted transfer into a motor vehicle. **A,** The caregiver protects the person's knees and assists him in standing; chair is prepositioned and locked. **B,** The knees are protected as the person pivots. **C,** The caregiver uses the safety belt to assist the person in sitting. **D,** The lower extremities are placed into the car.

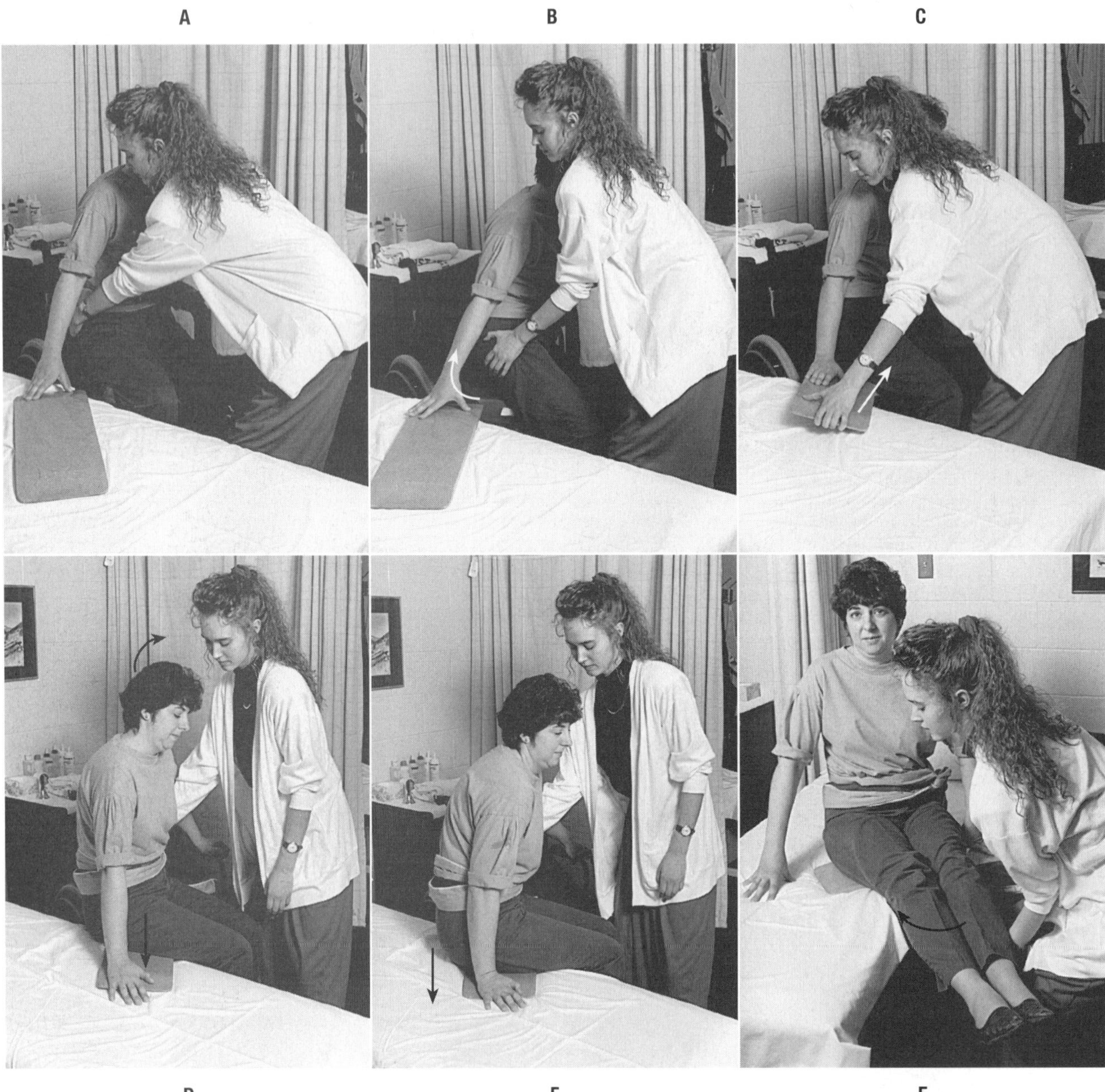

Fig. 7-17 Sitting transfer using a sliding board.

nearest to the bed. The person moves the buttocks to partially pivot the body so the back is toward the bed. If the patient is going to move to the right, the right hand is placed on the edge of the bed and the left hand is placed on the armrest on the seat of the chair or on the back of the chair, depending on the patient's strength, size, and skill. Instruct the patient to push with the upper extremities to elevate the body and to swing the buttocks onto the edge of the bed by moving the head quickly to the left and pushing toward the right with the left arm simultaneously, then reposition the hands and move farther onto the bed. The patient then stabilizes the body on the edge of the bed, places the lower extremities onto the bed, and lies on the bed. It may be necessary to assist some patients to place their lower extremities onto the bed and to lie down (Fig. 7-18).

The return to the wheelchair is performed by use of the same techniques in reverse order. The patient should learn to transfer to the left and right to maximize independence.

One-Person Dependent (Lift) Transfer The one-person lift transfer can be used when a patient is unable to stand or is unable to perform any type of sliding board transfer and when the assistant is sufficiently strong and skilled to perform the lift. The caregiver must use proper body mechanics and perform the lift over the shortest possible distance (Fig. 7-19).

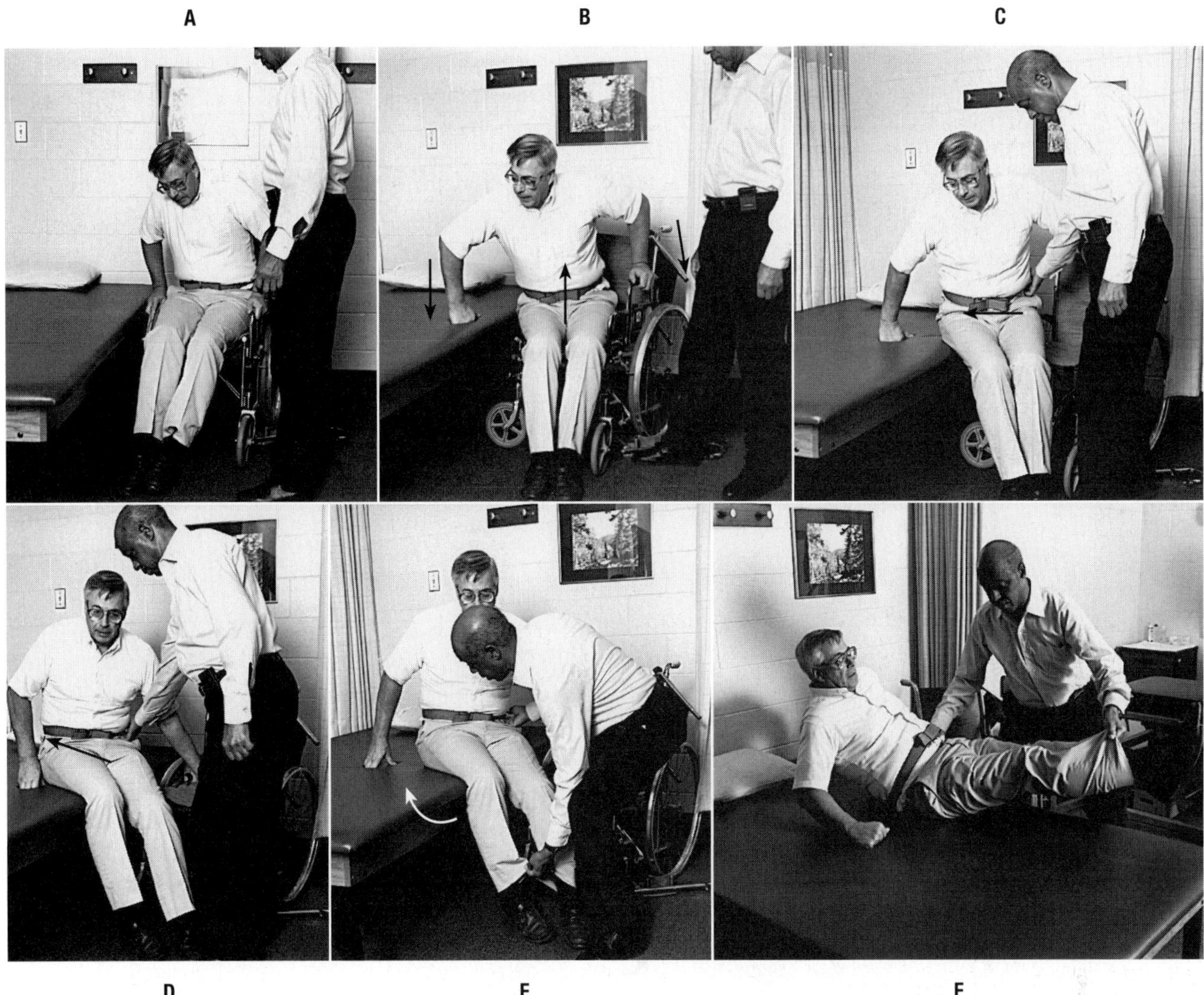

Fig. 7-18 Sitting transfer with an independent lateral swinging movement.

Caution: If you have not been taught how to perform this transfer or have not practiced it with an able-bodied person, do not attempt it with a patient. Position the wheelchair at an angle to and touching the other surface and apply a safety belt to the patient. Position the caster wheels forward, lock the chair, and remove the patient's feet from the footrests. Elevate the footrests or remove or swing away the front rigging and place the feet on the floor. Remove the armrest nearest to the object to which the patient is to be transferred and move the person forward to the front of the chair.

Stand in front of the patient, flex your hips and knees, and position your knees and feet on the outside, but next to, the patient's knees and feet. Lift the thighs and hold them between your knees or the lower area of the thighs so the feet are off the floor. Flex the patient's trunk with the head positioned on the side of your hip that is opposite to the direction of the transfer; the arms should be folded in the lap or across the chest (see Fig. 7-19, *A* and *B*).

Grasp the safety belt on each side of the patient and lift from the chair. Pivot your body by moving your feet and turn the patient's buttocks toward the transfer object (see Fig. 7-19, *C* and *D*). Lower the patient onto the transfer object, place the feet on the floor, and straighten the trunk to an upright, sitting position. Be certain to protect the patient while sitting and then reposition as necessary.

The return to the wheelchair is performed by use of the same techniques in reverse order. *Caution:* Do not leave the patient sitting unattended on the edge of the bed, mat, or plinth. If you have returned the patient into the wheelchair, be certain the hips are positioned back on the seat so the trunk will be supported by the chair back.

Two-Person Dependent (Lift) Transfer; Chair to Bed

The two-person lift transfer can be used when the patient is unable to stand, when the transfer is performed from two surfaces of unequal height, or when the patient is unable to assist with the transfer. The use of proper body mechanics for the persons performing the lift is extremely important. Each person should mentally review and plan how the lift will be performed and one person must assume the role of the leader.

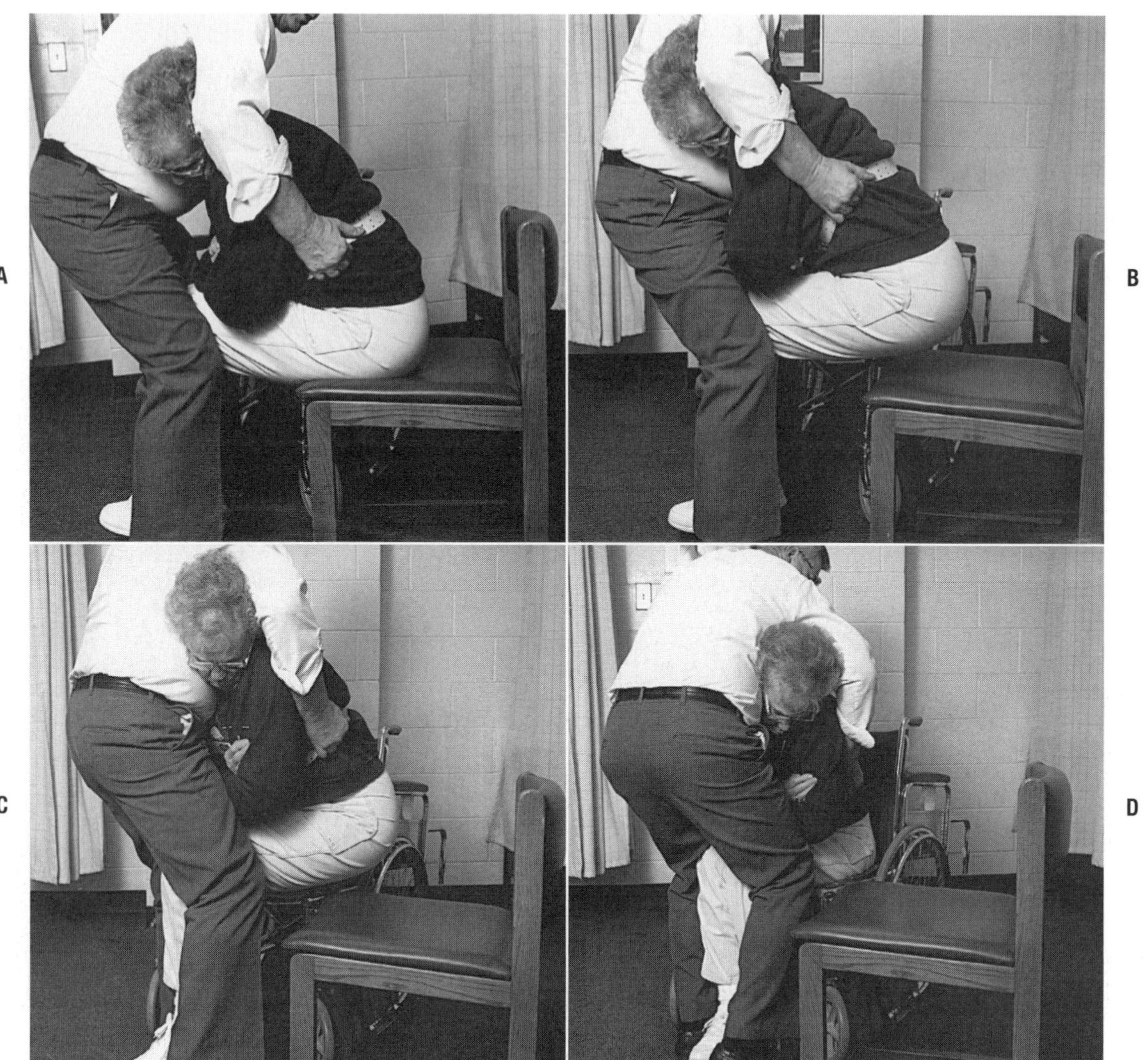

Fig. 7-19 One-person lift transfer.

The leader will instruct the patient and the other person so all three can work together. The transfer procedure should be explained to the patient and the person should understand what is planned and what to expect. This information should be provided before you perform any of the lifting transfers to reduce possible fears or apprehensions the patient may have. *Caution:* This transfer can cause back strain for the persons lifting and should be used only in an emergency or when mechanical equipment is not available.

Position and lock the wheelchair as described previously. The armrest nearest to the bed or mat should be removed only if it is higher than the surface of the bed or mat. The taller and stronger person stands behind the chair and the other person removes the patient's lower extremities from the footrests and swings away or removes the front rigging. The person standing behind the patient reaches through the patient's axillae, grasps the patient's opposite forearms with the hands, and folds the patient's forearms over the abdomen (Fig. 7-20). (*Note:* A safety belt can be used instead of the patient's forearms, but it must be secured tightly and firmly below the flair of the rib cage so that it will not slip upward when the lift occurs.) The other person stands facing the outer side of the patient's lower extremities, then stoops and places one forearm under the distal area of the patient's thigh and the other forearm under the patient's lower leg and extends the patient's knees. *Caution:* One forearm must be under the patient's thighs to assist in lifting the pelvis and to avoid strain to the posterior aspect of the knees.

The person standing behind the patient instructs the patient to push down and hold the position with the shoulder muscles. The other person is instructed when to lift (for example, "One, two, three, lift"; "Ready, lift";

One person elevates the patient's trunk so the person is long sitting and the patient's forearms are grasped as described previously. The other person cradles the patient's lower extremities as described previously, keeping the patient's knees straight. One person gives the command to lift and the patient is transferred to the wheelchair. *Caution:* Both persons performing the transfer must use proper body mechanics to lower the patient into the chair by flexing at the hips and knees and avoiding excessive trunk flexion. Some trunk rotation may be required by the person who stands behind the patient during the lift and this person must be prepared to pivot using the hips and feet to avoid lower back strain. The patient's body is moved to the rear of the chair seat and the feet are positioned on the footrests. If necessary, a lap or chest belt is applied to protect or stabilize the patient.

Alternative Method The wheelchair is positioned as described previously and the patient is positioned sitting on the edge of the bed with the lifters positioned on each side of the patient.

The patient is supported by the lifters as described previously. One lifter gives the command to lift and the patient is lifted and carried to the wheelchair. The patient is lowered into the chair and positioned as described previously. The lifters must use proper body mechanics to lower the patient into the chair. The armrests and front rigging are replaced, the feet are positioned on the footrests, and a lap or chest strap is applied, if necessary, to protect or stabilize the patient.

Two-Person Dependent (Lift) Transfer; Chair to Floor Position the wheelchair parallel to the area on the floor to which the patient is to be transferred. One person stands behind the patient and other person stands at the near side of the lower extremities. The patient is lifted from the chair as described previously and the lifters move sideward away from the chair. On command, both lifters stoop to lower the patient to the floor (Fig. 7-22). *Caution:* The lifters must flex their hips and knees and avoid trunk flexion as the patient is lowered to the floor. The patient is assisted to a lying position or maintains a sitting position, using the upper extremities to form a tripod with the hips.

To return the patient to the chair, the person is positioned long sitting. The two lifters stoop and grasp the patient as described previously. On command, the lifters stand simultaneously to lift the patient; then they step toward the chair. The patient is lowered into the chair and properly positioned.

Three-Person Dependent (Lift) Transfer; Bed to Stretcher The three-person lift transfer can be used to transfer a patient from one flat surface to another (as from a wheeled stretcher to a bed, or vice versa) while leaving the patient supine. It is used when no other type of transfer can be used, in an emergency, when mechanical equipment is not available, and when the patient cannot sit or stand. The two stronger and taller of the three persons should be positioned at the patient's head, shoulders, and pelvis. The third person is positioned to control the lower extremities. One person becomes the leader to instruct and give commands to the lifters.

Proper body mechanics must be used to prevent possible injury to the lifters. They should flex their hips and knees before lifting and when lowering the patient, and they should be close to the patient and cradle the patient's body in their arms by flexing their elbows to use short lever arms when lifting or lowering the patient.

The stretcher is positioned and locked at a right angle to the bed with either the foot of the stretcher nearest to the head of the bed or the head of the stretcher nearest to the foot of the bed. *Note:* Rather than lift a patient, a plastic spine board placed under the patient may be used to slide the patient to or from a stretcher or bed when they are positioned parallel (side by side) (Fig. 7-23).

The lifters place their upper extremities under the patient's head and upper trunk, just above and below the pelvis and under the upper thigh and lower leg to maintain the knees straight (Fig. 7-24, *A*). The patient is moved to the near edge of the bed with the upper extremities positioned along the sides of the body. Moving the patient close to the near edge of the bed will allow the lifters to use their upper extremities as short lever arms and will position the patient's COG closer to their COGs. The leader commands the lifters to roll the patient to side lying and cradled in their flexed elbows (Fig. 7-24, *B*). Next, the leader commands the lifters to lift the patient, keeping the person on one side; to step back from the bed; to pivot so the patient's back is toward the other surface onto which the person is to be placed; and to sidestep to carry the patient to the stretcher (Fig. 7-24, *C*). The lifters should use short steps and should sidestep rather than use a crossover step to avoid stepping on another person's foot. Once the patient is positioned over the stretcher, the leader commands the lifters to lower the patient by flexing their hips and knees until their elbows contact the stretcher top (Fig. 7-24, *D*). The patient should remain side lying until the lifters' elbows contact the top of the stretcher (Fig. 7-24, *E*). The leader commands the lifters to slowly release their elbows to position the patient supine onto the stretcher. The patient is properly positioned toward the center of the stretcher and side rails or body straps are applied, if necessary, for protection or stability.

To transfer the patient from the stretcher to the bed, the process described previously is performed in reverse sequence. It is important to properly position the stretcher in relation to the bed or item to which the patient is to be transferred before lifting the patient (Procedure 7-6).

PROCEDURE 7-6

Three-Person Lift Transfer

BED TO A NEW SUPPORT SURFACE (SUCH AS STRETCHER, BED, TILT TABLE)

Position the head of the new support surface perpendicularly (that is, at a right angle) to the foot of the bed; move the patient close to the near edge of the bed; select one person to lead.

One of the stronger lifters slides the forearms under the patient's head and upper trunk, another strong lifter slides the forearms under the patient above and below the pelvis, and the third lifter slides the forearms under the thighs and lower legs near the ankles.

On command from the lead lifter, roll the patient to a side-lying position.

On command from the lifter at the patient's head lift the patient, cradle the body between your forearms and upper arms.

Carry the patient to the second surface using short side steps.

On command from the lead lifter, lower the patient to the new support surface by bending your knees and hips; keep the body cradled until your elbows rest on the support surface.

On command, lower your forearms to the support surface to place the patient flat.

Move the patient toward the center of the support surface; position the body for comfort and safety; and apply security straps, pillows, and towel rolls, as necessary.

RETURN TO BED

Reverse the sequence of the transfer from bed to a new support surface to return the patient to the bed.

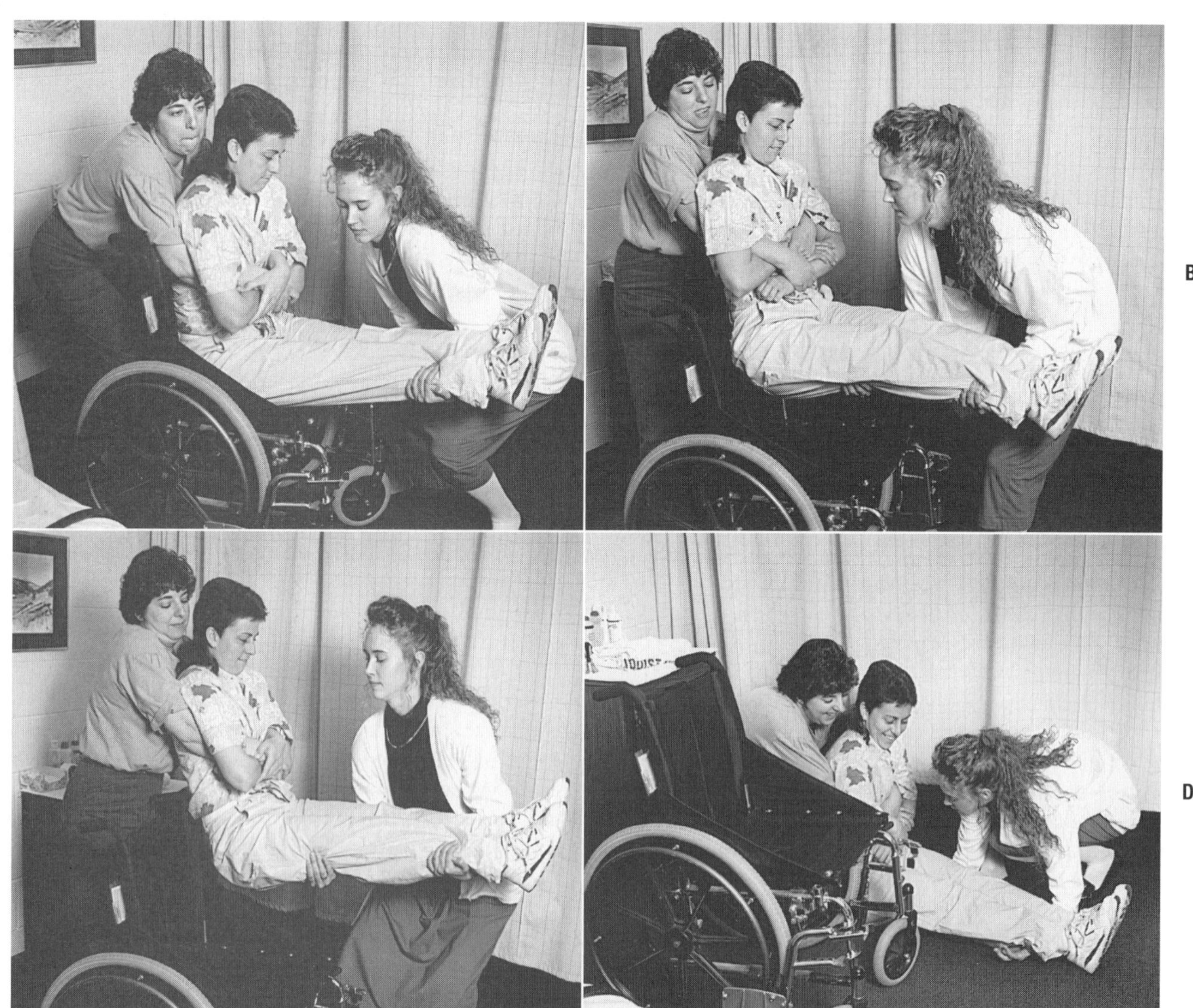

Fig. 7-22 Two-person lift transfer from the wheelchair to the floor.

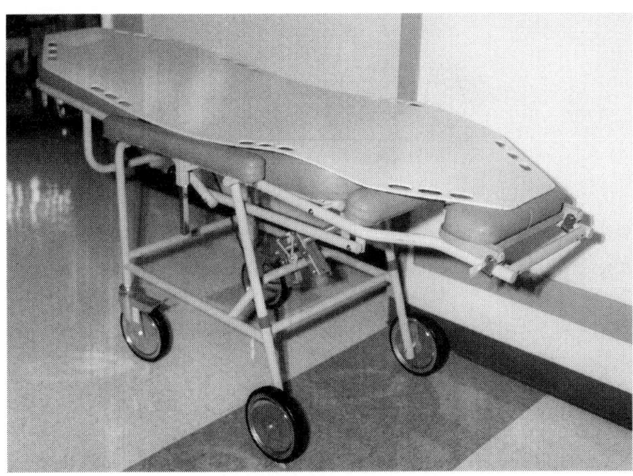

Fig. 7-23 The flexible plastic item on the stretcher is used to transfer a supine patient to or from a bed or stretcher.

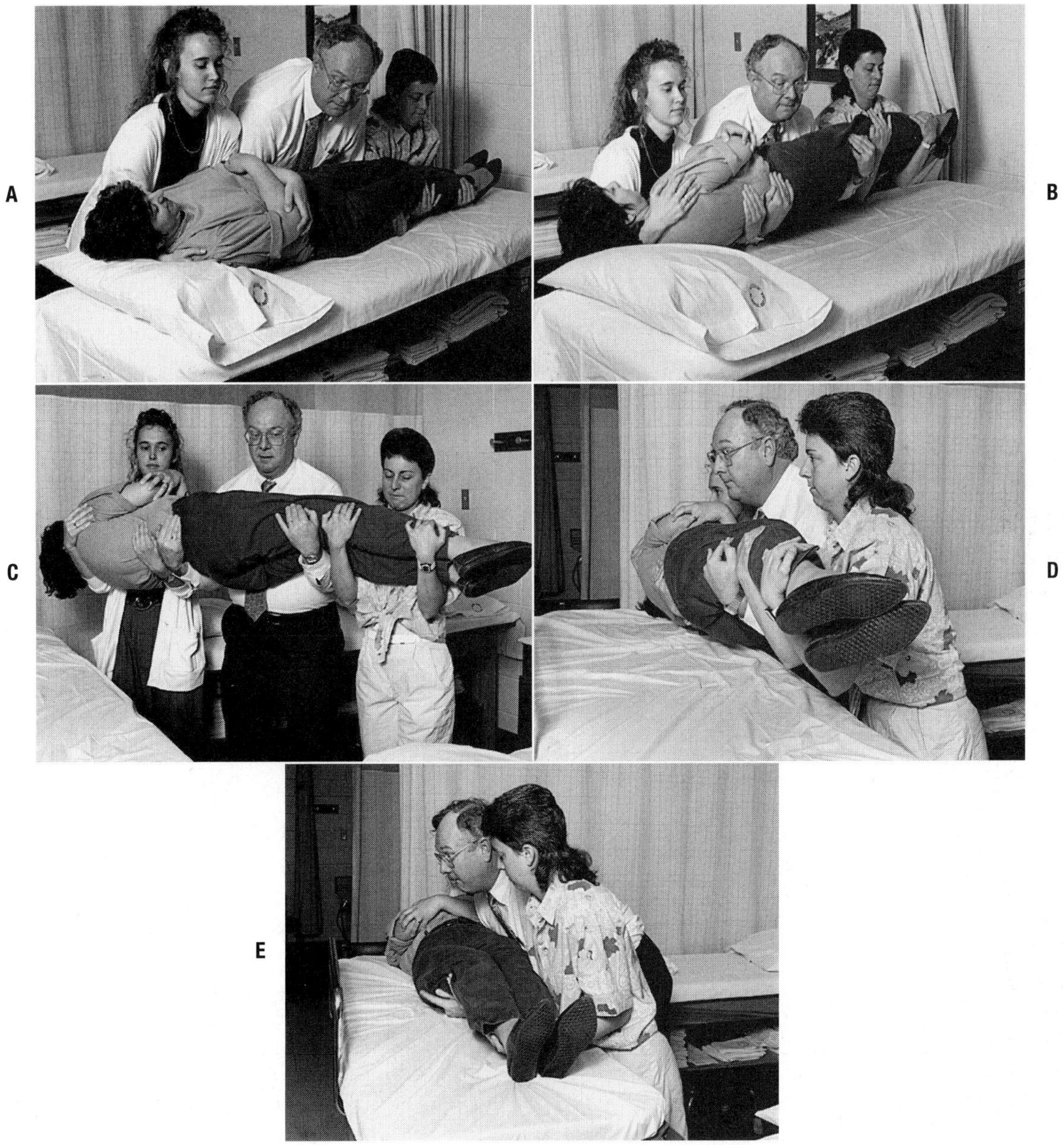

Fig. 7-24 Three-person lift transfer from the bed to a stretcher.

MECHANICAL EQUIPMENT

When a large or very dependent patient needs to be lifted and transported, a hydraulic or pneumatic lift is the safest and most effective device to use. This device has a U-shaped base supported by four caster wheels, at least two of which usually can be locked. A tubular metal support column is attached to the base, which contains the controls for the adjustable lift column with its attached overhead spreader bar (Fig. 7-25, *A*). A body seat or wide support slings can be attached to the adjustable overhead bar by chains or web straps, which are sewn directly or attached to the seat or slings by metal S-shaped hooks. The base can be narrowed for storage or widened to increase its BOS or to allow it to be positioned around a wheelchair or the end of a bathtub. A long control lever attached to the base of the lift is used to widen or narrow the base (Fig. 7-25, *B*).

A valve on the tubular support column controls the release or containment of air or fluid from a closed chamber (cylinder). When the valve is closed (tightened), the adjustable bar is raised by means of a handle to compress the air or hydraulic fluid in the chamber (Fig. 7-25, *C*). This raises the adjustable bar and elevates the patient. When the valve is opened (loosened), the adjustable bar will descend to lower the patient as the air or fluid pressure is released. The amount the valve is opened and the patient's weight will affect the rate of descent. It is important to remember to close the valve whenever the patient is elevated and when the unit is not in use. *Caution:* When the patient has been lowered to the proper level, the valve must be closed to prevent the adjustable bar from continuing to descend and striking the patient's head.

This device is very safe for one person to use to lift and transfer a very large (up to 250- to 300-pound) patient or a patient who is extremely dependent, provided the device is operated correctly.

Transfer from Bed to Wheelchair

Roll the patient onto one side and slide the slings under the upper trunk and thighs. Next, roll the patient onto the other side and pull the slings completely under the body so the sling attachments are exposed, with the outside seams of the sling, directed away from the patient (Fig. 7-26, *A* to *C*).

Position the base of the lift perpendicularly to the patient and the edge of the bed and with the spreader bar directed across the patient's upper body. *Caution:* Be certain the valve that controls the adjustable arm is closed as you position the lift. Open the valve and carefully lower the adjustable arm so that the spreader bar is close enough to the patient to attach the sling (Fig. 7-26, *D*). *Be certain to close the valve when the proper position of the adjustable arm is attained.*

Apply the rings of the web strap or the S hook of the chain to the sling. Attach the shortest segment of the chain or web strap to the upper part of the sling and attach the longest segment to the lower part of the sling. These positions will ensure that the patient will be lifted into a sitting position. Direct the open end of the S hook away from the patient to prevent injury to the skin (Fig. 7-26, *E*).

Before you attempt to lift the patient, check all the attachments, fold the arms over the abdomen, and check the position of the slings (Fig. 7-26, *F*). Caution the patient not to reach for or grasp the spreader bar when being raised.

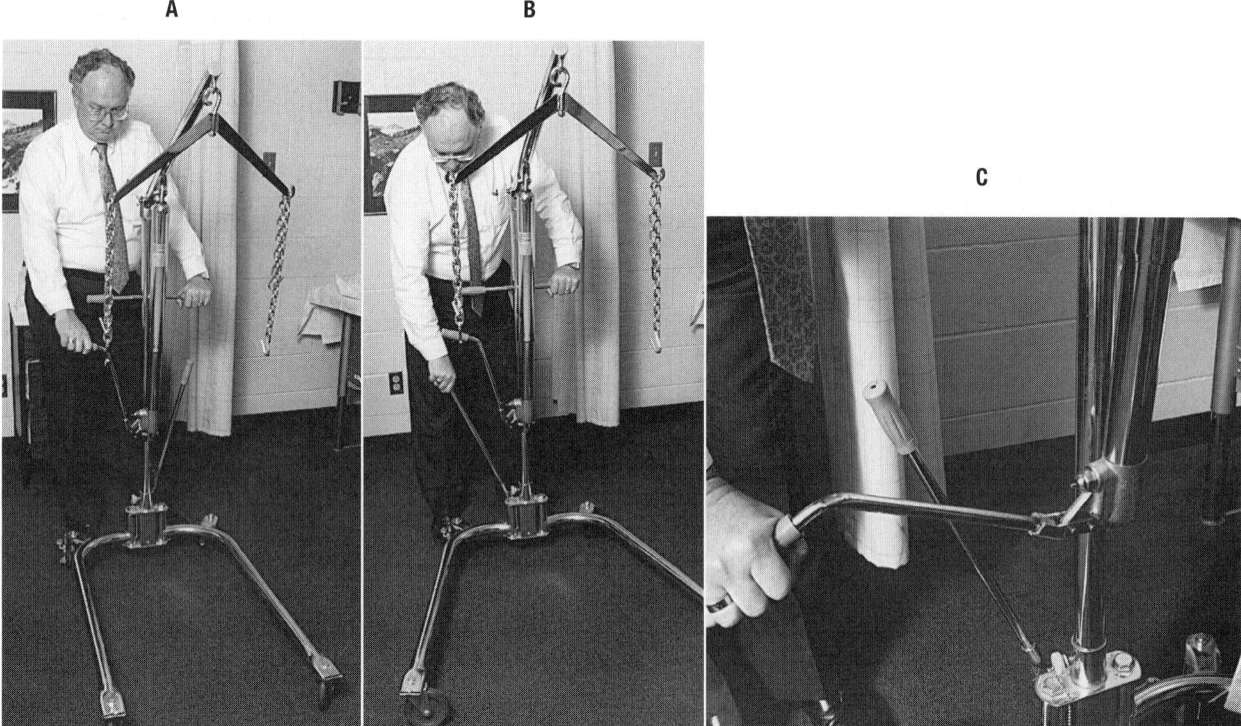

Fig. 7-25 Mechanical lift to transfer large or very dependent patients.

A B C D E F

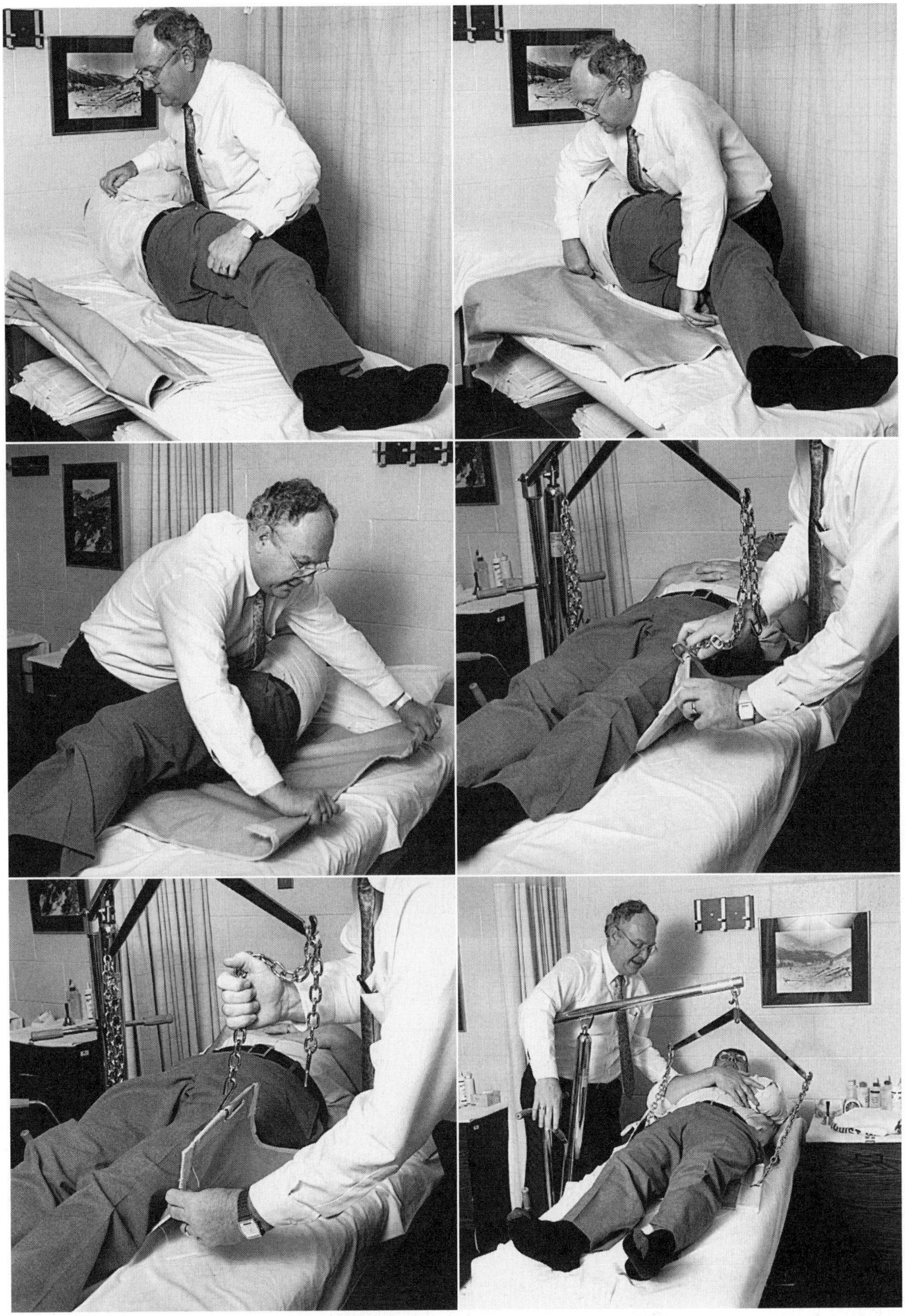

Continued

Fig. 7-26 Transfer from the bed to the wheelchair using a hydraulic lift device.

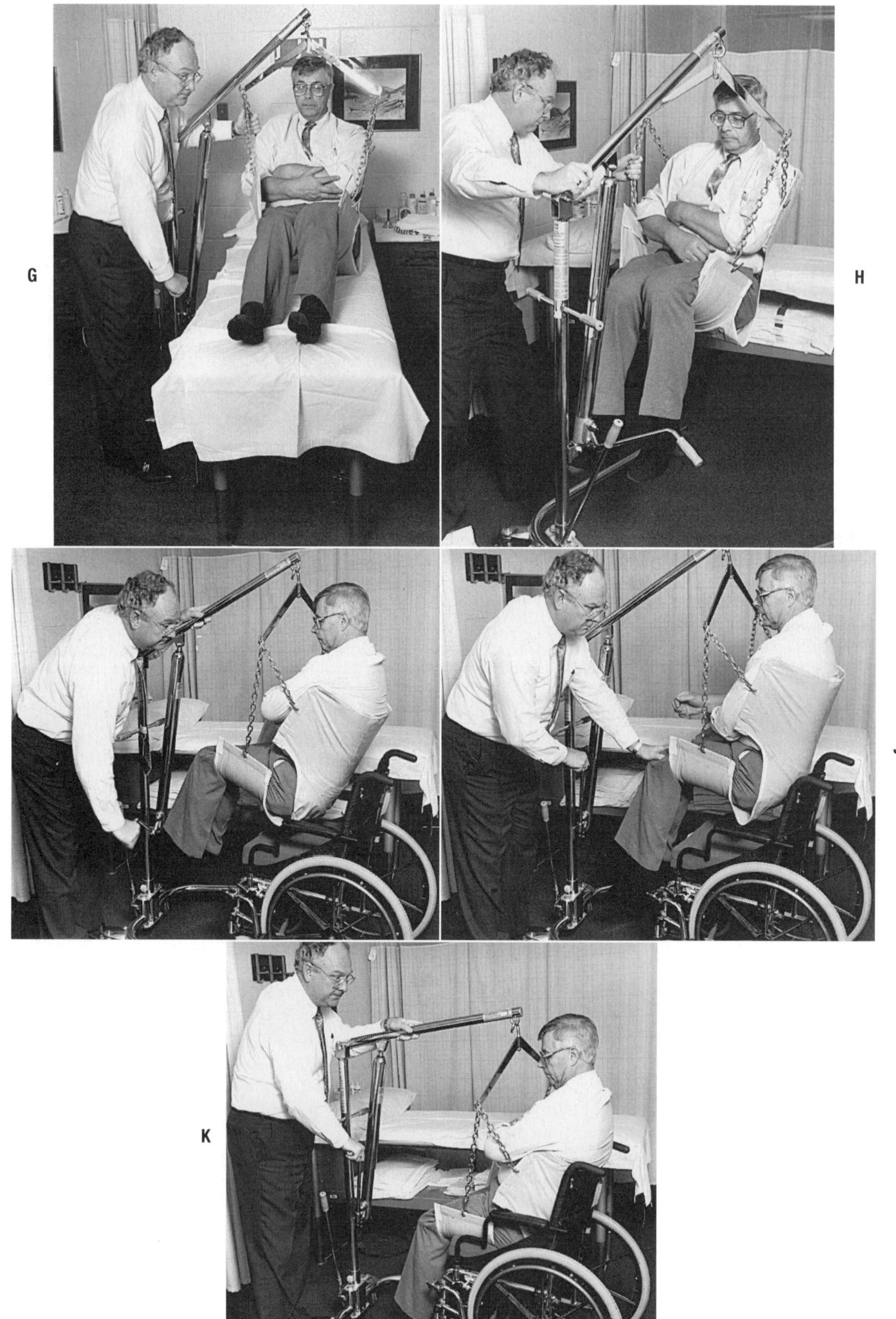

Fig. 7-26, cont'd For legend see p. 157.

Elevate the patient until the buttocks clear the surface of the bed; reevaluate the position, the location of the slings, and the security of the attachments before moving away from the bed (Fig. 7-26, G). Continue to elevate the patient and assist by moving the lower extremities from the bed so the person sits properly in the slings. The knees can be allowed to flex or can be kept extended as you carefully move the lift away from the side of the bed and then turn the patient to face the support column (Fig. 7-26, *H*). Transport the patient to the wheelchair by using the cross handles on the support column. *Caution:* Be certain the floor is free of objects and there is sufficient space to maneuver the lift. Objects that could interfere with or block the caster wheels from moving smoothly, such as a throw rug, a door threshold, or a line cord, should be avoided. Maneuver the patient so the buttocks are over the front or the middle of the seat of the locked wheelchair and open the valve to lower into the chair (Fig. 7-26, *I*). As the patient is lowered, you may need to push against the knees to position the hips back into the chair (Fig. 7-26, *J*). *Caution:* Be certain to close the valve as soon as the patient is properly positioned in the chair so that the adjustable bar does not continue to lower and strike the patient's head (Fig. 7-26, *K*).

Remove the sling attachments and move the lift away from the chair; however, the slings remain under the patient to permit a transfer back to bed. If the slings are removed, they will be difficult to reposition under the patient while seated. Position the feet on the footrests, and apply a lap or chest strap, if necessary, to protect or stabilize the patient (Procedure 7-7).

Movement from Wheelchair to Bed

Transfer from the wheelchair to the bed is accomplished by reversal of the sequence described for transferring the patient from the bed to the wheelchair. After the patient has returned to the bed, the slings are removed.

It will be helpful to have multiple slings available if this equipment is to be used for several patients. In addition, it will be necessary to launder the slings periodically; therefore more than one sling should be available to use when one of them is being laundered.

Patients are apt to be apprehensive the first few times this device is used. To help overcome any fear or apprehension, explain the procedure to the patient and provide information about the safety of the unit before using it. It may be helpful to allow the patient to observe the unit being used for another person before it is used for him or her.

PROCEDURE 7-7

Mechanical Lift Transfer

BED TO WHEELCHAIR

Explain the activity to the patient the first time it is performed.

Place the slings under the upper trunk and buttocks and upper thighs by rolling the patient onto one side and then onto the other side.

Position the lift perpendicularly and close to the bed with the spreader bar over the chest; attach the chains or web straps to the spreader bar.

Partially open the control valve to slowly lower the spreader bar until the chains or web straps can be attached to the sling or slings. *Close the valve* so that the spreader bar does not continue to lower.

Attach the chains or web straps to the slings; attach the shorter segment of the chains or web straps to the trunk sling. When S hooks are used, they should be directed away from the body.

Adjust the sling or slings and attachments as necessary, fold the arms onto the chest, and elevate the body using the pump handle.

Check all attachments and the position of the slings; continue to elevate the patient until the buttocks are off the mattress.

Move the lift away from the bed using the cross handles on the center post. The knees can be allowed to flex or be supported by the caregiver; maintain the patient within the base of the lift.

Transport the patient to the wheelchair. Turn the body so the back is toward the front of the chair; position the buttocks over the center of the chair seat.

Partially open the control valve to slowly lower the patient into the chair; move the body toward the back of the seat by pushing on the knees before the buttocks contact the seat. *Close the valve* when the person is seated.

Remove the chains or web straps from the sling or slings; leave the slings in place so the patient can be transferred back to the bed.

WHEELCHAIR TO BED

Reverse the sequence of the activities of the transfer from the bed to chair. Position the patient on mattress; remove sling.

Be certain to check the position of the sling or slings and security of the chains or web straps before lifting the patient from the chair.

Remember to *close the valve* after the spreader bar has been positioned to attach or remove the chains or web straps.

OTHER TYPES OF TRANSFERS

Movement from Stretcher to Bed or Bed to Stretcher, Totally Dependent Patient

When the two surfaces are at approximately the same height, position the stretcher parallel to and touching one edge of the bed. *Caution:* Be certain the stretcher and the bed are locked or secured so they will not separate during the transfer.

If the stretcher has a loose pad, slide it and the patient onto the bed and then remove the pad; if a draw sheet is available, use it to slide the patient from the stretcher onto the bed.

The patient can be rolled from the stretcher toward you onto the bed, or you can segmentally slide the patient from the stretcher to the bed, as you kneel on the bed using your forearms to support under the patient to avoid skin irritation.

Caution: Extreme care must be used when any of these techniques are attempted because the stretcher and bed could separate and the patient could fall. Another person may be needed to hold the two objects together or to assist with the transfer.

Caution: You are advised not to use bed linen to lift and carry a patient from one object to another because the linen could tear and the patient could fall. This technique should be used only in an emergency when no other technique is possible or when the situation requires a rapid transfer. It is relatively safe to use a sheet to transfer a patient by sliding because even if the sheet tears, the patient remains supported by a firm surface. Do not use this technique if there are contraindications to sliding the patient or when the shear forces associated with sliding are likely to cause skin irritation (such as a burn or sutures).

Standing Transfer, Assisted, for a Patient with Total Hip Replacement

There are special precautions or considerations that should be used with a patient after surgery for a total hip replacement. Each surgeon will have instructions or preferences for the amount of weight bearing, the movement or activities to be permitted, and the alignment of the trunk in relation to the surgically replaced hip. The person who assists the patient must be aware of these specific precautions, instructions, and preferences. Most of the precautions or contraindications are designed to reduce the possibility of hip dislocation during the first 10 to 14 days of postoperative care. Some of the generally and widely accepted precautions or contraindications for this patient condition are listed in Box 7-4.

Movement from the Bed to a Walker

A walker is frequently used initially for hip replacement patients to improve stability and support, though bilateral axillary crutches may be used. Before allowing the patient to stand, measure and adjust the walker (refer to Chapter 9) for the patient, apply a safety belt, apply footwear, lock the bed, adjust the height of the bed slightly higher than its lowest position, and partially elevate the head of the bed to assist the patient to come to sitting before standing. Instruct the patient to move to the edge of the bed by using the upper extremities and the normal lower extremity to elevate the body. The patient should move toward the normal lower extremity to maintain the surgically replaced hip in abduction. The trunk should be maintained unaffected in no more than 60 degrees of flexion by semireclining on the arms, which are positioned behind the body. You should help to control the surgically replaced hip and its lower extremity and the trunk as the patient pivots and positions the lower extremities over the edge of bed. Instruct the patient to place the normal foot on the floor as you assist in lowering the surgically affected lower extremity to the floor. The patient maintains a semireclining position of the trunk by resting on the extended upper extremities, which are placed posterior to the hips. *Caution:* The patient may need to sit on the edge of the bed for a short time to avoid dizziness or syncope and to accommodate to being upright before standing. Do not allow the patient to sit unattended or unprotected.

Box 7-4 Precautions for Patients With a Total Hip Replacement

Maintain the surgically replaced hip slightly abducted from the midline of the body and in neutral rotation (patella and toes positioned toward ceiling) when the patient is supine. The hip should not be adducted beyond the midline of the body when the patient lies, sits, or stands.

Maintain the surgically replaced hip in neutral extension. The hip should not be extended beyond a midposition of flexion and extension.

Maintain hip abduction and neutral rotation while the patient is in a side-lying position on the unaffected hip by supporting the affected lower extremity on pillows, powder board, or a bolster. The affected extremity should be in the uppermost position.

Avoid external hip rotation when an anterior or anterolateral surgical approach was used.

Avoid internal hip rotation when a posterior or posterolateral surgical approach was used.

Avoid rotating or twisting the upper body with the lower extremity fixed or immobile (as when reaching for an object on a bedside stand while lying in bed); such activity indirectly causes hip rotation.

Avoid hip flexion beyond a range of 60 to 90 degrees when a posterior or posterolateral surgical approach was used. This means the patient should not sit erect in a wheelchair or in bed; bringing the trunk closer to the thigh produces hip flexion.

Avoid excessive trunk flexion while the patient is sitting; an elevated toilet seat and an elevated chair seat should be used for most patients.

Instruct the patient to push up from the bed, stand, and grasp the hand grips on the walker while you maintain control of the safety belt and shoulder. You may guard or stabilize the patient's normal foot so that it does not slide as the person rises. The patient maintains balance and takes time to accommodate to standing before ambulating. Monitor the pulse rate and ask the patient about any reaction to standing.

Instruct the patient to ambulate using a three-one pattern (refer to Chapter 9); instruct to turn by pivoting on the normal lower extremity and stepping around the normal lower extremity with the surgically affected lower extremity. (For example, a patient with a right hip replacement will be taught to turn toward the left.) These procedures are explained in Chapter 9. *Caution:* The patient must not pivot or twist the hip while standing on the surgically affected lower extremity.

Return to Bed Be certain the bed is locked and will not roll; elevate the bed so that it is slightly below the patient's buttocks. Instruct the patient to back toward the bed until the posterior area of the thigh of the normal lower extremity touches the edge of the mattress; the surgically affected lower extremity should remain slightly forward of the opposite lower extremity.

Instruct the patient to reach back to the mattress and shift the body weight onto the normal lower extremity while allowing the surgically affected lower extremity to slide forward. The patient sits on the edge of the bed in a semireclining position as you control the surgically affected lower extremity.

Instruct the patient to pivot toward the center of the bed, leading with the normal lower extremity and keeping the surgically replaced hip abducted. Assist in controlling the surgically affected lower extremity to maintain abduction and to limit flexion of the hip.

The patient uses the normal lower extremity and the upper extremities to shift the body toward the center of the bed, while you guide the surgically affected lower extremity, until a proper position is attained.

Note: Some patients may return to the center of the bed leading with the surgically affected lower extremity so that it moves in abduction. The position of the bed and the ability to have access to either side of the bed may dictate how the return-to-bed transfer is accomplished.

Standing Transfer; One Nonweight Bearing Lower Extremity

This transfer is described in Procedure 7-8.

Transfer from Wheelchair to Floor and Return

Initially the patient will need to be protected or guarded using the general guarding principles and techniques described previously. The activity should be practiced in an area free of hazards and mats may be placed on the floor to

PROCEDURE 7-8

Standing Transfer; One Nonweight Bearing Lower Extremity

Note: NWB, nonweight bearing; *FWB,* full weight bearing.

BED TO WHEELCHAIR

Position wheelchair at an angle on the side next to the hip of the FWB lower extremity, facing the foot of the bed; lock the chair and swing away the front rigging or elevate the foot plates.

Assist the patient to move to the edge of the mattress and sit up; apply a safety belt.

Position yourself in front of the patient to guard and protect; assist in moving the NWB extremity to the edge of the mattress. *Caution:* Avoid excessive hip flexion and adduction if the patient has had a total hip replacement.

Assist the patient to stand on the FWB lower extremity; assist in controlling or supporting the NWB lower extremity.

Instruct the patient to reach for and grasp the far armrest of the wheelchair and pivot on the FWB foot to position the hips in preparation to sit.

Instruct the patient to use the upper extremities and FWB lower extremity to slowly lower the body into the chair; maintain control and support of the NWB lower extremity.

Position the NWB lower extremity on an elevated legrest as necessary; place the other foot on the foot plate.

Position the patient for safety and comfort; remove the safety belt.

WHEELCHAIR TO BED

Position the wheelchair at an angle next to the bed, facing the foot of the bed and midway between the head and foot of the bed; either lower extremity can be nearest the bed. Lock the chair, swing away the front rigging, and apply a safety belt.

Assist the patient to move forward in the chair; maintain control of and support the NWB lower extremity. Position yourself in front of the patient to guard and protect throughout the transfer.

Instruct the patient to stand by pushing with the upper extremities and FWB lower extremity.

Instruct the person to pivot so that the buttocks are toward the bed. Control and support the NWB lower extremity as the patient sits on the edge of the mattress.

Assist in lifting the NWB lower extremity onto the mattress as the patient lifts the FWB lower extremity. *Caution:* Avoid excessive hip flexion and adduction if the patient has had a total hip replacement.

Instruct the patient to move toward the center of the mattress and lie down.

Position the patient for safety and comfort; remove the safety belt.

protect the patient. Some patients may benefit from the use of incremental steps or small platforms when they initially perform and practice this transfer. Eventually the patient should be taught how to move down to the floor and return to the chair without any additional equipment, to maximize independence.

Wheelchair to Floor: Strong Right Upper and Lower Extremities and Weak Left Upper and Lower Extremities Instruct the patient to position the caster wheels forward, lock the chair, remove the feet from the footrests, and remove or swing away the front rigging or elevate the footrests. The patient moves forward in the chair with the body pivoted or turned slightly so the right extremities are forwardmost (Fig. 7-27, A).

Instruct the patient to shift the weight onto the right lower extremity and to reach toward the floor with the right upper extremity (Fig. 7-27, *B*). When the right hand is on the floor, the patient uses the right upper and lower extremity to lower the body to the floor and sit on the right buttock (Fig. 7-27, C). The body position can be adjusted as desired.

Floor to Wheelchair: Strong Right Upper and Lower Extremities and Weak Left Upper and Lower Extremities Instruct the patient to sit on the right hip facing the locked wheelchair with its caster wheels forward. The lower extremities should be flexed at the hips and knees (Fig. 7-28, A).

Instruct the patient to reach to the back of the seat or the armrest and to pull up to a kneeling position. The patient moves to a half-kneeling position with the right foot forward and flat on the floor and kneeling on the left knee (Fig. 7-28, *B* and *C*). Instruct the patient to place the right upper extremity on the near armrest or on the seat of the chair. The patient uses the right extremities to push to a partial or full standing position facing the wheelchair (Fig. 7-28, *D*). *Note:* The caster wheels may pivot or turn to one side when the patient uses the chair for support. That movement does not cause a safety problem and the patient can continue to perform the transfer. However, the caster wheels should not be permitted to be directed backward during these transfers because that position reduces the stability of the chair. The patient should be informed and taught not to allow the caster wheels to be directed backward or a chair with caster wheel locks may be recommended.

Instruct the patient to reach for the far armrest with the right upper extremity and to pivot on the right lower extremity so the back is toward the chair. Then the patient lowers into the chair using the right extremities.

Wheelchair to Floor, Forward or Sideward: Strong Upper Extremities and Weak or Paralyzed Lower Extremities Instruct the patient to position the chair with the caster wheels forward, lock the chair, remove the feet from the footrests, and remove or swing away the front rigging. The patient moves to the front of the chair and the lower extremities are positioned to one side with the knees extended or flexed and positioned under the chair.

Instruct the patient to maintain one hand on the armrest or chair seat rail and to reach toward the floor with the other upper extremity while flexing the head and trunk (Fig. 7-29, A). After the hand has contacted the floor, the patient releases the grasp on the wheelchair and lowers onto the floor (Fig. 7-29, *B*). The patient repositions the body as desired.

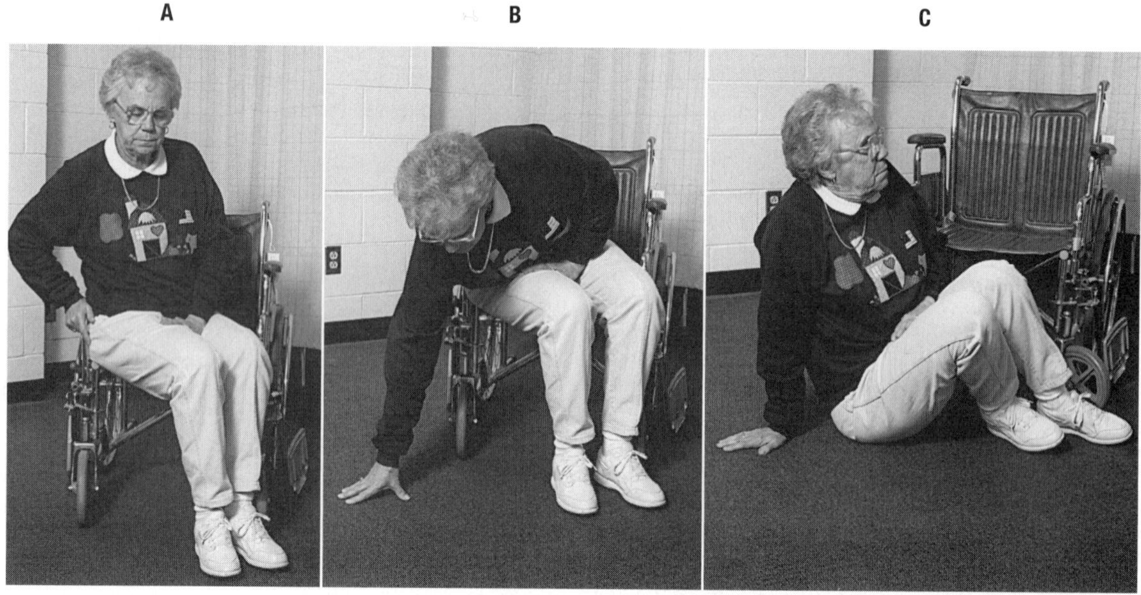

Fig. 7-27 Transfer from the wheelchair to the floor for a patient with strong right upper and lower extremities.

A

B

C

D

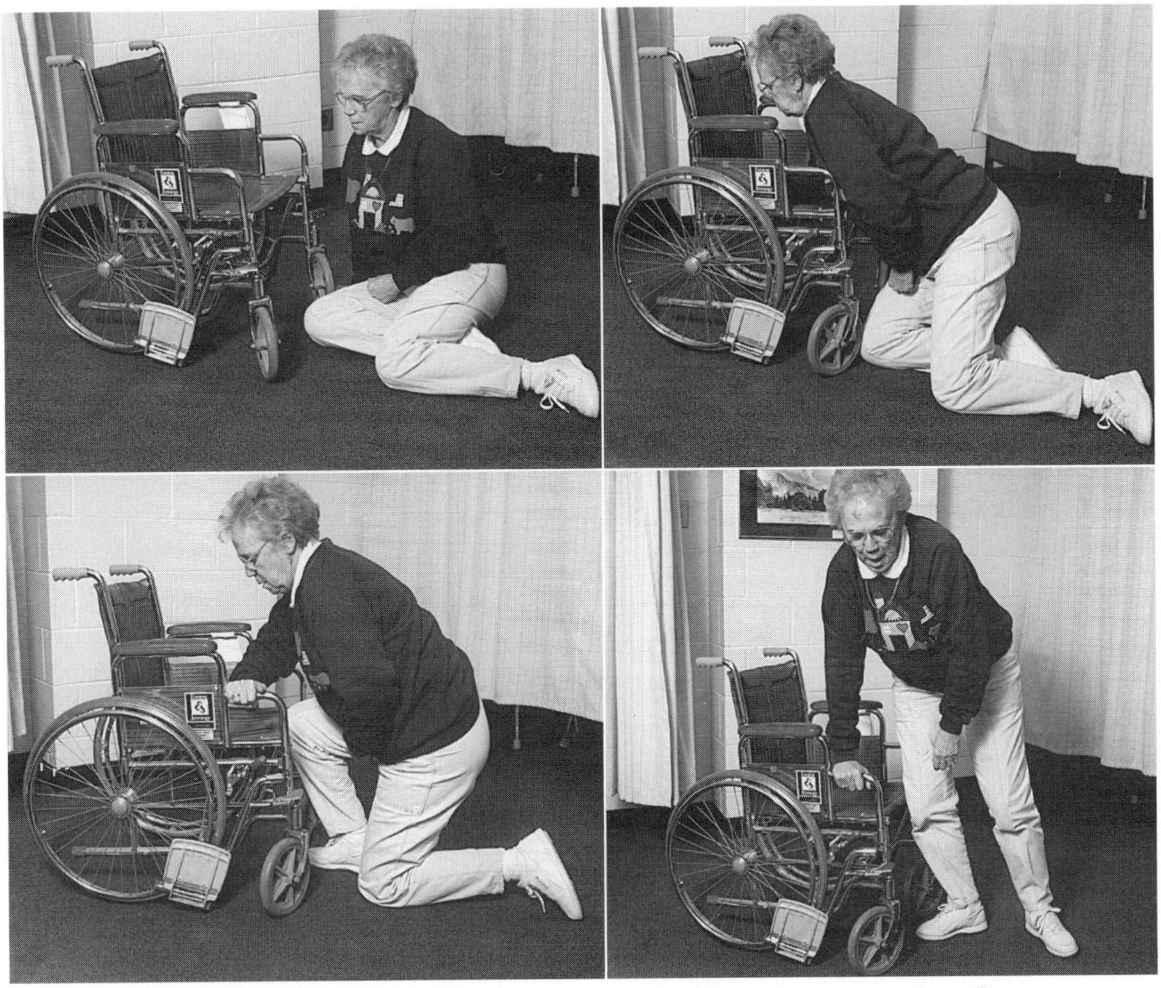

Fig. 7-28 Transfer from the floor to the wheelchair for a patient with strong right upper and lower extremities. *Note:* For transfers from the chair to the floor and return to the chair, the caster wheels will probably pivot or turn to one side when the patient uses the chair for support unless the wheels can be locked in the forward position. If the caster wheels pivot, there is no safety problem, and the patient can continue to perform the transfer. However, the patient should not allow the caster wheels to be directed backward because that position reduces the stability of the chair.

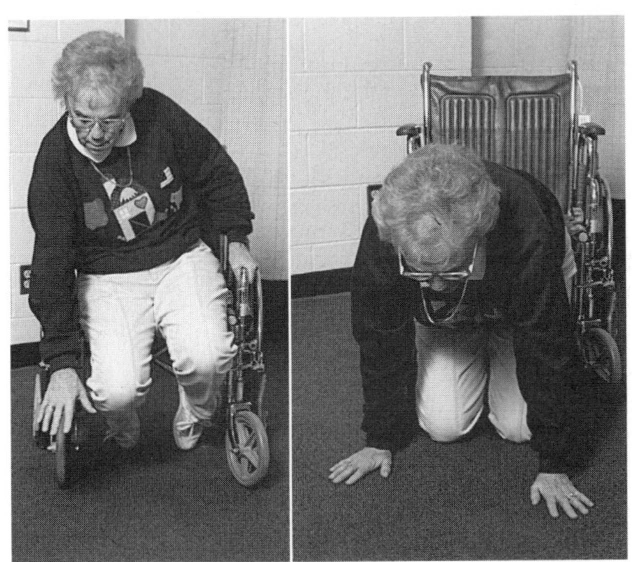

Fig. 7-29 Transfer from the wheelchair to the floor, forward, for a patient with strong upper extremities.

Floor to Wheelchair Forward: Push-Up, Strong Upper Extremities, Weak or Paralyzed Lower Extremities Instruct the patient to sit on one hip close to and facing the wheelchair with the hips and knees flexed (Fig. 7-30). The chair must be locked, the front rigging swung away, and the caster wheels positioned forward or turned to one side. Some patients may prefer to initiate this transfer from an all-fours position (that is, on hands and knees). Instruct the patient to move to the front of the chair and to place one hand on the armrest or on the seat (Fig. 7-30, *B*). The patient grasps the armrest or the seat of the chair and pulls to a high kneeling position and maintains balance (Fig. 7-30, C). Instruct the patient to grasp both armrests or to place one hand on the seat of the chair and one hand on the armrest and then to perform a push-up to elevate the hips above the seat level (Fig. 7-30, *D*). At the peak of the lift, the patient pivots so that one hip is over the seat and releases the innermost hand to lower one hip into the chair (Fig. 7-30, *E*). The patient repositions the hands on the armrests and performs a push-up to position the body in the chair (Fig. 7-30, *F*).

This method requires exceptional upper extremity strength and trunk control and the patient must have the ability to maintain balance while in a high kneeling and push-up position. However, this is a safe and secure method and many patients will be able to perform it efficiently.

Wheelchair to Floor Backward: Strong Upper Extremities, Weak or Paralyzed Lower Extremities Instruct the patient to position and prepare the wheelchair as described previously. Instruct the patient to move to the front of the chair, pivot onto the right or left side of the hip, and grasp the armrests. If sitting on the right side of the hip, the right hand grasps the left armrest and the left hand grasps the right armrest to rotate the upper body so the person now partially faces the back of the chair.

Instruct the patient to perform a partial push-up to clear the pelvis from the seat and then to use the upper extremities to lower onto the knees in a high kneeling position facing the front of the chair. Then instruct the patient to lower to a side-sitting position or onto all fours and then onto one hip.

This method is the reverse of moving from the floor to the chair forward. It requires exceptional upper extremity strength, trunk control, and balance and the patient must be flexible and agile. Some patients will be able to lift their buttocks onto the front edge of the chair seat using an initial push-up with one hand on the chair seat and one hand on the front rigging. The patient can reverse this method to move from the wheelchair to the floor.

Wheelchair to Floor Forward: Strong Upper Extremities, Weak or Paralyzed Lower Extremities Instruct the patient to position and prepare the wheelchair as described previously. The patient moves forward in the chair and positions the feet under the wheelchair by flexing the knees. The front rigging must be swung away or removed before the patient continues.

Instruct the patient to lean forward and to reach toward the floor with both upper extremities so the hands will contact the floor as he or she falls toward the floor onto all fours (see Fig. 7-29, A). Alternatively, the patient can reach forward with one hand and grasp an armrest with the other hand; when the first hand is on or close to the floor, the person releases the armrest and reaches toward the floor to be positioned on all fours. The patient can side sit or alter the body position as desired.

Alternative Method Instruct the patient to position and prepare the wheelchair as described previously, except one or both front riggings remain in place with the footrests elevated (Fig. 7-31, *A*). The patient moves forward in the chair and positions the lower extremities away from the chair with the knees extended. Instruct the patient to place one hand on the front rigging and one hand on the chair seat; then perform a push-up with the upper extremities to elevate the buttocks from the chair seat while extending the head and upper trunk (Fig. 7-31, *B*). The patient lowers the body to the floor with the buttocks between the footrests of the front rigging (Fig. 7-31, C). A patient with wide hips will need to swing away, but not remove, one front rigging to have sufficient space for the hips when they descend to the floor. (*Note:* This method is the reverse of moving from the floor to the wheelchair backward.) The patient must have excellent flexibility in the shoulders and maximal strength in the upper extremities to perform this technique.

Caution: Many inactive or paralyzed patients may have osteoporosis in their lower extremities and vertebral bodies. Some of these transfer methods may be unsafe for these patients because of the floor reaction force that the patient may experience when dropping onto the knees or hip. This force may be sufficient to cause a fracture in weakened bone. Therefore the patient may need to be assisted down to the floor to avoid injury.

The wheelchair-to-floor-and-return transfer methods described may be interchanged to meet the needs, strength, preference, flexibility, agility, balance, size, and skill of a given patient. For example, a patient may prefer or find it easier to transfer to the floor forward and return to the chair backward, or to transfer to the floor backward and return to the chair forward. The patient should be given the opportunity to attempt any of the methods to determine which is most suitable, safe, and efficient. Guard and assist the patient during practice sessions until the patient is able to perform the transfer independently with safety. A safety belt should be used and you should not use the patient's clothing or upper extremities to control or guard as these transfers are performed for the reasons cited elsewhere in this text.

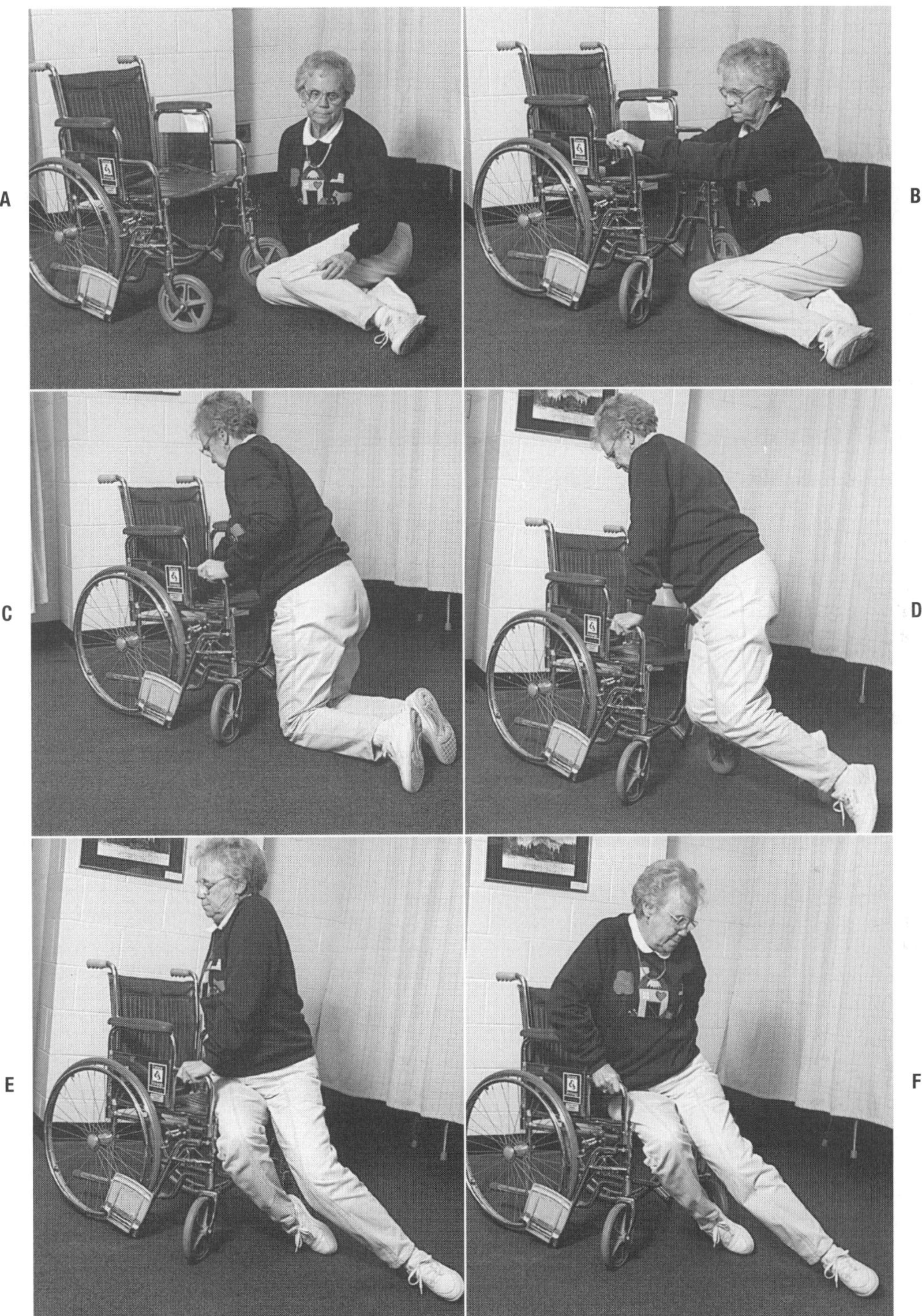

Fig. 7-30 Transfer from the floor to the wheelchair, forward push-up, for a patient with strong upper extremities. The procedure is reversed to move from the wheelchair to the floor. *Note:* The caster wheels may pivot during this transfer if they cannot be locked in a forward position. The transfer can be performed safely provided that the caster wheels do not pivot completely rearward.

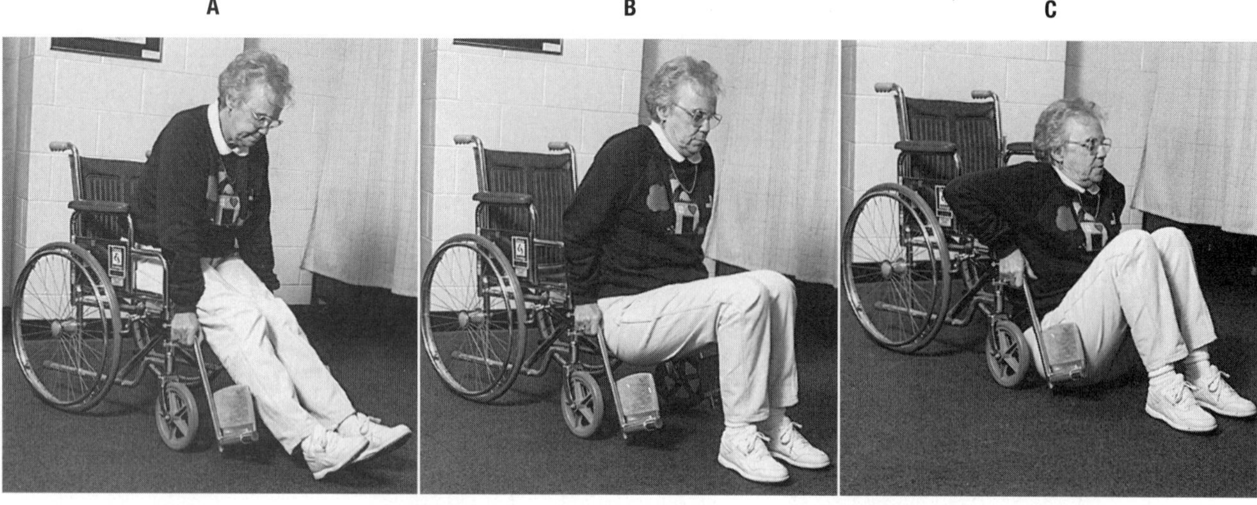

Fig. 7-31 Transfer from the wheelchair to the floor (alternative method). The procedure is reversed to move from the floor to the wheelchair.

SUMMARY

Transfer activities are necessary to alter a patient's position, move a patient from one surface to another, and promote independent functional activities. Some patients may require various amounts of assistance or may be dependent on other persons or mechanical equipment to perform or complete a transfer. Other patients will be able to accomplish their transfers without assistance or with only standby assistance. Transfers can be performed with the patient lying, standing, or sitting; some patients may need to be lifted by other persons or mechanical equipment. Regardless of the technique used, the caregiver must guard and protect the patient during all transfers. A safety belt should be used with all patients when they transfer until they can perform the transfer safely and independently.

The procedures or techniques used to assist or teach the patient will vary depending on the person's condition, abilities, and needs. The philosophy and preferences of the caregiver may also affect the way the transfer is taught or performed. The caregiver and patient may need to problem solve together to develop the most efficient and safest transfer technique. Observing other patients as they perform a specific transfer may assist the patient in understanding how to perform the transfer. Practicing the transfer and using the same technique consistently should improve the patient's skill and efficiency.

self-study ACTIVITIES

- Describe five different types of transfers.
- Explain the rationale for teaching a patient bed-mobility activities.
- Describe at least five specific precautions that should be followed when you are transferring a patient who has recently undergone a total hip replacement.
- Explain the wheelchair positions you might use for a standing and a sliding board transfer and indicate why these positions are necessary and important for the transfer.
- Demonstrate two different methods to move from a wheelchair to the floor and return for a person with lower extremity paralysis.
- Describe how you would reduce friction between a patient's body and the surface of the bed or mat, center the patient's weight, reduce the effects of gravity, and use gravity as an assistive force.

problem SOLVING

1. You are to assist a patient with right-sided *hemiplegia* to transfer from the bed to chair. What directions will you give the patient to assist you? What precautions should be performed before the transfer?
2. You are to move a patient status post abdominal exploratory surgery from a bed to a stretcher. Explain to the patient the procedure and give directions for the other two caregivers who will assist you.

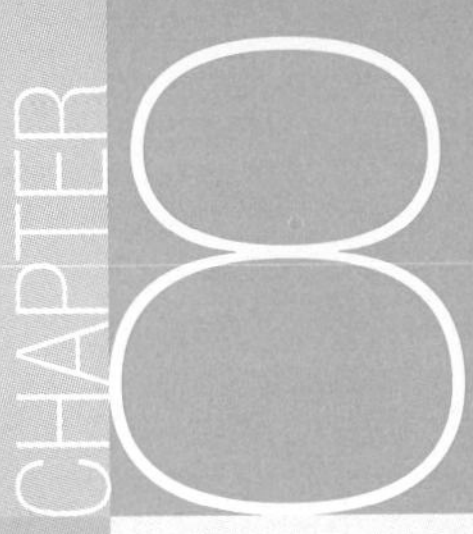

Wheelchair Features and Activities

objectives *After studying this chapter, the reader will be able to:*

- List the standard measurements for an adult wheelchair.
- Measure a patient for a wheelchair and confirm the fit of the chair.
- Teach a person to propel a wheelchair using both upper extremities or one upper extremity and one lower extremity.
- Name the components of a standard wheelchair and describe the purpose of each.
- Teach a wheelchair user various functional activities.
- Perform various wheelchair functional activities with a person in the chair by providing assistance.

key terms

Condyle A rounded projection on a bone.
Crash bar The metal bar on a door that disengages the door latch when it is pushed.
Descend To go down; proceed from a higher to a lower level.
Femoral Pertaining to the femur (thigh bone).
Independent Able to function or perform without assistance from another.
Locomotion The ability to move from one place to another.
Pedal Pertaining to the foot or feet.
Pneumatic Of or containing air or gases.
Popliteal Pertaining to the area behind the knee.
Propulsion The act of propelling; movement of a wheelchair by the person in the chair or by another person.
Restraint The forcible confinement or restriction of movement of a person through the use of belts, straps, or other similar items.
Self-closing device A device attached to a door that closes the door through the use of compressed fluid or air.
Semipneumatic Partially containing air or gases.

INTRODUCTION

Persons who use a wheelchair as their primary mode of mobility should have a chair that fits properly to provide maximum function, comfort, stability, safety, and protection of body structures. The initial measurement and subsequent confirmation of fit must be done carefully. Information about special seating needs, chairs designed for special activities (such as chairs for recreation or sports participation), or chairs designed to fulfill special patient needs is not presented. However, it may be important to consider whether the person will require a cushion, a reclining back, an elevating or swing-away front rigging (leg rests), adjustable armrests, or other similar adaptations.

The type of wheelchair selected and its components will depend on the patient's disability, functional ability, size, weight, and functional needs or activities; the expected use of the chair; and the prognosis for change in the patient's condition. Proper fit of the chair becomes more important if the patient has decreased sensory awareness; limited ability to alter a position; decreased subcutaneous soft tissue,

Table 8-1 Types of Wheelchairs

Type	Description
Standard adult	Designed for persons who weigh less that 200 pounds and for limited use on rough surfaces or for vigorous functional activities.
Heavy-duty adult	Constructed for persons weighing more than 200 pounds or those who perform vigorous functional activities.
Intermediate or junior	Designed for persons with a body build smaller than an adult but larger than a child.
Growing	Designed to permit adjustments in the frame to accommodate the growth of the user.
Child or youth	Designed for persons up to the approximate age of 6 years.
Indoor	Constructed for use indoors, with the larger drive wheels placed at the front of the chair and the caster wheels at the rear. It functions better in confined areas but is more difficult to propel or for the user to perform many functional activities.
"Hemiplegic"	The seat is lowered approximately 2 inches to allow better use of the user's lower extremities to propel the chair; however, the lower seat may make it more difficult for the user to perform a standing transfer.
Amputee	The rear wheel axles are positioned approximately 2 inches posterior to their normal position to widen the base of support of the chair and compensate for the loss of the weight of the user's lower extremities.
One-hand drive	Two handrims are fabricated on one drive wheel, and the two drive wheels are connected by a linkage bar. The smaller handrim propels the near drive wheel; the large handrim propels the far drive wheel; and when both rims are moved simultaneously, both wheels are propelled.
Externally powered	The chair is propelled by a deep-cycle battery system, and there are various types of controls to operate the chair (such as joystick, chin piece, or mouth stick).
Sports	A low-profile chair with features such as a low back, canted rear wheels, small handrims, and adjustable axles. It can be used for various sports activities, and some users prefer the type of chair for day-to-day activities.
Reclining	Used for persons who need to partially or fully recline at some time when they are in the chair. The chair may be a semireclining or fully reclining chair. Semireclining chairs recline to approximately 30 degrees from vertical, and fully reclining chairs can recline to a horizontal position. Elevating leg rests and headrest extensions are necessary components for these chairs.

Table 8-2 Standard Wheelchair Measurements for Proper Fit

Measurement	Instructions	Average Adult Size
Seat height/leg length	Measure from the user's heel to the popliteal fold and add 2 inches to allow clearance of the footrest.	19.5 to 20.5 inches
Seat depth	Measure from the user's posterior buttock, along the lateral thigh, to the popliteal fold; then subtract approximately 2 inches to avoid pressure from the front edge of the seat against the popliteal space.	16 inches
Seat width	Measure the widest aspect of the user's buttocks, hips, or thighs and add approximately 2 inches. This will provide space for bulky clothing, orthoses, or clearance of the trochanters from the armrest side panel.	18 inches
Back height	Measure from the seat of the chair to the floor of the axilla with the user's shoulder flexed to 90 degrees and then subtract approximately 4 inches. This will allow the final back height to be below the inferior angles of the scapulae. (*Note:* This measurement will be affected if a seat cushion is to be used. The person should be measured while seated on the cushion or the thickness of the cushion must be considered by adding that value to the actual measurement.)	16 to 16.5 inches
Armrest height	Measure from the seat of the chair to the olecranon process with the user's elbow flexed to 90 degrees and then add approximately 1 inch. (*Note:* This measurement will be affected if a seat cushion is to be used. The person should be measured while seated on the cushion or the thickness of the cushion must be considered by adding that value to the actual measurement.)	9 inches above the chair seat

Box 8-1 Factors Associated with the Selection of a Wheelchair Type and Components

Patient's disability and functional ability
Patient's age, size, stature, and weight
Expected use or patient needs of the wheelchair (such as indoors, outdoors, recreation, transfer needs, ability to transport the chair)
Temporary versus permanent use of the wheelchair
Potential or prognosis for change in the patient's condition, especially as it affects mobility
Mental and physical condition or capacity of the patient

especially over bony prominences; impaired peripheral circulation in the lower extremities; abnormal skin integrity or condition; or if the chair is required for use for extended periods. Any of these factors individually or in combination could cause a serious secondary problem or complication for the patient (Box 8-1).

There are several wheelchair types and designs (Table 8-1). The more common or frequently prescribed types are described briefly. Product and accessory catalogs can be obtained from the manufacturers of wheelchairs. These catalogs will contain information about the styles and types of wheelchairs each company manufactures.

STANDARD WHEELCHAIR MEASUREMENTS

The initial measurements should be made with the user seated on a firm, flat surface such as a wood chair or on a piece of plywood placed on a mat platform. The user should wear clothing similar to the clothing usually worn. The person should sit with the trunk erect in a comfortable position and posture. If a seat cushion or backrest (such as a cushion or posture panel) is going to be used, it should be in place when the measurements are made. A tape measure that can be read easily is recommended for measurements (Table 8-2).

The patient's age, weight, disability, or condition; the expected use of the chair; the functional and recreational activities to be performed; and specific features such as adjustable armrests, desk arms, reclining back, swing-away front rigging, elevating leg rests, and caster wheel locks should be specified when the chair is ordered.

CONFIRMATION OF FIT

The fit of a wheelchair should be determined with the user seated in the wheelchair and wearing usual clothing, including shoes. Any cushions or other components that would affect the fit should be in place. The importance of proper fit of the chair must be assured to enable the user to attain maximal comfort, stability, function, and safety. You should be able to confirm the fit of the wheelchair within approximately 1 to 2 minutes.

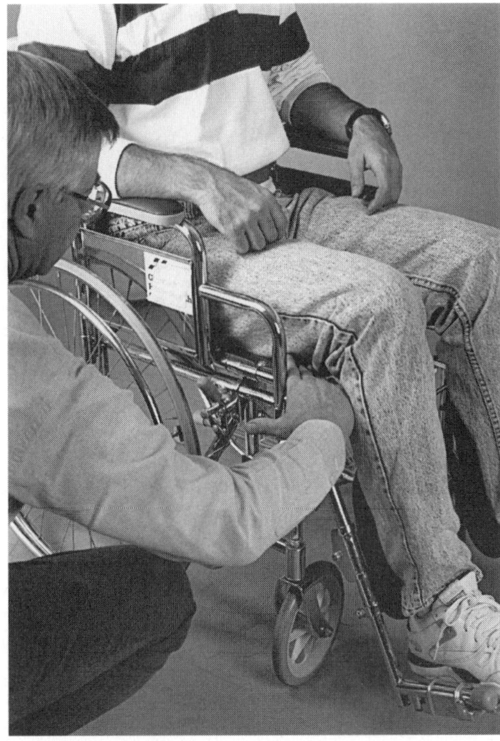

FIG. 8-1 Proper fit allows two or three fingers to be placed under the thigh from the front seat edge.

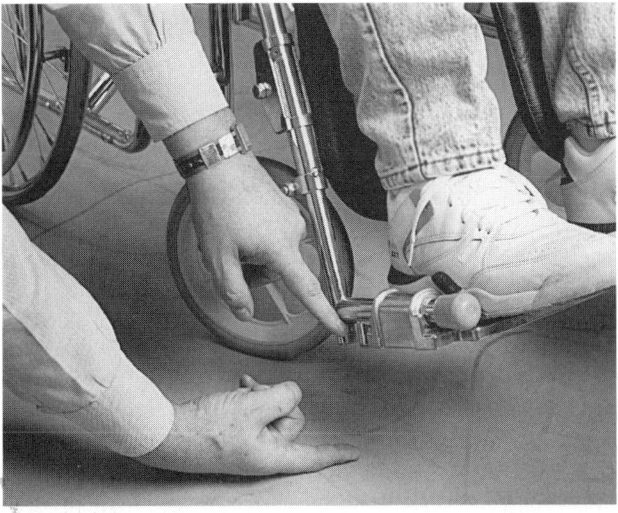

FIG. 8-2 The footrest must be at least 2 inches from the floor.

METHODS TO EVALUATE THE FIT

Seat Height and Leg Length Proper fit will allow you to place two or three fingers easily under the thigh from the front edge of the seat to a depth of approximately 2 inches (Fig. 8-1). The bottom of the footrest must be at least 2 inches from the floor with the chair on a level surface when this evaluation is performed (Fig. 8-2). The 2 inches provide adequate

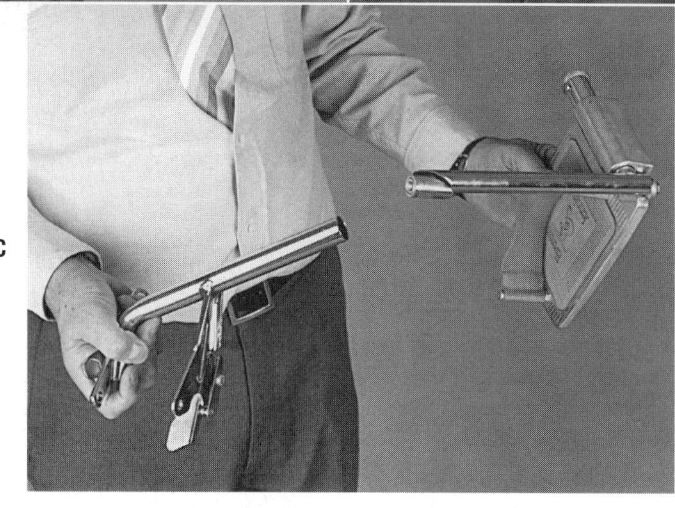

FIG. 8-3 The footrest can be adjusted for proper fit.

distance from the bottom of the footplate to the floor so the chair can be maneuvered easily and safely on most surfaces. The footplate can be adjusted to the proper position by means of the adjusting bolt or nut located at the bottom of the shaft of the front rigging (Fig. 8-3).

Seat Depth Proper fit will allow three or four fingers to be placed between the front edge of the seat and the user's *popliteal* fold with your palm horizontal to the seat. It is important the person is seated well back in the chair with the posterior area of the pelvis in contact with the seat back when this component is evaluated. If the person is not positioned back in the chair, the seat will appear to be too short, and there may not be sufficient support for the thighs (Fig. 8-4).

Seat Width Proper fit will allow the placement of your hand between the user's trochanter, hip, or thigh and the armrest panels with your hand positioned vertically to the seat. Your hand should be in slight contact with the user and the armrest panel when the user is seated in the center of the seat. Both hands should be used, one hand on the side of each hip, to assure there is sufficient space between each hip and each armrest panel when the user is in the center of the seat (Fig. 8-5).

Back Height Proper fit for a standard seat back will allow you to place four fingers, with your hand held vertically, between the top of the back upholstery and the floor of the user's axilla. The inferior angles of the scapulae should be positioned approximately one fingerbreadth above the back upholstery when the user sits with an erect posture (Fig. 8-6).

Armrest Height The user should be able to sit with the trunk erect and the shoulders level when bearing weight on the forearms as they rest on the armrest (Fig. 8-7). While the user is in this position, a triangle should be formed by the

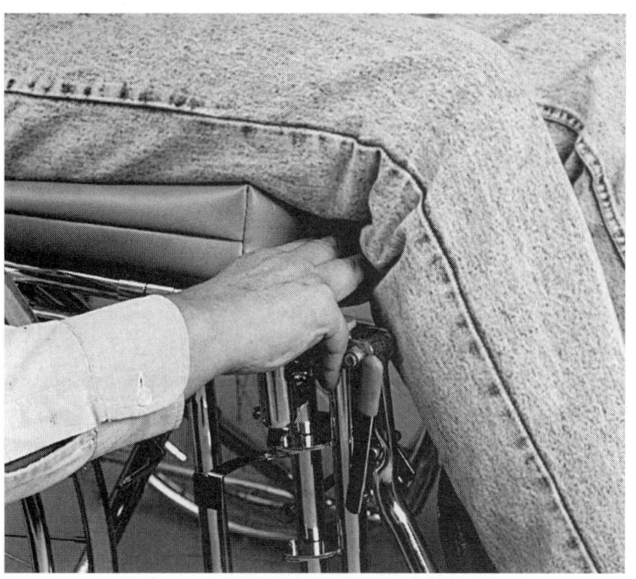

FIG. 8-4 Proper fit of seat depth.

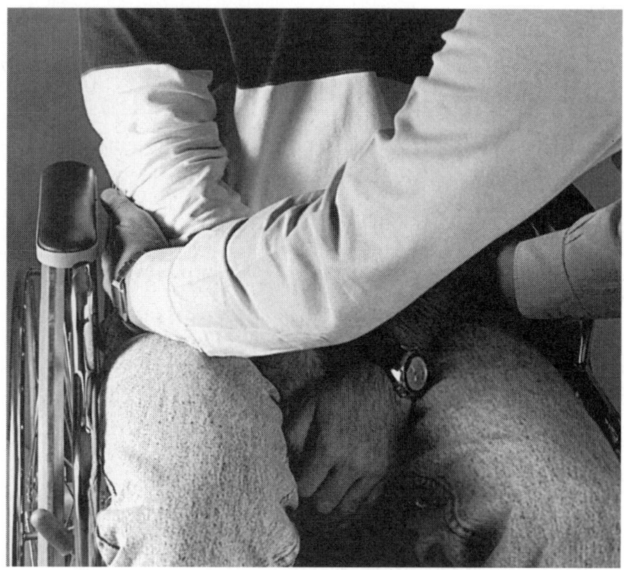

FIG. 8-5 Proper fit of seat width.

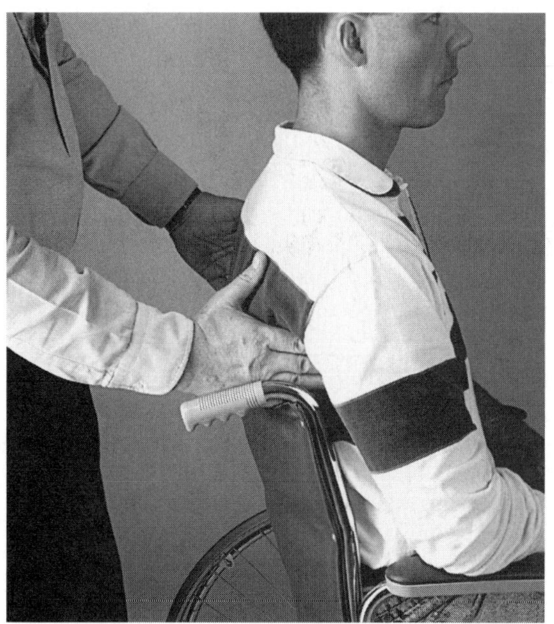

FIG. 8-6 Proper fit of back height.

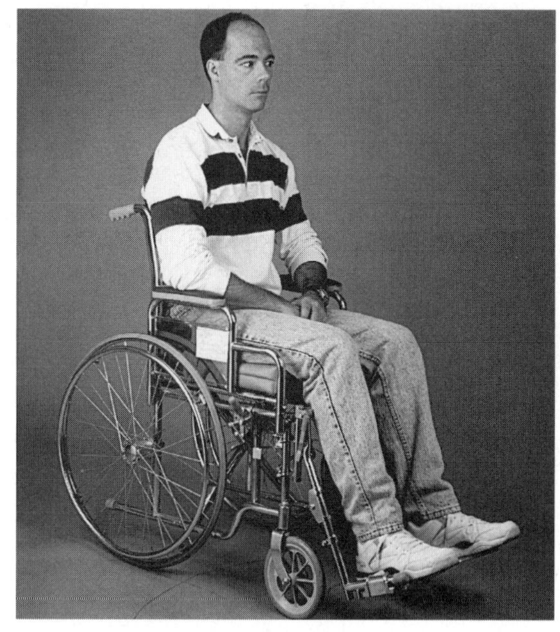

FIG. 8-7 Proper fit of armrest height.

PROCEDURE 8-1

Wheelchair Fit Confirmation

The chair should be on a level, smooth surface and the patient must sit erect with the pelvis in contact with the back upholstery.

SEAT HEIGHT AND LEG LENGTH

With your hand parallel to the floor, you should be able to insert two or three fingers lengthwise between the posterior area of the patient's thigh and the seat upholstery to a depth of approximately 2 inches.

The bottom of the footplate must be at least 2 inches above the floor.

SEAT DEPTH

With your hand parallel to the floor, you should be able to place the width of three or four fingers between the front edge of the seat and the popliteal fold.

SEAT WIDTH

With your hands vertical to the floor, you should be able to slide each hand between the patient's hips and the clothing guard of the chair with minimal contact.

BACK HEIGHT

With your hand vertical to the floor, you should be able to place the width of four fingers between the top of the back upholstery and the floor of the axilla.

ARMREST HEIGHT

Observe the angle made by the posterior aspect of the upper arm and the back post when the elbows rest on the armrest approximately 4 inches in front of the back post.

Observe the position of the shoulders; they should be level.

Observe the position of the trunk; it should be erect.

posterior aspect of the user's humerus, the top of the armrest, and the frame of the chair back (Procedure 8-1).

POTENTIAL ADVERSE EFFECTS OF IMPROPER FIT

Although there may be deviations in the proper fit that do not cause a problem for the patient, some deviations may cause or create serious problems. Thus each component of the fit must be evaluated to ensure that comfort, security, stability, and safety are maintained. By observing the user when maneuvering the wheelchair or performing functional activities, you may be able to detect problems associated with the fit of the chair.

Seat Height If the seat is too high, the user may experience insufficient trunk support because the back upholstery will be too low; difficulty positioning the knees beneath a table or desk because they are too high; difficulty propelling the wheelchair because of the difficulty reaching the handrims on the drive wheels; or poor posture when the forearms rest on the armrests.

If the seat is too low, the user may experience difficulty performing a standing or lateral swing type of transfer because the center of gravity (COG) is lowered, making it difficult to elevate the body, and may cause improper weight distribution. If the footplates are lowered to compensate for the low seat, they may contact objects on the floor or ground, leading to decreased mobility and unsafe use of the chair.

Seat Depth If the seat is too short from the front to the back, the user may experience decreased trunk stability because there will be less support under the thighs; increased weight bearing on the ischial tuberosities because the body weight will be shifted posteriorly because of the lack of support to the thighs; or poor balance because the base of support (BOS) has been reduced.

If the seat is too long from the front to the back, the user may experience increased pressure in the popliteal area, leading to skin discomfort or compromise of circulation because the seat upholstery is longer than the thighs.

Seat Width If the seat is too wide, the user may experience difficulty propelling the chair when using the upper extremities because the distance to the handrims is increased; difficulty performing a standing or lateral swing type of transfer because the distance between the armrests is increased and the user will have to move the body over a greater distance; difficulty moving through narrow hallways or doorways or using public restroom facilities because the overall width of the chair is increased; or postural deviations because it may be necessary to lean to one side of the chair for support.

If the seat is too narrow, the person may experience difficulty changing position because there is not sufficient space to adjust a position; excessive pressure to the greater trochanters because they are likely to contact the armrest panel; and difficulty wearing bulky outer garments, orthoses, or braces because there will not be sufficient space for the object to fit between the user's hip or thigh and the armrest panel.

Back Height If the back is too high, the user may experience difficulty propelling the chair because it will be more difficult to use the arms comfortably; excessive irritation to the skin over the inferior angles of the scapulae may occur as they rub against the upholstery; or difficulty with balance because the trunk may be inclined forward by the high back.

If the back is too low, the user may experience decreased trunk stability or postural deviations because there will be less support from the chair back. (*Note:* The current trend in many wheelchair styles is to have a low back to maximize function, as in Fig. 8-8. However, many patients may require and desire the traditional higher back for safety, stability, and support.)

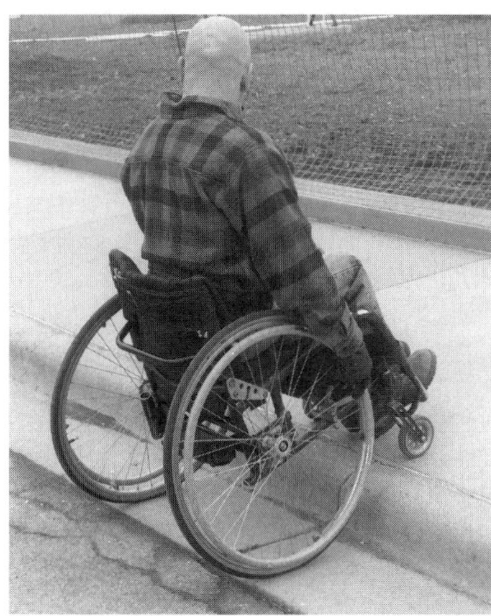

FIG. 8-8 Wheelchair with low back height.

Armrest Height If the armrest is too high, the user may experience difficulty propelling the chair because it will be difficult to reach over the high armrest to grasp the handrims; difficulty performing a standing transfer because the armrest height will require the arms to be positioned in a poor functional position to push to stand; postural deviation as a result of elevated shoulders when resting the forearms on the armrest; or limited use of the armrests caused by discomfort when trying to use them, leading to decreased trunk stability and fatigue.

If the armrest is too low, the user may experience poor posture or back discomfort caused by excessive forward trunk inclination when leaning forward to place the forearms on the armrest; less efficient respiration because of the decreased function of the diaphragm when leaning forward; inadequate balance; or difficulty rising to stand from the chair because the armrests are too low to offer support when pushing to a standing position.

Leg Length If the footplates are too low, the user may experience increased pressure to the distal posterior aspect of the thigh and decreased function and unsafe mobility because of lack of sufficient clearance of the footplate from the floor or ground surface.

If the footplates are too high, the user may experience increased pressure to the ischial tuberosities, difficulty positioning the chair beneath a table or desk, or decreased trunk stability caused by lack of support by the posterior area of the thighs.

PATIENT AND FAMILY EDUCATION

The wheelchair user and the family should be educated to inspect the skin after periods of prolonged sitting. Inspection of the skin that overlies bony prominences such as the vertebral spinous processes, inferior angles of the scapulae, ischial tuberosities, greater trochanters, lateral *femoral condyles*, sacrum, and medial humeral epicondyles is particularly important. Instructions should be given to the patient, family, or personal care attendant so each person will know how and when to relieve weight bearing. The importance of pressure relief must be emphasized and compliance with a relief schedule or program should be encouraged. Some users will need to perform several sitting push-ups each hour and some will need to elevate one buttock at a time by leaning to one side several times each hour they are in the wheelchair to relieve pressure from the ischial tuberosities. Other patients will need to adjust their position by shifting the trunk forward, backward, or to each side several times each hour they are in the chair. Some users may have to be removed from the chair after sitting for 1 to 4 hours or lifted briefly from the seat by another person several times per hour. The user and the family member should be informed that sitting on a cushion or pillow does not eliminate the need to relieve pressure on the buttocks frequently by any of the methods described.

The patient and family should be instructed to observe signs or symptoms of decreased circulation in the lower extremities. Ankle edema; color changes in the toes, feet, or legs; decreased sensory response to surface stimuli; loss of hair follicles; or other similar observations that cannot be explained or are not associated with the person's illness or condition should be reported to a physician. If any of these signs or symptoms occur, it may be necessary to reduce the amount of time the person sits in the wheelchair. Prevention of a severe secondary problem is extremely important and should supersede the user's desire to sit in the wheelchair. Evaluation of the femoral, popliteal, and *pedal* pulses and observation of the legs should be performed frequently. Evidence of venous stasis or ischemic skin (such as dark skin over the malleolus) and soft-tissue ulcers should be reported to a physician. These activities are particularly important to perform for the person whose illness or condition may lead to circulatory changes, such as the person with a spinal cord injury, diabetes mellitus, a kidney disorder, or who uses nicotine or alcohol excessively.

WHEELCHAIR COMPONENTS AND FEATURES

There are several styles and types of wheelchairs with similar features, but the operation of these features may vary. The more common features and their operation are described and some are illustrated in this section. The components or features that are appropriate and necessary for one patient may be unnecessary or inappropriate for another patient. Decisions about the components and features selected for a patient's chair will depend on the criteria described previously. (See Fig. 8-30, p. 187, which illustrates the major components of a standard wheelchair and provides the nomenclature of these components.)

Wheel Locks

Toggle Lock Forward movement of the lever engages the lock and backward movement of the lever disengages it (Fig. 8-9). The lock should be engaged before any transfer to stabilize the chair and add to patient safety, but persons who become very proficient with the performance of a transfer may not engage the locks before a transfer. The device should not be used as a brake to stop the chair or to retard the motion of the chair, as when ascending or *descending* an incline. A special device can be added to the wheelchair to slow the chair's motion when the user ascends or descends an incline (Fig. 8-10).

A vertical extension can be attached to the lock to assist persons with poor trunk control or limited function of an upper extremity to operate the lock without leaning or reaching excessively (Fig. 8-11).

Z or Scissors Lock The Z lock is located beneath the chair seat (Fig. 8-12) toward the front of the seat rail. The wheelchair user must be able to reach under the seat to operate the lock. Because of the location, *propulsion* of the chair can be performed without interference from a lock positioned on the side of the seat rail and in front of the drive wheel.

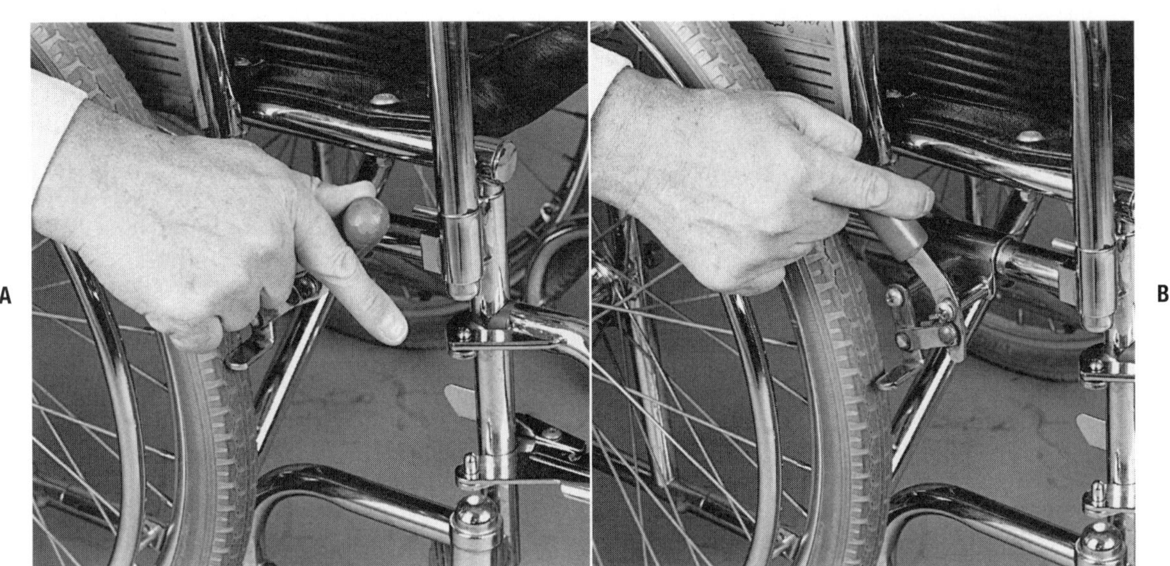

FIG. 8-9 Toggle lock for the wheels. **A,** Moving the lever forward engages the lock; **B,** moving it backward disengages the lock.

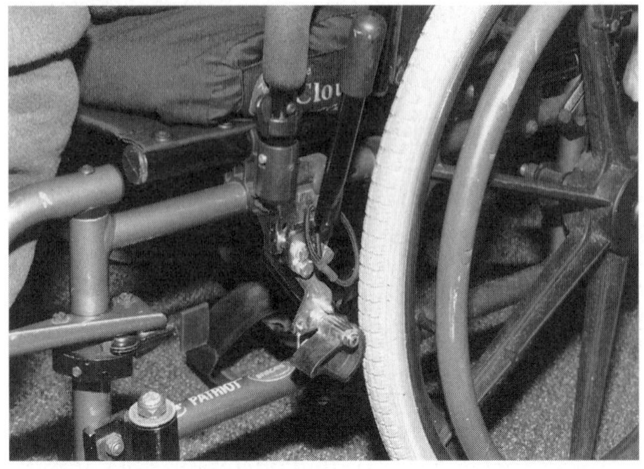

FIG. 8-10 Accessory to retard speed of the wheelchair when on a ramp or incline.

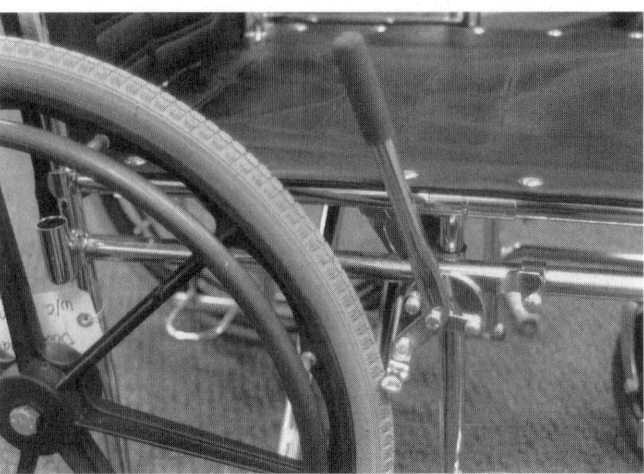

FIG. 8-11 Toggle lock extension.

Auxiliary Lock for a Reclining Back Chair An auxiliary lock is necessary to release the back and to increase the wheelbase when the back is reclined. An attendant is needed to engage and disengage the lock, unless a custom electric wheelchair with a reclining back system is used (Fig. 8-13).

Caster Locks Caster locks are used to lock the caster wheels before a transfer. Usually, these locks have a pin or small flat metal bar that engages a hole or notch located in a metal ring attached to the caster wheel. This is an optional item for most wheelchairs.

Body Restraints

Lap (Waist) Belt The lap belt (that is, *restraint*), attached to the frame of the chair, is designed to prevent the user from falling out of the chair. As the name implies, this strap crosses the user's lower abdomen or pelvis, similar to an airplane or automobile lap belt. The buckle may be located in back of the chair to prevent patient access to it.

Chest Belt The chest belt is attached to the frame of the chair at midchest level to increase trunk stability, prevent the user from falling out of the chair, and maintain the body upright. It may be combined with a lap belt for greater security. The buckle may be located in the back of the chair to prevent patient access (Fig. 8-14).

(*Note:* These belts are provided to protect the patient who has inadequate balance or trunk stability while seated. They are not appropriate for use as a method to restrain a patient in the chair for a prolonged time. Federal, state, and accrediting agency regulations and guidelines regarding the use of belts or straps as restraints must be followed.)

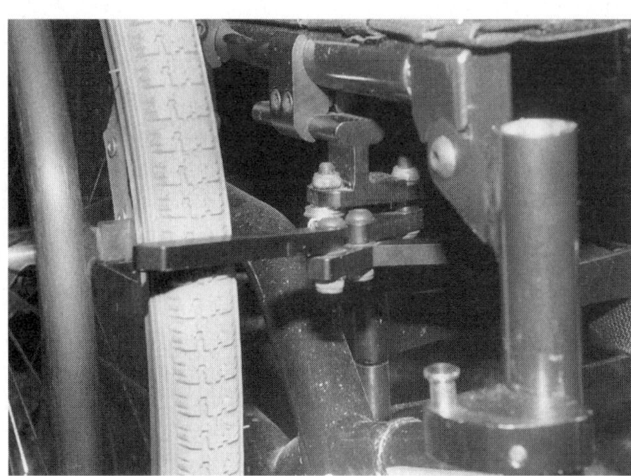

FIG. 8-12 Z or scissors lock.

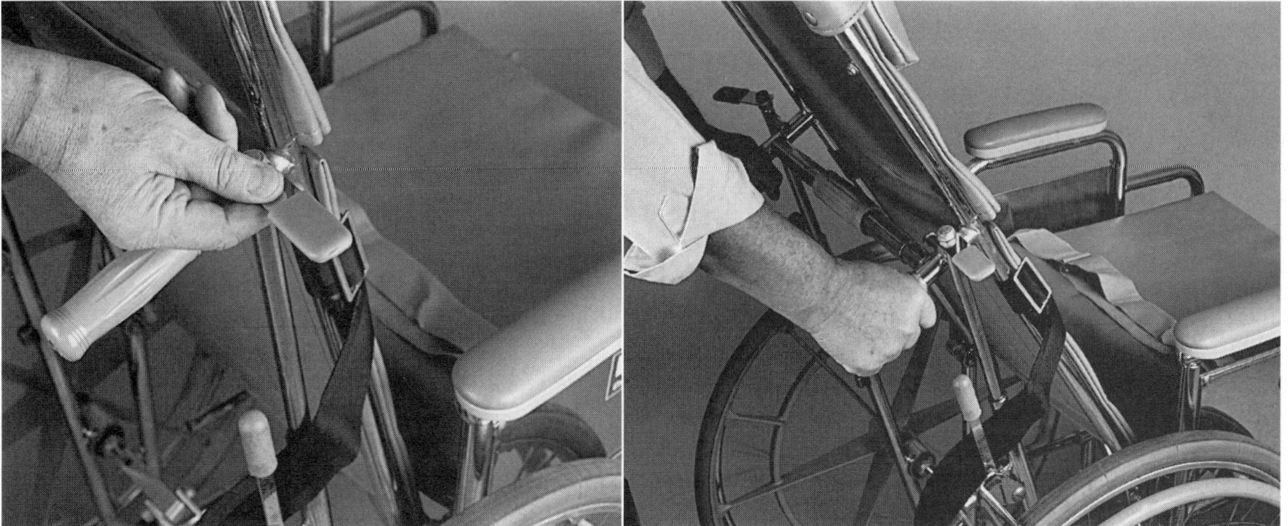

FIG. 8-13 Auxiliary lock for the back of a reclining wheelchair.

Wheels and Tires

Caster Wheels Caster wheels are usually located at the front of the chair to permit changes of direction and turns. They are usually 5 or 8 inches in diameter and may have solid rubber, *pneumatic* (air-filled), or *semipneumatic* (partially air-filled) tires (Fig. 8-15). Pneumatic or semipneumatic tires provide a smoother, more comfortable ride and function better on rough and soft surfaces such as sand, gravel, and grass, but they may require greater energy expenditure by the user to propel the chair because they are wider than solid tires and create more friction.

Drive or Rear Wheels Drive wheels are used to propel the chair. They may have solid rubber, semipneumatic, or pneumatic tires (Fig. 8-16). Some pneumatic tires are manufactured to specifically reduce or prevent the occurrence of a flat tire. The handrim may be molded to the wheel rim or separated from the rim. In addition, the handrim may have verti-

A

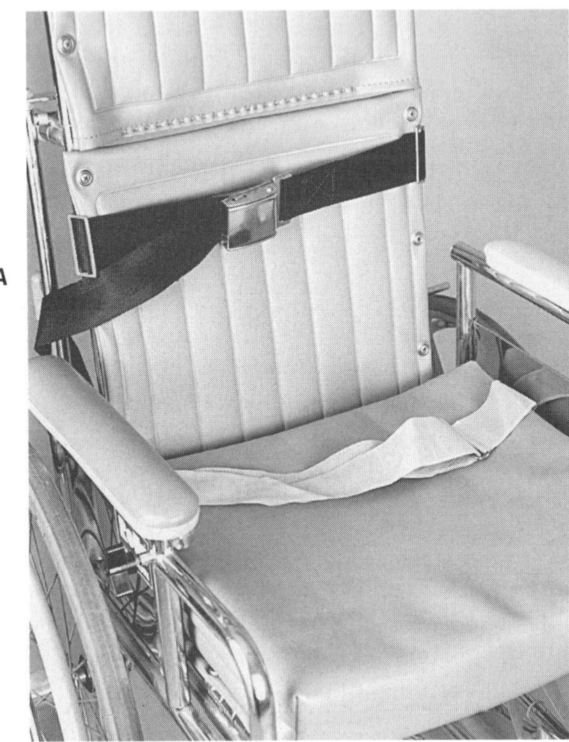

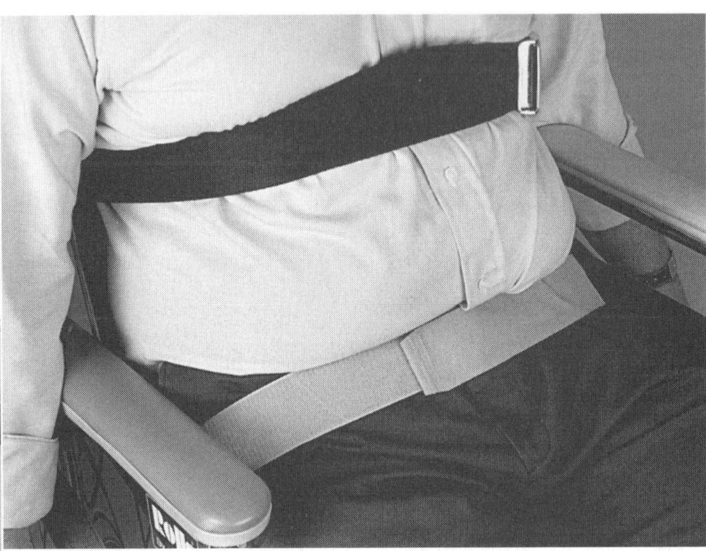

B

FIG. 8-14 Lap and chest belts of a wheelchair.

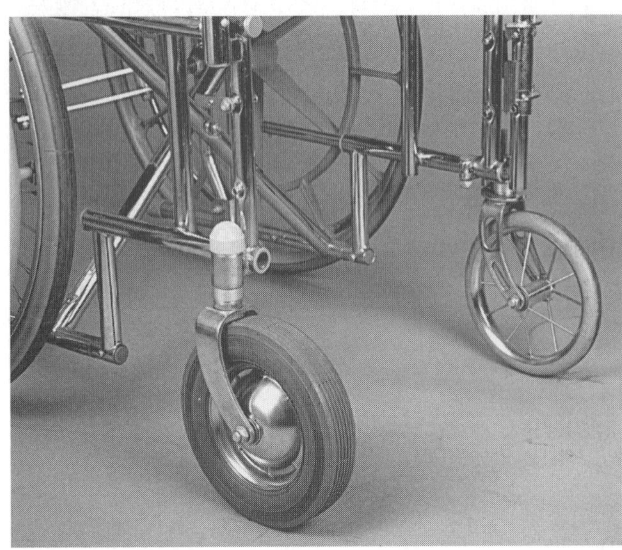

FIG. 8-15 Caster wheels of a wheelchair.

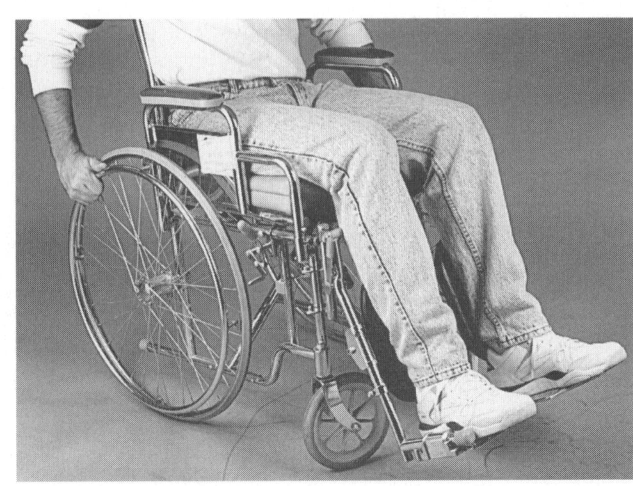

FIG. 8-16 Drive wheels of a wheelchair.

cal, horizontal, or angled projections, or it may be coated with plastic to enable the user to propel the chair with greater ease when there is decreased hand function.

One-Arm-Drive Chair The one-arm-drive chair may be used for *independent* propulsion when the user has only one functional upper extremity and no functional lower extremities. Two handrims are attached to the same wheel (Fig. 8-17, A). The outer, larger rim propels the far-drive wheel and the inner, smaller rim propels the near-drive wheel. When the user grasps and moves both handrims simultaneously, the chair is propelled in a straight line forward or backward (Fig. 8-17, *B*). Use of one handrim independently causes the chair to turn. A linkage bar connects the two drive wheels (Fig. 8-17, C). This chair is heavier than a standard chair and more difficult to fold.

Armrests

Fixed Armrests Fixed armrests are permanently attached to the chair frame. They are recommended for users who will be performing standing transfers and have no need to remove the armrest.

Removable or Reversible Armrests Removable or reversible armrests are recommended for users who will perform a lateral swinging or sliding transfer in a sitting posture. The armrest can be reversed to temporarily narrow the distance between the armrest panels and is usually secured to the frame by a pin-in-hole lock (Fig. 8-18).

Desk or Cut-Out Armrests Desk armrests are recommended for persons who desire to position the wheelchair close to a permanent surface such as a desk, table, or countertop.

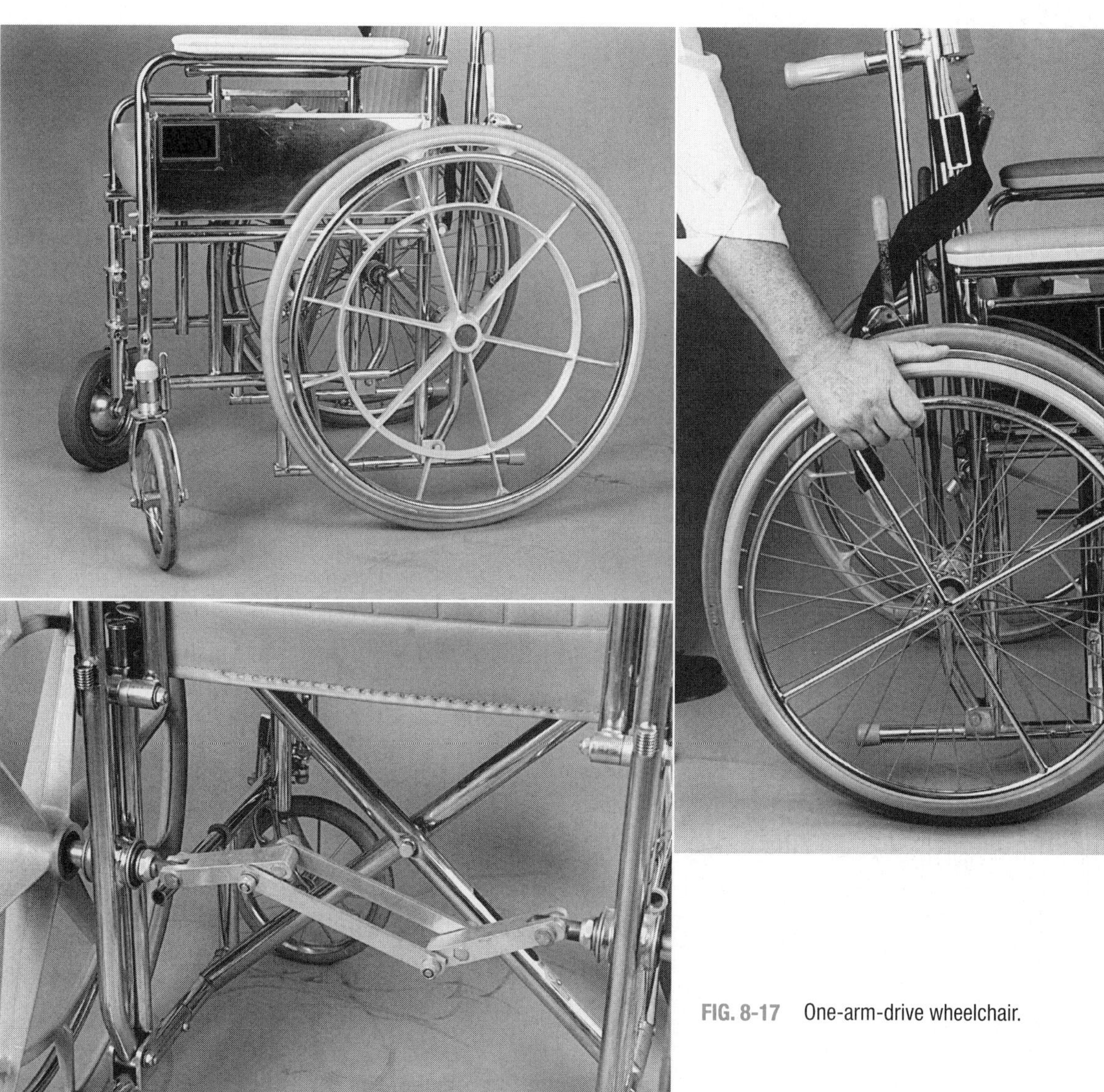

FIG. 8-17 One-arm-drive wheelchair.

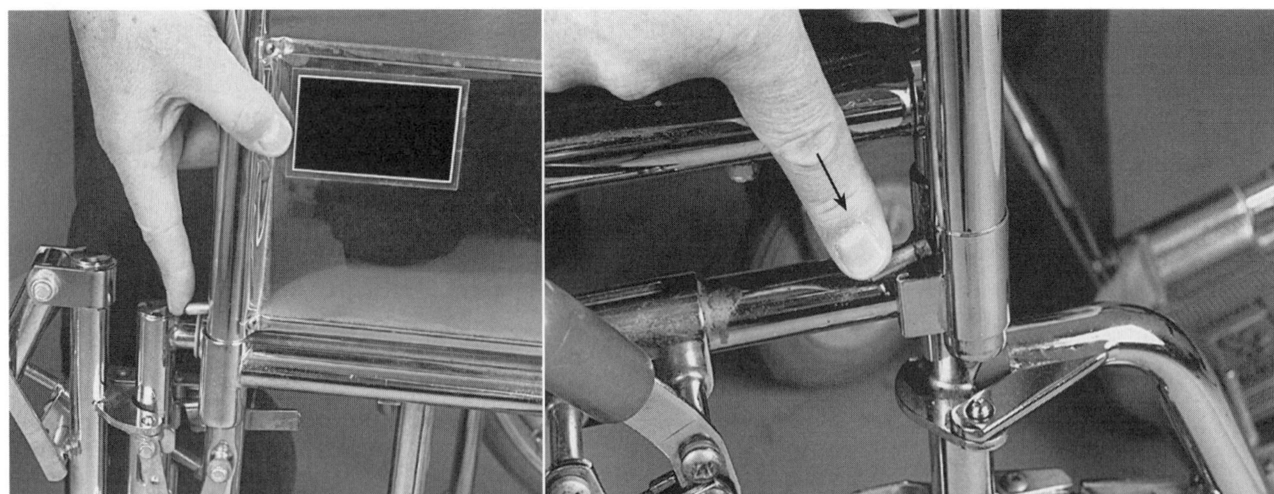

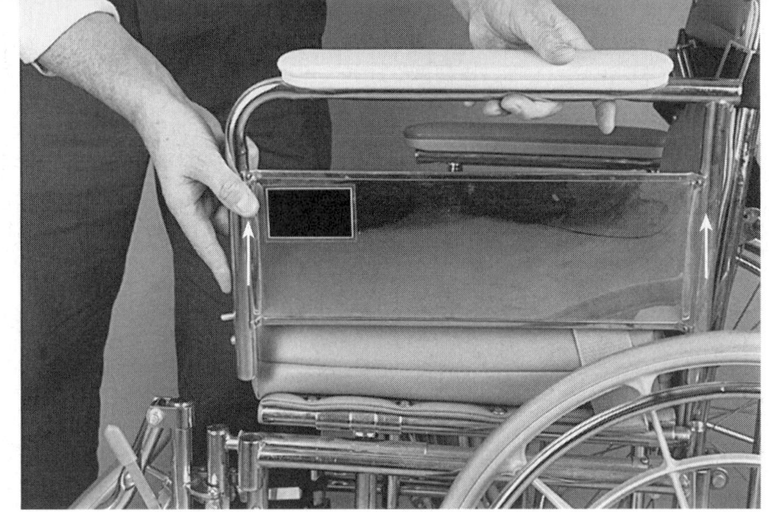

FIG. 8-18 Removable arm, with pin lock and release.

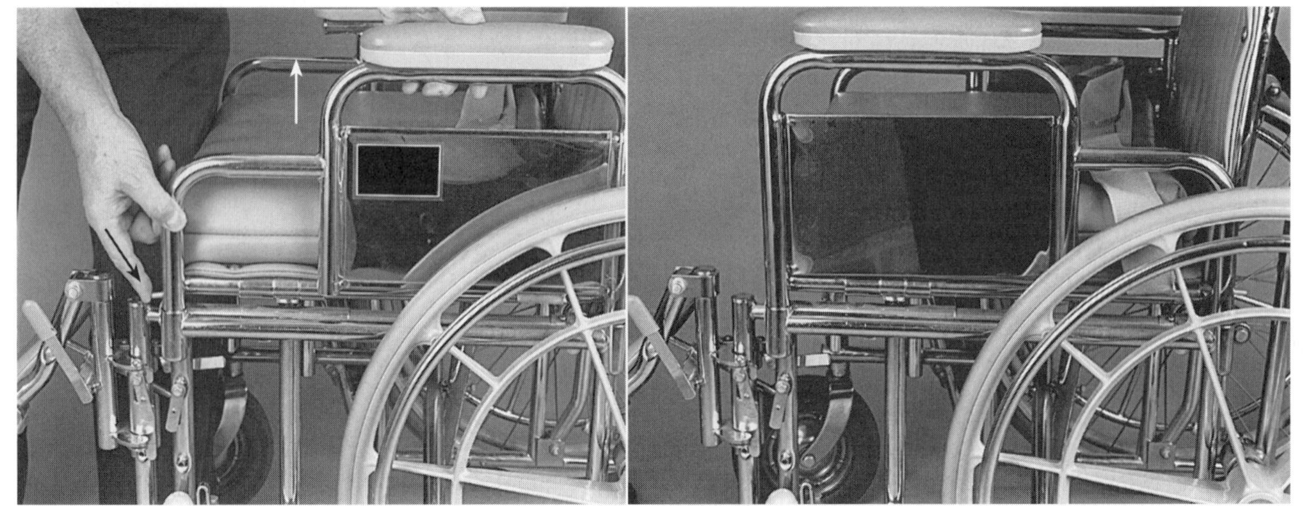

FIG. 8-19 Desk (or cutout) arm, with pin lock and release.

The armrests can usually be reversed to improve anterior support when the user performs a standing transfer (Fig. 8-19).

Adjustable Armrests Adjustable armrests are used by persons who need to adjust the armrest height for different activities or when cushions with different thickness or bulky outer garments are used. Typical adjustments include a friction adjustment, accomplished by loosening and tightening of a knob or by a pin-in-hole adjustment. Hand function is necessary to adjust the armrest height (Fig. 8-20).

Front Rigging, Leg Rest, and Footrest Components

Fixed Footrests Fixed footrests are attached permanently to the chair frame. The footrest or footplate can be elevated or raised from a horizontal to a vertical position when the user rises, sits, or desires to place the feet on the floor.

Swing-Away or Removable Leg Rest Release of a locking mechanism allows the front rigging to be pivoted outward and lifting the leg rest removes the front rigging from the chair frame (Fig. 8-21). There are several different locking mechanisms available, including a pin lock and a pressure release lever. This feature is used to allow the user to position the chair closer to objects and to provide greater unimpaired space at the front of the chair for the feet during transfers.

Elevating Leg Rest The entire front rigging can be elevated and maintained at different heights. This is useful for

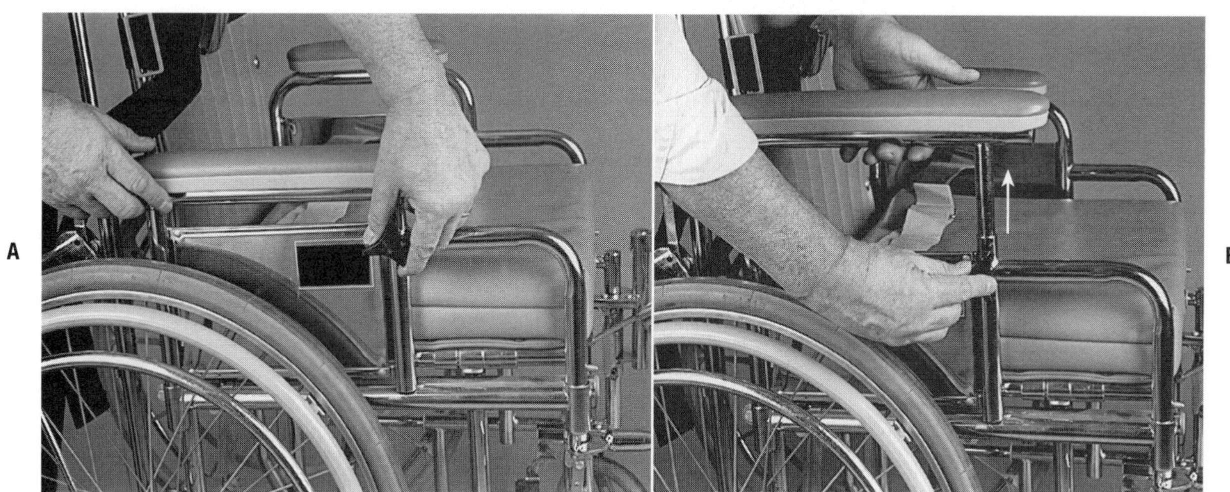

FIG. 8-20 Adjustable armrest.

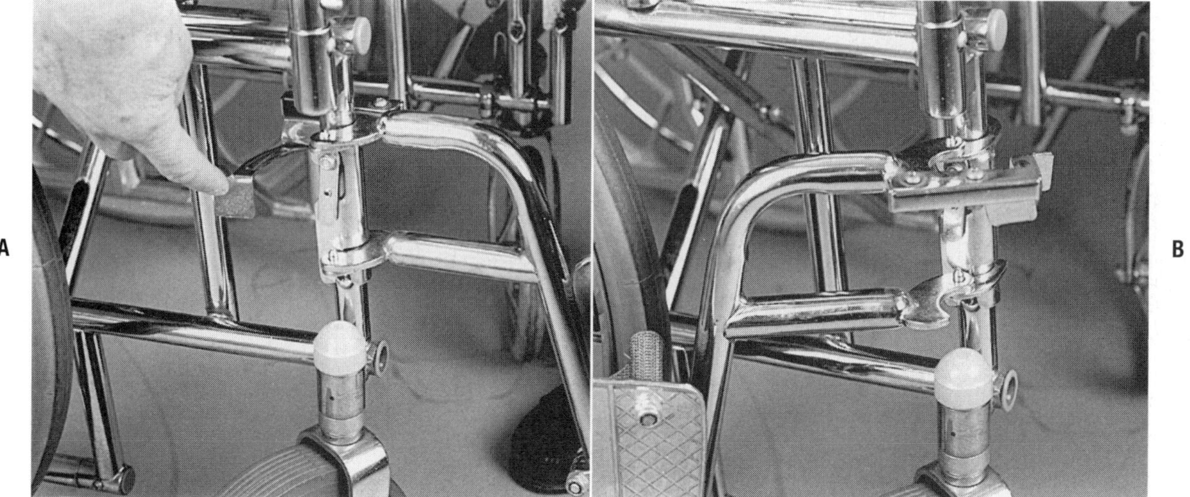

FIG. 8-21 Swing-away leg rest, with release and lock control.

A

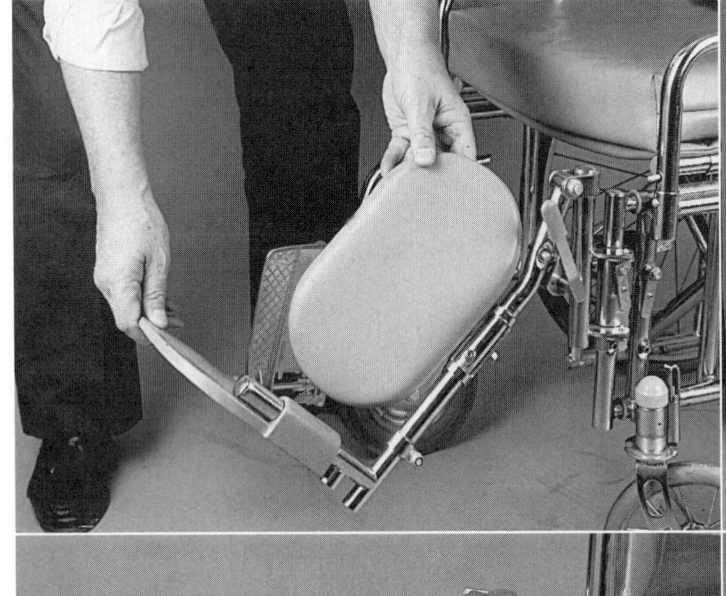

B

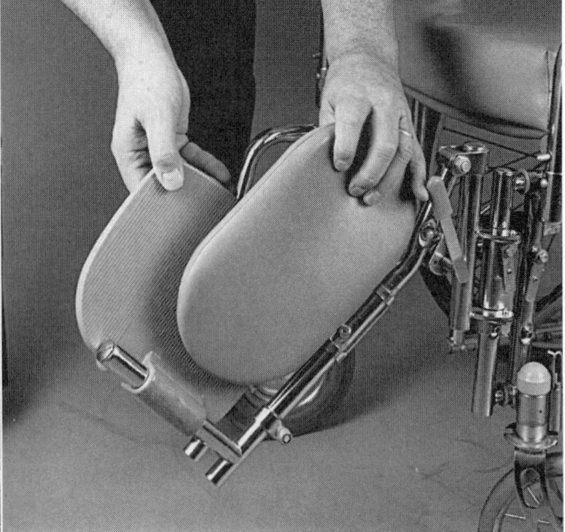

C

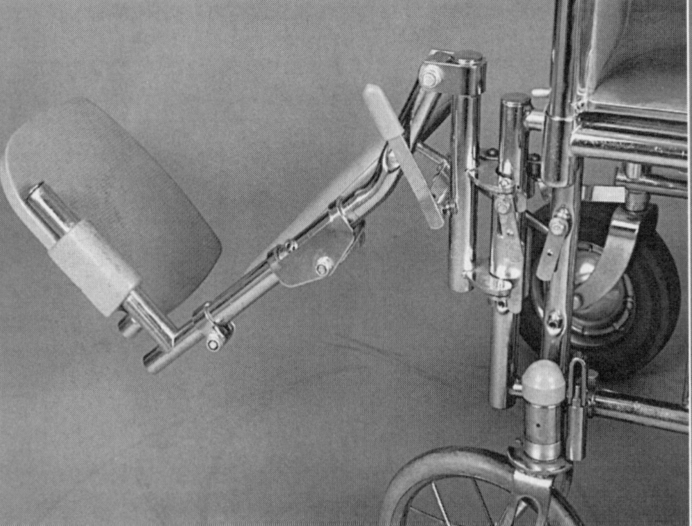

D

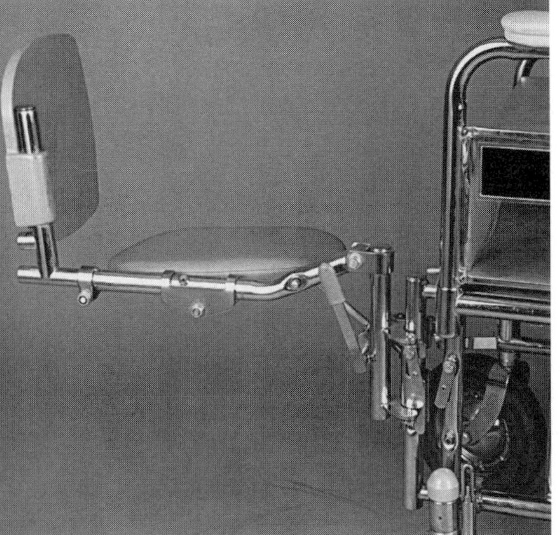

E

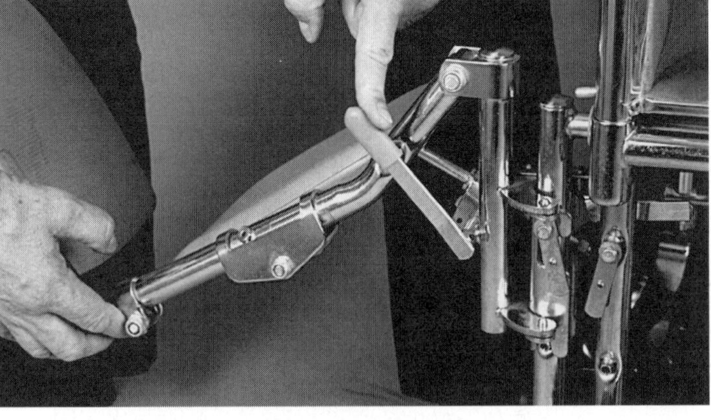

FIG. 8-22 Elevating leg rest.

the patient who is unable to fully flex the knees or when knee flexion must be avoided (such as, fused knee, long leg cast). A calf panel is attached to the leg rest to support the lower leg (Fig. 8-22, *A* and *B*). The leg rest remains elevated by a serrated cam or small gear, which engages a serrated piece of metal on the leg rest (Fig. 8-22, *C* and *D*). Lowering of the leg rest is usually accomplished by operating a lever that releases the adjustment lock (Fig. 8-22, *E*). The speed of the leg rest as it lowers must be controlled by supporting the leg rest as it descends. Be careful to protect the patient's lower extremity when the leg rest is lowered because the weight of the leg will cause it to descend rapidly if the patient cannot control its descent. This precaution is especially important when a lower extremity has a cast applied.

The front rigging can usually be pivoted outward or removed from the chair to aid transfer activities and the length of the leg rest can be adjusted to accommodate the patient's lower extremity when it is elevated. When one or both lower extremities are elevated, the chair will have a greater tendency to tip backward because the COG of the chair is altered; therefore the user must be careful when propelling the chair up an incline. Too strong or too rapid movement of the rear wheels is likely to cause the caster wheels to be lifted from the surface. A weight added to the front of the chair frame may help to reduce this problem.

Footrest The footrest, also called a footplate, is available in various shapes and sizes depending on the patient's needs. It may have a toe or heel loop to help maintain the foot on the footrest (Fig. 8-23, *A*). The heel loop prevents the foot from sliding backward and the toe loop prevents the foot from moving forward. The heel loop should be moved forward before the footrest is raised to prevent damage to the heel loop fabric and allow the footrest to be fully raised before a standing transfer or folding the chair is attempted (Fig. 8-23, *B* and *C*). *Caution:* The footrests should always be elevated before a standing transfer and before movement of a patient into or out of the chair.

A strap may be used between the two leg rests instead of heel loops to prevent posterior movement of the patient's legs. These straps may have various shapes or configurations (such as a single strap, a double strap, or an H strap).

Reclining Wheelchairs

Semireclining Semireclining wheelchairs allow the back of the chair to be adjusted to various positions from fully upright to 30 degrees of extension. Usually there are two adjustment knobs on either side of the back frame that are used to release and adjust the position of the back. The chair back will usually be higher than that on a standard chair and a removable head component is necessary to support the user's head when reclining. Elevating leg rests are necessary components of this chair for user comfort and to maintain stability of the chair. If the leg rests do not elevate, the chair will tend to tip

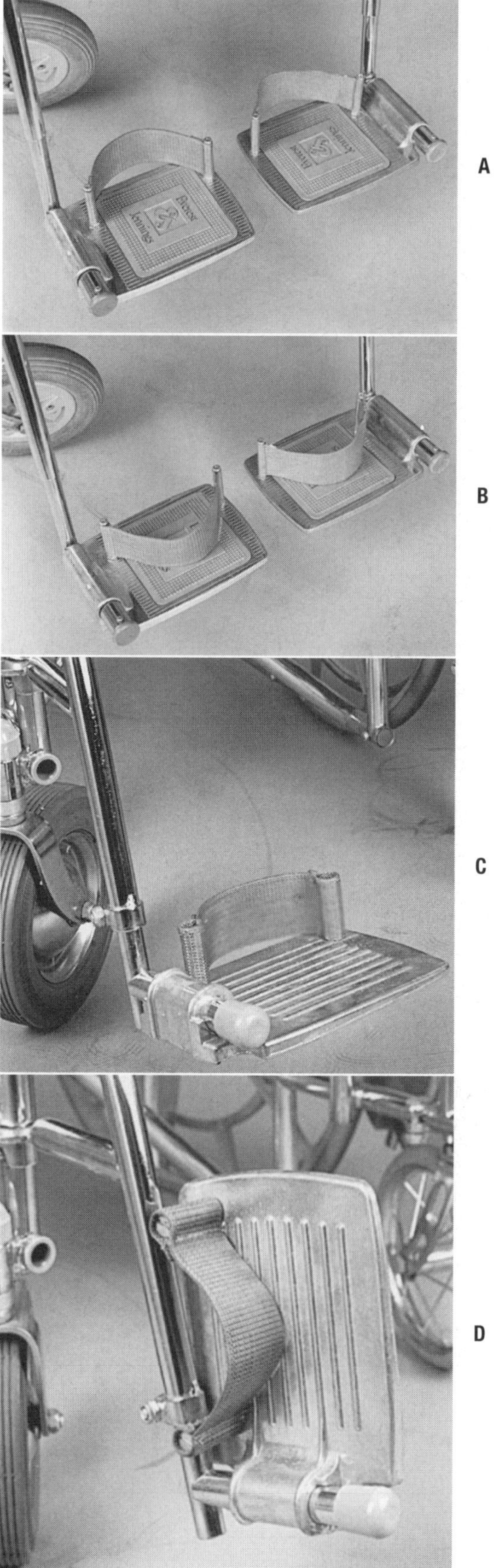

FIG. 8-23 Footrests (footplates).

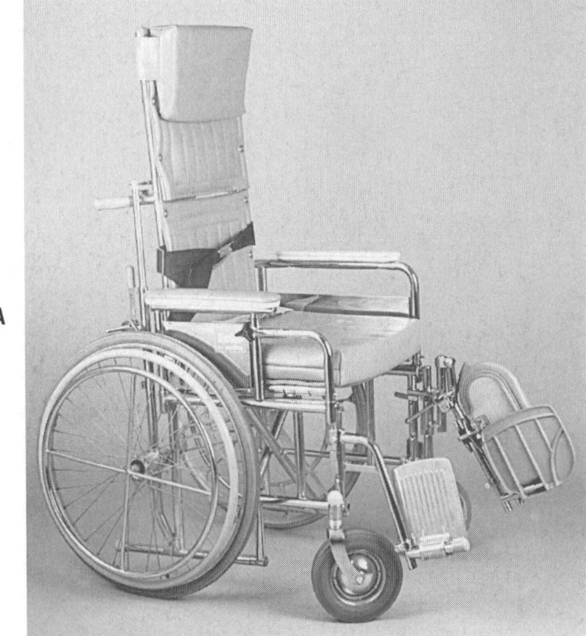

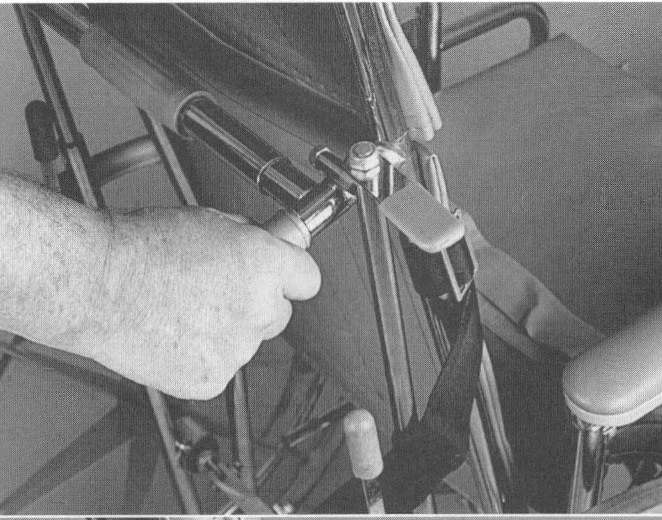

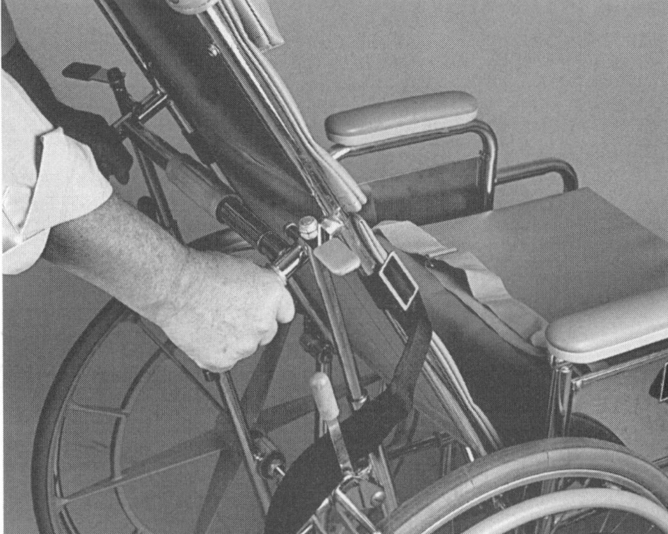

FIG. 8-24 Semireclining wheelchair.

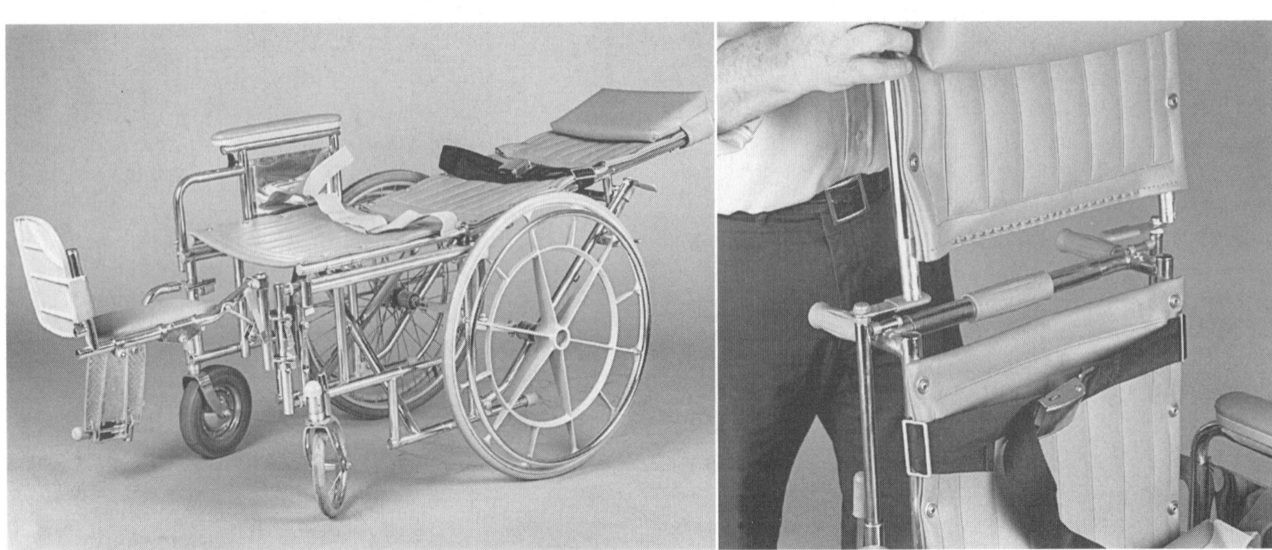

FIG. 8-25 Fully reclining wheelchair.

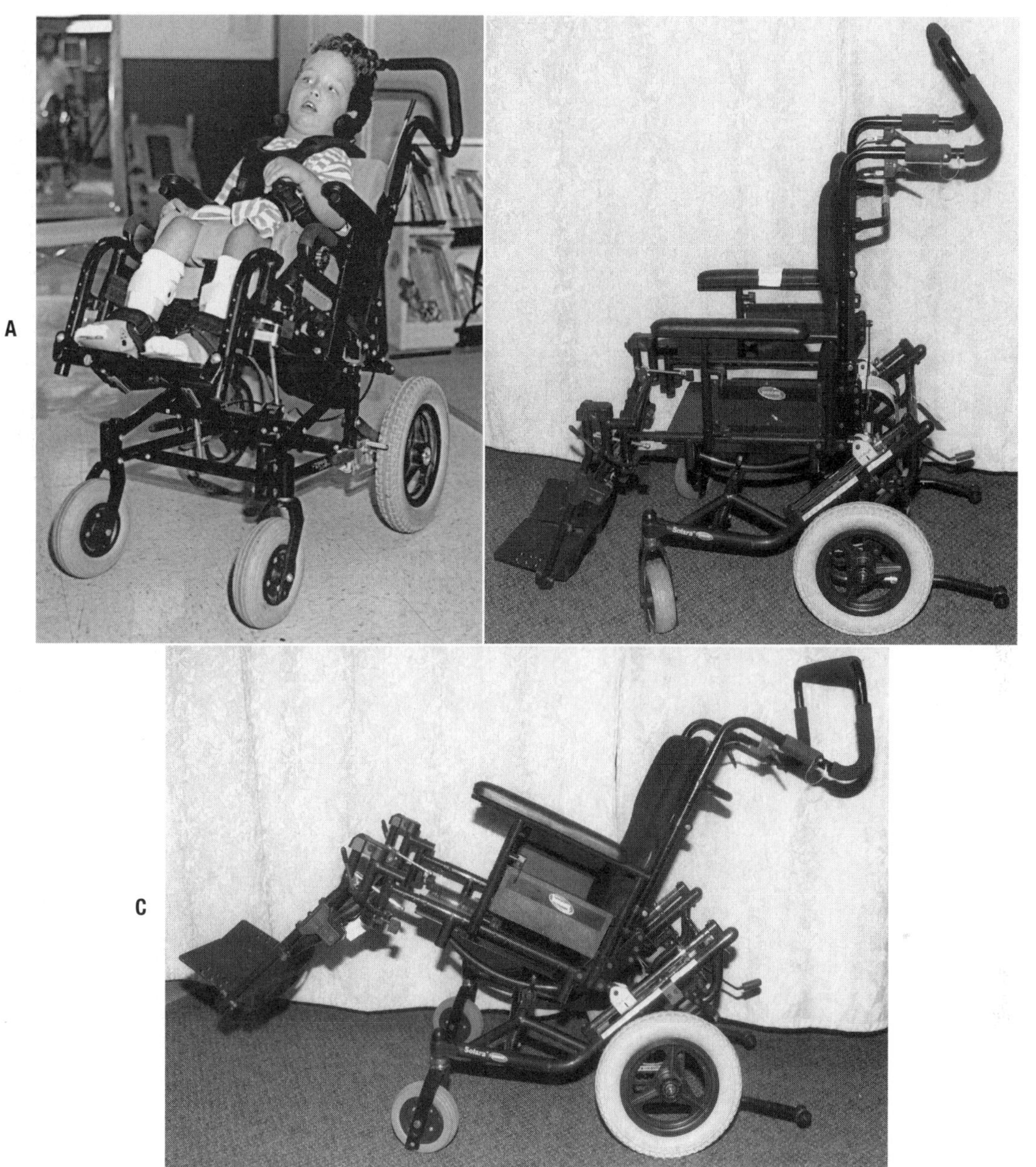

FIG. 8-26 Tilt-in-space wheelchairs.

backward when it is reclined because of a shift in the relative position of the user's COG and the BOS of the chair. A bar across the back adds support to the back frame (Fig. 8-24).

Fully Reclining Fully reclining wheelchairs allow the back to be adjusted to various positions from vertical to fully horizontal (Fig. 8-25, *A*). Adjustment knobs or levers located on either side of the back frame are used to adjust the position of the back. A headrest and elevating leg rests are necessary components as described previously (Fig. 8-25, *B*). In addition, the rear wheels will be located more posteriorly than on a standard chair, or they may move back as the chair is reclined to increase the BOS and stability of the chair. (*Note:* The reclining wheelchair is used for the person who must recline periodically while seated in the chair. Persons with lower extremity circulatory problems who cannot tolerate an upright position because of decreased circulation or who need to relieve skin pressure, but cannot perform pressure relief independently may find a reclining or Tilt-in-Space chair beneficial.) The Tilt-in-Space wheelchair can be adjusted to position the user at various angles. The chair can be wheeled with the person positioned at any angle (Fig. 8-26).

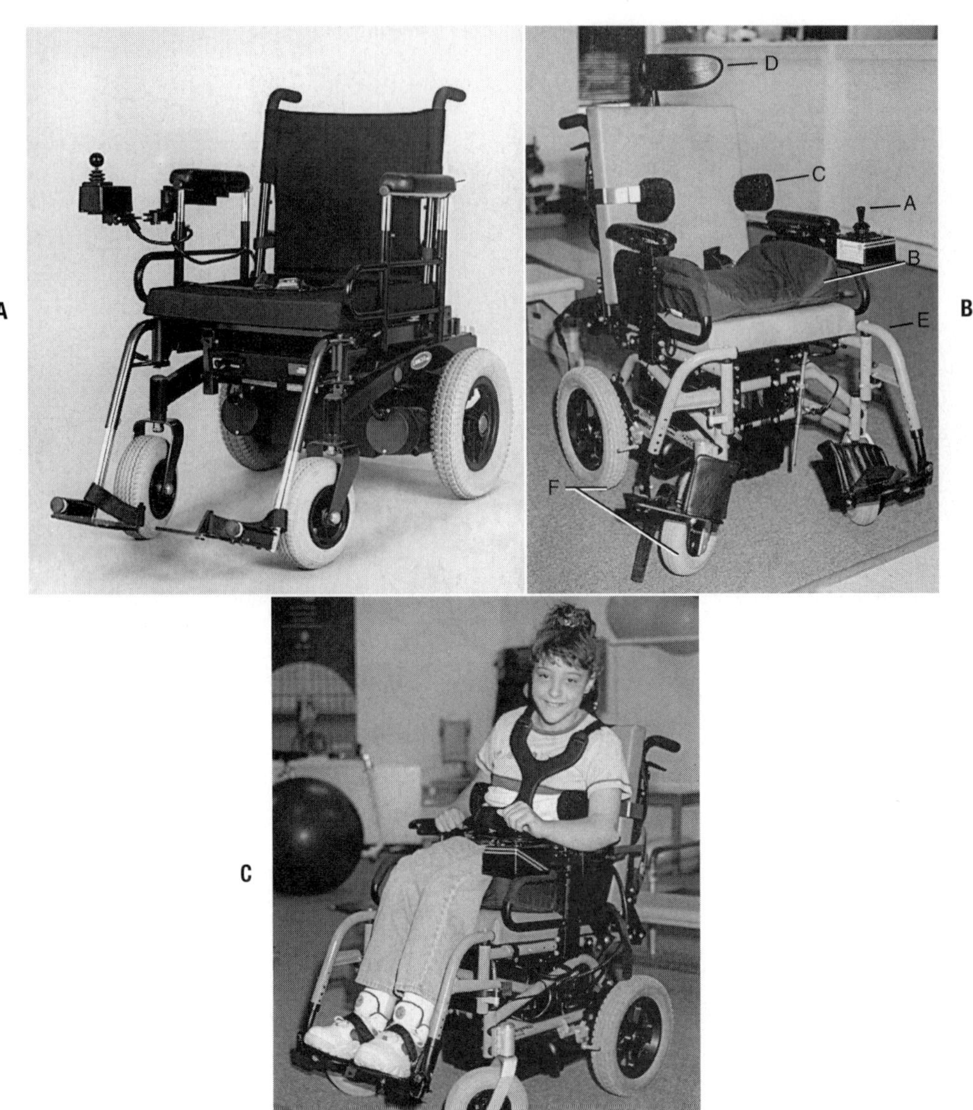

FIG. 8-27 **A,** Externally powered wheelchair. **B,** A youth-sized, externally powered wheelchair with *(A)* "joystick" control, *(B)* molded seat cushion, *(C)* side panels, *(D)* head support, *(E)* swing-away leg rests, and *(F)* semipneumatic tires. **C,** Youth seated in chair shown in **B,** showing yoke type of trunk restraint.

Externally Powered Wheelchair

The externally powered wheelchair is powered by one or more deep-cycle batteries that provide stored electrical energy to one or more belts that drive or propel the chair. The motorized chair is available for persons with insufficient strength or motor control of the extremities to propel a standard chair. Various controls are available to operate the chair, including those operated by the patient's hand, chin, head, tongue, or mouth; some sophisticated microprocessor control systems are available. The chair may have a proportional drive system, in which the speed is directly related to the pressure applied to the control device (that is, as more pressure is applied, there is greater speed), or it may have a microswitch system, in which the speed is preset so the chair will move only at a fixed speed regardless of the amount of pressure applied to the control (Fig. 8-27).

Sport, or Recreational, Wheelchair

The sport, or recreational, wheelchairs have specific features such as low backrests; solid, lightweight frames; canted (angled) rear wheels; lower and narrow seats; and an overall low profile to make the chair more functional for the user. Many of these chairs are custom fabricated, depending on the sport or recreational activity in which the user participates. One feature of this chair may be an adjustable back (Fig. 8-28). *Note:* Some users may select an ultralight wheelchair to reduce the amount of energy required for propulsion and to

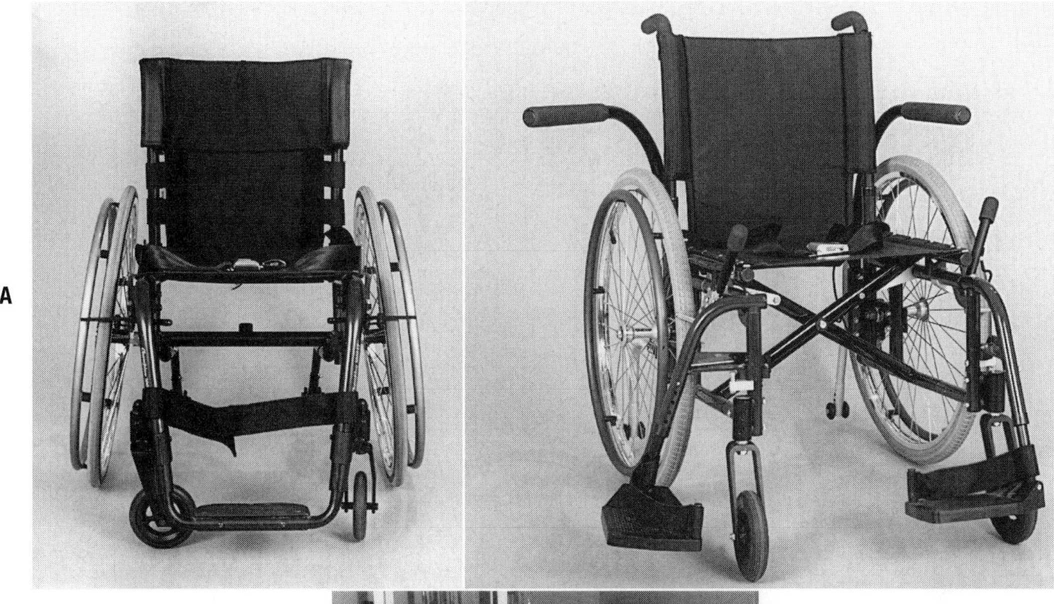

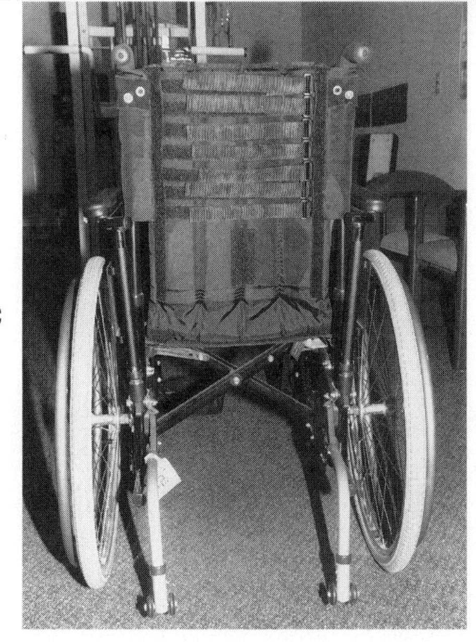

FIG. 8-28 **A,** Sport style of wheelchair with the angled (canted) drive wheels, solid frame, low backrest, and lack of armrests. **B,** Current use, lightweight wheelchair with swing-away front rigging *(left),* swivel armrest *(left),* and wheel lock applied *(left).* **C,** Adjustable back upholstery.

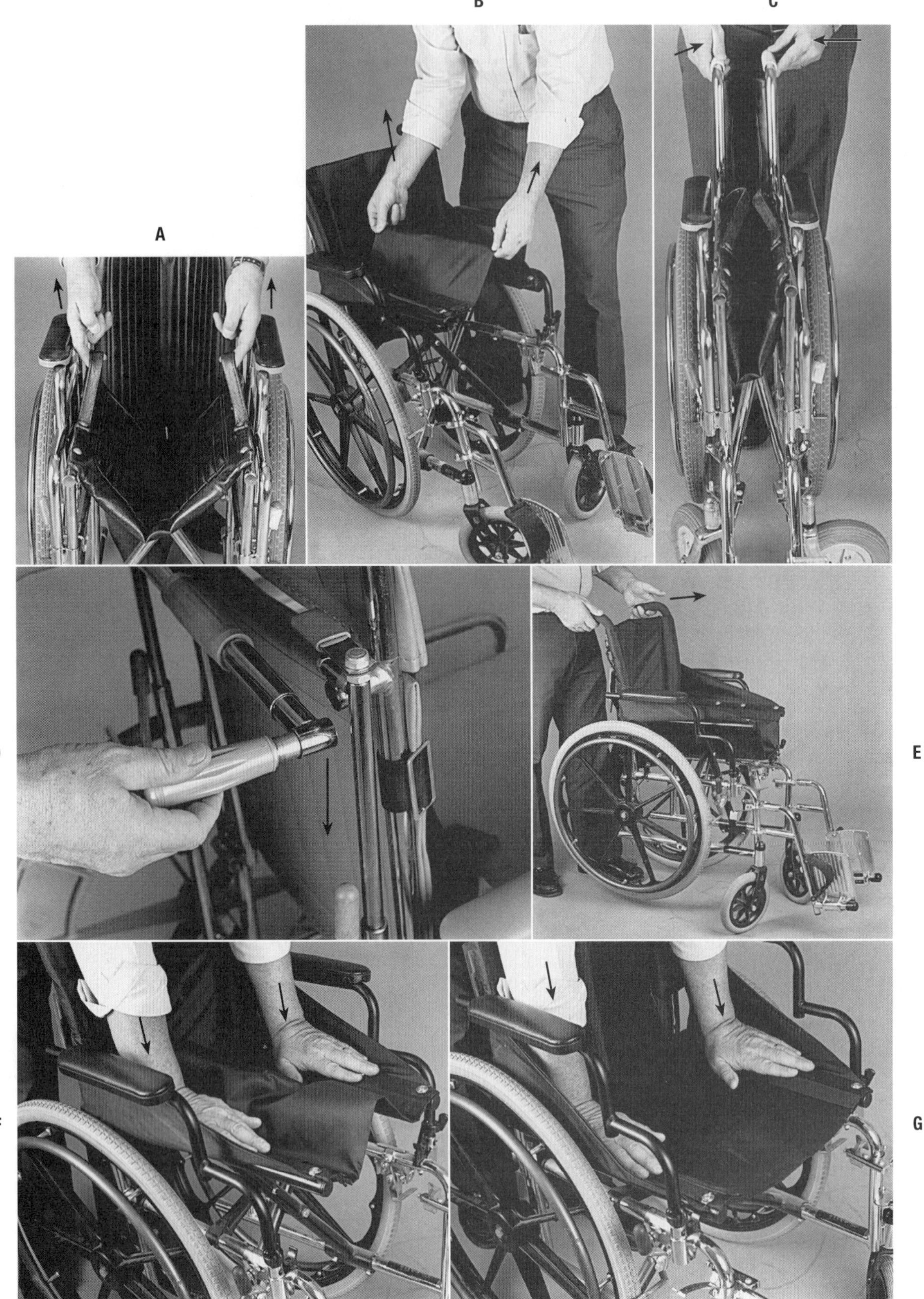

FIG. 8-29 Folding and unfolding the wheelchair.

make it easier to manage the chair. This type of chair is very durable, has higher quality wheel bearings, and has several adjustment features.

Folding Wheelchairs

Many wheelchairs can be folded for storage or transport. To fold the chair, the footrests must be raised after the heel loops have been moved forward. One can fold the chair by pulling up on the seat rails or on hand loops attached to the seat rails (Fig. 8-29, A). An alternative method is to grasp the midline of the front and back of the seat upholstery and lift upward (Fig. 8-29, *B* and C). However, this method may cause damage to the upholstery if it is used excessively. After the chair has been folded, the seat upholstery can be positioned downward between the seat rails.

The back support bar of the reclining chair must be released or removed before this chair is folded (Fig. 8-29, *D*). You will need to examine the bar to determine how to release it. The bar must be replaced and secured in place before a patient is placed into the chair.

To unfold the chair, lift the rear wheels from the floor by lifting on the push handles and gently begin to move the push handles away from each other (Fig. 8-29, *E*). When the chair is partially unfolded, replace the rear wheels on the floor and complete the unfolding by pushing down evenly on each seat rail (Fig. 8-29, *F* and G). If the chair is to be unfolded on a carpet, it may be necessary to unfold it with the rear wheels elevated throughout the entire process because the rear wheels will be difficult to separate when they are on carpet.

A folded chair can be wheeled (transported) most easily by elevation of the caster wheels and wheeling of the chair on the rear wheels using the push handles for control.

When the folded chair is to be lifted, the fixed or solid portion of the frame should be used. *Caution:* Do not lift the chair using any of the removable components, such as the armrests or front rigging, because they may disengage from the chair.

FUNCTIONAL ACTIVITIES

The person who uses a wheelchair for mobility should be instructed in the proper use and care of the chair. The projected use of the chair should be based on the person's goals, needs, and anticipated life-style. The many functional activities the person will need to learn should be practiced with use of proper safety and protective or guarding techniques. It may be necessary to visit the environment where the person will function to identify the usual, unusual, and special activities the person should be taught.

Figure 8-30 illustrates the major components of a standard wheelchair and the nomenclature of these components.

Operation of Wheelchair Components

Each wheelchair user should be taught to operate the wheel locks; remove and replace the armrests; swing away, remove, and replace the front rigging; and elevate and lower the footplates before performing other activities. The instructions may be oral, demonstrated, written, or illustrated; a videotape can also be used. The user should not be expected to inherently understand how to perform these activities and instructions should be given to each user along with an opportunity to practice and demonstrate the ability to perform these activities. The person with functional use of the upper and lower extremities, normal trunk control, and normal balance should not experience difficulty learning and performing

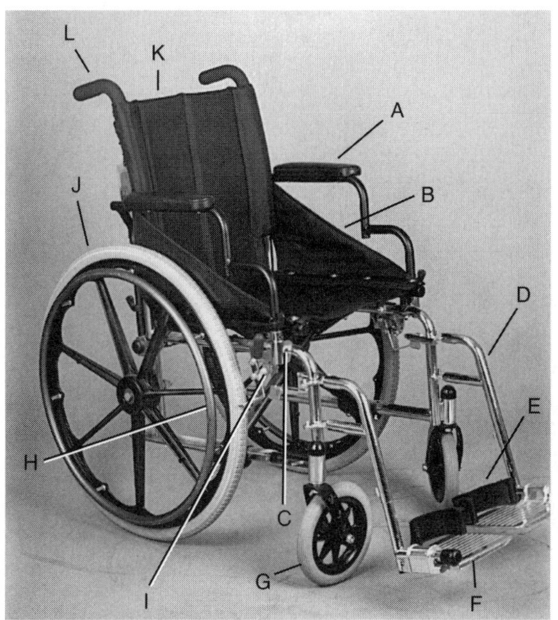

FIG. 8-30 Wheelchair components. *A*, Armrest. *B*, Clothing guard. *C*, Front rigging release. *D*, Front rigging. *E*, Heel loop. *F*, Footplate (footrest). *G*, Caster wheel. *H*, Handrim. *I*, Wheel lock. *J*, Drive wheel. *K*, Back upholstery. *L*, Push handle.

these tasks. However, the person with functional loss of use of the extremities, decreased trunk control, and decreased balance may require several practice sessions to learn to perform these tasks safely and proficiently.

Independent Propulsion

Bilateral Upper Extremities The user grasps the handrims at the top of the wheels (the 12 o'clock position) and pushes forward or pulls backward with equal force on each wheel (Fig. 8-31, *A*). To turn, instruct the user to hold one hand-rim and pull or push on the opposite handrim; to turn more quickly, simultaneously push forward on one handrim and pull back on the opposite handrim.

One Upper Extremity and One Lower Extremity The user grasps the handrim at the top of the wheel and pushes forward or pulls back, using the functional foot to pull or push simultaneously (Fig. 8-31, *B*). The foot also serves as a rudder to assist with turning while the user holds the handrim (Fig. 8-31, *C*). The use of one upper extremity and one lower extremity, usually on the same side, is an excellent method for a patient with hemiplegia.

Bilateral Lower Extremities The user uses the heels and soles of the feet or shoes to propel the chair forward and backward and as a rudder to turn to the left or right. This method is rarely used, but would be of value for any user with reduced function of both upper extremities, poor trunk control, and who is unable to ambulate.

The user should be instructed orally and by demonstration how to propel the chair forward and backward, turn to the left and to the right, and turn the chair in a half or complete circle. Practice of these techniques will be required for the user to become independent and safe. These activities

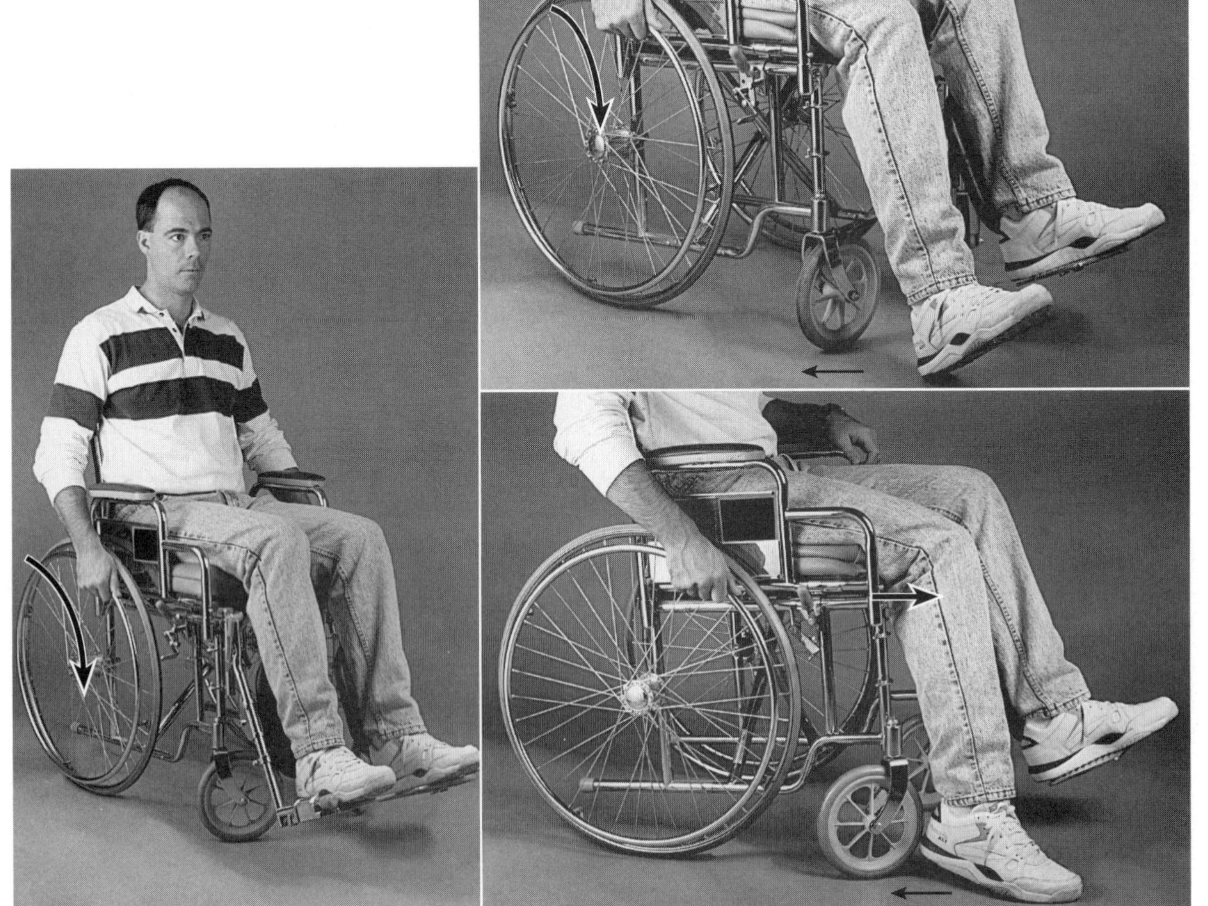

FIG. 8-31 **A,** Independent propulsion by a patient using both upper extremities. **B** and **C,** Independent propulsion by a patient using one upper and one lower extremity.

should be practiced initially on a smooth, flat surface rather than on a carpet and in a space free of objects. Eventually, the person should practice on carpeting or a rough surface and should attempt to maneuver around objects, in a congested area, and on a sidewalk, or other outdoor surfaces.

Assisted Functional Activities

Assisted Level-Surface Propulsion When propelling a patient in a wheelchair, use the push handles to move and control the chair. To turn the chair, hold one push handle and push or pull on the other push handle. For example, to turn to the left, hold the left push handle and push on the right push handle, or hold the right push handle and pull on the left push handle. Do not push the chair and then release the push handles; always maintain control of the chair when it is moving and you are propelling it, particularly when moving down an incline or ramp. Start and stop chair movement smoothly and avoid a sudden or abrupt start or stop. In most settings and environments, use the right side of the corridor or sidewalk when propelling the chair. Use caution when you reach the corner of a wall, especially when there is no mirror to view oncoming traffic or hazards that might be around the corner. Also use caution when you move the chair through any doorway because the patient's feet and chair footrests project in front of the chair, making them susceptible to being struck and injured.

In those situations when it is necessary or desirable to tip the patient and propel the chair on its rear wheels, be certain to inform the patient of your intentions before you tip the chair.

Finally, be certain the chair is secure and stable, with the footrests elevated, before the patient enters or exits the chair using a standing transfer. The chair wheels should be locked, or you should hold the push handles if the patient can enter or exit the chair independently and safely.

Elevation of the Caster Wheels To elevate the caster wheels, stand behind the chair and push down and forward with one foot on one tipping lever while pushing down and back with both hands on the push handles (Figs. 8-32 and 8-33). Once the caster wheels are elevated, you will need to control the chair with the push handles. The chair can be

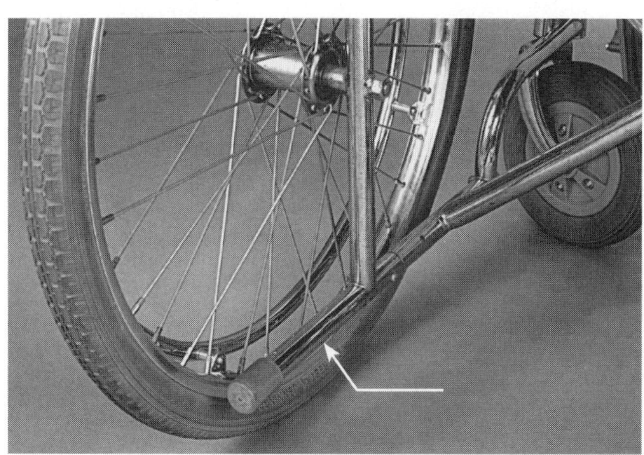

FIG. 8-32 Tipping lever for elevation of caster wheels.

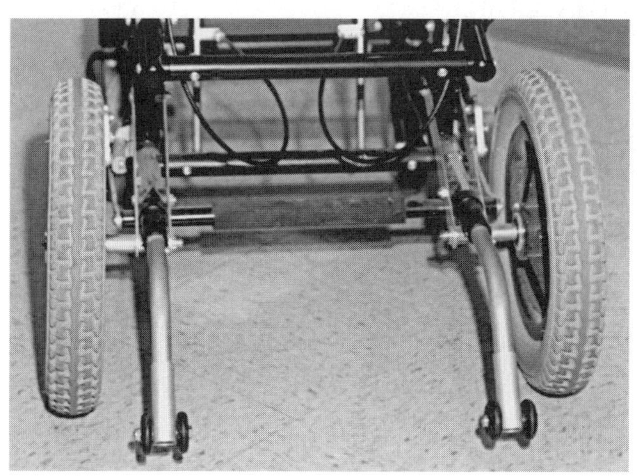

FIG. 8-33 Anti-tipping extensions in position to prevent the chair from tipping backward. The extensions can be rotated upward or removed.

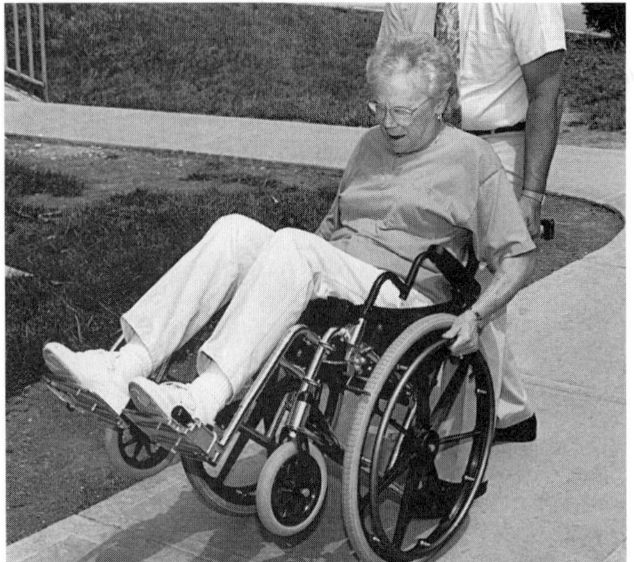

FIG. 8-34 Propelling a wheelchair while it is reclined on the drive wheels.

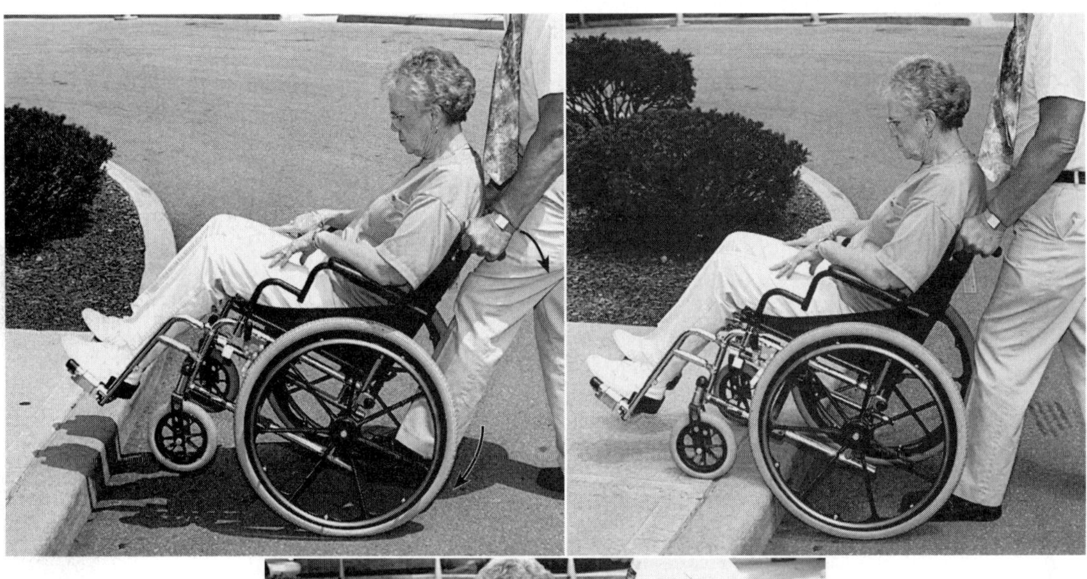

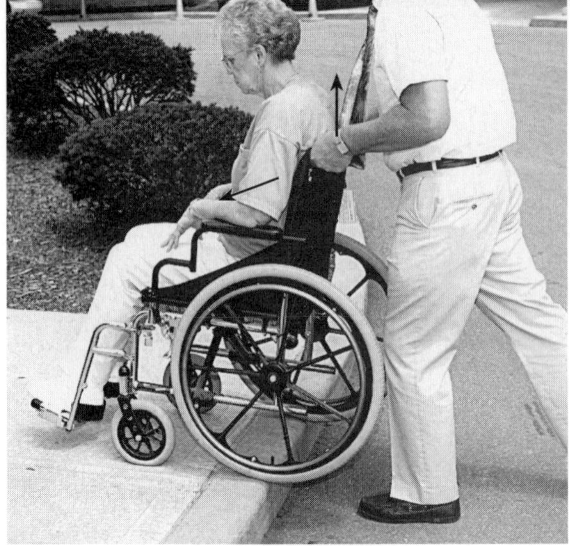

FIG. 8-35 Ascending a curb forward.

propelled while the caster wheels are elevated (Fig. 8-34). *Caution:* The person in the chair should be warned before being tipped and the entire procedure should be described before it is performed. Reverse the procedure to lower the caster wheels to the floor and retard the effect of gravity as the caster wheels descend. You must be certain you have the physical strength to perform this procedure and control the chair when it is tipped and your use of proper body mechanics will be very important.

Ascending a Single Elevation (Curb) Forward Position the chair facing the curb and elevate the caster wheels as described previously (Fig. 8-35). Move the chair forward on its rear wheels until they contact the curb lip and the caster wheels are above the surface of the curb. Carefully lower the caster wheels, as described previously, onto the surface; then roll the chair forward so the rear wheels ascend the curb and all four wheels are on the upper level of the curb. (*Note:* The person in the chair can assist by leaning the trunk forward and pushing forward on the handrims as the chair is elevated and rolled up onto the curb. The person must have control of the trunk musculature, adequate balance, and functional use of the upper extremities to assist with this activity.) This method is the easiest to use, provides the greatest control of the chair, and requires the least effort by the caregiver.

Ascending a Single Elevation Backward Position the chair so the rear wheels contact the curb and tip the chair back so the caster wheels are elevated (Fig. 8-36). Pull on the push handles so the chair ascends the curb on its rear wheels; then turn the chair 90 degrees to the left or right or pull it backward until the caster wheels are positioned over the upper level of the curb. Gently lower the caster wheels using the tipping lever and push handles. (*Note:* The person in the chair can assist by pulling back on the handrims as the chair is pulled up and over the curb. Maintain the chair in a tipped position until all four wheels are positioned over the surface

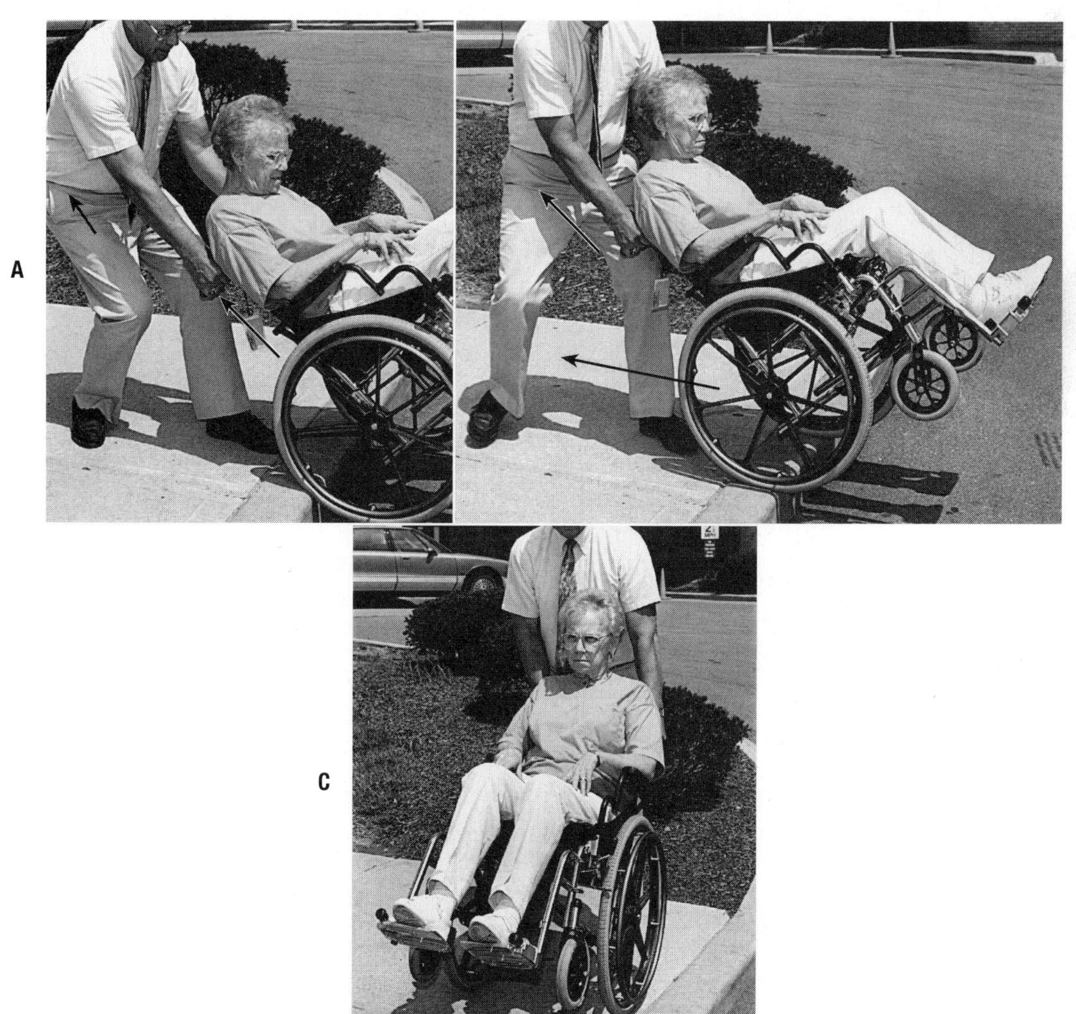

FIG. 8-36 Ascending a curb backward.

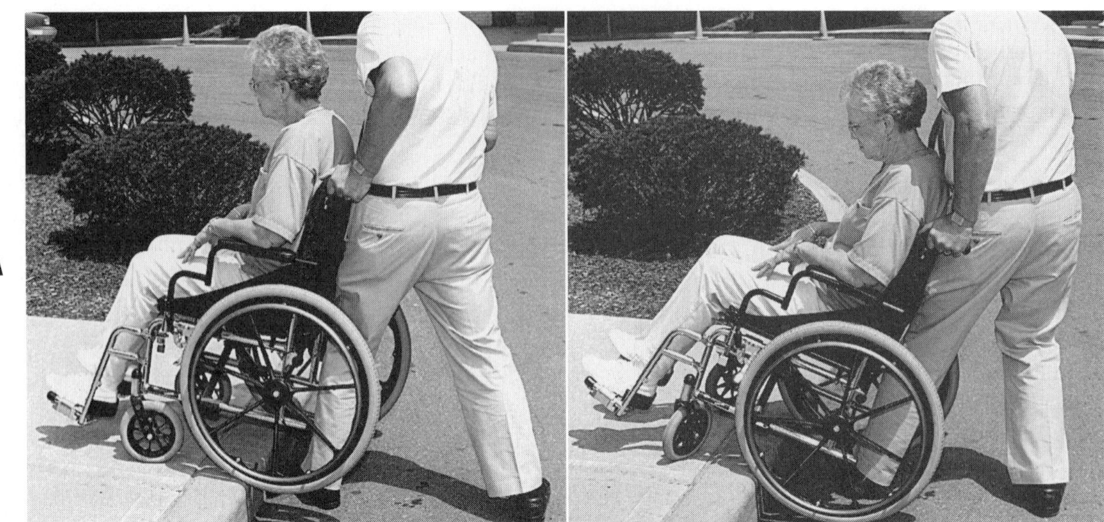

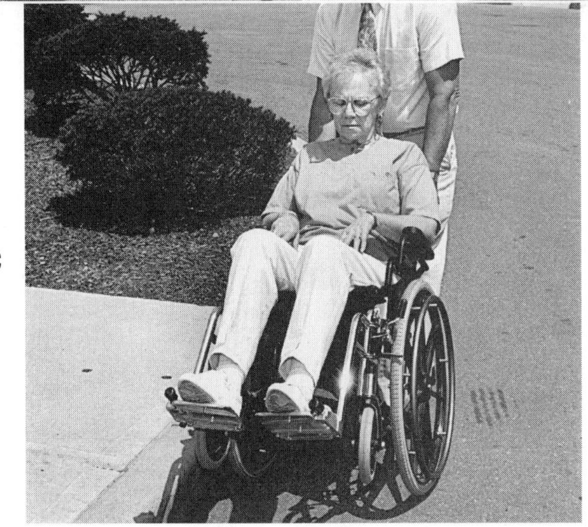

A B C

FIG. 8-37 Descending a curb backward.

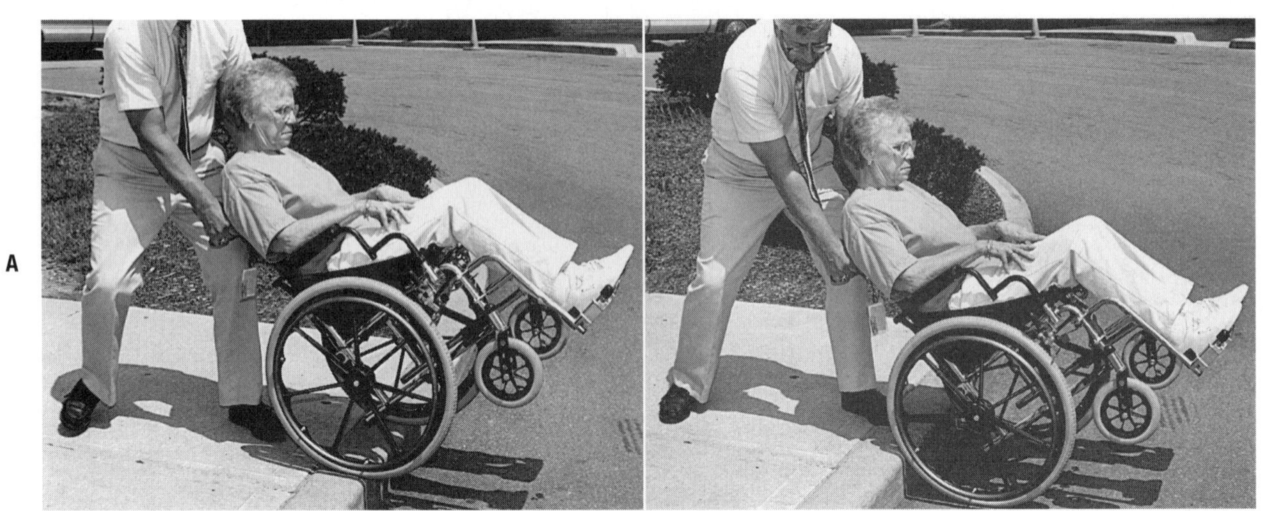

A B

FIG. 8-38 Descending a curb forward.

above the curb.) This method is more difficult to perform because the effort needed to pull the chair up the curb and to control the chair is greater than the forward method.

Descending a Single Elevation Backward Position the chair so the rear wheels are close to the edge of the curb (Fig. 8-37). Stand behind the chair and control the chair as it slowly rolls backward, rear wheels first, over the curb, while the caster wheels remain on the upper surface of the curb. The movement of the chair over and down the curb can be retarded if you use your thigh or the side of your hip against the back of the chair as it descends. When the rear wheels contact the street, turn the chair 90 degrees with the caster wheels elevated or roll it away from the curb until the caster wheels and front rigging clear the curb; then lower the caster wheels to the surface. *Caution:* Maintain the chair in a reclined position until the caster wheels and front rigging clear the curb. (*Note:* The person in the chair can assist by providing friction with the hands against the handrims and by leaning the trunk forward as the chair rolls over and down the curb.) This method is the easiest to perform because it provides greatest control of the chair and requires least effort by the caregiver.

Descending a Single Elevation Forward Position the chair with the caster wheels close to the edge of the curb. Tip the chair onto its rear wheels; control the chair as it rolls forward over the curb by pulling back on the push handles until the rear wheels are on the lower surface (Fig. 8-38). The chair must be maintained in a tipped position until the rear wheels are on the surface at the bottom of the curb. When the rear wheels are on the street, the caster wheels are lowered gently. (*Note:* The person in the chair can assist by providing friction with the hands against the handrims as the chair rolls over and down the curb.) This is a difficult procedure and you must be certain you have the strength and ability to control the chair. Your use of proper body mechanics will be very important when you perform this procedure.

Practice each of these methods to determine which is the most efficient and safest for you to perform. Perform each method with persons of different sizes and weights in the chair. By trying each method, you will be able to offer alternatives to a family member or other person who may eventually assist the user. Usually, the movements that are the easiest to control and the safest to use are the ascending forward and descending backward movements (Procedure 8-2).

PROCEDURE 8-2

Assisted Ascending and Descending a Curb with a Wheelchair

For these activities, explain the activity to the patient, instruct how and when to assist, and alert the person as you begin the activity.

DESCENDING FORWARD

Position the chair with the caster wheels at the edge of the curb; the patient should be seated back in the chair.
Stand on the sidewalk surface.
Tip the chair onto its rear wheels using the push handles and tipping lever.
Wheel the chair forward and allow it to roll over the edge of the curb as you pull back on the push handles; the patient can assist to control the movement of the chair by providing friction to the handrims with the hands.
After the rear wheels are on the street, lower the caster wheels using the push handles and tipping lever.

DESCENDING BACKWARD

Position the chair with the rear wheels at the edge of the curb; the caster wheels remain in contact with the sidewalk surface.
Stand on the street surface.
Allow the rear wheels to roll over the edge of the curb until they contact the street; control the movement of the chair with one hip against the back of the chair.
The patient can assist to control the movement of the chair by providing friction to the handrims with the hands.
Elevate the caster wheels until they have cleared the curb as you back up or turn the chair to one side.
Lower the caster wheels onto the street surface using the push handles and tipping lever.

ASCENDING FORWARD

Position the chair facing the curb with the foot plates about 6 inches from the curb face.
Stand on the street surface.
Tip the chair back using the push handles and tipping lever.
Wheel the chair forward until the rear wheels contact the curb and lower the caster wheels to the sidewalk surface.
Wheel the chair forward over the curb.
The patient can assist by leaning forward slightly and pushing on the handrims until the rear wheels are on the sidewalk surface.

ASCENDING BACKWARD

Position the chair so the back is toward the curb and the rear wheels contact the curb.
Stand on the sidewalk surface.
Tip the chair back using the push handles; maintain this position.
Pull the chair over the curb on its rear wheels.
The patient can assist by pulling on the handrims as the chair ascends.
Back or turn the chair to one side until the caster wheels are above the sidewalk surface.
Lower the caster wheels using the push handles and tipping lever.

Ascending Multiple Elevations (Steps) Backward

Caution: This activity is performed most safely using at least two persons other than the patient; three persons may be required for a heavy or severely incapacitated patient. Position the rear wheels so they contact the bottom step and elevate the caster wheels (Fig. 8-39, *A*). The chair must be maintained in this tipped position as it is moved up the stairs. Pull the chair up onto each step as described for ascending a curb backward. The persons who assist should stand on one or both sides of the chair and grasp the frame of the chair (Fig. 8-39, *B*). *Caution:* The assistants should not grasp any of the removable items of the chair such as the armrests or front rigging because these items could become disengaged from the chair. On command of the leader, all persons assist to roll the chair up the steps, one step at a time. The leader should indicate when the next step is to be ascended so all persons work together. (*Note:* The person in the chair can assist by pulling back on the handrims on command, for example, "Ready, pull"; Fig. 8-40.) At the top of the steps, turn the chair 90 degrees or roll it backward until it can be

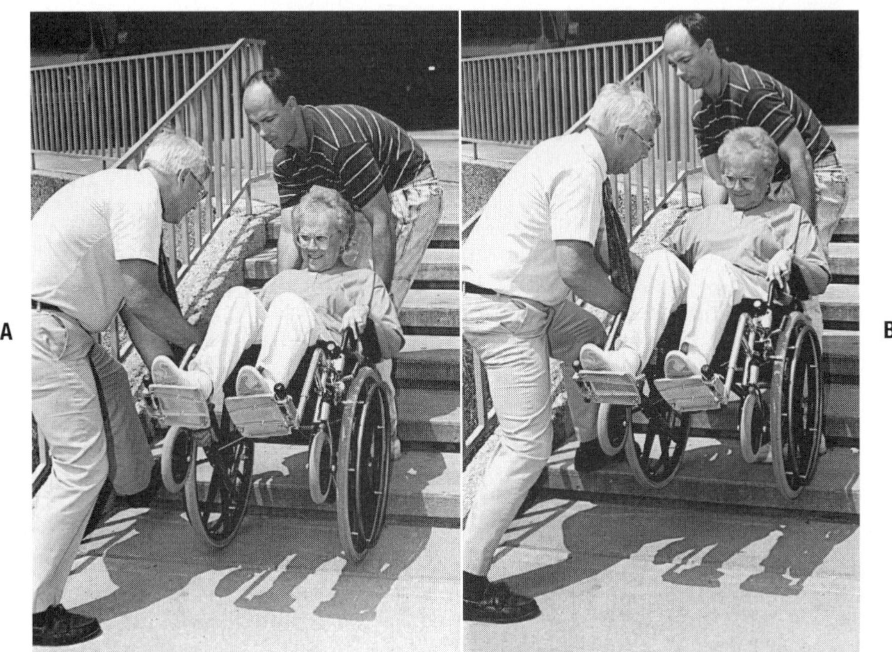

FIG. 8-39 Ascending steps backward or descending forward with two assistants.

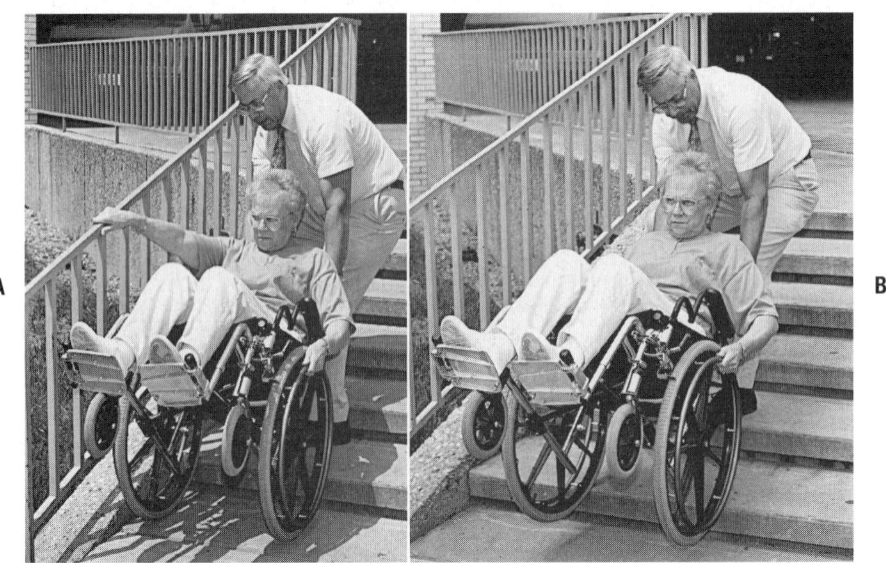

FIG. 8-40 Ascending steps with one assistant.

lowered onto its caster wheels. The person who controls the chair by grasping the push handles must use proper body mechanics by partially stooping, widening the BOS, and pulling rather than lifting, on the push handles.

Descending Multiple Elevations (Steps) Forward

Caution: This activity will be performed most safely if at least two persons assist and three persons will be required for a heavy or severely incapacitated patient. Position the caster wheels at the edge of the top step and tip the chair onto its rear wheels. Then slowly and carefully roll the chair until its rear wheels are at the edge of the step. The persons who assist should stand on one or both sides of the chair and grasp the frame of the chair. They should not grasp any of the removable items of the chair. On command of the leader, all persons retard the motion of the rear wheels down to the next step. The chair must be maintained in this reclined position as it moves down the stairs. Stop the chair on each step to avoid developing momentum. (*Note:* The person in the chair can assist by providing friction against the handrims as the chair descends each step.) Lower the chair onto its caster wheels at the bottom of the steps. The person who controls the chair by grasping the push handles must use proper body mechanics as described previously (see Fig. 8-40).

Ramps, Inclines, and Hills

Ascending a Slope. You can push the chair forward on all four wheels or elevate the caster wheels and propel it forward or backward on the rear wheels up the slope (Fig. 8-41). Pulling the chair up the slope backward with all four wheels in contact with the surface is not recommended because the patient may fall forward. *Note:* For steep elevations, it may be necessary to zigzag up or down the incline by angling the chair to the left and then to the right up or down the incline. The person in the chair can assist in propelling the chair as described previously.

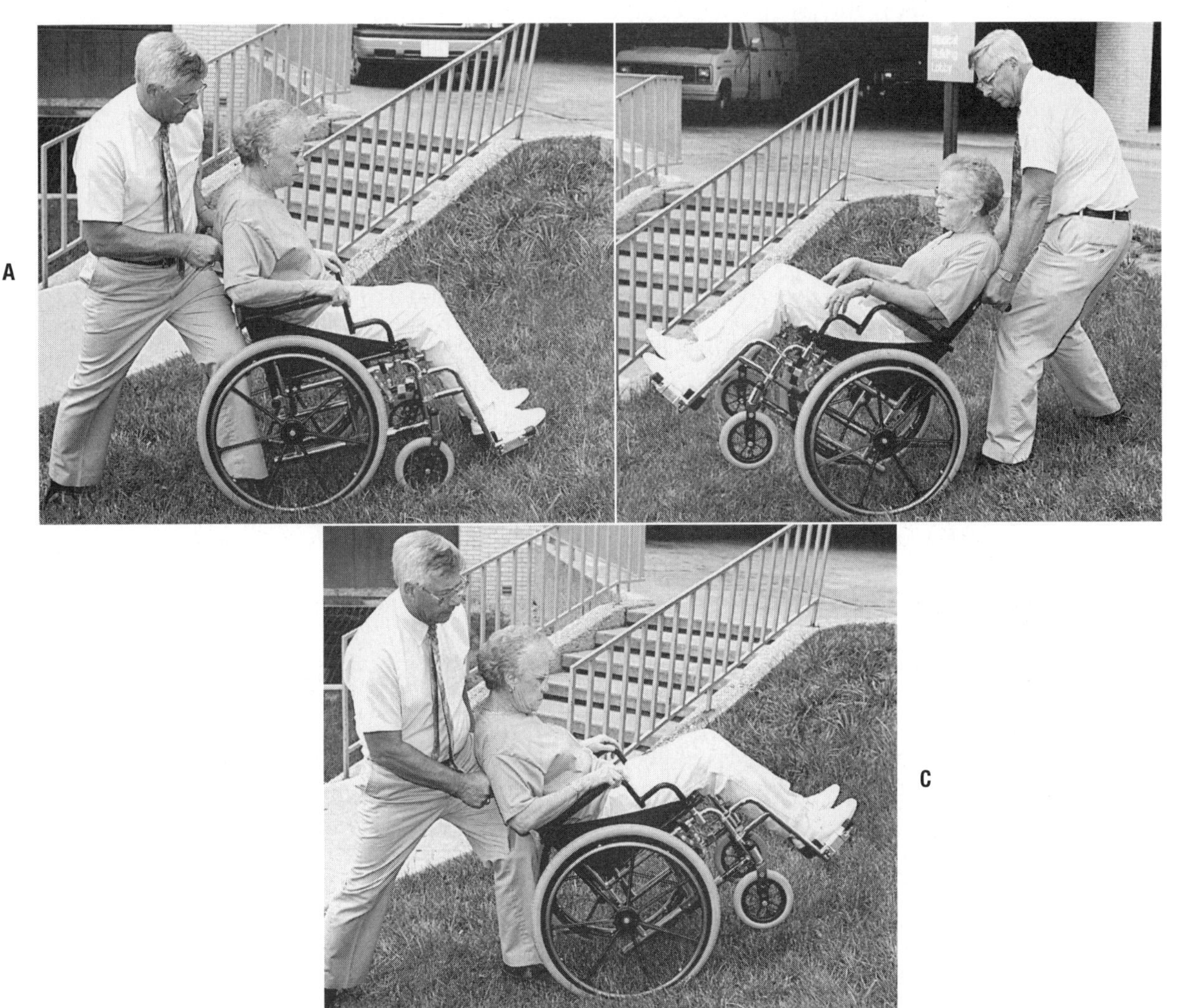

FIG. 8-41 Ascending and descending a slope. **A,** Forward or backward on all four wheels. **B,** Backward or forward on two wheels. **C,** Forward or backward on two wheels.

Descending a Slope. Elevate the caster wheels and retard the motion of the chair by holding the push handles as the chair descends forward, or leave all four wheels in contact with the ground and allow the chair to descend backward while retarding the motion of the chair with the side of your body against the back of the chair and your feet in a widened BOS. Allowing the chair to descend a steep slope forward with all four wheels in contact with the surface is not recommended because the patient may fall forward. The person in the chair can assist in retarding the motion of the chair by providing friction with the hands against the handrims.

Rough or Soft Surfaces The most effective method to control and propel the chair over an uneven or soft surface is to elevate the caster wheels so only the rear wheels are in contact with the surface. The chair must be maintained in this tipped position as it is propelled over the surface.

Elevators You can enter the elevator forward or backward. Many persons prefer to enter backward to access the selector panel, to avoid facing the back wall of the car, and to avoid turning the chair around to exit the car. However, entering the elevator backward and leaving the elevator forward places the lower extremities at risk if the door panels close prematurely or if there is limited access to the corridor into which the person exits. Furthermore, the caster wheels may lodge in the space between the elevator floor and the corridor surface and the traffic in the corridor cannot be observed until the patient has completely left the elevator. When the patient exits the car backward, the lower extremities are still at risk of being struck by the door panels and it may be difficult to turn in the corridor because of limited space or traffic. However, the patient will be able to view the traffic in the corridor easily and it will be easier to move the rear wheels over the space between the surface of the floor and the elevator car surface. Be certain the chair is completely out of the elevator car before you attempt to turn it. This is particularly important when one or both of the patient's lower extremities are elevated. You may need to position your body against the edge of the door or to request someone in the car to use the control button to keep the door open as the patient enters or leaves the car.

Many elevator locations have exterior wall mirrors to view the corridor before you exit. You should be familiar with the safety devices in the elevator car, such as the panel control to maintain the door open, and the emergency door-opening items, such as a photoelectric beam or pressure sensors in the edge of the door. You should observe whether the floor of the elevator car and the corridor surface are level. If the two surfaces are not level, you may need to elevate the caster wheels to safely enter or leave the car.

Escalators The person in a wheelchair should avoid using an escalator except in an extreme emergency. If the escalator is the only means to ascend or descend from one level to another, extreme caution will be required to maintain the person's safety.

The person, assisted by a caregiver, can ascend forward so the caster wheels are on the step above the rear wheels. Instruct the person to lean forward and grasp the moving handrails if the width of the escalator permits. The caregiver remains behind the chair to prevent it from tipping backward. When the level surface at the top of the escalator is reached, the caster wheels will contact it so the chair can be propelled forward (Fig. 8-42).

The person, assisted by the caregiver, can descend backward by positioning the rear wheels on the first step and positioning the caster wheels on the step above the rear wheels (Fig. 8-43). The user grasps the escalator handrails and leans forward; the caregiver remains behind the wheelchair for protection. At the bottom of the escalator, the person wheels backward until the front rigging clears the side of the escalator and turns the chair toward the direction to proceed.

Caution: This should not be considered to be an ordinary activity for a person in a wheelchair and extreme care must be used to prevent possible injury. The caregiver remains behind the wheelchair as the person ascends or descends to provide control and protection.

Doors and Doorways You can move a patient through a doorway forward or backward. *Remember:* problems or situations similar to those described for entering and leaving an elevator may occur with moving through a doorway.

Entering Forward. If the door opens toward you, position the patient at a slight angle so the person is nearest to and faces the edge of the door that will open (that is, faces the farthest door frame). Open the door wide enough so the chair will pass between the doorframe and the door edge. If the door has a *self-closing device*, use one foot or one hand to hold the door open as the chair moves through the doorway. Before you move the patient into the room or corridor, observe the area for traffic or other hazards.

If the door opens away from you, position the patient at a slight angle near the door facing the nearest doorframe (that is, faces the door frame opposite to the frame with the hinges attached). Open the door wide enough for the chair to pass through; hold the door open if it has a self-closing device. Follow the other precautions described previously to protect the patient.

Entering Backward. If the door opens toward you, position the patient so the back is toward the opening edge of the door with the chair at a slight angle away from the door edge. Open the door wide enough for the chair to pass through; pull the chair through the doorway. After the chair has passed completely through the doorway, turn the chair so the patient faces forward.

If the door opens away from you, position the patient so the back is toward the opening door edge with the chair at a slight angle toward the doorframe. Open the door

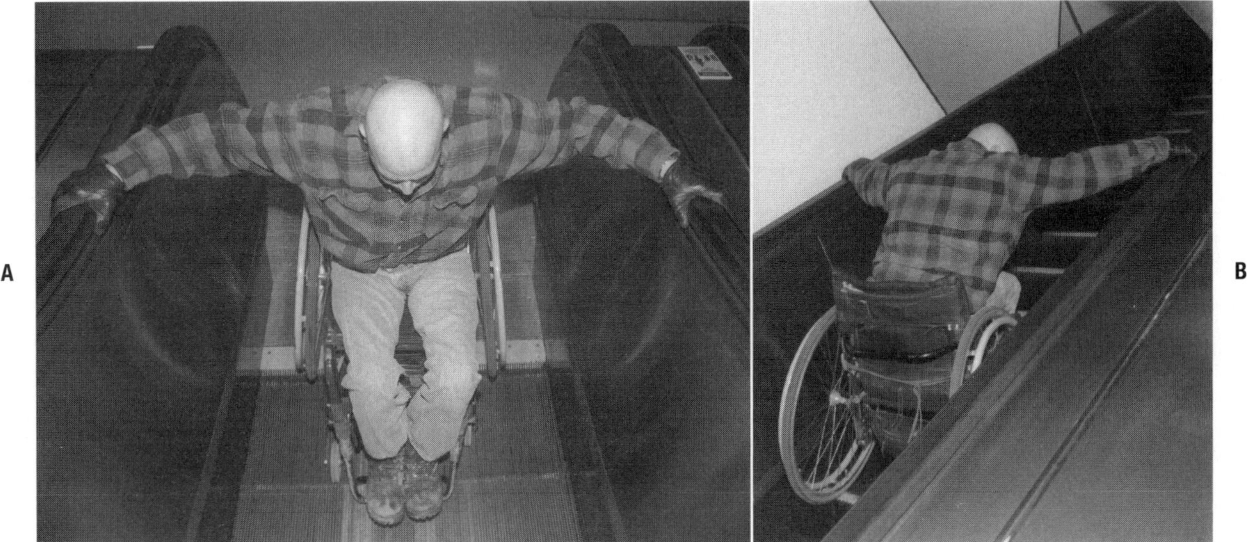

FIG. 8-42 Ascending an escalator. **A,** Ascending forward. **B,** Riding the escalator.

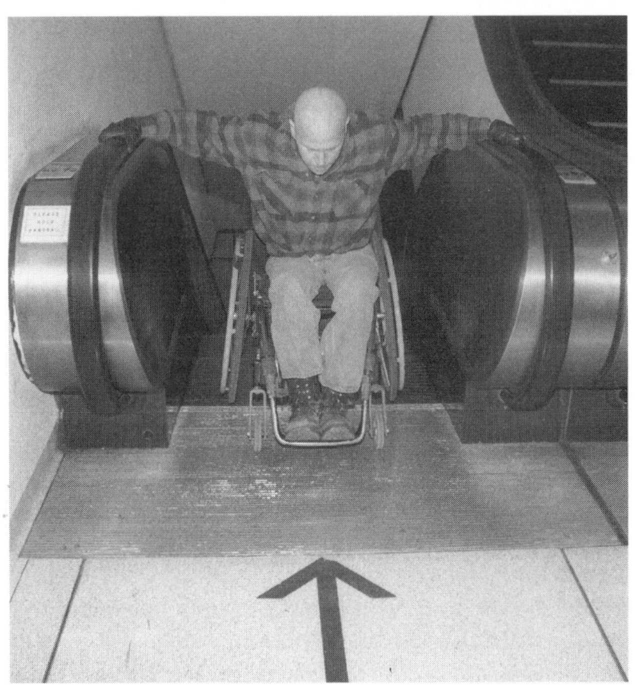

FIG. 8-43 Descending an escalator backward.

wide enough for the chair to pass through; pull the chair through the doorway. Follow the other precautions described previously to protect the patient. (*Note:* If there is a raised threshold, it may be easier to move the chair through the doorway backward because the larger rear wheels will roll over the threshold better than the caster wheels. If you move the chair leading with the caster wheels, it may be necessary to elevate the caster wheels to clear the threshold.)

Independent Functional Activities

Elevation of the Caster Wheels ("Wheelie" or "Pop-up") Elevation of the caster wheels is necessary so the wheels can clear objects on the floor, sidewalk, or ground and to ascend or descend curbs and curb cutouts. The patient must have sufficient upper extremity strength and coordination and the ability to maintain sitting balance when performing the activity. Practice will be required and the patient should be protected to prevent falling backward during practice sessions. A demonstration of the technique by another patient or by you is usually helpful and should be performed for all patients.

During practice sessions, stand behind the patient initially, tip the chair to find the balance point, and protect the person from falling backward. You must be alert when the patient performs the wheelie independently so you are always prepared to prevent the chair from tipping back too far. A rope properly measured to prevent the chair from tipping backward too far, attached to the push handles and running through a ceiling pulley or eye bolt, can be used to protect the person as this activity is practiced. A patient with only one functional upper extremity probably will not be able to perform this activity because it will not be possible to generate sufficient force to generate rearward momentum of the chair frame and still safely control the chair.

One way for a person to begin a wheelie is to instruct the user to pull back quickly and equally on both handrims and then abruptly stop the rearward motion of the rear wheels by firmly grasping the handrims (Fig. 8-44, *A*). The person should not attempt to propel the chair backward, but should develop a rearward movement momentum of the chair. The caster wheels will lift off the floor because of the abrupt stopping of the rearward motion of the chair. This action will occur because of the principles associated with Newton's first

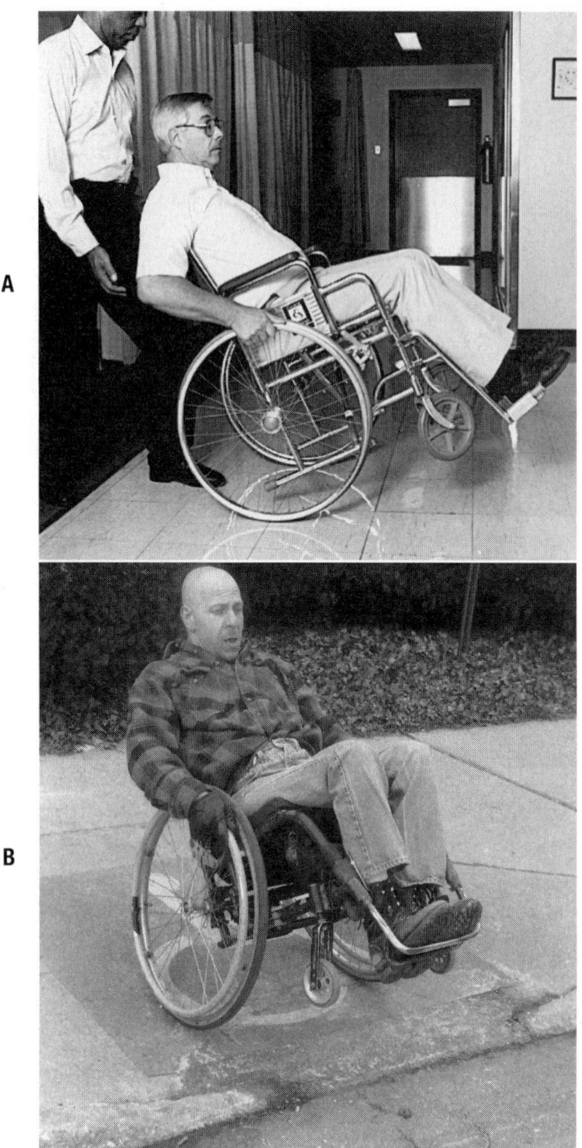

FIG. 8-44 **A,** Elevation of the caster wheels by the person in the wheelchair (a wheelie). **B,** Descending a cutout using a wheelie.

law of motion. This law indicates a body will remain at rest or in motion in a straight line until acted on by a force. Once the chair and the person in it start in motion backward, they will continue to move backward even when a force (that is, the hands grasping the handrims) stops the motion. The person will continue to move backward, with the axles of the rear wheels acting as a fulcrum, and the chair frame, with the person seated in it, will rotate backward, causing the caster wheels to become elevated. The patient's first attempts may only briefly lift the caster wheels a few inches. Over time and with continued practice, while being guarded and protected, many patients will be able to balance on the rear wheels and may be able to propel the chair in this position.

When the caster wheels are elevated, small forward movements of the handrims will cause a rearward movement of the chair frame and seat and small backward movements of the handrims will cause a forward movement of the chair frame and seat. The patient should be taught and should practice these motions by sliding the hands forward or backward on the handrims and using slight head movements to maintain a balanced position.

Eventually many patients will be able to perform a wheelie without the initial rearward motion of the chair. To do so, the person positions the hands on top of the handrims or tires slightly posterior to the hips (that is, a 2 o'clock position) with the trunk inclined forward slightly. The patient simultaneously leans the trunk back and pulls forward on the handrims or tires by bending the elbows and without propelling the chair forward; the head can be moved backward slightly to assist in elevating the caster wheels.

A proficient wheelchair user will be able to perform a wheelie while the chair is moving and maintain the wheelie to descend a curb, cutout, or ramp or to clear an obstacle on the ground or floor (such as threshold, uneven sidewalk, hose) (Fig. 8-44, *B*). To elevate the caster wheels when the chair is moving, the user must grasp the handrim or tire at a point well behind the hips and pull forward with the upper extremities as described previously.

The user may lean the trunk and head backward slightly to help to elevate the caster wheels. This activity requires a great deal of practice and the person must be guarded from behind the chair continuously. If the patient is unable to master this procedure, teach the person to perform the wheelie from a stationary position and then propel the chair with the caster wheels elevated.

Ramps or Inclines

Ascending Forward. When the patient propels the chair with both upper extremities, instruct the person to move the hips forward in the chair, lean the trunk forward, and push equally on the handrims using a smooth forward motion (Fig. 8-45). The hands will need to be repositioned on the handrims to progress up the ramp. It is important for the patient to lean forward to move the COG forward and to decrease the possibility of tipping backward.

When the patient propels the chair using one upper extremity and one lower extremity, instruct the person to move the hips forward in the chair seat and lean the trunk forward (Fig. 8-46). Instruct the patient to use the upper and lower extremities the same as they are used on a level surface, though it will be necessary to use the lower extremity for more power than is required on a level surface. The chair is likely to move to the left or right depending on the position of the caster wheels and the extremities used to propel the chair. If the patient propels the chair with the right extremities, the chair may deviate to the left; it may deviate to the right if the patient's left extremities propel the chair. This activity can be performed more easily by pa-

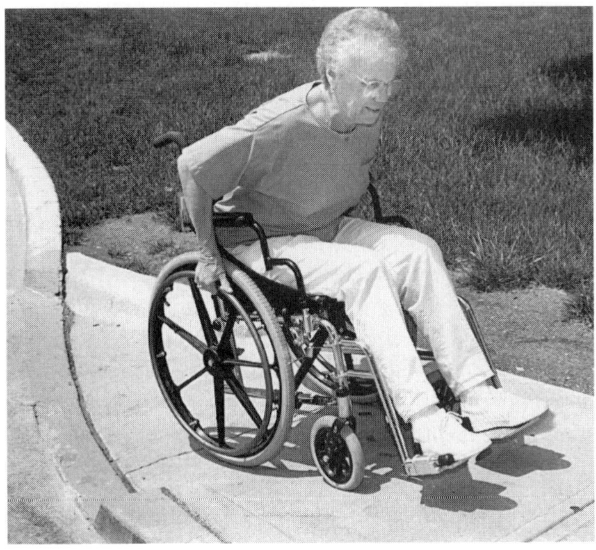

FIG. 8-45 Ascent of a ramp by the person in the wheelchair using both upper extremities.

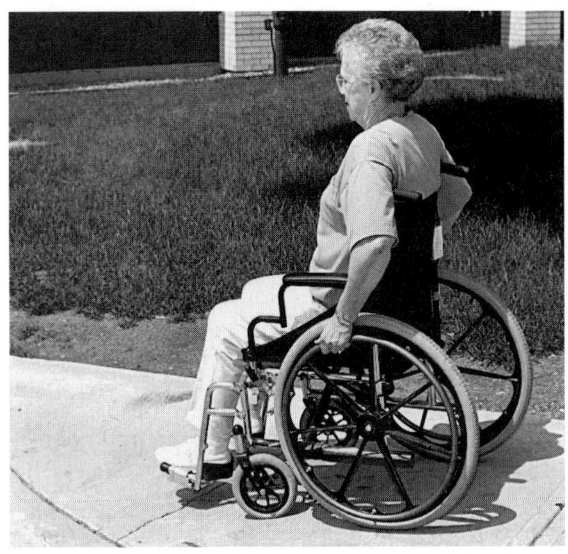

FIG. 8-47 Descent of a ramp by a patient using both upper extremities.

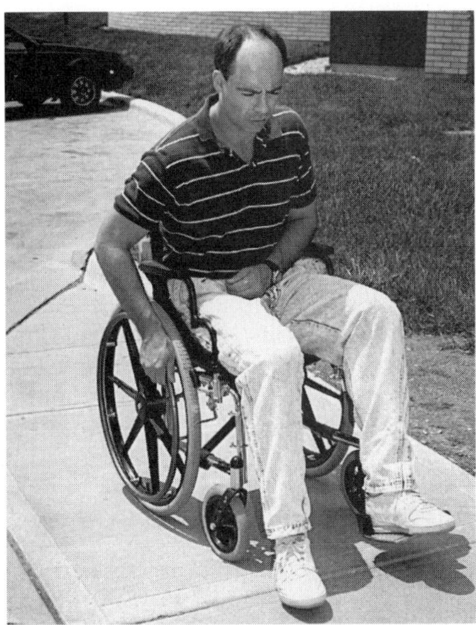

FIG. 8-46 Ascent of a ramp by a patient using one upper and one lower extremity.

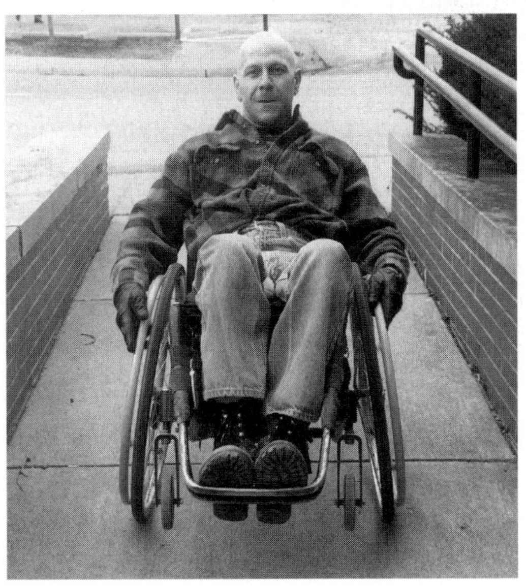

FIG. 8-48 Descending a ramp using a wheelie.

tients if they ascend backward or if a handrail is available to grasp and pull on.

Descending Forward. When the patient propels the chair with both upper extremities, instruct the person to position the hips to the rear of the seat and to maintain the trunk erect to avoid falling forward (Fig. 8-47). The person must be instructed to retard the forward motion of the chair by applying equal friction with the palms of the hands on the handrims and to avoid catching the fingers in the spokes of the wheel. The person can accomplish this by using only the palms against the side of the handrims and keeping the fingers extended. If uneven pressure is applied by the person's hands on the handrims, the chair will turn toward the wheel to which the greatest pressure is applied. Some persons may be able to descend using a wheelie position. This is an advanced technique and you must guard the patient during all practice sessions (Fig. 8-48).

When the patient propels the chair using one upper extremity and one lower extremity, instruct the person to position the hips to the rear of the seat and maintain the trunk erect. Instruct the person to retard the forward motion of the chair by applying friction of the palm of the hand against the handrim. Some additional friction may be applied when the sole of the shoe is applied to the surface. The person will need to use the functional foot to guide the chair because friction on only one handrim will cause the chair to drift or roll toward the side to which the friction is applied. For example, when friction is applied to the right handrim, the chair will tend to deviate to the right; when the friction is applied to the left handrim, it will deviate to the left. Therefore this may be a difficult activity for a patient to perform and master safely because of this problem.

Ascending Backward. Ascending backward is recommended for the person who uses one upper and one lower extremity for propulsion. Instruct the person to pull back on the handrim and push with the functional foot and lower extremity (Fig. 8-49). The person should maintain the trunk erect with the back positioned in the chair seat. One complication with this procedure is the patient is unable to see the rearward progress of the chair directly. The patient can be instructed to look behind the chair periodically or to locate a fixed object in front and use it as a guide to maintain the chair's direction.

Ascending or Descending Steep Inclines. It may be necessary to instruct the person to zigzag or angle up or down the incline; that is, propel up or down the incline at an angle to the right for several feet and then propel at an angle to the left for several feet. This pattern is continued until the top or bottom of the incline is reached.

Curbs

Ascending Forward. The person who is able to perform a wheelie can be instructed to position the chair close to and facing the curb and perform a partial wheelie to elevate the caster wheels onto the upper surface of the curb (Fig. 8-50, A). The person should lean forward and propel the chair onto the curb by pushing strongly and equally on the handrims (Fig. 8-50, *B* and C).

Occasionally, only one drive wheel ascends the curb. When this occurs, the person must shift the body weight to the side opposite to the trailing drive wheel and push forward on both handrims to propel the trailing drive wheel onto the curb (Fig. 8-51). *Caution:* If the caster wheels are not elevated high enough or if they are not placed on the upper level of the curb, the footrests are likely to strike the front of the curb. When this happens, the person's body will move forward and he or she may fall out of the chair. When the caster wheels are placed on the upper level, the person must maintain the body weight forward to avoid tipping backward.

Descending Forward. Instruct the person to approach the edge of the curb and, when the caster wheels reach the edge, perform a wheelie (Fig. 8-52). The rear wheels roll over the edge of the curb until they rest on the surface below the curb; then the caster wheels are lowered onto the support surface. *Caution:* This technique creates a risk that the person may tip backward or the chair may drop forward if the wheelie position is not maintained; thus it should be attempted only by those persons who are able to control the balance and position of the chair. You must guard the person very carefully when descending or ascending the curb forward.

Descending Backward. Instruct the person to turn the chair so the curb edge is behind the chair; wheel the chair to the edge of the curb; lean the trunk forward and allow the rear wheels to slowly and gradually roll over the edge of the curb by retarding the movement of the chair with hand friction on the handrims (Fig. 8-53). When the rear wheels are

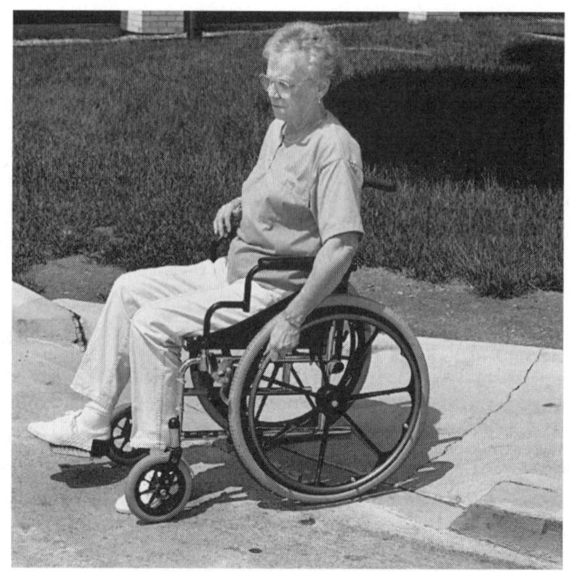

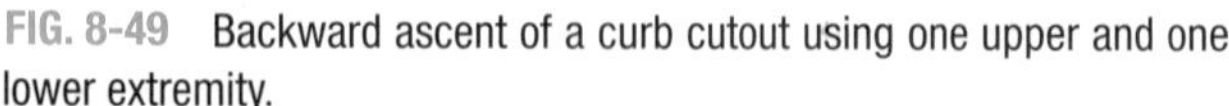
FIG. 8-49 Backward ascent of a curb cutout using one upper and one lower extremity.

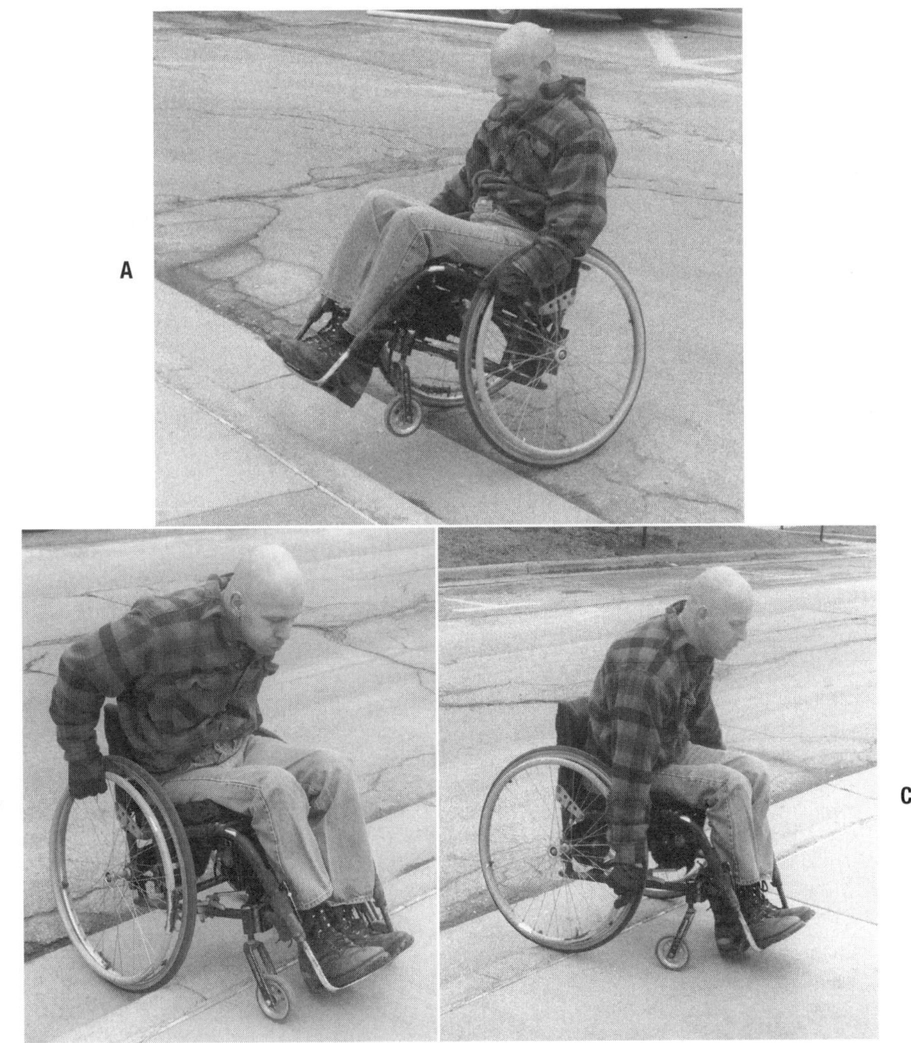

FIG. 8-50 Ascending a curb forward; **A,** Elevation of the caster wheels; **B,** Preparing to ascend the curb; **C,** Ascension of the curb.

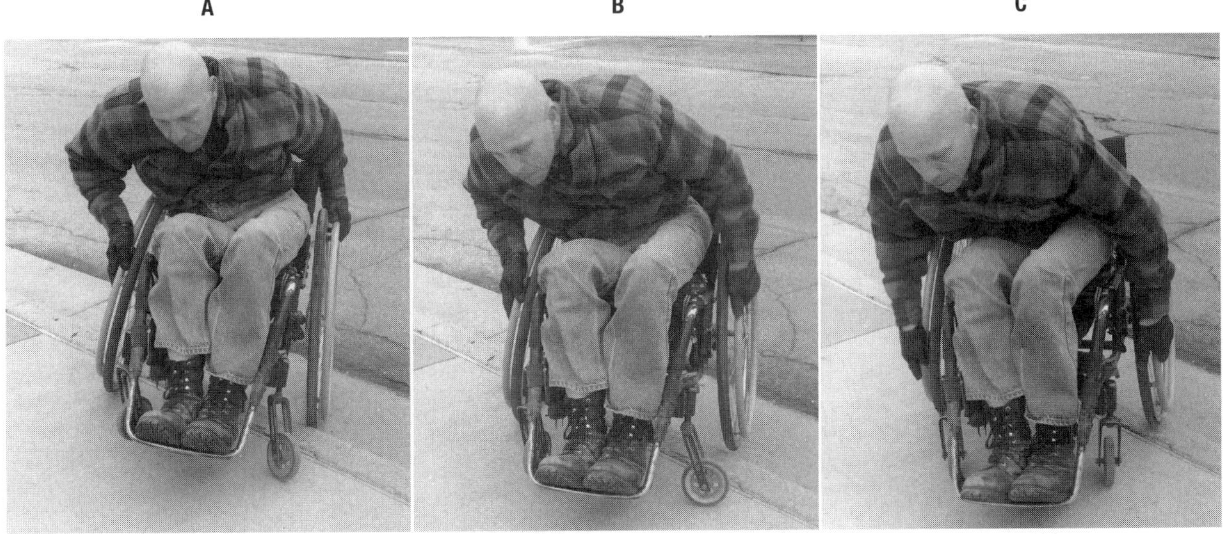

FIG. 8-51 Ascending a curb one wheel at a time. **A,** Ascent of one drive wheel; **B,** Weight shift; **C,** Ascent of the other drive wheel.

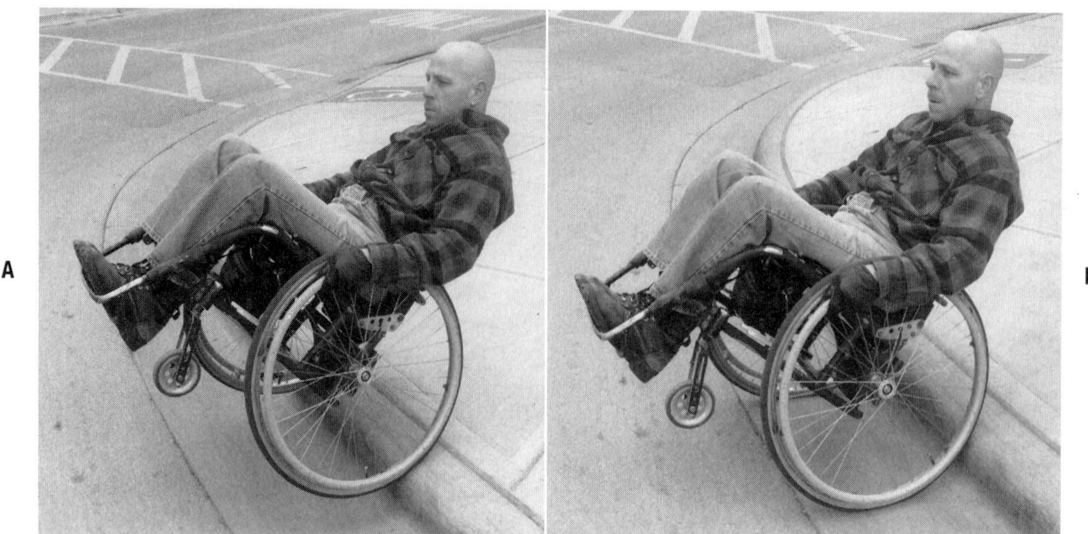

FIG. 8-52 Descending a curb forward using a wheelie.

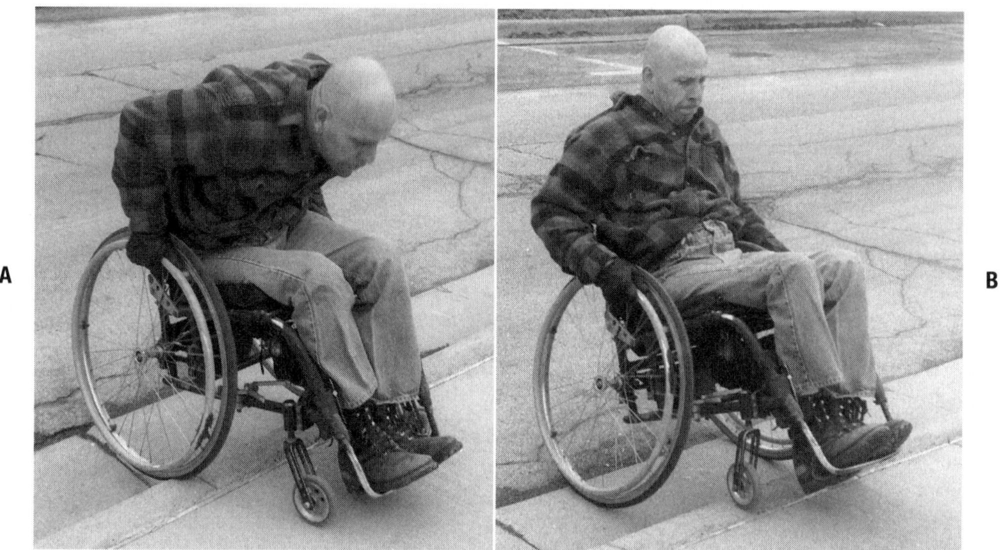

FIG. 8-53 Descending a curb backward.

on the lower surface, the person performs a wheelie and rolls back from the curb to clear the footrests from the curb; then lowers the caster wheels to the surface. If the patient is unable to perform a wheelie, the person can wheel the chair backward until the caster wheels are on the same level as the rear wheels. When this technique is used, the footplates will probably strike and rest on the curb as the chair is moved away from the curb. This can damage or cause malalignment of the footplates. *Caution:* There is a danger that the person may tip backward as the wheelie is performed or when the footrests are on the upper level of the curb. The person must lean the body forward to reduce this danger.

(*Note:* Independent ascent and descent of a curb requires excellent strength, balance, and coordination and a great amount of practice before the person is able to perform the activity safely and independently. You must guard the patient during the practice sessions by remaining behind the chair and being ready to react to excessive forward or backward movement of the chair or the person to prevent a fall or injury.) Persons who use one upper extremity and one lower extremity to propel the chair probably will not be able to ascend or descend a curb independently.

Curb Cutouts Many curb cutouts have a relatively narrow area where the cutout meets the street. If the person does not align the caster wheels of the chair properly with this area, it may be difficult to ascend the cutout forward because the footrests may contact the surface, the chair may tip back

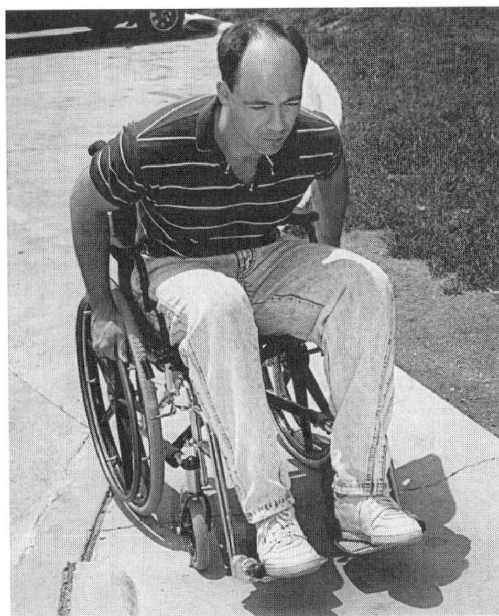

FIG. 8-54 Forward ascent of a curb cutout using both upper extremities.

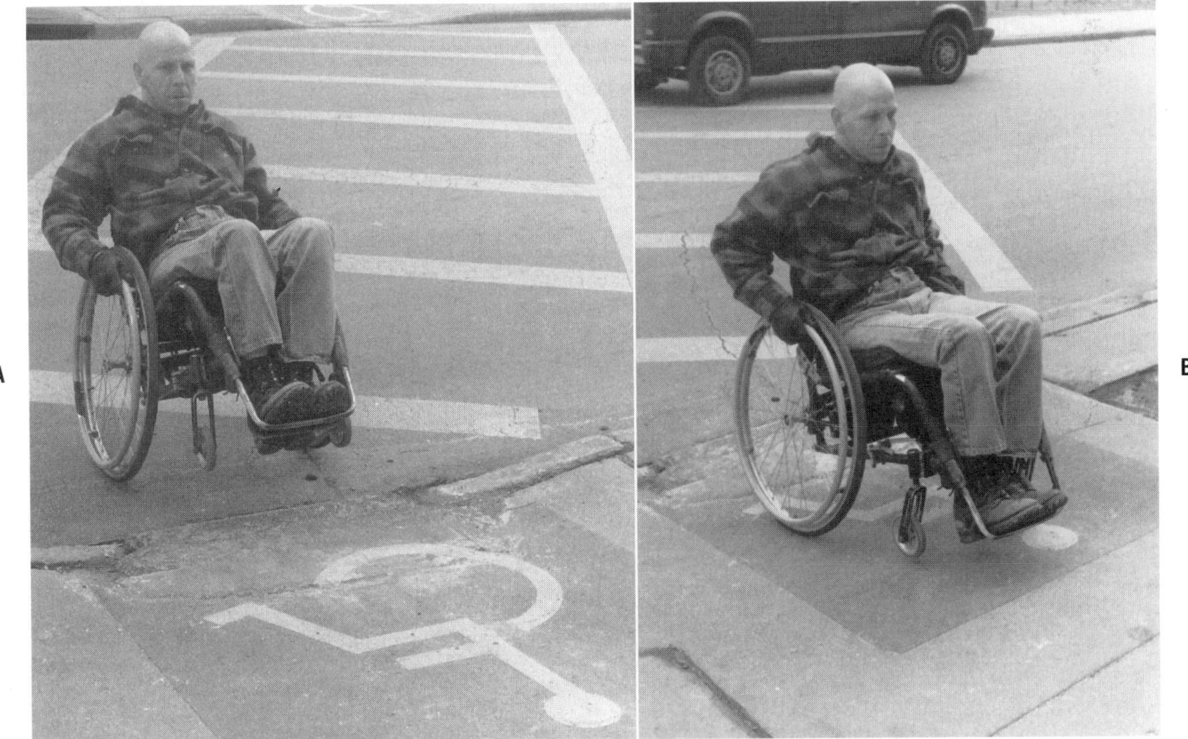

FIG. 8-55 Ascending a cutout using a wheelie to clear the base of the cutout.

when the caster wheels contact the surface, or the chair may stop abruptly when the footplate or caster wheels contact this area. The person should be instructed to observe the cutout before attempting to use it to prepare for the difficulties that could occur because of the construction of the cutout.

Ascend Forward. Instruct the person to use the same positions and techniques described for ascending an incline or ramp (Fig. 8-54). Some persons may be able to perform a wheelie and ascend the cutout on the rear wheels. This is an advanced method and you will need to guard the person during practice sessions. If the cutout is steep or uneven with the street surface, it may be necessary for the person to perform a partial wheelie to elevate the footplates over the edge of the cutout so the caster wheels will rest on the cutout surface (Fig. 8-55). The person who uses one upper and one lower extremity to propel the chair may find it easier to ascend backward. *Caution:* If the person ascends forward and the footplates strike the cutout surface before the caster wheels rest on it, a fall or loss of balance forward may occur.

Descend Forward. Instruct the patient to use the same positions and techniques described for an incline or ramp (Fig. 8-56). Some persons may be able to perform a wheelie and descend on the rear wheels of the chair (Fig. 8-57). This is an advanced technique and you will need to guard the person during practice sessions. If the cutout is steep or uneven with the street surface, the footplates may strike the street surface before the caster wheels rest on it; this may cause the person to fall or lose balance forward.

Descend Backward. Instruct the person to use the same positions and techniques described for descending a curb or incline backward by keeping all four wheels in contact with the cutout (Fig. 8-58). (*Note:* Patients who use one upper extremity and one lower extremity to propel the chair should use the same techniques as described for an incline or ramp.) If the cut out is steep, the person should lean forward during the descent.

Stairs

Descending Forward. Some persons may be able to descend multiple steps using a wheelie. This is a very advanced technique and the person must be guarded closely during all practice sessions. The same techniques that were used to descend a curb are used; balance and control of the chair must be maintained (Fig. 8-59).

Doors The user of a wheelchair should be taught to open a door, proceed through a doorway, and close a door with and

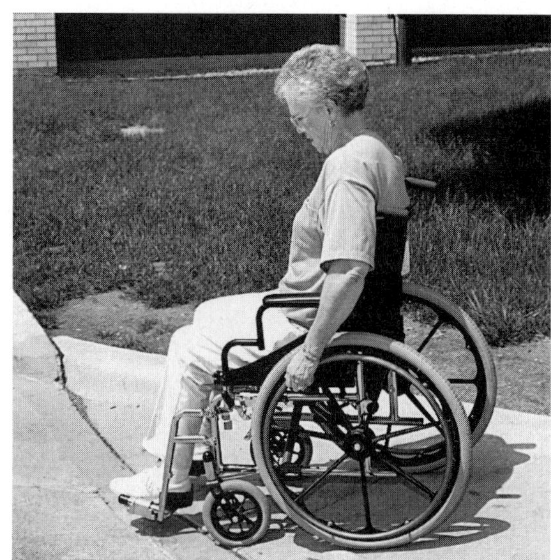

FIG. 8-56 Forward descent of a curb cutout.

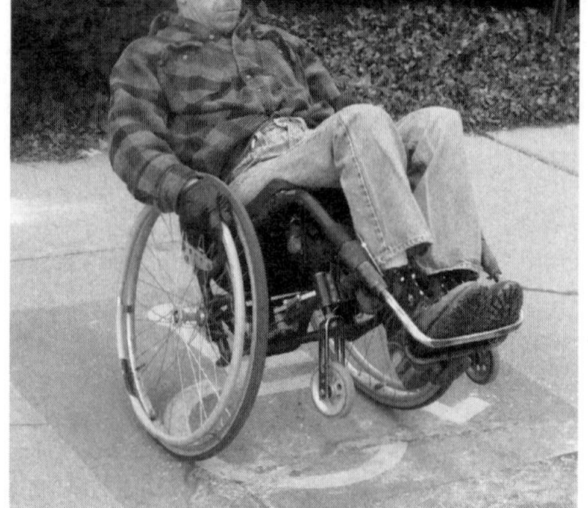

FIG. 8-57 Descending a cutout using a wheelie.

without a self-closing device. Propelling the chair through the doorway should be practiced until the activity can be accomplished safely and efficiently.

The door with a self-closing device poses problems for the wheelchair user because it offers resistance when it is opened and will be closing as the chair proceeds through the doorway. Therefore the user will need to learn specific techniques to open the door, keep it open while moving through the doorway, and avoid personal injury from the force of the self-closing device. If the resistance of the self-closing device or the size or weight of the door is excessive, or if the space available to open the door and maneuver the chair is limited, it may be necessary for the user to request assistance with this task.

If the user intends to pass through an automatic, self-opening door (that is, an electronically operated door) that swings on its hinges and opens toward the user, the person must be cautioned to remain far enough away from the door so the front rigging of the chair or the feet will not be struck by the door as it opens. The person should practice propelling the chair over a raised threshold, which is often associated with exterior doors. It may be necessary to have the patient enter and leave backward to lead with the rear wheels of the chair and make it easier to cross the threshold. When

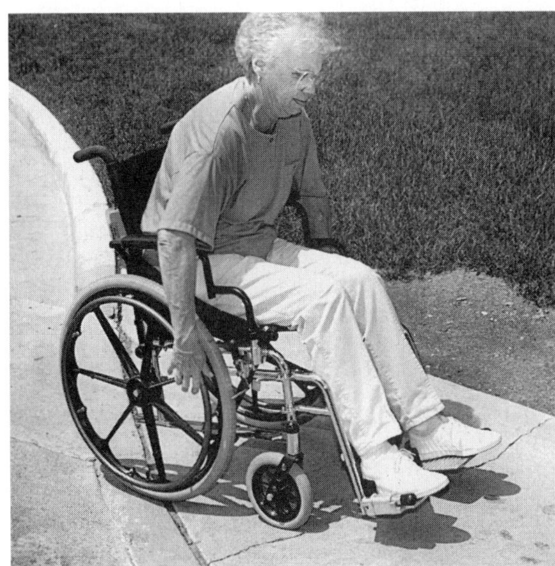

FIG. 8-58 Backward descent of a curb cutout.

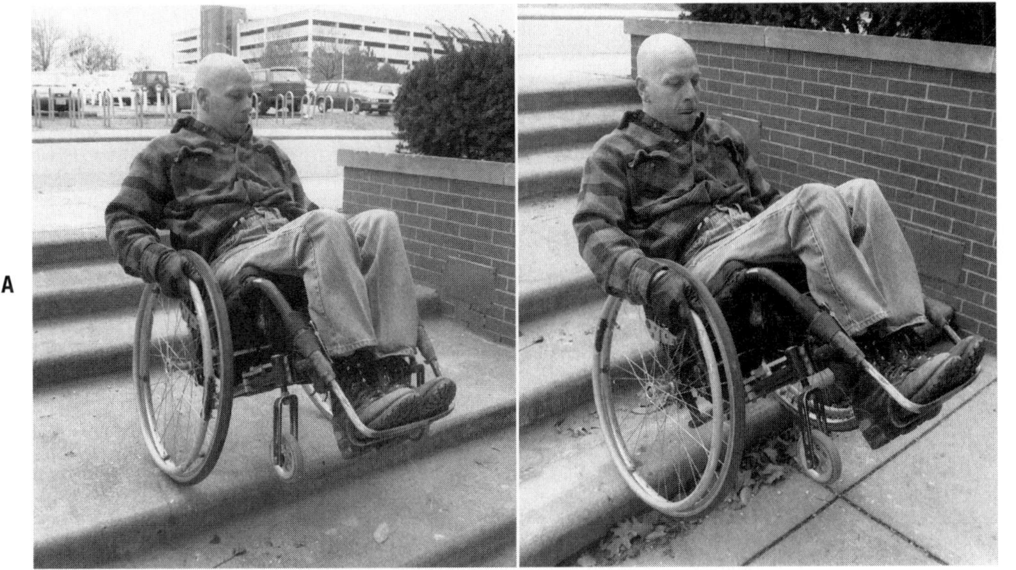

FIG. 8-59 Descending stairs forward using a wheelie.

A

B

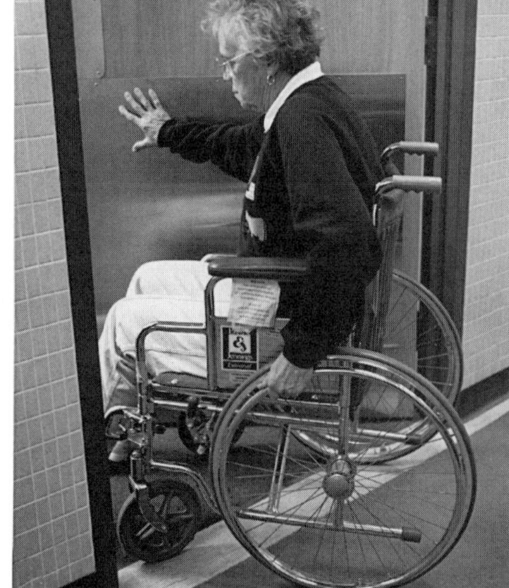

C

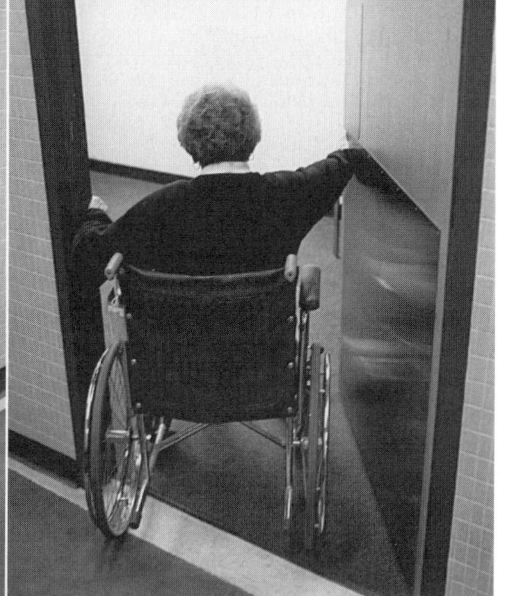

D

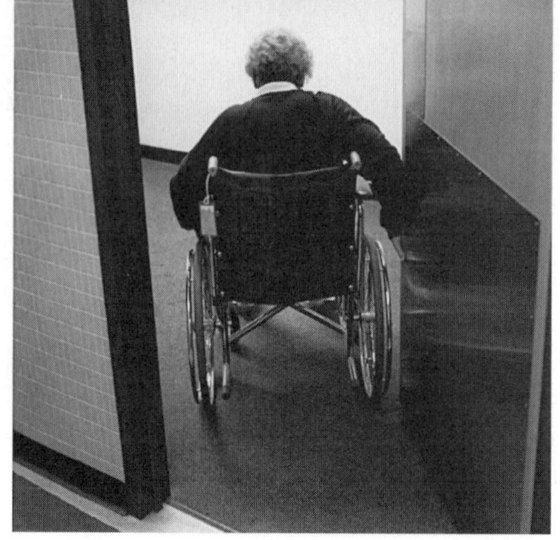

E

FIG. 8-60 Patient in a wheelchair negotiating a self-closing door that opens away from her.

entering forward, it may be necessary to perform a partial wheelie to elevate the caster wheels over the threshold.

Self-Closing Door Opening Outward (Away from the Person). Instruct the person to position the wheelchair to face the door at an angle toward the frame of the doorway containing the latch (Fig. 8-60, A). If space does not permit the person to angle the chair, instruct the person to approach the door forward and as near as possible to the edge that will open. (*Note:* The door will not need to be opened as far if the person can propel through the doorway at an angle.) The person reaches for the doorknob, latch, or *crash bar* to open the door with a quick, firm push (Fig. 8-60, *B*). The door may be opened wider than necessary with one push, but it may need to be opened with a series of short pushes until it is opened wide enough for the chair to pass through the doorway. (*Note:* Some self-closing devices provide greater resistance when a forceful push is used to open the door.)

Because of the resistance offered by the self-closing device, the patient may need to stabilize the wheelchair so it does not roll backward before pushing on the door; this can be done by holding one handrim, locking one wheel, or holding onto the doorframe (Fig. 8-60, C). The patient may be able to quickly propel the chair through the doorway before the door closes, but it is more likely the door will need to be kept open to move through it (Fig. 8-60, *D*). The person can do this by using the distal portion of the front rigging, by holding the crash bar, or by using a series of pushes on the door or crash bar to keep the door open to pass through the doorway (Fig. 8-60, *E*). The patient must protect the foot and hand nearest to the door when proceeding through the doorway.

Self-Closing Door Opening Inward (Toward the Person). Instruct the patient to position the wheelchair to face the door at an angle toward the frame of the door with the hinges (Fig. 8-61, A). If space does not permit the patient to angle the chair, instruct the person to approach the door forward and near to the edge that will open. The person reaches for the doorknob or latch to open the door with a quick, firm pull; it may need to be opened with a series of short pulls until it is opened wide enough for the chair to pass through the doorway (Fig. 8-61, *B*). The same techniques and precautions described previously to keep the door open, stabilize the chair, and propel the chair through the doorway can be applied to this activity. The person can use one hand on the door frame to pull the chair quickly through the doorway and the rear wheels can be used to prevent the door from closing until the chair is completely through the doorway (Fig. 8-61, C to *E*). (*Note:* This will be an extremely difficult task for the patient who does not have functional use of both upper extremities and good trunk control.)

Regular Door, No Self-Closing Device. Instruct the patient to position the wheelchair as described for the door that opens outward or inward. Because there is not a self-closing device, the patient will not need to use strong force to open the door and should open the door only wide enough for the chair to pass through the doorway. It will be necessary to turn the chair or the patient will need to turn the body to close the door once the chair has passed through the doorway. If the patient can move through the doorway at an angle, the door will not need to be opened as wide as it would if moving straight through the doorway. However, if there is a wall or other obstruction in the area where the person enters, it may be necessary to open the door fully to provide adequate space for the wheelchair.

Elevators The user should be taught and should practice entering and leaving an elevator car. The person may enter and exit forward or backward depending on the space available in the car and in the area outside the car, such as the corridor or entryway. You should caution the person to observe and be aware of some specific problems associated with an elevator. For instance, the floor of the elevator and the surface of the corridor or entryway may be uneven; that is, the car may stop slightly above or below the outside surface. This may make it difficult for the person to enter or exit the car because the caster wheels may not roll over the elevated surface, or the chair could stop abruptly or tip forward. If this problem occurs, the person should enter and leave by leading with the rear wheels.

A second problem occurs when there is a large space between the front edge of the car floor and the outside surface. The caster wheels may drop into this space if they are turned to the side and it may be difficult for the patient to extract them. If this problem occurs, the person should enter and leave the car with the caster wheels directed straight forward. Most of the information provided previously in the section on assisted propulsion of a wheelchair regarding use of an elevator also applies to the independent use of it; the person will need to decide whether to enter and exit forward or backward. Instruct the person to approach the external panel with the control pads or buttons with the wheelchair positioned at an angle or parallel to the wall containing the panel to be able to reach the control pads or buttons more conveniently. If the person approaches the wall directly forward, the front rigging will prevent the chair from being close to the control panel and the person will need to lean forward to reach the panel. Furthermore, it may not be possible to reach the pads or buttons that are located at the top of the panel and assistance from another person may be required.

Once the person is inside the car, it may be necessary to request another passenger to press the desired floor pad and to activate the door open control so the person can have more time to exit safely.

The person should be taught to recognize automatic door-opening devices such as a photoelectric beam or pressure sensors in the edge of the elevator doors. Remind the person that the feet and lower extremities project in front of the chair and are relatively unprotected from various objects in the environment, including the doors of an elevator.

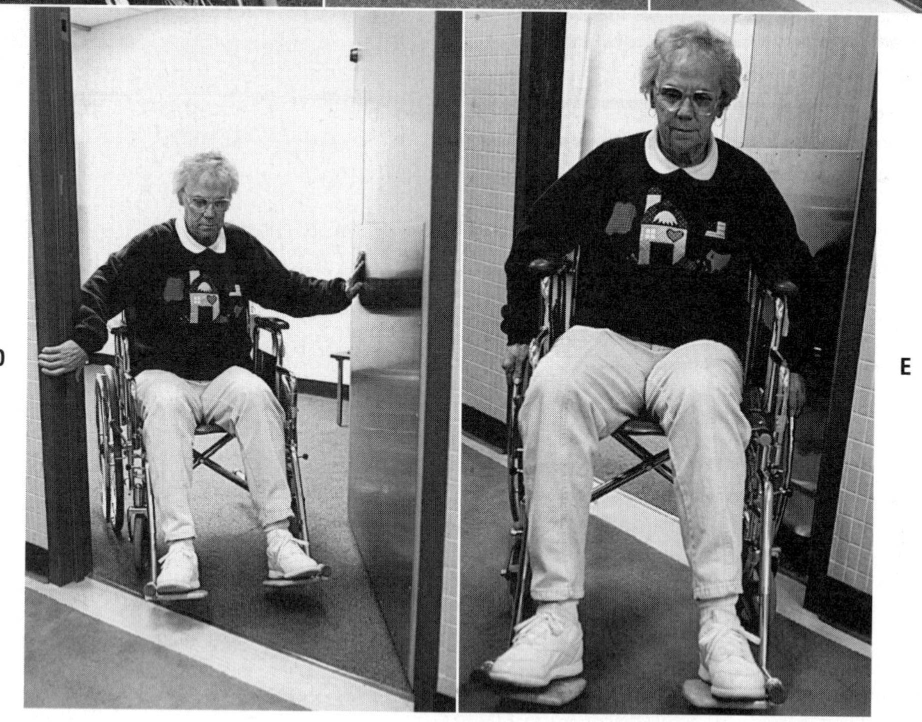

FIG. 8-61 Patient in a wheelchair negotiating a self-closing door that opens toward her.

Therefore the patient must be aware of the potential hazards or objects that could cause an injury to the feet and lower extremities. Also remind the patient that the handrims and rear wheels can provide protection, when the hands and arms are placed within the area between the two wheels (as in the lap or on the armrests). The rear of the chair is protected by the push handles and by the posterior position of the rear wheels. The front of the chair is somewhat protected by the distal portion of the front rigging; however, the feet may project beyond the foot plate.

Reaching an Object on the Floor in Front of the Chair Instruct the person to position the caster wheels in a forward position to increase the BOS of the chair (Fig. 8-62, *A* and *B*), lock the rear wheels, and shift the hips forward in the chair. Some persons may prefer to place their feet on the floor, but it is possible for the feet to remain on the footplates while the activity is performed and the person can reach forward for the object (Fig. 8-62, *C* and *D*). *Caution:* Instruct the person how to position the caster wheels and how to maintain trunk control while reaching forward. The caster wheels can be positioned by maneuvering the chair until they face forward to increase the distance between the back of the caster wheel and the front of the rear wheel. The person may need to control the trunk by holding onto a push handle, the back frame, the seat frame, the armrest, or the upper position of the front rigging. The specific site chosen will depend on the patient's condition and abilities.

If the object weighs more than 5 to 10 pounds, the chair is likely to tip forward onto the footplates when the object is lifted from the floor, or the person may have difficulty lifting the object and returning to an erect posture. This activity should be considered relatively unsafe and should be used primarily in an emergency. It is imperative to have the caster wheels positioned *forward* before the patient attempts this

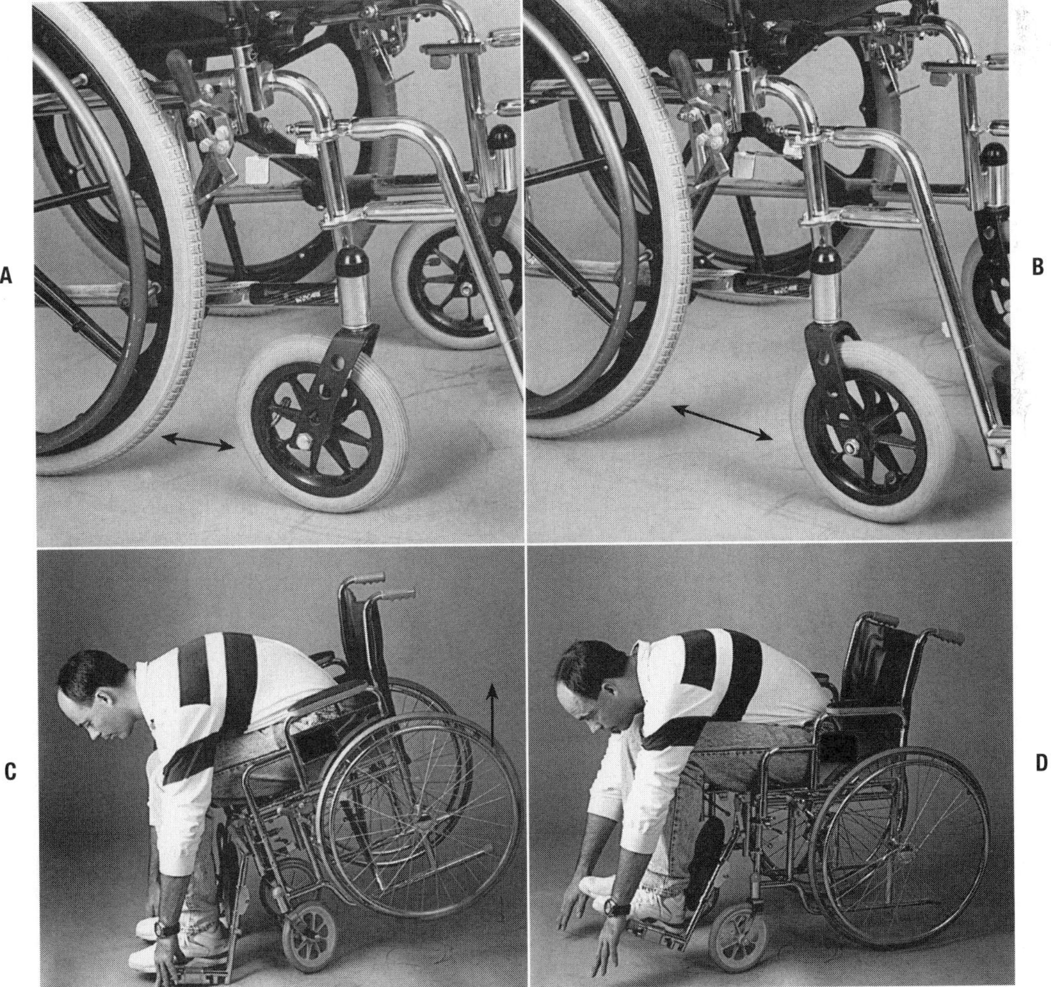

FIG. 8-62 Patient in a wheelchair reaching for an object on the floor. **A,** Improper position of wheels. **B,** Proper position of wheels. **C,** Person reaching forward with wheels in improper position. **D,** Person reaching forward with wheels in proper position.

task. A safer procedure is to teach the patient to reach for and lift the object with the chair positioned to the side and parallel to the object.

Falling Backward When the chair tips backward, instruct the person to prevent the knees and thighs from hitting the face by placing one forearm across them with the hand holding the opposite armrest (Fig. 8-63, *A*). The person should flex the neck and reach forward with the free arm to promote trunk flexion (Fig. 8-63, *B*). The person should not attempt to reach backward for protection because this will increase the speed of the fall and the possibility of injury to the upper extremities and head. The push handles of the chair will strike the ground before the back of the chair, but it is important for the person to keep the head and trunk forward. Grasping an armrest with one hand will help to keep the body in the chair. The feet are likely to fall off the footrests and the lower legs may dangle below the seat when the chair tips back.

Returning to an Upright Sitting Position. Instruct the person to remain in or return to the chair and lock the rear wheels, place one hand on the floor behind the chair, and reach with the other arm across the body to the opposite seat rail or armrest (Fig. 8-64). The person uses the hand on the floor to "walk" forward, keeping the head and trunk flexed to move the chair to an upright position. When the chair has been elevated to its highest point, a rapid, strong push with the hand on the floor while reaching forward with the other arm and flexing the head and neck will assist in tipping the front of the chair down. (*Note:* This is an advanced activity that will require a great amount of practice. A lap belt may be necessary during the practice sessions and an assistant may be needed to help the patient attain an upright position. Many patients may not be able to perform this activity independently.) Some persons may fall out of the chair when it tips; therefore it may be necessary to instruct the person to place the chair upright and enter the chair forward or backward as described in Chapter 7.

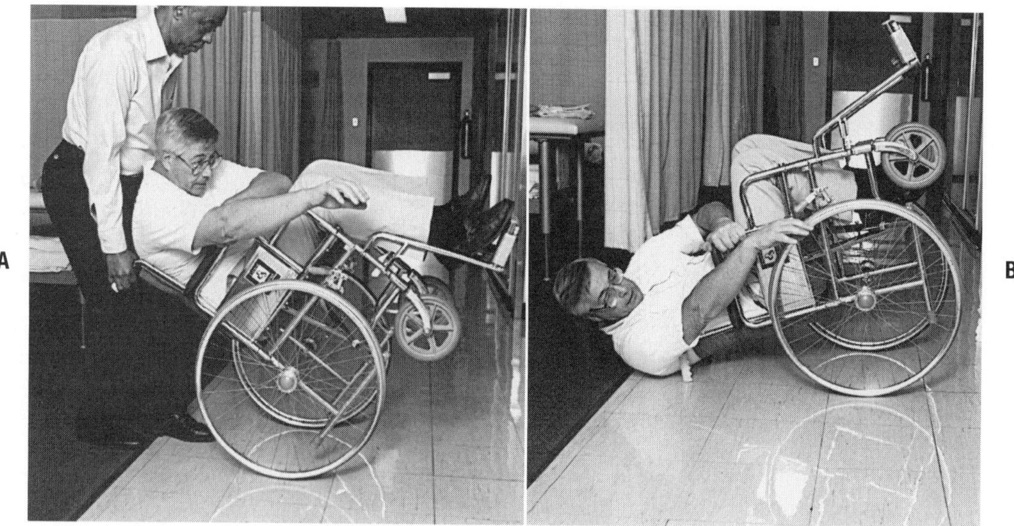

FIG. 8-63 Instructing a patient in a wheelchair how to fall backward.

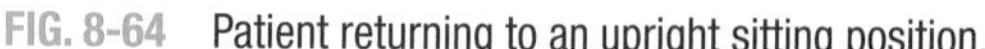

FIG. 8-64 Patient returning to an upright sitting position.

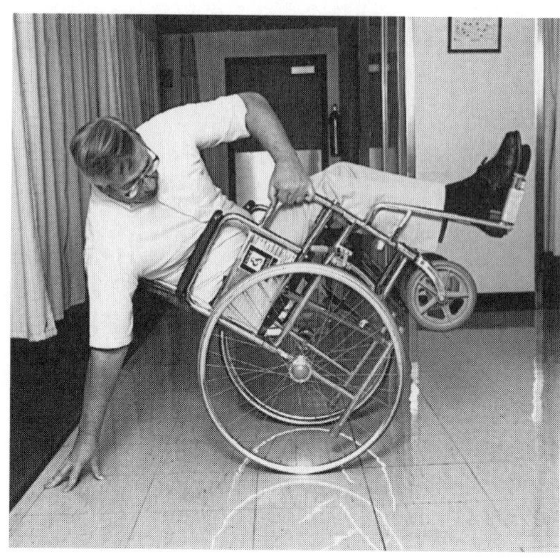

Falling Forward If the caster wheel strikes an object while the chair is moving, the patient may fall forward. If this occurs, instruct the person to hold an armrest with one hand and reach toward the floor with the other hand. This technique may cause the chair to fall on top of the person if the armrest is held too long; therefore some patients prefer to reach forward with both hands simultaneously for protection. Instruct the patient to absorb the force of the fall by flexing the elbows when the hands strike the floor. The knees may strike the floor with excessive force and injury may result unless the person is taught to turn the body to land on the lateral area of a hip (Procedure 8-3).

Moving from the Wheelchair to the Floor and Returning to the Wheelchair Techniques for the patient to move from the wheelchair to the floor and return to the wheelchair are presented in Chapter 7. These techniques allow the patient to plan and somewhat control the movement from the wheelchair to the floor and return to the wheelchair. They should not be confused with the information related to falling forward or backward while seated in a wheelchair. However, a review of that material may provide some ideas you could offer the patient to assist in developing methods of self-protection should a fall from the chair occur.

PROCEDURE 8-3

Protected Fall from a Wheelchair

These procedures should be described and demonstrated by the caregiver before the patient attempts them; guard closely when the patient practices the activity and protective mats should be placed on the floor.

BACKWARD FALL

The patient quickly grasps an opposite armrest with one hand, allowing the forearm to rest on the thighs.

The chin is lowered toward the chest and the free upper extremity reaches *forward.*

A semiflexed position is maintained and the push handles contact the floor.

To return to an upright position, the person remains in the chair, locks the rear wheels, places one hand on the floor behind the chair, grasps an opposite armrest with the free upper extremity, and "walks" the hand on the floor forward while keeping the head and trunk flexed.

The fingers are used to push strongly and the opposite upper extremity reaches forward to move the chair to an upright position.

An alternative method is to remove the body from the chair, position the chair on all four wheels, and reenter the chair using one of the techniques presented in Chapter 7, provided no serious injury has occurred.

FORWARD FALL

The patient reaches forward with both upper extremities.

When the hands contact the floor, the elbows are flexed to absorb some of the force of the fall.

The person attempts to turn or pivot the pelvis to land on one hip or, if the knees contact the floor first, attempt to side sit on one hip.

To return to the chair, the chair is positioned on all four wheels and the person reenters the chair using one of the techniques presented in Chapter 7, provided that no serious injury has occurred.

GENERAL CARE AND MAINTENANCE

A wheelchair will function best when it is maintained properly. The user should be encouraged to read and follow the instructions contained in the maintenance manual supplied by the manufacturer or distributor. Periodic cleaning of exposed metal with a nonabrasive metal polish or automobile wax and cleaning of the upholstery by use of an appropriate fabric cleaner or damp cloth is recommended. The chair should not be immersed in water or sprayed with a hose and it should be wiped dry after exposure to rain, snow, or other types of moisture. The cross-brace center pin should be lubricated with a molybdenum-based grease every 6 months. Do not use light oil because it will collect dirt particles and will not provide long-lasting lubrication. The armrest insert posts and the front and rear post slides (that is, the open tubing into which the armrest posts insert) should be lubricated periodically with a silicone spray such as WD-40 or with a small amount of paraffin. The wheel bearings can be lubricated only if they are removed from the wheels. A high-quality bearing grease should be used as the lubricant. Do not oil the bearings because oil will decrease the effectiveness of the grease that is in the bearings and the overall lubrication will be decreased. It may be best to have these items inspected and lubricated by a reputable dealer or repair service.

Frequent visual inspection of the frame, upholstery, wheels, joints, tires, and other parts of the wheelchair will enable early detection of signs of wear or disrepair. Pneumatic tires should be checked for proper inflation at least monthly. Wheel spokes should be tested for tightness and loose ones should be tightened to maintain proper rim shape and support. *Caution:* Improper tightening of the spokes may distort the shape of the rim and it may be best to have this adjustment performed by a reputable dealer or repair service. The user and family members should be encouraged to read the owner's manual periodically for information about proper maintenance. The facility where the chair was purchased and the manufacturer are additional sources of information about proper chair maintenance. In many large cities, wheelchair repair or service facilities are available and can be found in a telephone directory; additional information may be available from a health care facility. The patient and the family should be encouraged to perform proper maintenance and repair the chair promptly to enhance its function and longevity.

SUMMARY

When a wheelchair is a person's primary means of *locomotion*, it must fit and function properly to enhance independence. The caregiver should evaluate and confirm the fit of the wheelchair and determine its mechanical and functional condition. The potential adverse effects of an improperly fitting wheelchair should be recognized by the caregiver and explained to the user. These problems should be corrected or modified as soon as possible to avoid injury, discomfort, or reduced independent function.

The caregiver should become competent in the management and handling of the chair to be able to demonstrate and instruct others in proper techniques or procedures. The person using the chair should be instructed to use the chair independently, including how to perform as many functional activities as possible within established abilities. Instruction in the proper maintenance and care of the chair should be provided.

self-study ACTIVITIES

- Discuss the potential adverse effects on the user of an improperly fitted wheelchair in relation to seat width, seat depth, leg length, armrest height, seat height, and back height.
- Describe how you would teach a patient to propel a standard wheelchair on a level surface using both upper extremities; one upper extremity and one lower extremity. Consider how the person will turn and move backward.
- List the primary components of a standard wheelchair.
- Describe how you would confirm the fit of the wheelchair with the patient seated in the chair.
- Describe how you would teach a patient to elevate the caster wheels (that is, perform a wheelie or pop-up).
- Outline what type wheelchair and components are required and explain your rationale for your selection for persons with hemiplegia of the left upper and lower extremities; paralysis below the level of T10; bilateral midthigh amputations (no prostheses); paralysis below the level of C3.

problem SOLVING

1. You are preparing a wheelchair user for reentry to her job and she informs you that she will need to use an elevator and must be able to turn the wheelchair using a small radius. What instructions or directions would you provide to enable her to perform these activities safely and effectively?
2. One of your patients who uses a wheelchair must be able to perform a wheelie to ascend and descend curbs and maneuver over rough terrain. He is a 20-year-old patient with a spinal cord injury at the T10 level. How would you teach him to perform these activities safely and effectively from initial instructions to independent function?

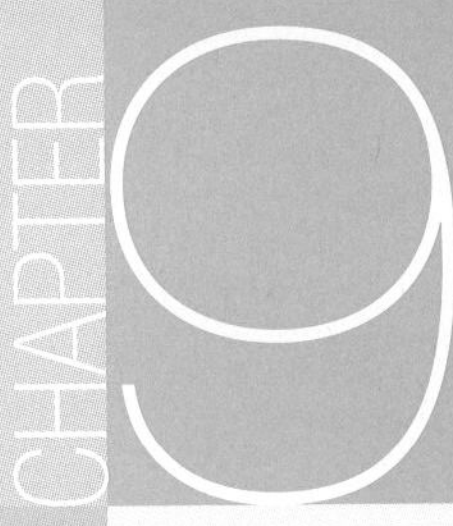

Ambulation Aids, Patterns, and Activities

objectives *After studying this chapter, the reader will be able to:*

- Identify various types of ambulation aids.
- Describe the advantages and disadvantages of various types of ambulation aids.
- Describe and perform the two-point, four-point, three-point, three-one–point, and modified gait patterns.
- Describe the advantages and disadvantages of the previously cited gait patterns.
- Teach a patient to perform any of the gait patterns cited, using appropriate equipment for the person's condition.
- Describe and perform various functional activities when using ambulation aids.
- Teach a patient to perform the functional activities appropriate for the person's condition, using proper ambulation aids.

key terms

Affected Attacked by disease; afflicted.
Ambulation Act of walking or being able to walk.
Ambulation aid A piece of equipment (such as crutch, cane, or walker) used to provide support or stability for a person when walking.
Anteroposterior From the front to the rear of an object or living being.
Axilla Armpit.
Axillary crutches Wooden or metal crutches, adjustable or nonadjustable, that fit under a person's upper arms and into the axilla with a handpiece to grasp.
Bilateral Pertaining to two sides.
Crab cane A cane with three or four feet that forms a wider base of support than the single crutch tip; also referred to as a *three-* or *four-footed, quad,* or *hemi cane.*
Dorsiflexion Backward flexion or bending, as of the hand or foot; for example, when the top of the foot (dorsum) approaches the lower leg or ankle, *dorsiflexion* has occurred.
Forearm crutches Wooden or metal crutches with a full or half cuff that fits over a person's forearms and with a handpiece to grasp; also known as *Lofstrand* or *Canadian crutches.*
Four-point gait The repetitive, alternate, reciprocal forward movement of an ambulation aid (such as a crutch or cane) and a person's opposite lower extremity.
Functional activities Activities identified by an individual as essential to support the person's physical and psychologic well-being and to create a personal sense of well-being.
Gait The manner or style of walking.
Immobilizer An object or apparatus that immobilizes or prevents motion, such as a cast or brace.
Monitor To check constantly on a given condition or phenomenon, such as blood pressure or heart or respiration rates.
Parallel bars Wooden or metal bars, adjustable or nonadjustable, that are horizontal and parallel to each other and attached to vertical uprights to provide a stable, nonmobile support for a person who requires an ambulation aid.
Pelvis The lower portion of the trunk of the body.
Platform attachment Wooden or metal crutches with an adjustable or nonadjustable platform for a person's forearm to rest on and aid in weight bearing.

key terms—cont'd

Reciprocal Corresponding but reversed on both sides.
Riser A vertical piece of wood joining two steps; the back of the step.
Scapular Pertaining to the scapula.
Styloid process Long and pointed bony projection.
Three-one–point gait One lower extremity is full weight bearing and the opposite lower extremity is partial weight bearing; bilateral canes, crutches, or a walker are used to partially support the body weight as the person bears weight on the partial weight-bearing lower extremity; the full weight-bearing lower extremity advances independently and the ambulation aids and partial weight-bearing lower extremity advance simultaneously.
Three-point gait One lower extremity is full weight bearing and the opposite lower extremity is nonweight bearing; bilateral crutches or a walker are used to support the person's weight when the weight-bearing lower extremity advances.
Tripod position The use of three points as supports, such as a cane or crutch tips and a person's feet, with the tips in front of and to the side of the person's feet to form a base of support when the person stands.
Trochanter A broad, flat surface on the femur at the upper end of its lateral surface (greater trochanter).
Two-point gait The repetitive, simultaneous, reciprocal forward movement of an ambulation aid (such as a crutch or cane) and a person's opposite lower extremity.
Ulnar Pertaining to the ulna, one of the two bones of the forearm.
Unilateral Pertaining to one side.
Walker An ambulation aid, usually with four contacts that are placed on the floor and a frame to support the patient's weight and provide stability during ambulation.

INTRODUCTION

An individual may require *ambulation aids* or devices to compensate for impaired balance, decreased strength, alteration in coordinated movements, pain during weight bearing on one or both of the lower extremities, absence of a lower extremity (with or without prosthetic replacement), or altered stability; to improve functional mobility; to enhance body functions; and to assist with fracture healing. Selection of the proper ambulation devices or aids and *gait* pattern is important to provide optimal security, safety, and function with the least expenditure of energy.

ORGANIZATION OF AMBULATION ACTIVITIES

It is important that planning and organization occur before initiating *ambulation* activities. The caregiver must be aware of the patient's disability and abilities; the goals and expectations of ambulation; the selection, measurement, and fit of the equipment; and the selection, practice, and progression of specific gait patterns and functional activities required by each patient (Box 9-1). The caregiver must provide safety and protection for each patient through the use of proper guarding techniques, precautions, and instructions (Box 9-2). The caregiver may need to prepare the patient physically or mentally to perform the activities the patient and caregiver decide are important.

PREAMBULATION EQUIPMENT, PROCEDURES, AND ACTIVITIES

Usually it is beneficial and necessary to provide a period of preparation and training for a patient who will ambulate with assistive aids. This is especially true for persons who have been immobile; whose condition has affected their balance, coordination, strength, flexibility, or ability to tolerate an erect position; who are elderly; or whose physical capacity to learn or perform motor skills has been diminished. The purposes of preambulation procedures and activities are to provide safe and stable practice sessions; improve the patient's ability to use assistive ambulation aids safely and effectively; determine the type of assistive aids and functional skills the patient will require; and allow the patient to develop confidence in the use of the assistive aids. Equipment such as a tilt table to assist the patient to accommodate to an erect position, parallel bars for safety and security when practicing a gait pattern or to improve balance, and various ambulation aids to allow mobility and functional tasks can be used. Methods to strengthen muscles of the upper and lower extremities, to improve cardiopulmonary function and endurance, to train in sitting and standing balance, and to teach and practice ambulation patterns and functional skills may need to be performed. The selection of specific equipment, including ambulation aids and the procedures or activities to be used, is based on the findings of the patient's examination and evaluation and the goals of treatment

Box 9-1 Preparation for Ambulation Activities

Review the patient's medical record for information to assist in planning the ambulation activities. What information will be particularly important to you?

Assess, examine, and evaluate the patient to determine limitations and capabilities to assist in planning the preambulation activities and gait pattern.

Determine the appropriate equipment and pattern based on the medical record, your assessment, and the goals of intervention.

Prepare the patient for ambulation (for example, explain the pattern, obtain consent, and improve physical abilities).

Remove items in the area that may interfere with ambulation to maintain a safe environment.

Verify the initial measurement of the equipment to ensure a proper fit and determine that the equipment is safe (for example, tighten loose nuts and bolts, be certain spring adjustment buttons are secure, and examine rubber tips for dirt or cracks in the rubber).

Always apply a safety belt to the patient.

Be certain the patient is mentally and physically capable of performing the selected gait pattern.

Explain and demonstrate the gait pattern for the patient; ask the patient to describe the pattern, how it is to be performed, and what is expected to be performed. Require an explanation of the procedure or activity to verify the person truly understands and comprehends your instructions.

Use the safety belt and the patient's shoulder as points of control when guarding the patient.

Maintain proper body mechanics for yourself and the patient.

Box 9-2 Precautions for Ambulation Activities

Be sure the patient wears appropriate footwear; do not allow the patient to ambulate while wearing slippers or loosely fitting shoes or while not wearing shoes. These conditions can lead to patient insecurity and injury.

Monitor the patient's physiologic responses to ambulation frequently and evaluate vital signs, general appearance, and mental alertness during the activity. Compare your findings with normal values to determine the patient's reaction to the activity.

Avoid guarding or controlling the patient by grasping clothing or an upper extremity. These items are insufficient for protection.

Anticipate the unexpected and be alert for unusual patient actions or equipment problems; anticipate that the patient may slip or lose stability or balance at any time.

Guard the patient by standing behind and slightly to one side and maintain a grip on the safety belt until the patient is able to ambulate independently and safely.

Do not leave the patient unattended while standing; the patient may not be totally stable.

Protect patient appliances (such as cast, drainage tubes, intravenous tubes, and dressings) during ambulation.

Be certain the area used for ambulation is free of hazards, such as equipment or furniture, and the floor or surface is dry. Safe conditions must be maintained to reduce the risk of injury to the patient.

related to the patient's functional outcomes. The caregiver must be aware of the home, workplace, and social environments to which the patient will return to be certain all functional needs can be determined and practiced. Often it will be helpful for a family member or coworker to observe the patient perform the ambulation pattern and primary functional activities before discharge. If necessary, the family member should be instructed in and should practice guarding techniques. Specific oral or written instructions regarding safety, precautions, or contraindicated activities should be given to the patient and family member.

PREAMBULATION EQUIPMENT

Ambulation aids are designed to improve a person's stability by expanding the base of support (BOS), to reduce weight bearing on one or both lower extremities, and to permit mobility. Stated another way, they help the patient compensate for decreased balance, strength, coordination, or a decreased ability to bear weight on one or both lower extremities, and they assist to relieve pain during ambulation. Although it is not an ambulation aid, a tilt table can be used for patients who must physiologically accommodate to an erect position before they can initiate ambulation.

The basic categories of ambulation aids, given in order from greatest to least in their amount of support or stability, are parallel bars, *walkers*, bilateral crutches, single crutches, bilateral canes, *crab canes*, and single canes. A patient may need to initiate ambulation with an aid that provides maximal stability or support, but restricts mobility. As the patient's ability or condition improves, the person may be able to progress to an aid that provides less stability or support and allows greater mobility. Decisions regarding which type of aid to use, when to change to a different aid, and the type of gait pattern to use are made by the caregiver. Criteria to consider include information on the referral, the persons present mental and physical abilities, the environment in which the patient will ambulate, the expected or desired ambulation activities, and the prognosis for improvement or regression of the patient's condition and abilities.

Tilt Table

A tilt table may benefit persons who need to physiologically accommodate to an upright position because of a variety of conditions, such as prolonged recumbence; disturbance in balance, proprioception, kinesthesia, or lower extremity circulation; or generalized weakness. A tilt table is particularly useful because it can be elevated gradually and maintained at any position between horizontal and completely vertical. Changes in elevation levels are accomplished manually or mechanically; an angular scale or protractor attached to the frame can be used to measure the elevation angle the person attains and tolerates. The ability to gradually elevate a person from a horizontal to an upright position and to allow the person to adapt or adjust to any given elevation provides a safe method for the body to accomplish physiologic accommodation for upright activities (Fig. 9-1).

The person's vital signs should be measured before treatment to establish baseline values, especially for blood pressure and pulse rate, and each time there is a progression to a higher elevation; a log of the values should be maintained. Excessive increases or decreases in the blood pressure and pulse rate are usually indicators the person is experiencing difficulty adapting to an upright position. Other indicators of the person's intolerance include changes in consciousness, excessive perspiration, edema formation in the lower legs, decrease in or loss of pedal pulses, complaints of nausea or numbness, change in facial or limb color (flushed or pale), tingling in the lower extremities, and dizziness. A person whose condition limits the capacity or ability to return venous blood from the lower extremities or abdomen to the heart may benefit from the application of elastic bandages or elastic hose to the lower extremities or from an abdominal binder.

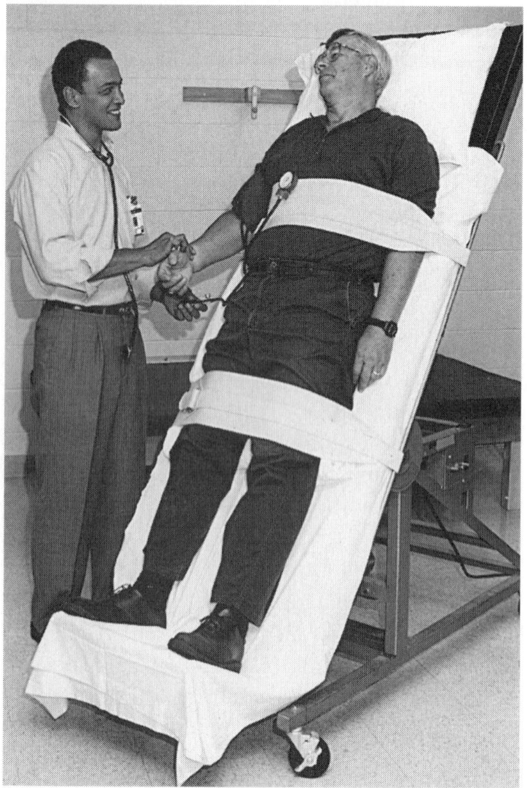

Fig. 9-1 Use of a tilt table; caregiver measures pulse rate and blood pressure.

Although it is the circulatory system that is primarily conditioned, bowel and bladder function may also be affected because of the effect of gravity. In addition, it has been theorized that standing on a tilt table may assist in promoting or maintaining bone density in the lower extremities, especially for the person with a complete spinal cord injury. However, research studies have not provided conclusive evidence that this effect occurs.

Many persons who have used a tilt table have indicated that their mental outlook was improved because they were able to assume a semiupright or fully upright position even if only for a brief period. Other activities can be performed by the person while standing, depending on the amount of function of the upper extremities, mental status or capacity, and the maximum elevation tolerated. An adjustable over-the-bed table or a lap board attached to the frame of the tilt table can be used to support items such as reading or writing materials, food and utensils, communication devices, personal hygiene materials, games, cards, and similar items. Thus the person can be somewhat active while erect rather than merely standing. Strengthening and range-of-motion exercises can be performed and some lower extremity muscle groups can be positioned so a prolonged passive stretch force can be applied to them.

Usually it will not be necessary to elevate the table to 90 degrees to assist the person to adapt to or accommodate to an upright position. An elevation of approximately 70 to 80 degrees for 15 to 20 minutes should be sufficient; however, you must consider each person individually. When the person is elevated above 80 degrees the sensation of falling forward may occur. This occurs because the person's center of gravity (COG) will be shifted forward because of the pressure from the surface of the table against the back. The compensatory function of the *anteroposterior* curves of the body is negated by the table surface; thus the person senses a forward position change has occurred. The frequency and duration of treatment sessions with a tilt table vary depending on the person's condition or diagnosis, the response to the treatment, and the ability or capacity to adapt to, accommodate, or tolerate an upright position. A session may be as brief as 5 or 10 minutes or as long as 1 hour and sessions may occur once or twice per day or on alternate days (Procedure 9-1).

Parallel Bars

Parallel bars are used when the patient requires maximal stability, support, and safety. Balance training and gait patterns can be initiated in parallel bars and the evaluation of the fit of the ambulation aids is frequently performed in bars. The bars severely limit mobility and the patient must progress to another ambulation aid to be mobile. The bars should be adjusted so the patient's hips and trunk pass though them with clearance on each side and at the height of the person's greater trochanters when the person stands erect.

Walkers

Walkers are used when maximal patient stability, support, and mobility are required. Various styles are available and most have four support legs or feet; some may have two or more wheels, and most can be adjusted for proper fit. Walkers are lightweight and some can be folded for storage. Disadvantages of a walker include the following:

- It may be difficult to store or transport.
- It is difficult or impossible to use on stairs.
- It reduces the speed of ambulation.
- It may be difficult to perform a normal gait pattern.
- It can be difficult to use in narrow or crowded areas.

Types include standard (adjustable, nonadjustable), *reciprocal*, stair-climbing, wheeled, folding, and one-handed ("hemiplegic") (Fig. 9-2).

PROCEDURE 9-1

Tilt Table

Explain the procedure to the patient and obtain consent; measure the person's vital signs.

Position the patient supine on the table; place a rolled towel beneath each knee; position the feet flat on the footboard approximately shoulder width apart. The upper extremities may be positioned parallel to the sides of the body; they may be placed beneath or remain free from the chest strap or they may rest on an over-the-table support or be supported by slings attached to the table frame. A pillow under the head will add to the patient's comfort until elevated to approximately 75 degrees, at which time it may be more comfortable to remove it.

Apply one restraint strap over the lower thighs (just proximal to the patellae) and one strap across the mid or upper thorax; a towel may be placed beneath each strap for protection and comfort; the strap buckles should be positioned so they do not contact the patient. *Note:* When the lower strap is applied over the distal thigh rather than directly over the patellae, pressure to the patellae can be avoided. If desired, a third strap can be applied over the abdomen or pelvis. *Caution:* An abdominal strap should not be used in place of a chest strap, especially for a person who lacks functional trunk and hip extensors. An abdominal strap, without a chest strap, will not prevent the upper body from falling forward at elevations at which gravity has a forward force effect (that is, approximately 65 degrees and higher). If a chest strap is not in place, the person must have sufficient strength and control of the trunk and hip extensors to maintain the body erect.

Elevate the table to a position tolerated by the person; maintain that position for several minutes; measure and log the vital signs; inquire about his or her status (for example, "How do you feel?" "Are you comfortable?").

When the patient's condition is stable, raise the table to a new elevation; measure and log the vital signs; determine the tolerance to the new position; maintain the position for several minutes.

Repeat this process based on the person's ability to tolerate and accommodate to becoming more erect; continue to measure and log the vital signs; decrease elevation of the table when it is apparent a given elevation is not tolerated. *Caution:* Signs and symptoms of intolerance to being upright include loss of consciousness; excessive increase in pulse rate (tachycardia) or excessive decrease in blood pressure (hypotension); facial pallor; excessive perspiration; or complaints of nausea, dizziness, sensory or color changes in the lower extremities. Be observant for signs and symptoms of autonomic hyperreflexia and postural (orthostatic) hypotension. (Refer to Chapter 12 for information about these conditions.) *Note:* Several sessions may be required for the person to become tolerant to an upright position.

To conclude a treatment session, return the patient to horizontal; observe the person; measure and log the vital signs; observe and palpate the lower extremities for edema or circulatory responses (that is, pedal pulses, color, temperature). Document your activities and findings as necessary.

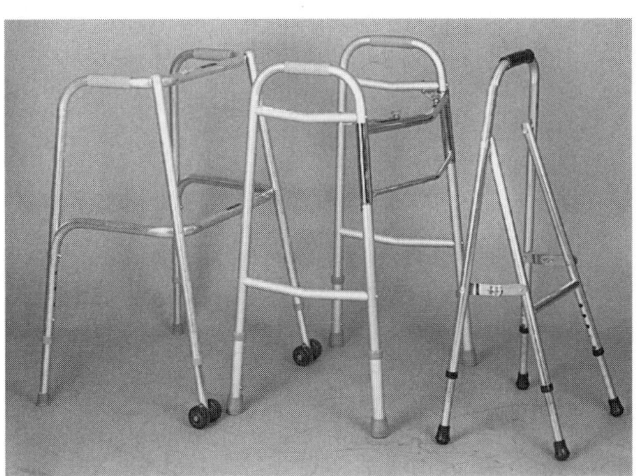

Fig. 9-2 Three types of walkers *(left to right):* the wheeled, folding, and "hemi" walkers. All are adjustable.

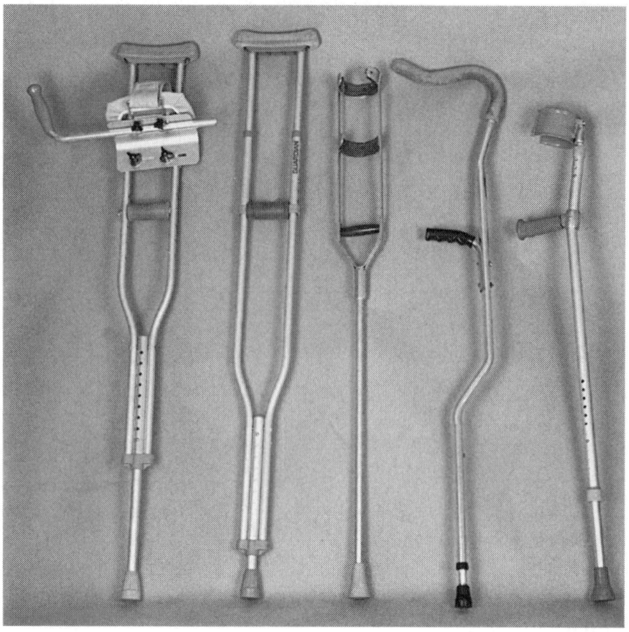

Fig. 9-3 Five types of crutches *(left to right):* the forearm attachment, adjustable aluminum, triceps, offset adjustable, and forearm adjustable (Lofstrand or Canadian crutches).

Axillary Crutches

Axillary crutches are used for persons who need less stability or support than is provided by parallel bars or a walker. They allow greater selection of gait patterns and ambulation speed and provide stability and support. Most crutches are composed of wood or aluminum and can be easily adjusted for proper fit. They can be stored and transported and can be used in narrow or crowded areas or for stairs. Disadvantages of axillary crutches include the following:

- They are less stable than a walker.
- They can cause injury to axillary vessels and nerves if used improperly.
- They require good standing balance.
- Elderly patients may feel insecure with them.
- Functional strength of the upper extremities and trunk muscles is required for selected gait patterns.

Types include standard (adjustable, nonadjustable), offset, and triceps (elbow extension) (Fig. 9-3).

Forearm Crutches

Forearm crutches, also referred to as *Lofstrand* or *Canadian crutches*, are used when the stability and support of an axillary crutch are not required, but more stability and support than can be provided by a cane are needed. They eliminate the danger of injury to axillary vessels and nerves and are more functional on stairs and in narrow, confined areas; are easy to store and transport; and the forearm cuff retains the crutch on the forearm when the patient reaches for an object. Disadvantages of forearm crutches include the following:

- They provide less stability and support than axillary crutches, a walker, or parallel bars.
- They require functional standing balance and functional upper body and upper extremity strength for many gait patterns.
- The forearm cuff makes it difficult to remove the crutch.
- Elderly patients may feel insecure with them.

Types include aluminum or wood, adjustable, nonadjustable (see Fig. 9-3).

Platform Attachment

A *platform attachment* is used for individuals who are unable to bear weight through their wrists and hands; who have severe deformities of the wrists or fingers, making it difficult to grasp the handpiece of a regular crutch; who have a below-elbow amputation; or who are unable to extend one or both elbows. Disadvantages of a platform attachment include the following:

- The patient loses the use of the triceps to elevate and maintain the body during the swing phase.
- Another person may need to apply them.
- They are less effective on stairs.

Types include a platform that can be attached to an axillary or forearm crutch or to a walker; it is sometimes referred to as a "trough" or "shelf" (see Fig. 9-3).

Cane

A cane is used to compensate for impaired balance or to improve stability. A cane is more functional on stairs and in narrow, confined areas, and it can be stored and transported more easily than crutches or a walker. Disadvantages of a cane include the following:

- A cane provides very limited support because of its small BOS.

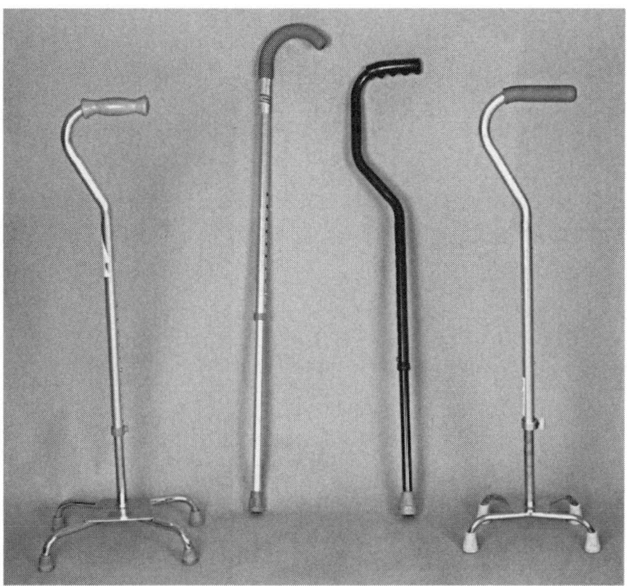

Fig. 9-4 Four types of canes *(left to right):* wide base four-footed adjustable ("crab" or "hemi"), J-top adjustable, offset adjustable, and narrow base four-footed adjustable ("crab" or "hemi").

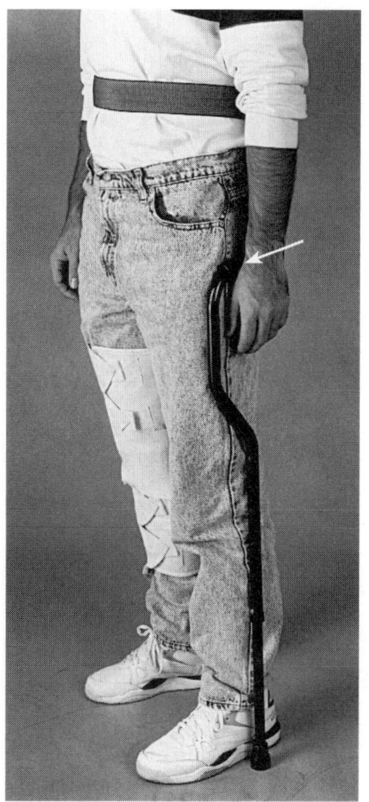

Fig. 9-5 Measurement for proper fit of a cane.

- Two canes do not provide sufficient stability and support to perform a *three-point gait* pattern, but they can be used to perform other gait patterns.

Types include "J," "T," pistol grip, offset shaft, three- or four-legged or -footed (sometimes referred to as a *quad, hemi,* or crab cane), and Walkane (walk cane) (Fig. 9-4).

MEASUREMENT AND FIT

Several methods can be used to initially measure the various ambulation aids. If the initial measurement is performed with the patient in a position other than standing, the fit of the aid must be evaluated and confirmed when the patient stands. An aid that does not fit the patient properly will adversely affect the patient's ability to perform a gait pattern and may result in an unsafe or unstable pattern. The position to use to confirm the fit of the aid is described in another section of this chapter.

Parallel Bars

Each bar should be adjusted to provide 20 to 25 degrees of elbow flexion when the patient stands erect and grasps the bars approximately 6 inches anterior to his or her hips. The bars should be approximately 2 inches wider than the patient's *greater trochanters* when the person is centered between the bars. Elbow flexion can be estimated by adjusting the bar so its top is even with the patient's greater trochanter or with the patient's wrist crease or *ulnar styloid process* when the patient stands erect and the upper extremity is straight along the side.

Canes

The length of the cane can be determined with the patient standing or supine. The handgrip of the cane should be placed at the level of the patient's greater trochanter or the wrist crease or the ulnar styloid process with the arm straight along the side. Place the cane parallel to the femur and tibia with the foot (tip) of the cane on the floor or at the bottom of the heel of the shoe (Fig. 9-5). A tape measure can be used to determine the distance from the patient's greater trochanter to the heel with the hip and knee straight, which determines the length of the cane when the patient is supine.

Forearm Crutch

The length of the crutch can be measured as described for the cane to determine the height of the handpiece with the patient supine or standing (Fig. 9-6, *A*). The top of the forearm cuff should be located approximately 1 to 1.5 inches distal to the olecranon process when the patient grasps the handpiece with the cuff applied to the forearm and the wrist in neutral flexion-extension (Fig. 9-6, *B*).

Axillary Crutch

Several methods can be used to measure this aid.

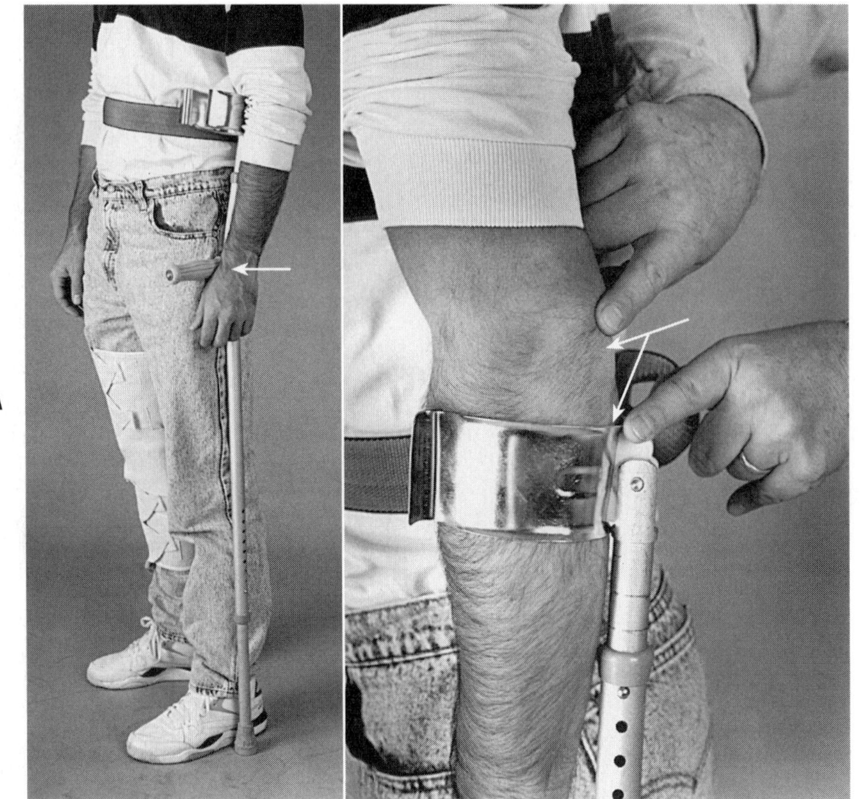

Fig. 9-6 Measurement for proper fit of a forearm crutch.

Length of Crutch

1. If the height of the patient is known, multiply the height by 77% (for example, 70 inches × 77% = 53.90, or 54 inches) *or* subtract 16 inches from the height (for example, 70 inches − 16 inches = 54 inches) and use the resulting value for the overall crutch length (that is, axillary rest to tip).
2. With the patient supine, use a tape to measure the distance from the anterior axillary fold (crease of the armpit) to a point approximately 6 to 8 inches lateral to the heel for the overall crutch length.
3. With the patient sitting and the upper extremities abducted at shoulder level, with one elbow extended and one elbow flexed to 90 degrees, measure from the olecranon process of the flexed elbow to the tip of the long finger of the hand of the opposite upper extremity; this determines the overall crutch length.

These methods should provide similar results, but there may be a difference in the measurements. You will need to select the method that provides the best result consistently. *Note:* These measurements are only estimates of the length of the crutch and need to be confirmed with the patient standing.

Handpiece Height With the patient supine, measure from the greater trochanter, from the wrist crease, or from the ulnar styloid process with the arm by the side, elbow extended, to the heel of the shoe; hold the tape next to the side of the lower extremity. Use this value to position the handpiece by measuring up from the rubber tip of the crutch to the handpiece. An alternative method is to measure from the anterior axillary fold to the patient's trochanter or ulnar styloid with the arm along the side, elbow extended. Use this value to position the handpiece by measuring downward from the center of the axillary rest to the handpiece.

Parallel Bar Method Stand the patient in parallel bars with the head erect, shoulders level and relaxed, upper extremities grasping the parallel bars, trunk erect, hips straight, *pelvis* level, knees slightly flexed, and feet flat on the floor. Use this position to measure from a point at the anterior axillary fold to a point on the floor approximately 2 inches lateral and 4 to 6 inches anterior to the patient's toes for the overall crutch length. *Note:* It will be necessary to ask the patient or another person to hold one end of the tape at the *axilla* as you extend the tape to the floor.

To determine the handpiece height, the crutch should be positioned in the patient's axilla with the tip forward and lateral to the patient's toes. The patient should have approximately 20 to 25 degrees of elbow flexion when grasping the handpiece while keeping the shoulders level and

Box 9-3 **Common Errors in Fitting of Axillary Crutches**

The patient elevates or hunches the shoulders and the crutches will be measured improperly; they will be too long when the patient stands properly.
The patient depresses or drops the shoulders or flexes the trunk at the hips and the crutches will be improperly measured; they will be too short when the patient stands properly.
The patient flexes or extends the wrist and the handpiece will be improperly positioned.
The measurements are made without the patient wearing shoes or without the crutch tips or axillary pads in place; the crutches will be improperly measured and will be too long as a result.
The crutch evaluation is made without the patient in the tripod position; the crutches may be too short or too long depending how the patient stood initially.

relaxed. The slight amount of elbow flexion will allow the patient to lift or support the body by extending the elbows during the nonweight-bearing (NWB) phase of the three-point gait pattern and to maintain a comfortable elbow position when other gait patterns are used. To obtain the most accurate measurement and fit, the axillary pad, handpiece pad, and crutch tip should be applied before all measurements are made and the fit is confirmed and the patient should wear shoes.

Alternative Method. Position the patient in the parallel bars as described previously. Using a crutch with push-button ("quick fit") length and handpiece adjustments, position the crutch in the axilla and along the patient's side. Adjust the handpiece at the level of the wrist crease, greater trochanter, or ulnar styloid process; then position the tip approximately 2 inches lateral and 4 to 6 inches anterior to the forefoot (toes), and adjust the length so that there are approximately two fingerbreadths between the axillary rest and the bottom of the axilla. Have the patient grasp the handpiece and evaluate the amount of elbow flexion and the length of the crutch with the crutch in the proper forward, *tripod position*. Readjust the crutch as necessary to obtain the proper length and handpiece position.

Any one of these methods should provide an initial measurement; do not rely on these measurements to be exact or final. The fit must be evaluated and confirmed with the person standing with the ambulation aid properly positioned.

Common errors associated with the measurement or evaluation of fit of axillary crutches are listed in Box 9-3.

Walker

The height of the walker can be determined with the patient standing or supine. The handgrip of the walker should be placed level with the patient's wrist crease, ulnar styloid process, or greater trochanter, with the walker positioned in front of and along the patient's sides and with the patient's arms straight along the sides (Fig. 9-7). The feet of the walker should be resting on the floor or even with the heels, the hips and knees should be straight, and shoes should be worn. A tape measure can be used to determine the distance from the patient's greater trochanter to the heel, with the shoe on and with the hip and knee straight. This value is used to adjust the height of the walker by measuring from the floor to the top of the handpiece with the walker resting on its feet on the floor or on a higher surface such as a treatment table for convenience.

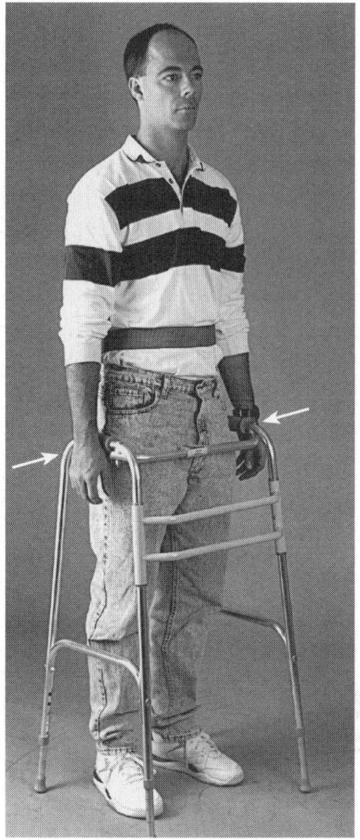

Fig. 9-7 Measurement for proper fit of a walker.

CONFIRMATION OF FIT

Improper fit is apt to cause decreased stability, increased energy expenditure, decreased function, and decreased safety for the patient.

The evaluation of the fit of axillary crutches can be performed only with the patient standing with the head erect, shoulders relaxed and level, trunk erect, hips in extension, pelvis level, knees slightly flexed, and feet flat on the floor. The crutch tips are positioned approximately 2 to 4 inches lateral and 4 to 6 inches anterior to the toes or forefoot; the elbows should be flexed approximately 20 to 25 degrees when grasping the handpiece with the wrists in a neutral

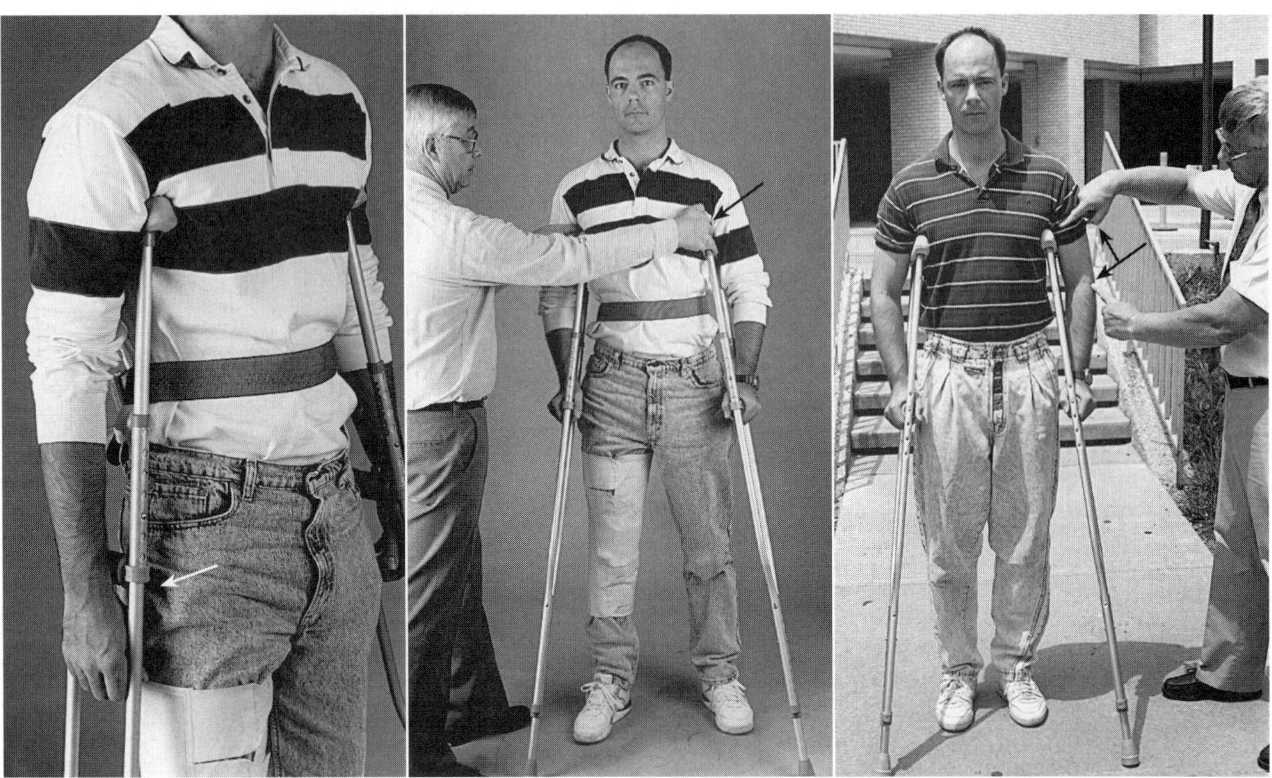

Fig. 9-8 Measurement and confirmation of the fit of axillary crutches.

PROCEDURE 9-2

Confirmation of the Fit of an Ambulation Aid

Each aid should be evaluated for fit with the patient standing with the head erect, shoulders relaxed and level, trunk erect, pelvis level, knees flexed slightly, and feet (foot) flat.

AXILLARY CRUTCHES

Position the axillary rest in the axilla; position the tips approximately 2 inches lateral and 4 to 6 inches anterior to the toe of the shoe(s).

Have the patient grasp the handpieces with the wrists straight (avoid wrist flexion or extension).

Evaluate for space between the top of the axillary rest and the floor of the axilla; it should be approximately 2 inches.

Observe the angle of elbow flexion; it should be approximately 20 to 25 degrees.

FOREARM CRUTCHES

Have the patient grasp the handpieces with the forearms inserted in the forearm cuffs.

Position the crutch tips approximately 2 inches lateral and 4 to 6 inches anterior to the toe of the shoe(s).

Observe the angle of elbow flexion; it should be approximately 20 to 25 degrees.

Observe the position of the upper edge of the cuff; it should be approximately 1 to 1.5 inches below the olecranon process.

WALKER

Position the walker in front of the patient so the rear feet are approximately opposite to the midportion of the shoes.

Have the patient grasp the handpieces.

Observe the angle of elbow flexion; it should be approximately 20 to 25 degrees.

CANE

Position the cane so the tip is approximately 2 inches lateral and 4 to 6 inches anterior to the toe of the shoe(s).

Observe the angle of elbow flexion; it should be approximately 20 to 25 degrees.

PARALLEL BARS

Position the patient standing erect between the bars.

Adjust the height of the bar (rail) so it is level with the greater trochanter or even with the wrist crease with the upper extremity by the side.

Observe the angle of elbow flexion when the person grasps the bars; it should be approximately 20 to 25 degrees.

Adjust the width of the bars, if possible, to provide approximately 2 to 4 inches of space between the patient's hip on each side and the bar.

position. This position forms a triangle of the crutch tips and the patient's foot or feet and is called the tripod position. This position provides the best BOS and starting position for most crutch gait patterns, especially the three-point and three-one patterns (Fig. 9-8).

The fit of a walker, a cane, and forearm crutches should also be confirmed with the patient standing. There should be approximately 20 to 25 degrees of elbow flexion when the patient grasps the handpiece and positions the device in preparation for ambulation. The tips of the forearm crutches and cane(s) are placed forward approximately 4 to 6 inches and approximately 2 to 4 inches lateral to each forefoot. The rear tips of the walker should be placed opposite to the midportion of the feet (foot). The patient's posture should be similar to that described for the crutch fit evaluation. The initial fit of the aid may need to be revised after the patient has ambulated several times. As the patient becomes stronger, more skilled, and more proficient, the initial fit of the aid may no longer be comfortable or efficient. It will be necessary to observe the patient during ambulation to determine whether the aid continues to fit properly. The aid should be readjusted if it does not provide proper function to avoid the development of bad gait habits or an unsafe gait pattern (Procedure 9-2).

Weight-Bearing Status

The patient may be required to perform the gait pattern with NWB, partial weight bearing (PWB), or full weight bearing (FWB) on one lower extremity. *Note:* The term weightbearing as tolerated (WBAT) may be used on some referrals. If only PWB is permitted, the patient must learn to judge the amount of weight placed on the restricted lower extremity. One method is to have the patient place the PWB extremity on a scale and bear weight up to the amount that has been predetermined. After this, the patient will need to rely on proprioception to remember and repeat using a similar amount of weight bearing during ambulation. It may be necessary to reevaluate the patient's ability to PWB with the proper amount of weight. For some patients, a temporary device with a microswitch connected to an audible alarm can be attached to the shoe. The microswitch can be adjusted to cause the alarm to sound when the predetermined amount of weight bearing is reached or exceeded.

If a "touch-down" or "toe-touch" gait is requested, the patient should be encouraged to use a heel-strike gait or place the foot flat with partial weight bearing rather than using a toe-touch gait. Although the toe-touch pattern can be used to decrease the amount of weight bearing a patient performs, it is an abnormal pattern because it positions the foot in plantar flexion at the beginning of the weight-bearing (stance) phase of the pattern. The normal gait pattern requires the heel to contact the floor first, so a heel-strike or foot-flat approach should be taught.

Box 9-4 Major Muscle Groups Used for Nonweight-Bearing Ambulation

Upper trunk: scapular depressors, scapular stabilizers
Lower trunk: trunk extensors, trunk flexors
Upper extremity: shoulder depressors, shoulder extensors and flexors, elbow extensors, finger flexors
Weight-bearing lower extremity: hip abductors, hip extensors, knee extensors, ankle dorsiflexors
Note: Strength, flexibility, endurance, and motor control of these groups should be evaluated before ambulation training and deficiencies should be corrected so the ambulation activity can be performed safely.

Muscle Activity

The primary phases of gait are the stance and swing phase. When a lower extremity is in contact with the floor or other surface (that is, weight bearing), it is in the stance phase; when it is not in contact with the floor (that is, NWB) it is in the swing phase. The upper extremities are used for support, stability, and movement when ambulation-assistive devices are used. The scapular stabilizers; shoulder depressors, flexors, and extensors; elbow flexors and extensors; and finger flexors are the primary muscles involved to support the body's weight and assist in propelling the body. In the weight-bearing phase, the hip extensors and abductors and the knee flexors and extensors are the primary muscles involved to support the body's weight. The hip flexors, knee flexors, and ankle dorsiflexors are used to elevate the extremity and, with momentum, move the extremity during the NWB (swing) phase. Other muscles of the upper and lower extremities are also used during gait and should not be overlooked during the assessment of the patient's strength. Trunk musculature, especially the trunk extensors, is necessary to maintain an erect position and proper posture (Box 9-4).

SAFETY CONSIDERATIONS AND PRECAUTIONS

Proper guarding techniques must be used to protect the patient during ambulation and associated *functional activities*. The caregiver must observe the patient and note any problems with balance, coordination, strength , or endurance and determine the ability to perform all activities safely. The judgment of the caregiver as to when the patient is able to ambulate independently and safely is a critical decision.

Patient Protection and Guarding Techniques

A safety belt must be applied before and during all ambulation and functional gait activities. The belt should be applied securely around the waist; if it has a buckle,

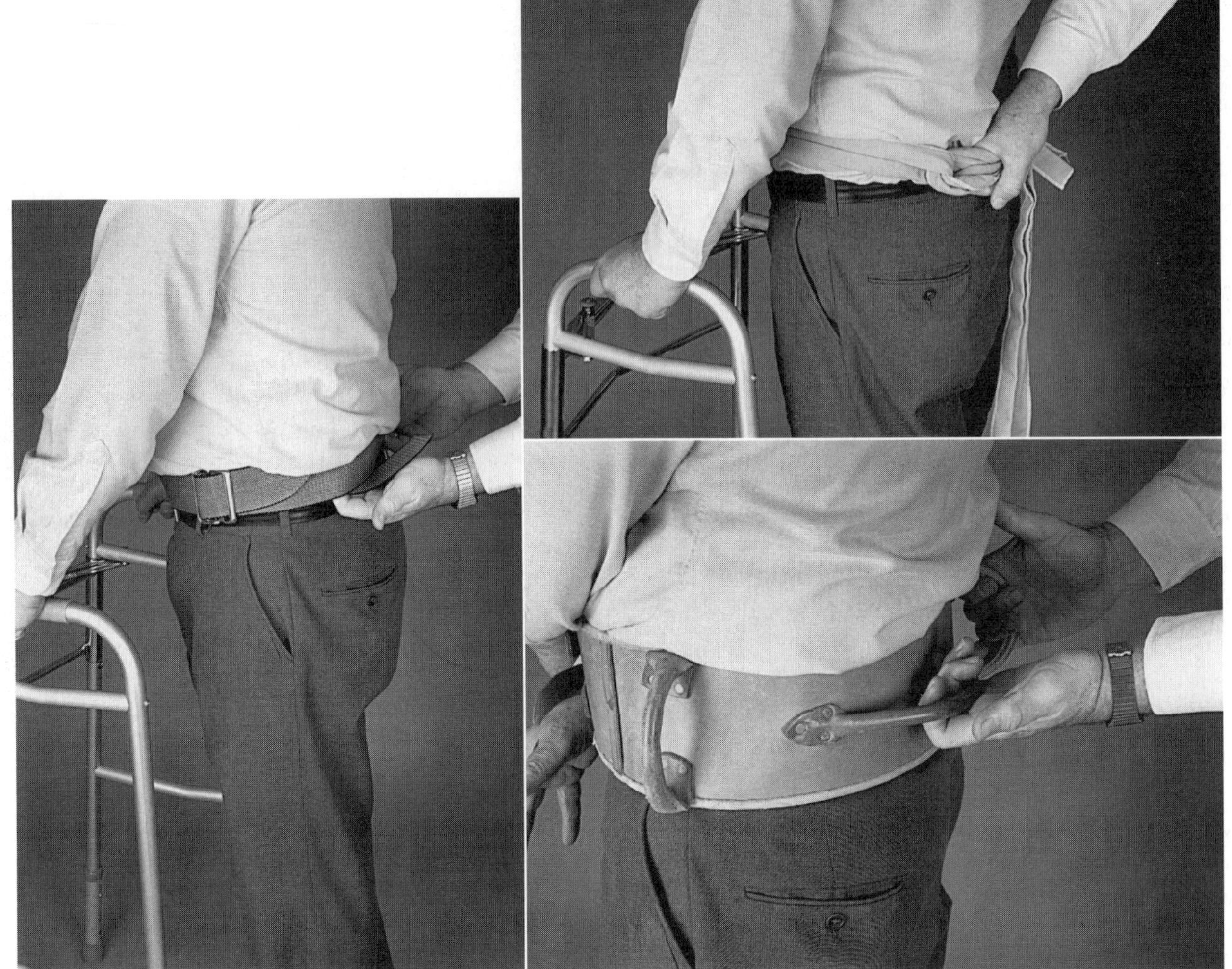

Fig. 9-9 Caregiver grasping a correctly applied safety belt.

position it so it will not injure the patient if tension is applied to it (that is, position the buckle to the side or at the back (Fig. 9-9). *Caution:* Do not use the patient's clothing, upper extremity, or personal belt for control. These items are not sufficiently strong or secure to provide a safe grasp site.

Position During Level-Ground Ambulation Stand behind and slightly to one side of the patient. Many clinicians recommend the caregiver stand to the side of the patient's affected or weakest side or lower extremity. However, a patient can be guarded safely and protected regardless of which side you stand. Your personal preference, sense of best control, or facility policy may be factors that determine the position you choose.

Use your hand nearest to the patient to grasp under the back of the safety belt with your palm up and forearm supinated. Position your other hand above the patient's nearest shoulder or allow it to rest lightly on it (Fig. 9-10). If you rest your hand on the shoulder you must not restrict the patient's movement or cause an alteration in balance. You must be prepared to control the shoulder and upper trunk quickly or move your forearm across the chest to maintain optimal control. *Caution:* Be certain your arm does not contact the anterior neck or throat. If the patient is much taller than you it will be better to slide your arm between the patient's upper extremity and chest when you need to control the trunk.

Place your feet in an anteroposterior stance with your most forward lower extremity between the patient's lower extremity and the ambulation aid; position your opposite

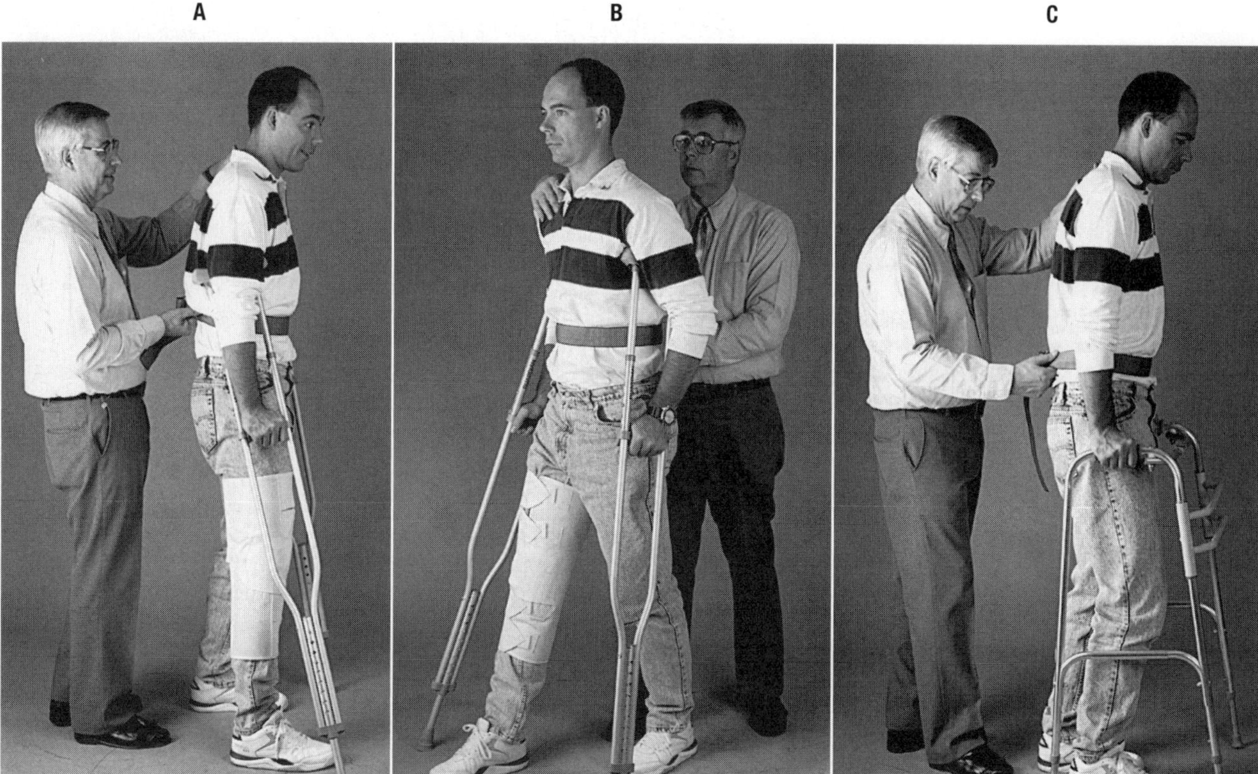

Fig. 9-10 The caregiver's hand nearest to the patient grasps the safety belt; the other hand controls the shoulder.

lower extremity posterior to the patient's nearest lower extremity. For example, if you stand behind and on the patient's right side, your right foot will be positioned forward, between the ambulation aid and the right foot; your left foot trails behind. You must learn to move forward in step with the patient; your most forward foot moves with the ambulation aid and your trailing foot moves forward as the patient moves (Procedure 9-3). Avoid "cross steps" with your feet by allowing one foot to trail the other foot.

Guarding from in front of the patient is not recommended because this position does not allow you to move smoothly with the patient, it blocks the patient's view, you cannot see objects or hazards behind you and you must stay too far from the patient so there is sufficient space to step (Procedure 9-4). You should be alert for unexpected or unusual movements by the patient (such as misplacement of the ambulation aid, slippage of the aid, or a misstep) and be prepared to prevent or control a forward, backward, or sideward loss of balance. It may not be possible to totally prevent a fall, but you must be prepared to reduce the possibility of patient injury by assisting the person to a safe, secure position (such as onto the floor, ground, or stair step). Additional specific instructions related to protection for loss of balance are presented elsewhere in this chapter.

PROCEDURE 9-3

Guarding Guidelines for Ambulation

Apply a safety belt on the patient before ambulation.

Stand behind and slightly to one side of the patient (that is, toward the weak or affected extremity); remain close.

Grasp the safety belt with one hand; use your other hand to guard at the patient's shoulder. DO NOT GRASP THE PATIENT'S ARM OR CLOTHING.

Position your feet anteroposterior; place your outside foot between the patient's foot and assistive aid and forward of your other foot; your inside foot trails your outside foot as the patient moves forward.

Move forward as the patient moves forward; maintain your outside foot forward of your inside foot as you move forward.

If the patient loses balance forward, pull the person toward you using the safety belt and your hand on the shoulder or chest; assist the patient to regain balance and stability.

If the patient loses balance backward, position your body behind the patient with feet anteroposterior; allow the person to lean against the side of your body; assist the patient to regain balance and stability.

PROCEDURE 9-4

Guarding Techniques: Standing and Level Surface Ambulation

GENERAL CONSIDERATIONS

The size, stature, weight, and strength of the patient and the caregiver may affect how the techniques presented are applied; modifications may be necessary.

For some situations, it may be necessary to have two persons guarding.

The patient should be instructed to release the ambulation aids and assist with self-protection when it is apparent the patient will not be able to remain in a balanced, upright position.

If you are unable to maintain the patient in a balanced, upright position, you should assist the person to a safe position (that is, on the floor, on a step, on the ground, into a chair, or onto another firm surface).

PATIENT STANDS WITH AMBULATION AIDS

Position yourself on the side opposite to the extremity with which the patient holds the aids and somewhat behind.

Grasp the safety belt with one hand; be prepared to use your other hand to control the trunk; maintain a wide BOS with your feet.

Balance Lost Forward

- Pull back on the safety belt; use your other hand to pull the trunk upward and back; do not pull on the patient's clothing or arm.
- It may be helpful to push forward against the pelvis as you pull back on the trunk.
- Assist the patient to regain a balanced position, or if unable to maintain an upright position, assist to the floor or chair.

Balance Lost Backward

- Push forward on the pelvis and trunk to assist the patient to regain a balanced position.
- If unable to maintain an upright position, assist to sit in the chair.

Balance Lost to One Side, Away from You

- Pull on the safety belt to move the patient toward you.
- Assist the patient to regain a balanced position or assist to sit.

Balance Lost to One Side, Toward You

- Move your body so you face the patient's side; widen your stance; use your body to support the patient.
- Assist the patient to regain a balanced position or assist to sit.

LEVEL SURFACE AMBULATION

Position yourself somewhat behind and toward one side of the patient; position your outside foot between the ambulation aid and the foot; position your other foot so it trails as you walk.

Grasp the safety belt with one hand; be prepared to use your other hand to control the trunk; do not use it to grasp clothing or an arm.

Note: Many caregivers prefer to be positioned to the side of the patient that is weakest or with the less functional extremity or extremities.

BALANCE LOST FORWARD

- Pull back on the safety belt; turn your body sideward; widen your stance.
- Use your free hand to pull back on the upper trunk (that is, shoulder or chest); position one hip against the pelvis.
- Assist the patient to regain a balanced position or assist to the floor or ground.

Balance Lost Backward

- Turn your body so one side is toward the patient; widen your stance; allow the person to be supported by your body.
- Use the safety belt and your other hand for control.
- Assist the patient to regain a balanced position or assist to the floor or ground.

Balance Lost to One Side, Away from You

- Pull on the safety belt to move the patient toward you.
- Allow the patient to lean against you for support.
- Assist the patient to regain a balanced position or assist to the floor or ground.

Balance Lost to One Side, Toward You

- Turn your body so the patient can lean on you; use the safety belt and your other hand for control.
- Assist the patient to regain a balanced position or assist to the floor or ground.

Caution: When you pull on the safety belt, you must not pull too quickly or use excessive force. You should attempt to correct the movement of the patient by using a firm, smooth pull on the belt. If you pull with excessive force, you may cause further disturbance of the patient's balance. It is recommended you practice with an unimpaired individual, who can simulate various loss-of-balance movements, to help develop a sense of the control needed when you use a safety belt.

PROCEDURE 9-5

Standing in Parallel Bars and Return to Sitting

To stand, prepare and instruct the patient to do the following:

Position and lock the wheelchair in front of the bars.

Remove the feet from the footrests, lift the footrests, and swing away the front rigging or remove it, if possible; position the caster wheels forward.

Position desk-type arms with the higher portion forward, if these are one of the features of the chair.

Move the body forward to the middle or the front edge of the seat by either alternately lifting each hip or side of the pelvis and moving it forward or by leaning against the back of chair and sliding the hips forward, then moving the trunk forward. If the patient can move each hip forward alternately, more independence in preparing to stand and adjusting the position of the body will occur.

Position the foot of the stronger lower extremity slightly posterior to the foot of the affected or involved lower extremity so the stronger extremity will be in the best position to help raise or elevate the patient from the chair seat. (*Note:* For some patients, it may be desirable to place their feet parallel to each other or to position the foot of the weaker lower extremity posterior to the other foot. You will have to try each position with some patients to determine which one is most effective.)

Place both hands forward on the armrests of the chair with the trunk inclined forward (that is, the "nose over the toes" position).

Simultaneously push down with the upper and lower extremities while leaning the trunk forward and continue to stand by extending the hips and knees, then alternately place each hand onto a bar. Do not allow the patient to use the bars to pull to a standing position because when the bars are not available, the patient will not have a stable object on which to pull. The ability to stand independently is enhanced when the patient is taught to stand by pushing on the chair armrests while simultaneously using the lower extremities to elevate the body.

To sit, prepare and instruct the patient to do the following:

Turn so the back is toward the chair; position the stronger lower extremity approximately 4 to 6 inches from the front edge of the seat.

Release one hand from the bar and reach to an armrest; simultaneously partially flex the hip and knee of the stronger lower extremity (or both lower extremities if they are both able to bear weight). *Note:* It may be easier to release the hand on the side of the stronger lower extremity.

Release the other hand and grasp the other armrest.

Flex both hips and knees and bend the trunk forward; use the upper and lower extremities to lower into the chair.

Move the pelvis and trunk back into the seat until they contact the back upholstery. *Note:* For a short patient, it may be necessary for the patient to use the footrests to move the body back into the back of the chair.

Reposition the front rigging and footrests and replace the feet on the footrests when the treatment session concludes.

PARALLEL BAR ACTIVITIES

For most patients, ambulation should be initiated with *parallel bars* to provide maximal security, stability, and safety. The gait pattern to be used should be explained and demonstrated to the patient before it is attempted. Ambulation is a motor skill and it is important to provide instruction and allow the patient to practice the activity to reduce anxiety and fear and to increase the safety of the activity. The equipment selected must fit properly and be in safe condition. When parallel bars are used, you should remain inside the bars to guard and assist the patient most effectively and to reduce the risk of injury to yourself.

Moving from Sitting to Standing and Return to Sitting

The necessary components of the activity of moving from sitting to standing are forward movement of the body to the center or front portion of the seat, proper foot placement, forward inclination of the trunk with flexion of the hips, flexion of the neck and spine, forward movement of the pelvis to initiate an erect posture, pushing with the upper extremities on the arms of the chair, extension of the head and trunk, and extension of the hips and knees to attain the final standing posture. These activities assist the individual to shift the COG over and within the BOS and to align the trunk and to move the COG from a lower to a higher position. To return to sitting, the patient needs to incline the trunk forward, combined with hip and knee flexion and flexion of the neck and spine; move the pelvis rearward toward the seat; grasp the arms of the chair; and flex the hips and knees to lower the body into the chair seat. These same principles should be applied to standing transfers (Procedure 9-5).

Balance and Initial Gait Pattern Activities

While standing in parallel bars, the patient:

- Slowly shifts the body from side to side and forward and back while maintaining the shoulders and pelvis in line and the trunk erect; hold each position change for 3 to 5 seconds and maintain the proper weight-bearing status on each lower extremity.
- Briefly and alternately lifts the hands from the bars to promote a sense of the decreased support that will be experienced when the ambulation aid is moved; later, both hands can be lifted simultaneously.
- Performs a "push-up" using the bars to improve arm strength and to experience the sense of effort required to

support the body when the lower extremities are not in contact with the floor or ground.

- Alternately or simultaneously lifts the opposite upper and lower extremities to simulate a particular gait pattern or to increase balance when support and stability are decreased. Other exercises to improve the patient's strength, endurance, and coordination can be performed with the patient in the bars. The selection of specific exercises should be based on the patient's disability and residual abilities and the particular gait pattern to be used and the exercises should be designed to improve his or her ambulation and coordination skills.
- Practices the selected gait pattern in the bars, including moving forward, backward, and sideward and turning to the right and to the left.
- Practices the selected gait pattern using the proper ambulation aids. The aids may be used with the patient inside the bars or the patient may use one bar and one ambulation aid.

Guard the patient using a safety belt and proper protective techniques. It is recommended you remain inside the bars with the patient for optimal control and safety.

BASIC GAIT PATTERNS

Selection of the appropriate gait pattern will depend on the patient's balance, strength, coordination, functional needs, weight-bearing status, and energy level (Procedure 9-6). The advantages and disadvantages of several patterns are presented.

Four-Point Pattern

The *four-point gait* pattern requires the use of *bilateral* ambulation aids. The pattern uses an alternate and reciprocal forward movement of the ambulation aid and the patient's opposite lower extremity (that is, right crutch, then left foot; left crutch, then right foot) (Fig. 9-11). This is a very slow, stable pattern and is the safest one to use in crowded areas. It requires low energy expenditure and can be used when the patient requires maximal stability or balance. It approximates a normal gait pattern, but the patient must ambulate slowly.

Two-Point Pattern

The *two-point gait* pattern requires the use of bilateral ambulation aids. The pattern uses a simultaneous, reciprocal forward placement of the ambulation aid and the patient's opposite lower extremity (that is, right crutch and left foot; left crutch and right foot) (Fig. 9-12). This is a relatively stable pattern and can be performed more rapidly than the four-point gait. It requires relatively low energy expenditure and is very similar to a normal gait pattern. However, it also requires coordination by the patient to move one upper extremity and its opposite lower extremity forward simultaneously. The patient can ambulate more rapidly, but with less stability than with the four-point pattern (Fig. 9-13).

Modified Four-Point or Two-Point Pattern

These patterns require only one ambulation aid and are used for the patient who has only one functional upper extremity

Text continued on p. 233

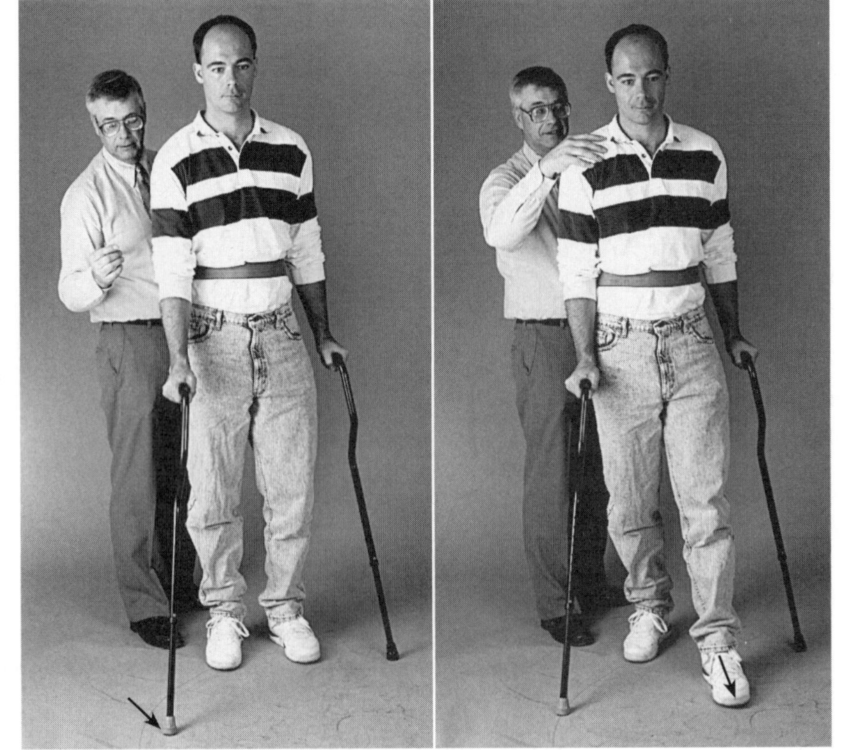

Fig. 9-11 Four-point gait pattern.

PROCEDURE 9-6

Ambulation Patterns with Assistive Aids

A. Four-point: Assistive aid (o) and opposite lower extremity (foot) advance *alternately;* bilateral canes, crutches, or reciprocal walker may be used.
B. Two-point: Assistive aid (o) and opposite lower extremity (foot) advance *simultaneously;* bilateral canes, crutches, or reciprocal walker may be used.
C. Three-point: Assistive aid (o) advances *simultaneously* with the NWB lower extremity; then the FWB lower extremity (foot) steps through the aids; bilateral crutches or walker may be used.

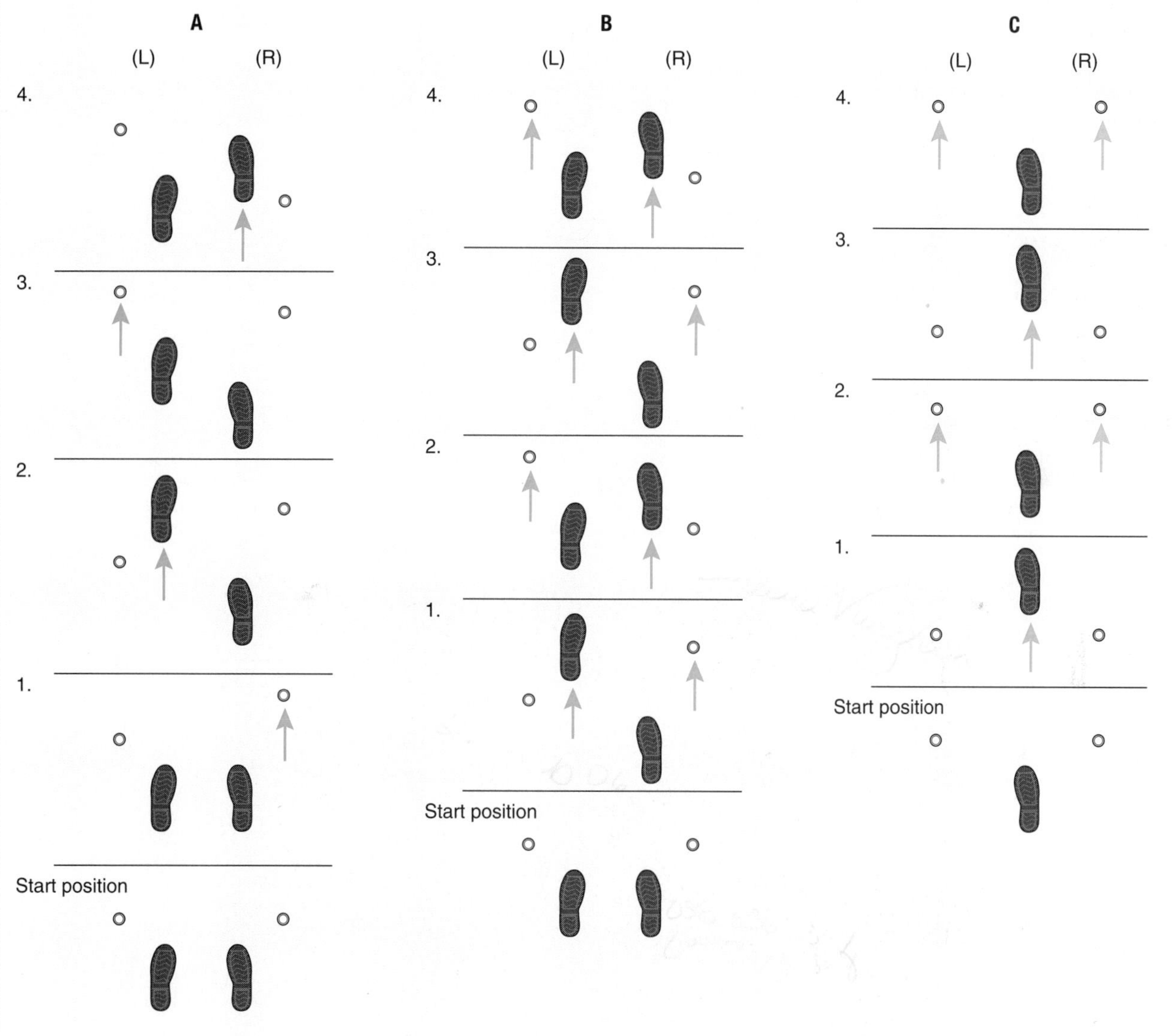

Continued

PROCEDURE 9-6

Ambulation Patterns with Assistive Aids—cont'd

D. Three-one–point: Assistive aid (o) and PWB lower extremity (foot) advance *simultaneously;* then the FWB lower extremity steps through the aids; bilateral cane, crutches, or walker may be used.

E. Modified four-point: Only one assistive aid (o) is used; the assistive aid and the opposite lower extremity (foot) advance *alternately;* the assistive aid is held in the hand opposite the affected lower extremity; one cane or crutch may be used.

F. Modified two-point: Only one assistive aid (o) is used; the assistive aid and the opposite lower extremity (foot) advance *simultaneously;* the assistive aid is held in the hand opposite the affected lower extremity; one cane or crutch may be used.

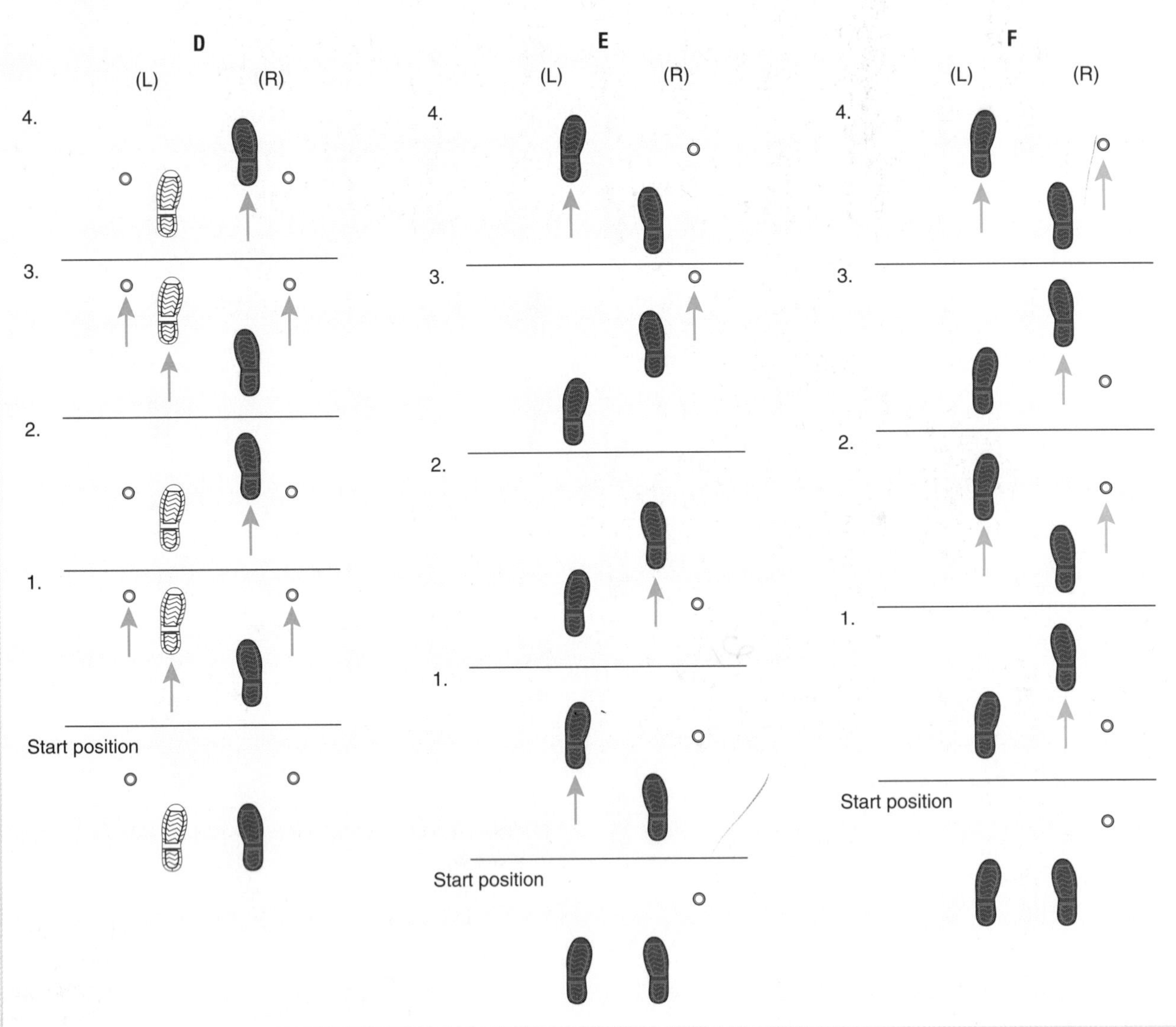

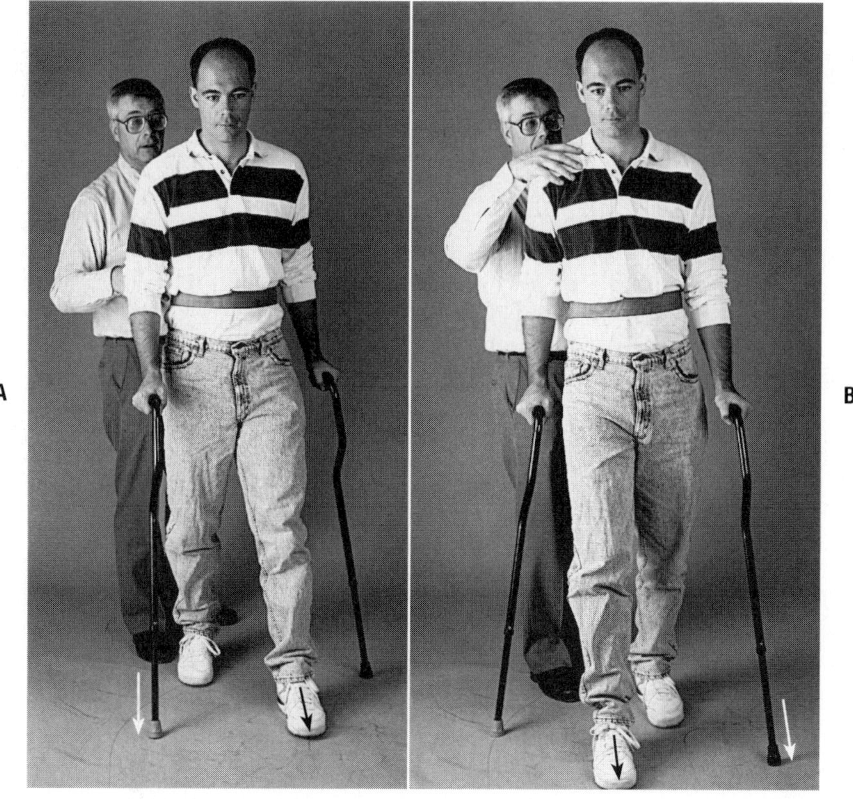

Fig. 9-12 Two-point gait pattern.

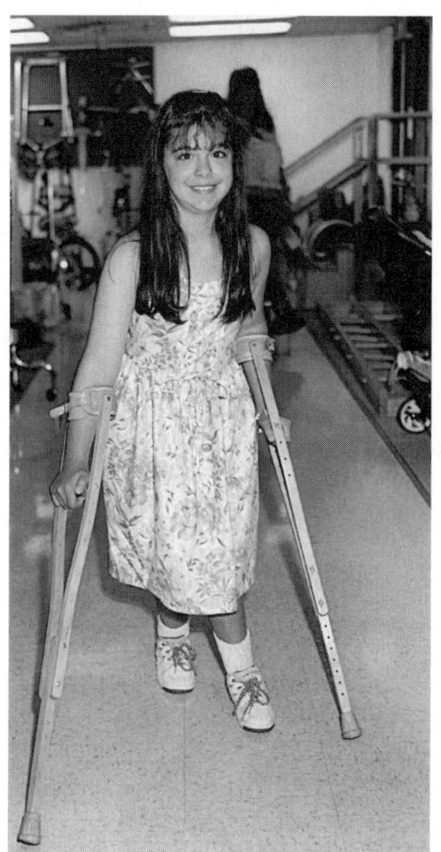

Fig. 9-13 Adolescent ambulating with forearm crutches; a two- or four-point pattern is demonstrated.

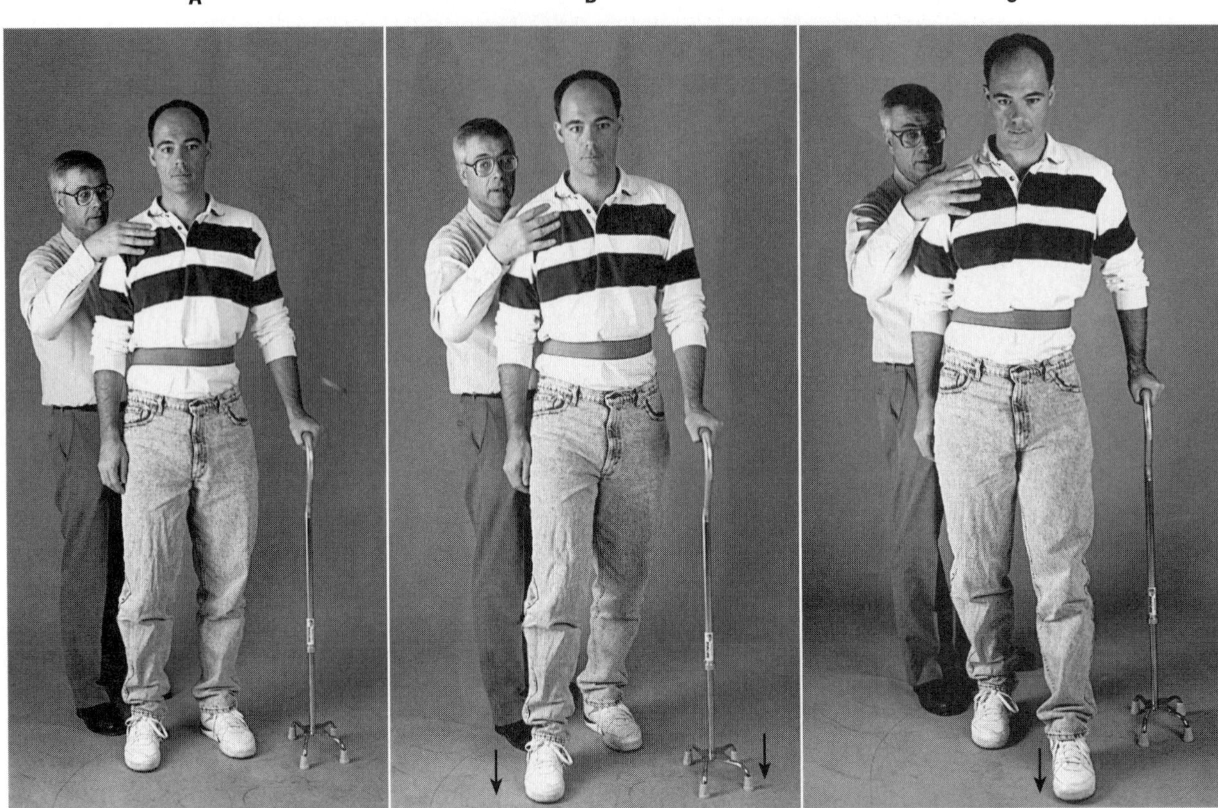

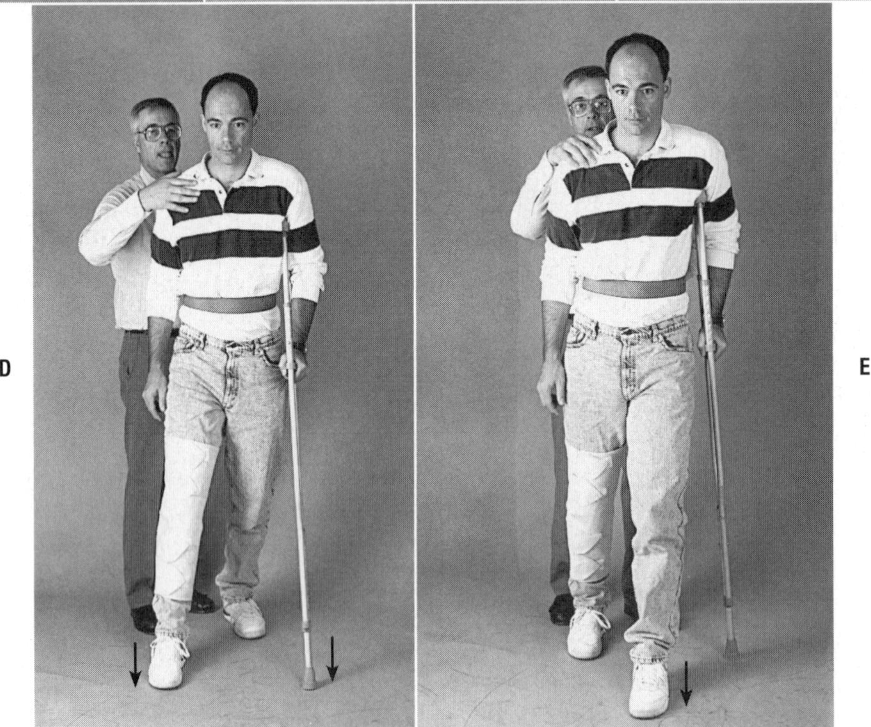

Fig. 9-14 Modified two-point gait patterns. **A** through **C,** Modified two-point gait with cane. **D** and **E,** Modified two-point gait with an axillary crutch.

or who uses only one ambulation aid. The aid is held in the upper extremity opposite to the lower extremity that requires protection. This widens the BOS and assists in shifting the patient's COG away from the protected lower extremity. This pattern is sometimes referred to as a "hemi" gait or "hemi" pattern. The patient performs the pattern in the sequences described for the four- and two-point patterns, but only one ambulation aid is used; thus the pattern is modified (Fig. 9-14).

Three-Point Pattern

The three-point gait pattern requires bilateral ambulation aids or a walker, but cannot be performed with bilateral canes. The pattern should be referred to as a "step-to" or "step-through" pattern rather than a "swing-to" or "swing-through" pattern. It is used when the patient is able to FWB on one lower extremity, but is NWB on the opposite lower extremity.

The walker or crutches and the NWB extremity are advanced and then the patient steps up to the front rail of a walker or through the crutches (Fig. 9-15). It is a less stable pattern than the patterns described previously or the *three-one–point gait* pattern, but rapid ambulation is possible. It requires good strength in the upper extremities, trunk, and one lower extremity, but energy expenditure is high because of the need to use the upper extremities to lift, support, and propel the body. The patient should be taught to step through rather than "swing through" the crutches and to control the movement of the trunk and lower extremities with his or her normally functioning musculature. This will reduce energy expenditure and increase the patient's balance and stability.

Note: It is recommended that the terms "swing-to" and "swing-through" not be used in conjunction with the three-point pattern. These terms are better suited for the patient who is unable to actively use the muscles of the lower trunk and lower extremities during ambulation and who must "swing" the trunk and lower extremities "to" or "through" the crutches to ambulate. These gait patterns are associated most frequently with the patient with a spinal cord injury or a developmental disability that requires the patient to use the upper extremities to support and provide the force necessary to lift and move the body forward without assistance from the lower extremities.

Three-One–Point or Modified Three-Point Pattern

The three-one–point gait pattern requires the use of bilateral ambulation aids or a walker. The pattern is used when the patient is permitted FWB on one lower extremity, but only PWB on the other lower extremity. The walker, crutches, or canes are advanced simultaneously with the PWB lower

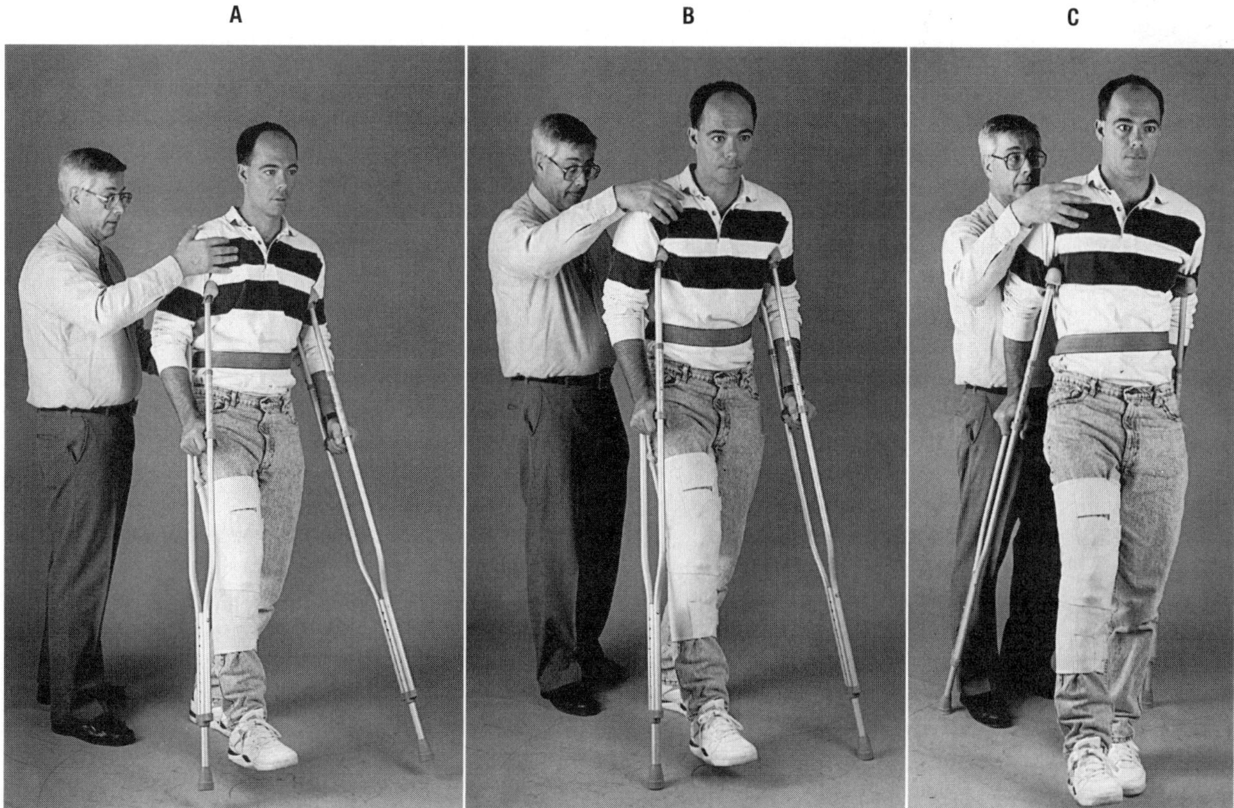

Fig. 9-15 Three-point gait pattern.

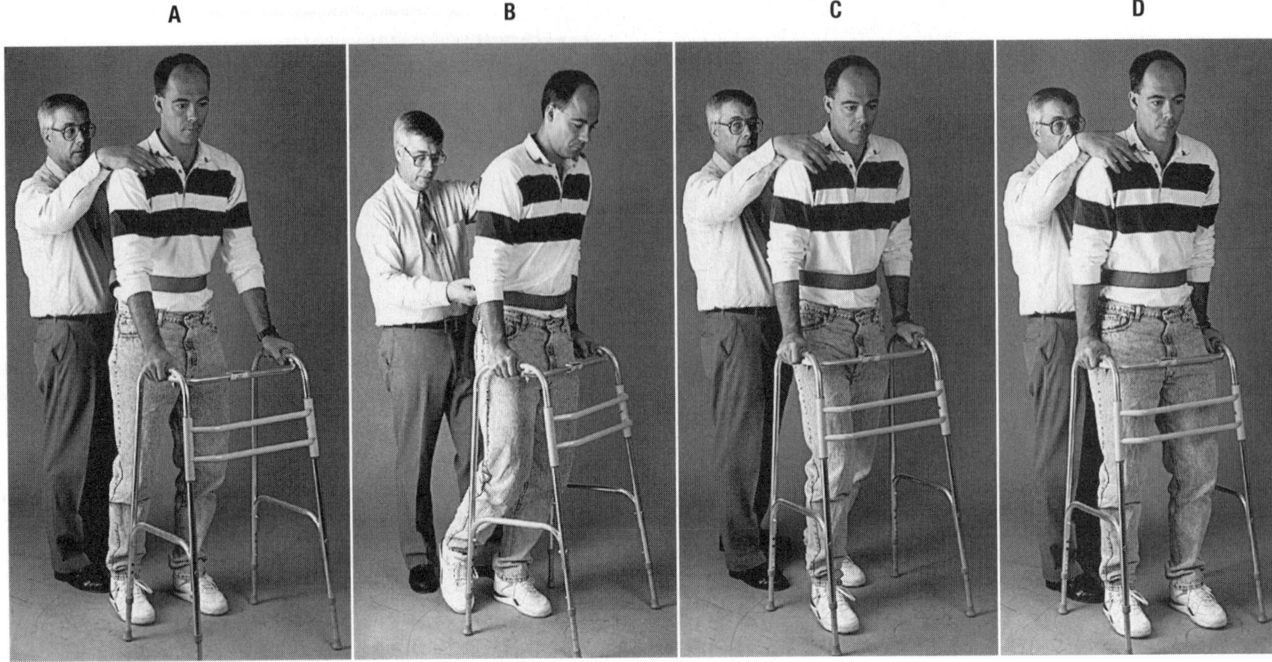

Fig. 9-16 Three-one, or modified three-point, gait pattern.

extremity (Fig. 9-16, *A*). Then the FWB lower extremity is advanced while the patient distributes the body weight onto the aid and partially bears weight on the protected lower extremity (Fig. 9-16, *B* through *D*). It is a more stable pattern than the three-point pattern and requires less strength and less energy expenditure than the three-point pattern, but it is a slower pattern. It allows the affected lower extremity to function actively while maintaining some weight bearing on it. These can be positive features and benefits depending on the patient's diagnosis or condition (see Procedure 9-6).

PREAMBULATION FUNCTIONAL ACTIVITIES

Each patient will need to be instructed how to perform the gait pattern to be used and how to perform various functional activities. Actual requirements may vary from patient to patient depending on each person's goals, needs, problems, and abilities. Instruction and practice in various functional activities such as using stairs, curbs, inclines, ramps, and doors; sitting into and standing from different types of chairs or other seating items (such as armless chairs, low chairs and sofas, soft chairs and sofas, toilets, automobile seats, theater seats, and benches); ambulating on rough, soft, or uneven surfaces (such as grass, carpeting, gravel, or concrete); sitting on the ground or floor and returning to standing; protecting himself or herself at the time of a fall and returning to standing; using public transportation; crossing a street during the walk cycle of the traffic control system; and using an elevator and escalator should be considered for inclusion in the gait training program. The specific activities selected will depend on the patient's needs, goals, anticipated activities, problems, ambulation aid used, and abilities.

The caregiver must explain and demonstrate the activities to the patient and protect or guard the patient during practice sessions to reduce the risk of injury (Fig. 9-17). Videotapes, instructional booklets or manuals, and observation of other skilled and competent patients are other methods of instruction that can be used.

The goal for most patients will be the safe and independent performance of the functional activities selected to be accomplished. However, some patients may not become independent. In such instances a family member, friend, or coworker should be instructed in the proper way to assist and protect the person. In addition, the patient should be made aware of any limitations and the risk of injury that would accompany an attempt at independent performance of an activity for which assistance is required. The caregiver should document the activities the patient is able to perform safely and independently. Any restrictions or limitations in the person's ambulation activities should be noted and the family should be informed of them. This information is especially important for family members of young or elderly patients or patients who have decreased mental competence, which would interfere with the ability to make a competent decision or judgment.

The amount of time available to instruct the patient and practice ambulation activities may be extremely limited because of restrictions on the patient's length of stay in the

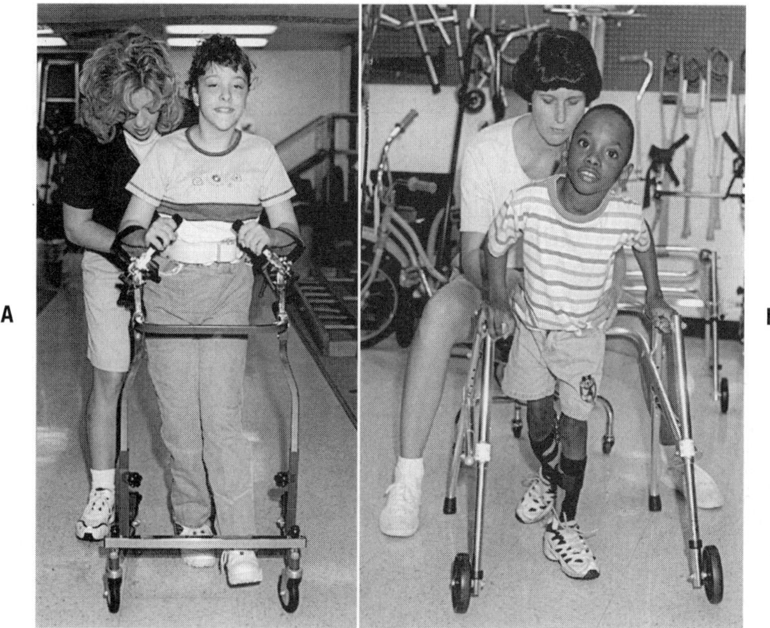

Fig. 9-17 Children ambulating with adjustable wheeled walkers.

hospital. Many patients may be hospitalized for only a few days before they are discharged and return to their home. Thus they may not have access to multiple treatment or practice sessions and their opportunities to become proficient in functional activities will be minimal. Therefore it may be necessary to provide written instructions and precautions related to functional activities for the patient and family.

These precautions may include suggestions for the proper maintenance of equipment, such as inspecting the support tips of the device for wear or damage or dirt in the grooves, checking wing nuts for tension, inspecting the item for cracks or broken parts, and checking all spring adjustment buttons to be certain they are securely positioned in the holes provided. The patient should be cautioned that moisture on the support tips or ambulation on a wet floor could cause the tips to slip or slide. Loose objects, such as small area rugs, and waxed or polished floor surfaces are also threats to safety and should be avoided if possible. Extra care should be taken during ambulation on grass or on rough or uneven surfaces and in an area crowded with furniture or other hazards or where there are many other persons (such as a busy hallway, store, or sidewalk).

Sidewalks that are wet or obstructed by rain or snow create special problems and only the most proficient and cautious person should attempt to ambulate with assistive devices in these conditions. The patient should be made aware of the potential problems associated with doorway thresholds, the change from one type of surface to a different surface (as from a linoleum surface to carpeted surface), and the stair tread overhang (stair lip).

These precautions are most important for the person who uses the assistive aid for maximal body support and stability, such as the person who is NWB on one lower extremity. However, all persons who use an ambulation aid should be provided with instructions to assist them in avoiding or reducing the risks to their safety caused by the conditions or factors cited. It is the caregiver's responsibility to discuss these precautions with the patient during the ambulation training program. In addition, you should inform the patient or the family how you can be contacted for advice or assistance after the patient has been released from the facility. This information should be written and given to the patient or the family.

STANDING AND SITTING ACTIVITIES

Each patient must be taught to stand and return to sitting using the ambulation aids so this can be done safely, efficiently, and independently. The entire program or technique used may differ among patients, but many components should be taught to all patients.

Before a patient attempts to stand, the body must be moved forward in the chair seat. This will position the COG nearer to the BOS (that is, the feet and lower extremities) so the person will be able to stand more easily and will have better balance once standing. Most patients find it easier to stand if they place the foot of the unaffected or stronger lower extremity slightly posterior to the foot of the opposite lower extremity. This anteroposterior position of the feet promotes a better "push-off" or lift from the stronger lower extremity as the person begins to stand. The position also provides a wide BOS when the person is standing and approximates the foot position most people use to stand from a chair. If both lower extremities have essentially equal strength and weight-bearing capacity, the foot of the dominant lower extremity is usually positioned most posteriorly (Fig. 9-18, *A*).

The patient uses the upper extremities to push simultaneously with the lower extremities to elevate the body. The hands should be placed on the chair armrests and positioned anterior to the hips. This allows the patient to push upward and forward to move the hips and trunk forward and toward the BOS (Fig. 9-18, *B*) and also enables the patient to use the most stable object for support as the movement to stand is initiated. The more advanced patient may be able to stand using the ambulation aid rather than the chair armrests. However, this method requires excellent strength, coordination, and balance to perform the activity safely (Fig. 9-18, *C* and *D*).

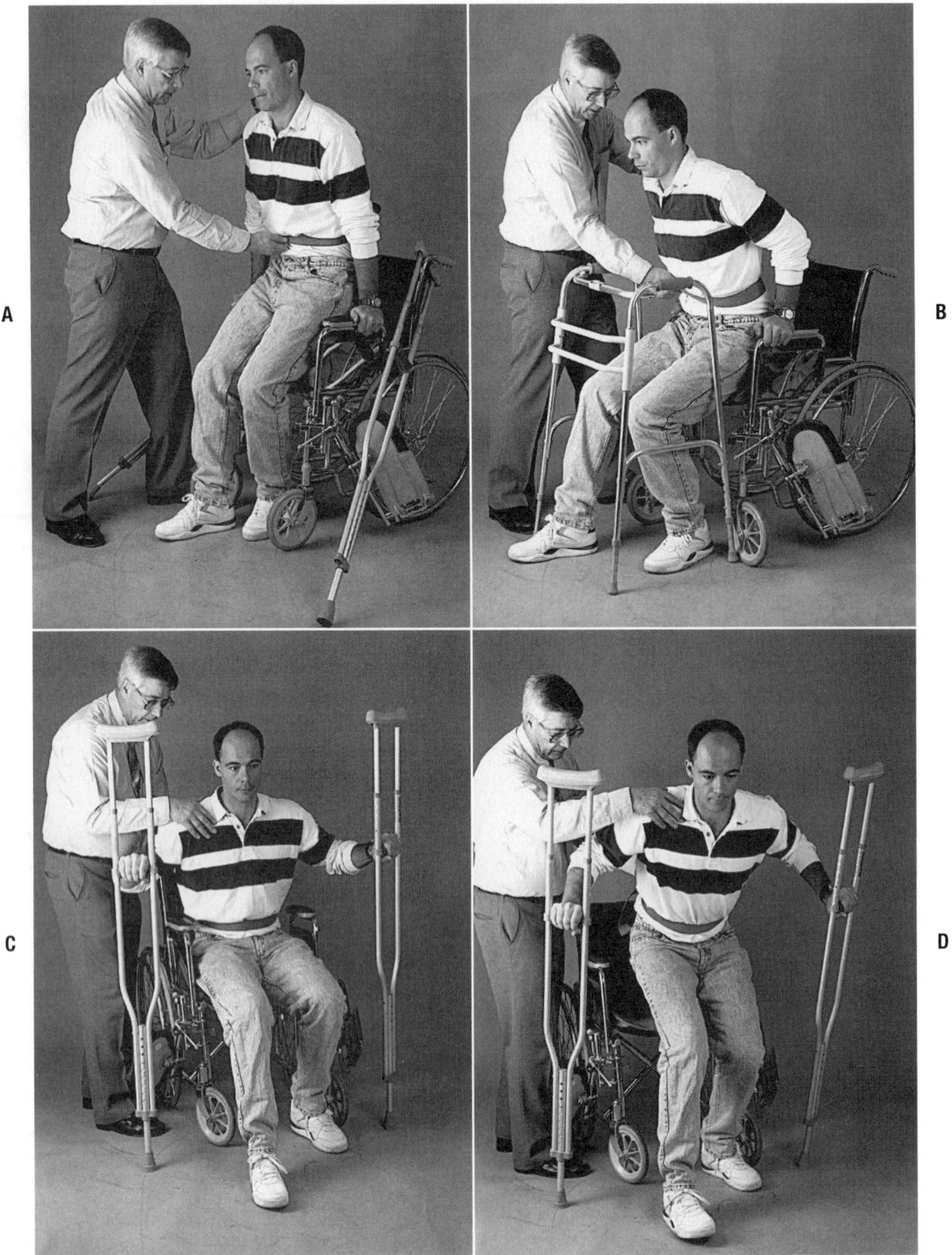

Fig. 9-18 Methods used to stand from a wheelchair.

The patient inclines the trunk forward and pushes with the upper and lower extremities. This shifts the COG forward and eventually over the BOS, leading to a relatively stable standing position. *Note:* When a patient stands from a wheelchair, the chair will be most stable when the caster wheels are positioned forward and the wheel locks are engaged as described in Chapter 8.

When the person returns to the chair, the process is reversed. The foot of the stronger lower extremity is positioned nearest to the chair seat, with the patient facing away from the chair. The patient lowers into the chair using the upper and lower extremities to control the movement. The trunk is inclined forward to maintain the COG over the BOS and to avoid striking the back of the chair with the upper back before the buttocks are on the chair seat. The person who attempts to sit without inclining the trunk forward will be unstable and will have difficulty controlling the movement of the body into the chair.

Axillary Crutches

For standing, instruct the patient to move the hips forward to the middle or front portion of the chair seat. The foot of the stronger or unaffected lower extremity is positioned slightly posterior to the foot of the other lower extremity. If the knee of the most affected lower extremity cannot be flexed, the patient should be taught to slide the heel forward before attempting to stand or the caregiver may have to support the lower extremity as the patient stands (Fig. 9-19, A).

The patient holds both crutches with the hand on the same side as the most affected lower extremity. The crutches are placed opposite to the foot of the stronger lower extremity. This widens the patient's BOS so when the patient stands, the body's vertical gravity line will be located between the crutches and the strong lower extremity (Fig. 9-19, *B*). The patient simultaneously pushes down with the upper extremities and the stronger or less affected lower extremity and leans forward to stand (Fig. 9-19, C).

After the patient is standing, the free hand reaches for one crutch, held in the opposite hand, and places it in the axilla on the side of the body of the hand that is not holding the crutches. The remaining crutch is positioned into the opposite axilla (Fig. 9-19, *D*).

An alternative method is to hold the crutches with the hand on the same side of the body as the unaffected lower extremity. This narrows the BOS, but increases the force the patient is able to use to stand. The ipsilateral upper and lower extremities function simultaneously to lift the patient upward. The patient pushes from the armrest, seat, or back of the chair with the opposite hand to assist with the stand (Fig. 9-20).

To return to sitting, the patient is instructed to approach the chair and then pivot on the stronger or less affected lower extremity so the back is toward the chair (Fig. 9-21). The person steps back until the posterior thigh of the stronger or less affected lower extremity touches the front of the chair seat (see Fig. 9-19, *D*).

The patient alternately removes the crutches from the axillae and holds them with the hand on the same side of the body as the most affected lower extremity to widen the BOS and increase stability (see Fig. 9-19, *B*). An alternative method is to hold the crutches with the hand on the same side of the body as the stronger or less affected lower extremity as described previously.

The patient uses the free hand to grasp the armrest of the chair and lowers the hips into the chair using the upper extremities and the least affected lower extremity. If the knee of the most affected lower extremity cannot be flexed, the patient should allow it to slide forward to sit. The crutches are placed on the floor and the body moves back in the chair. (*Note:* Instruct the patient to avoid placing the crutches against a wall, table, or chair because they are likely to slide and fall to the floor, which could damage the crutches or injure someone nearby.)

Forearm Crutches

To stand, instruct the patient to perform the process discussed for standing with axillary crutches. After the patient stands, the free hand reaches and grasps the handpiece of one crutch and positions the crutch lateral and anterior to the foot on the same side as the hand holding the crutch (Fig. 9-22). Then the person positions the second crutch lateral and anterior to the other foot. When each crutch is positioned, the forearm cuff is applied alternately to each forearm, unless the patient has reached through the cuff to grasp the handpiece.

An alternative method can be used for the patient with good strength, coordination, and balance, but usually cannot be performed by elderly, weak, unstable, or debilitated patients. For this method, the patient moves the hips forward to the middle or front portion of the chair seat. The foot of the stronger or less affected lower extremity is positioned slightly posterior to the foot of the other lower extremity. The patient grasps the handpiece of each crutch in each hand and the crutch tips are positioned lateral and anterior to each foot. The person simultaneously pushes down with the upper extremities and the stronger or less affected lower extremity, leans the trunk forward, and stands (Fig. 9-23).

To return to sitting, the patient is instructed to perform the same process discussed for axillary crutches. An alternative method is to instruct the patient to perform all activities described for sitting with axillary crutches before removing the crutches. Then the patient alternately removes the cuff from each forearm, but continues to grasp each handpiece. The patient lowers into the chair using the upper and lower extremities, places the crutches on the floor, and moves back into the chair seat.

Walker

To prepare for standing, instruct the patient to move the hips forward to the middle or front portion of the chair seat. The foot of the stronger or less affected lower extremity is

Text continued on p. 242

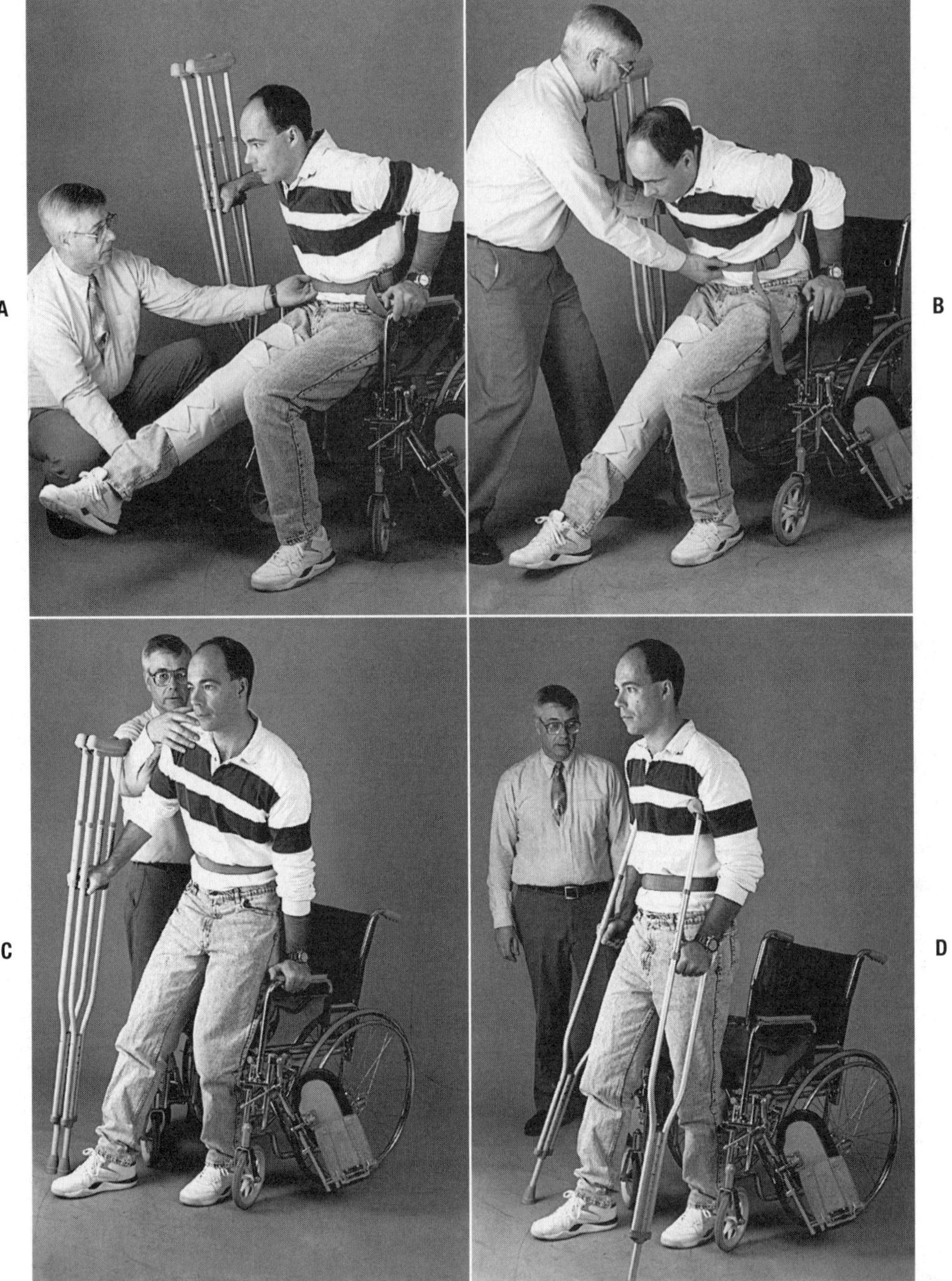

Fig. 9-19 Patient rising from a sitting position with axillary crutches.

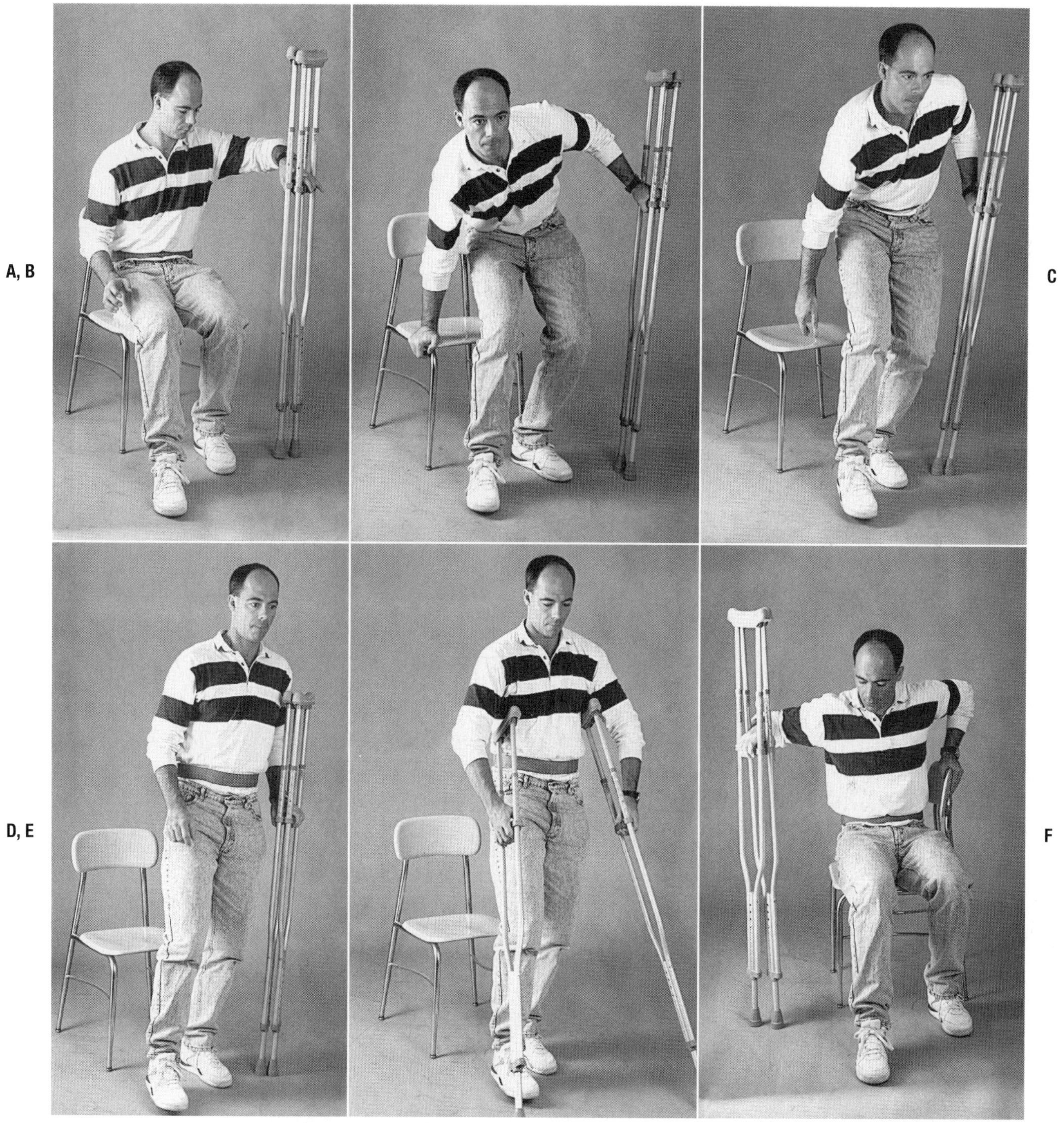

A, B

C

D, E

F

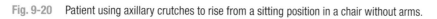

Fig. 9-20 Patient using axillary crutches to rise from a sitting position in a chair without arms.

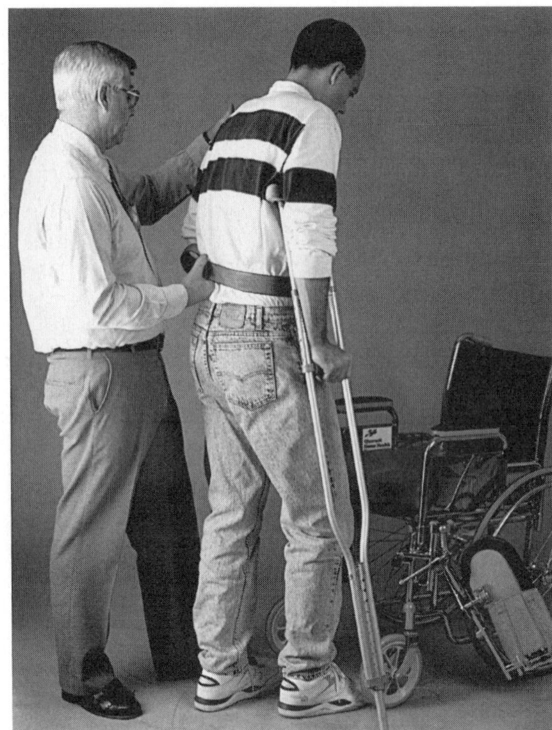

Fig. 9-21 Patient approaching a wheelchair using axillary crutches.

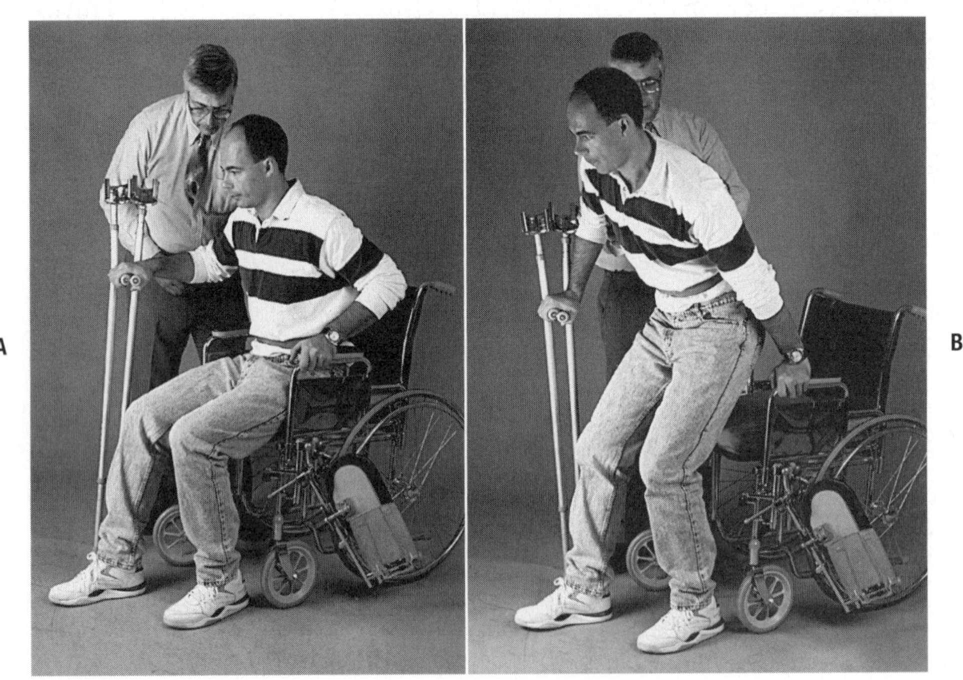

A B

Fig. 9-22 Patient standing from a wheelchair using forearm crutches.

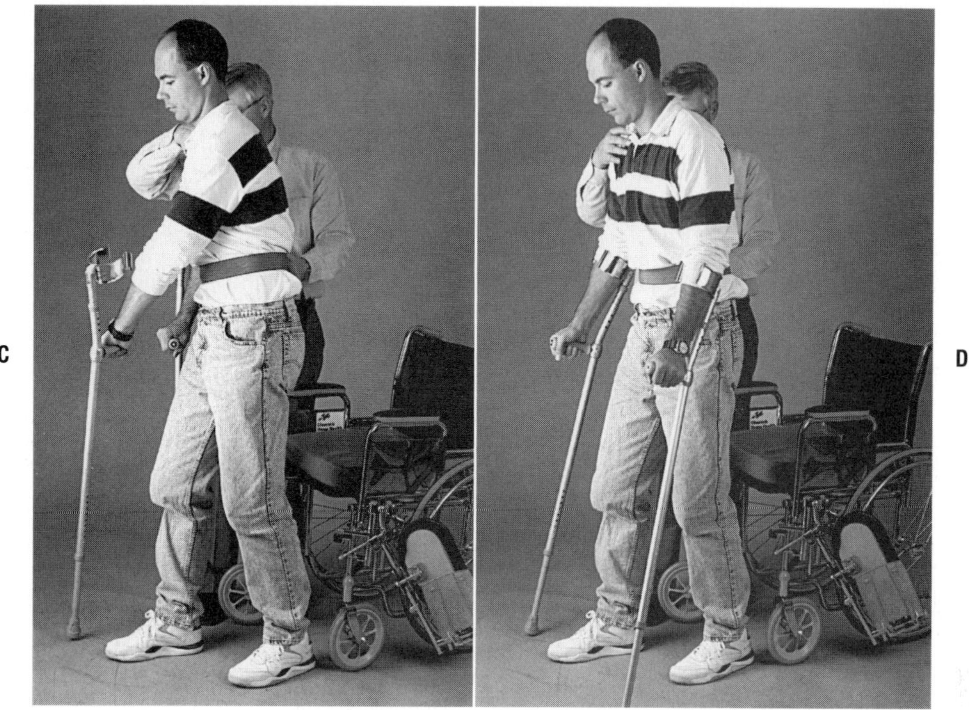

Fig. 9-22, cont'd See legend on opposite page.

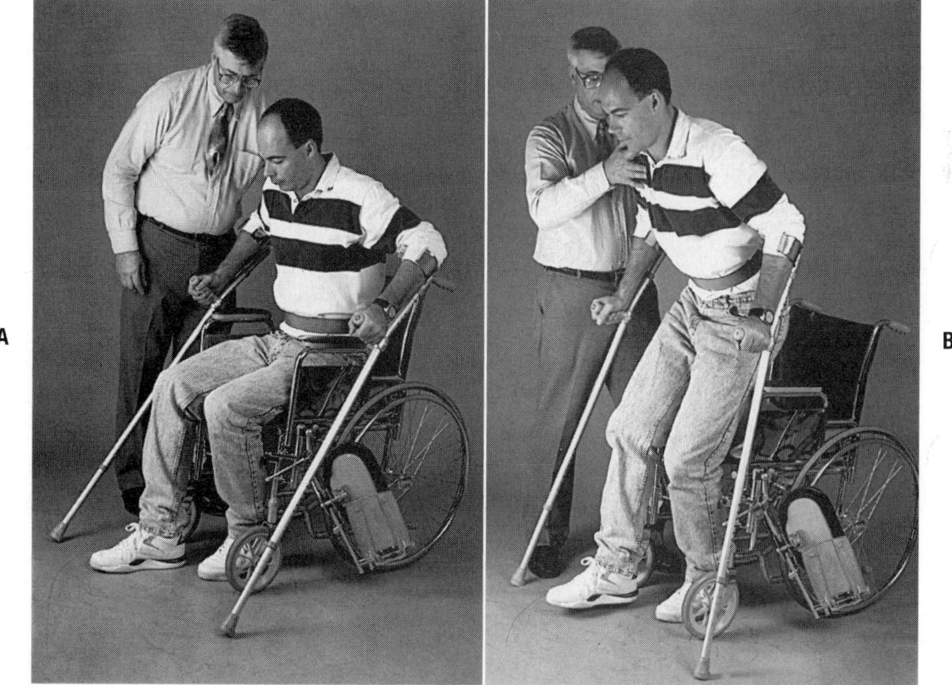

Fig. 9-23 Patient standing from a wheelchair using forearm crutches (alternative method).

positioned slightly posterior to the foot of the other lower extremity. The walker is positioned directly in front of the chair with the open side toward the patient. The patient grasps the chair armrests in front of the hips. This position provides the greatest stability and allows the patient to use the upper and lower extremities most effectively to stand.

To stand, the patient leans forward, simultaneously pushes down with the upper extremities and the strongest lower extremity, and stands. If the person has started with both hands on the chair armrests, one hand is moved onto the handgrip of the walker when partially standing and then the opposite hand moves to the other handgrip (Fig. 9-24, *A*, *B*).

An alternative method is to instruct the patient to preposition the body and feet as described previously and place one hand on one handgrip of the walker and the other hand on the chair armrest in front of the hips (Fig. 9-24, *C*). However, this position can be unsafe if the patient attempts to pull to a standing position using only the walker because the walker is not secure on the floor. Furthermore, if the person attempts to push down with both upper extremities on the handgrips, it may be difficult to stand because the upper extremities will be too high to exert a strong downward force and the walker may tip depending on how the patient pushes on the handpieces.

To return to sitting, the patient is instructed to approach the chair and pivot on the stronger or less affected lower extremity so the back is toward the chair and the walker remains in front (Fig. 9-25, *A* and *B*). The patient steps back until the back of the stronger or less affected lower extremity touches the front of the chair seat. One hand at a time reaches for each armrest of the chair. Once the patient has both hands on the armrests of the chair, the body can be lowered into the chair using the upper and lower extremities. This method provides the greatest stability for the patient because the chair is more secure and stable than the walker (Fig. 9-25, *C* through *E*).

An alternative method is to instruct the patient to reach one hand to the armrest while the other hand remains on the walker handgrip (Fig. 9-26). This method offers less stability than the previous method because the walker is not as secure as the chair. However, some patients may perform better using this method. The patient lowers the hips onto the chair using the upper extremities and the stronger or less affected lower extremity and then positions the body in the chair by moving the hips back into the seat. If the chair does not have arms, the patient can be taught to use the handgrips of the walker to help raise or lower the body using the alternative methods previously described. It is important to teach the patient to push down on the walker handgrips and to avoid pulling or pushing the walker when attempting to stand or return to sitting. These methods should not be considered safe to use with wheeled walkers or for patients who are weak or mentally confused or have poor balance or decreased strength in the upper and lower extremities.

Canes

To stand, instruct the patient to move the hips forward to the middle or the front portion of the chair seat. The foot of

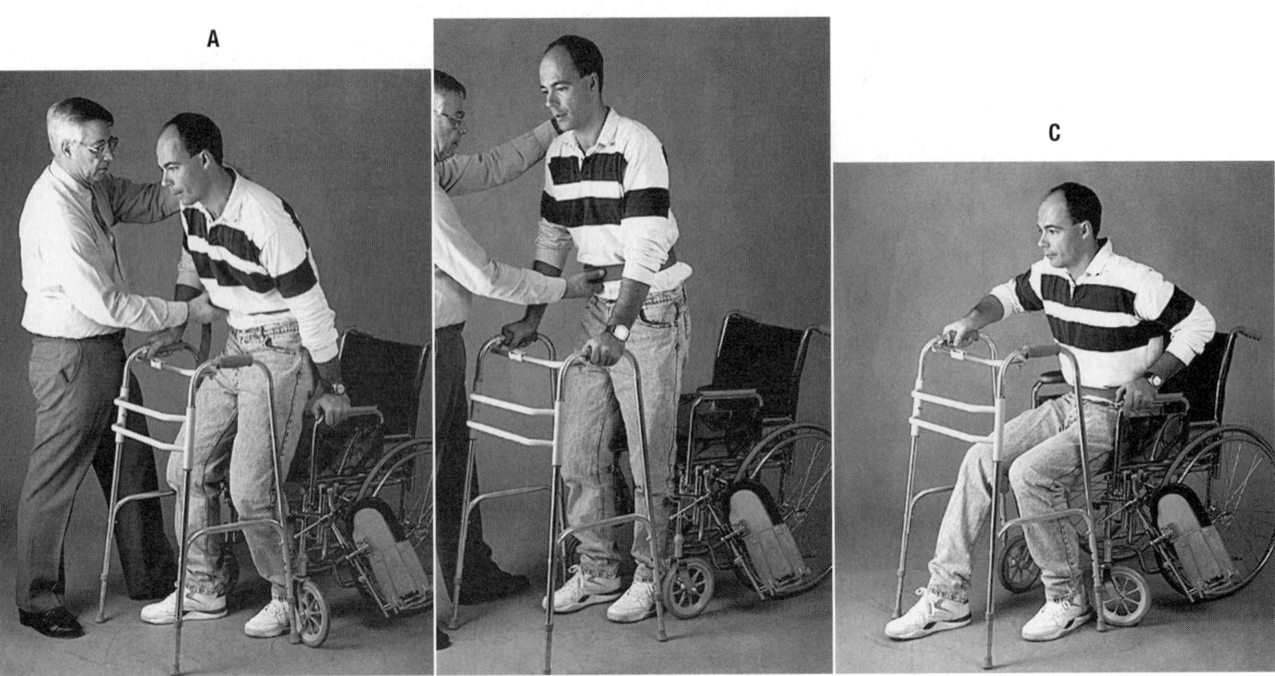

Fig. 9-24 Patient standing from a wheelchair using a walker.

the stronger or less affected lower extremity is positioned slightly posterior to the foot of the other lower extremity. The patient places the hands on the armrests in front of the hips to be able to push with them to lift the body from the chair.

The standard cane is hooked over the front portion of the armrest. If a *unilateral* cane is used, it is placed on the armrest on the side of the stronger or less affected upper and lower extremities. The self-standing (three- or four-footed, crab, or Walkane) cane is placed next to the front of the armrest of the stronger or less affected upper and lower extremities (Fig. 9-27, *A* and *B*). By positioning each cane as described, the patient will be able to use the aid with the upper extremity opposite to the weaker or more affected lower extremity. This positions the cane in the proper hand, widens the patient's BOS, and allows some weight shift from the weaker or more affected lower extremity onto the cane when both items are used during the weight-bearing (stance) phase of the gait pattern.

The patient simultaneously pushes down with the upper and lower extremities and leans the body forward to stand, then picks up the cane from the chair armrest or reaches for

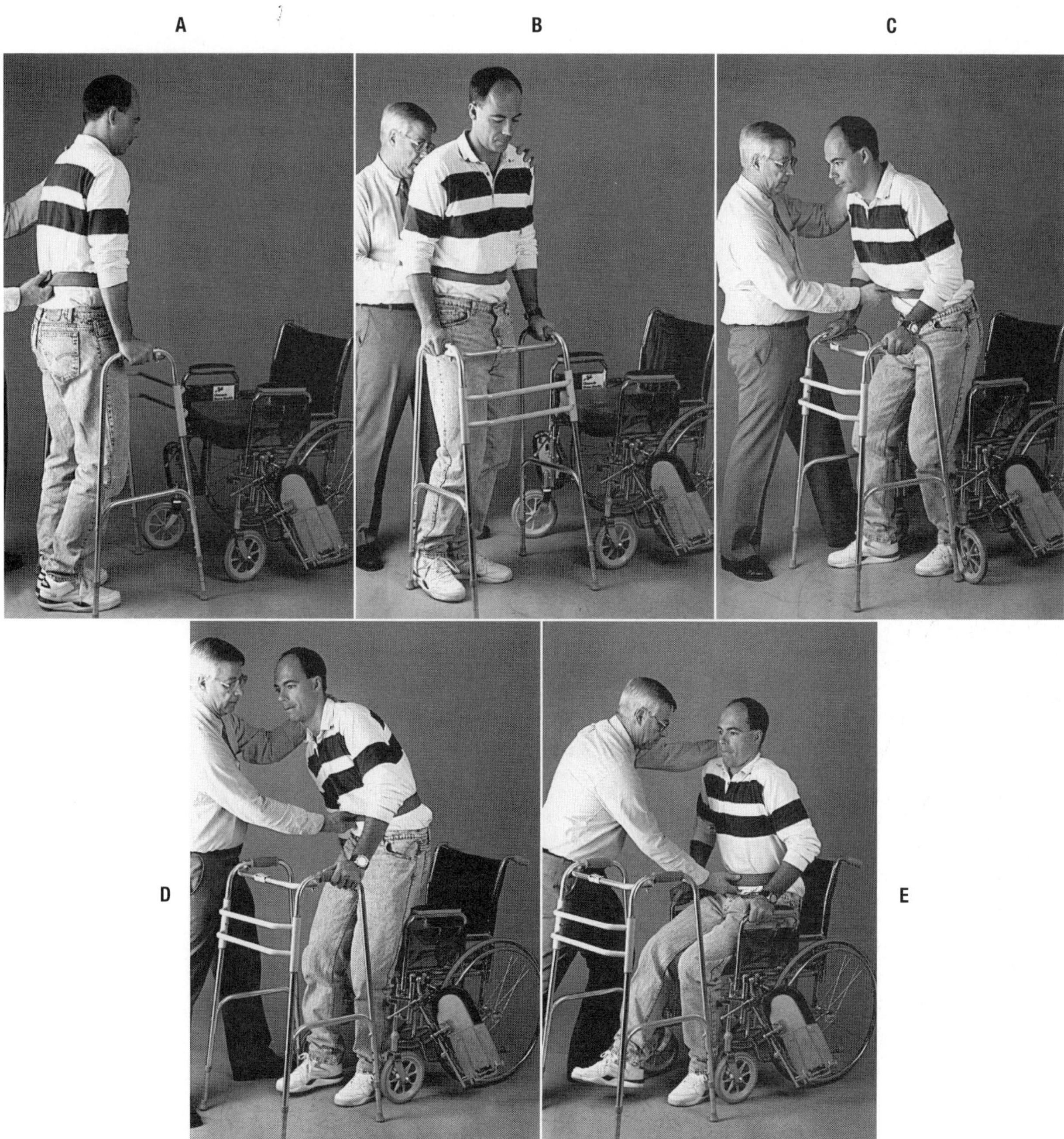

Fig. 9-25 Patient returning to a wheelchair from a walker.

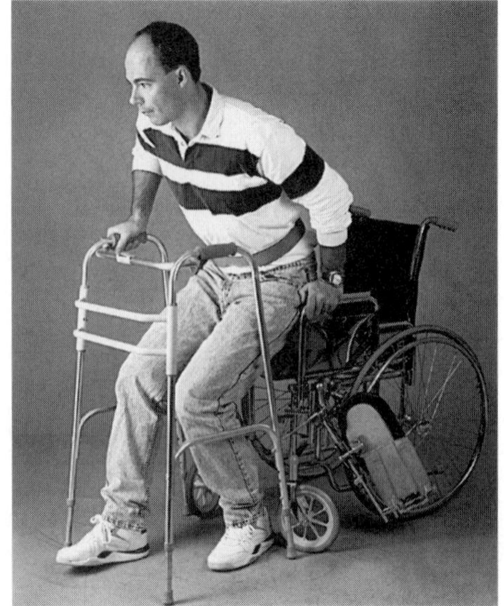

Fig. 9-26 Patient returning to a wheelchair from a walker (alternative method).

A, B

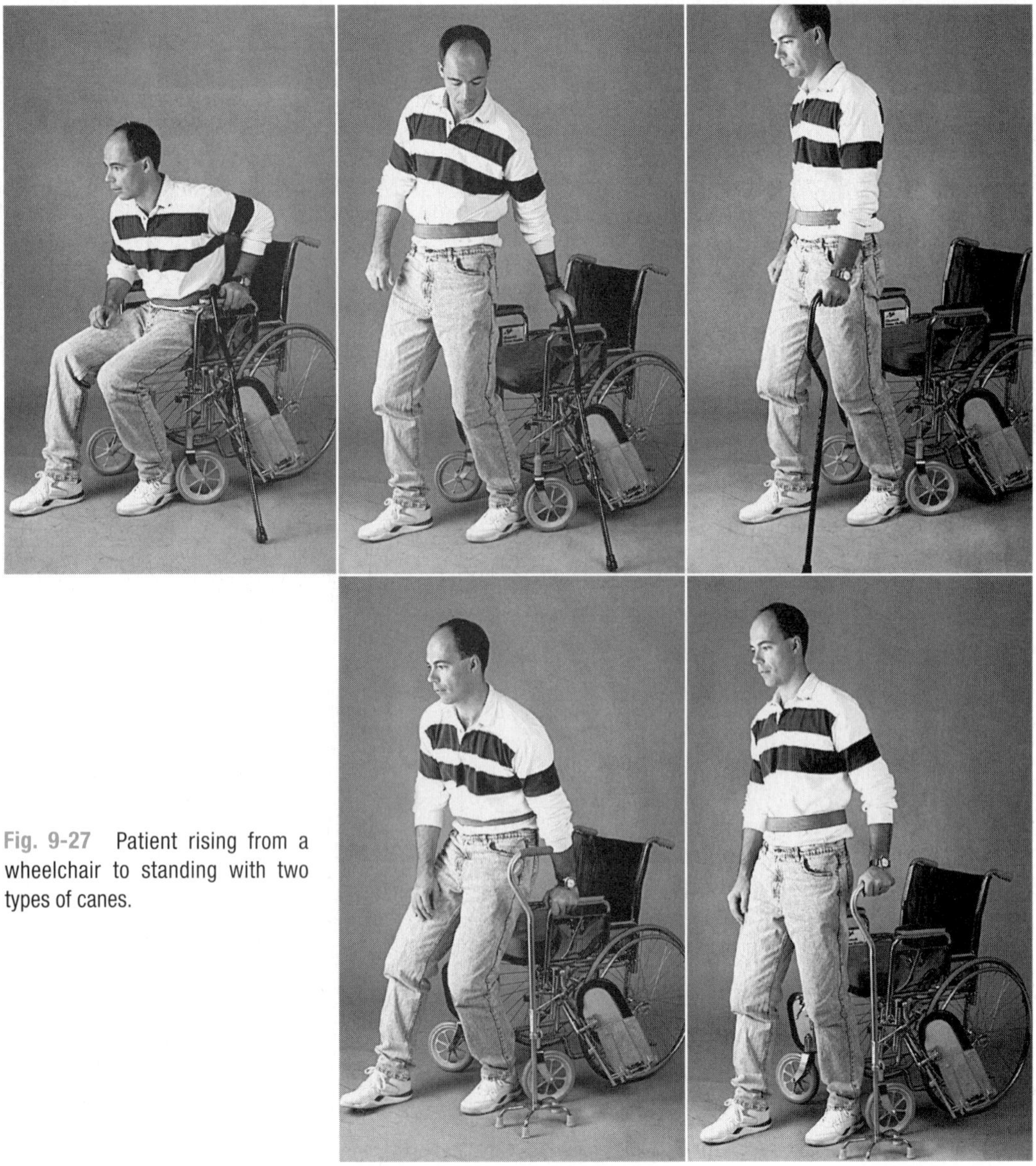

C

Fig. 9-27 Patient rising from a wheelchair to standing with two types of canes.

D, E

the self-standing cane (Fig. 9-27, C through *E*). (*Note:* If the chair does not have arms, the patient can be taught to hold the cane in the hand opposite to the weaker or more affected lower extremity and to use either or both upper extremities to push down on the chair seat or back to assist in standing.)

To return to sitting, instruct the patient to approach the chair and turn sideward, leading with the stronger or less affected upper and lower extremities. With the stronger or less affected extremities nearest to the chair, the cane is hooked over the armrest or the self-standing cane is placed to the side or in front of the armrest the patient faces.

The patient first grasps the near armrest and then, if able, grasps the far armrest and continues to pivot until the back is toward the chair. The hips are lowered into the chair seat using the stronger or less affected upper and lower extremities (Fig. 9-28), then moves the hips back into the chair. (*Note:* If the chair does not have arms, the patient can be taught to release the cane, allowing it to fall sideward to the floor, and

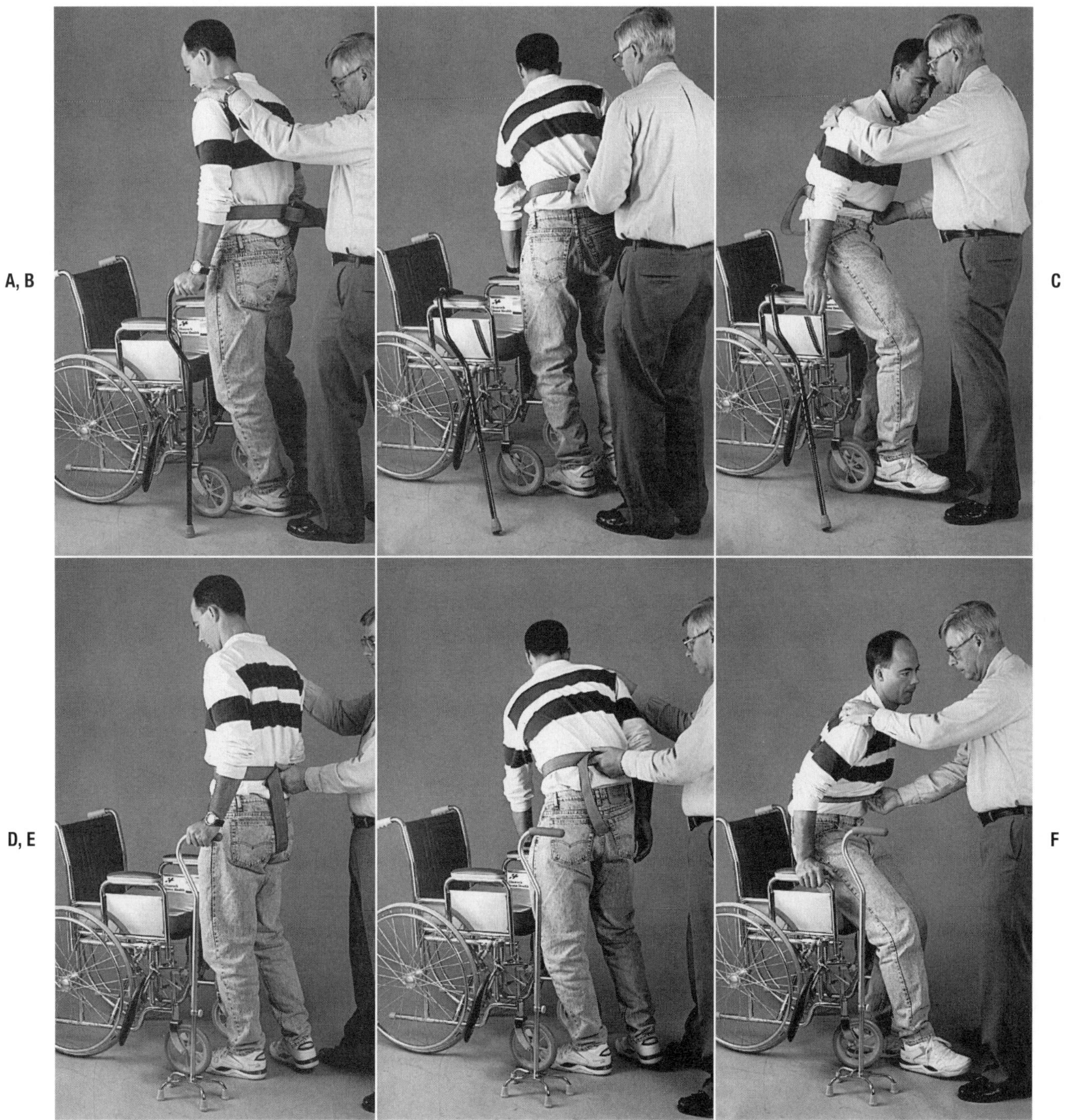

Fig. 9-28 Patient returning to a wheelchair from standing with cane.

to reach to the chair seat or the back of the chair with the free upper extremity to help lower the body into the chair.)

The methods described for standing from and sitting into a chair should be safe and effective for the majority of patients who have average or normal strength, coordination, and balance. However, some patients may require the assistance of another person or the use of a firm, stable object (such as a chair with arms; a table; a handrail or grab bars; or a vanity, bed, or counter) to help them to stand or sit. The patient who uses a wheelchair may need to be taught to turn toward the chair and to face the chair after standing to grasp the crutches, which have been hooked over the push handles or armrests. Observing the patient or attempting different methods may be necessary to determine which method will be the safest and most independent for the patient. You must protect the patient when any of these methods are taught by using proper guarding techniques, including the application and use of a safety belt (Fig. 9-29 and Procedure 9-7).

Guarding during Gait Training on Curbs, Stairs, and Ramps

Ascending Stairs Remain behind and slightly to the side of the patient in the area where there is the least protection for the patient. Use an anterioposterior stance with your outside foot on the step on which the patient is standing and your inside foot on the step below the step on which the patient stands. Grasp the safety belt with one hand and the handrail, if one is available, with your opposite hand (Fig. 9-30).

Advance your feet up one step after the patient has advanced one step, but maintain your feet in an anteroposterior position as described previously. This process is repeated to ascend all the steps. Teach the patient to stop and gain balance on each step before progressing to the next step (Procedure 9-8).

(*Note:* If there is no handrail, grasp the safety belt with one hand and position your other hand anterior and above, lightly touching the patient's shoulder as described for level-ground ambulation. In many instances, when no handrail is available, it is recommended two persons guard the patient. One person is positioned in front of the patient and another person is positioned behind or to the side. If you are alone with the patient, you should be prepared to use your free hand to gently push the patient's trunk forward if balance is lost backward.)

Descending Stairs Stand in front and to the side of the patient in the area where there is the least protection. Use an anteroposterior stance with your outside foot on the step to which the patient will step and your inside foot on the step that is one step lower. Some people prefer to widen their

Text continued on p. 250

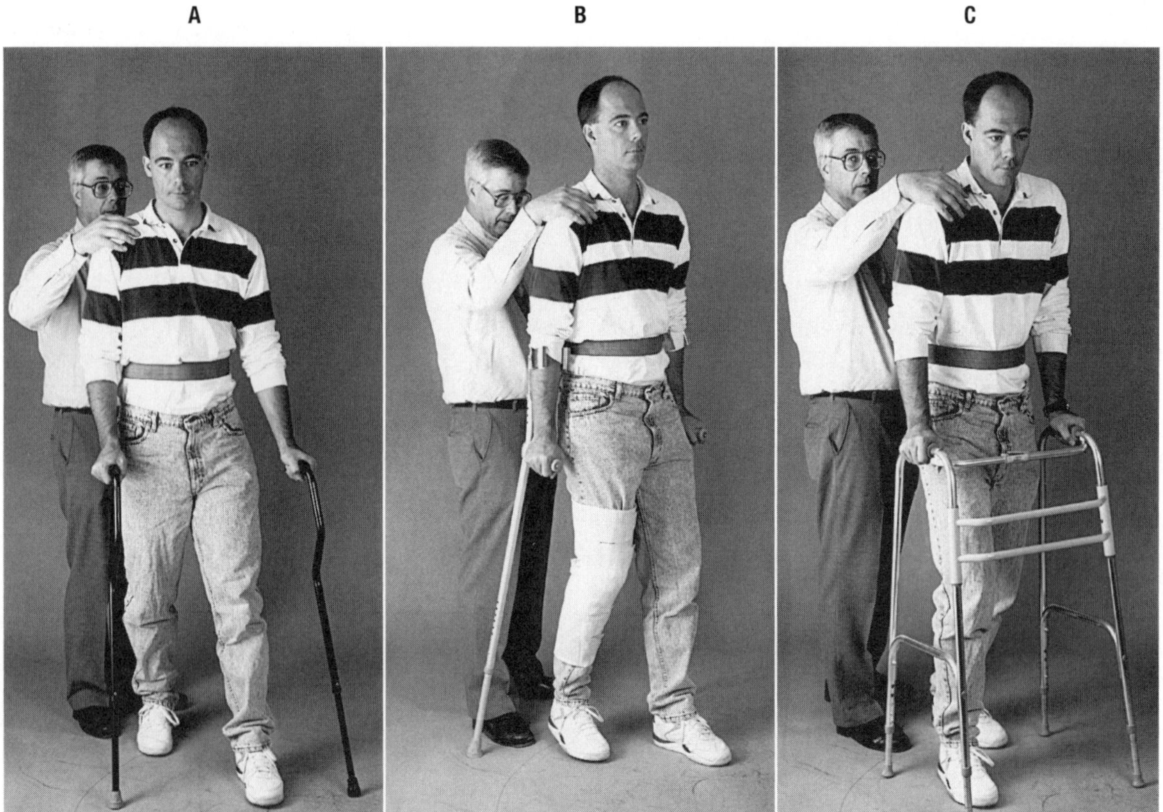

A B C

Fig. 9-29 Correct position of the caregiver behind a patient with an ambulation aid.

PROCEDURE 9-7

Independent Standing and Sitting with Assistive Aids

CANE

For descriptive purposes, assume the left upper and lower extremities are affected or weaker.

Rise to Stand

The cane is positioned on the right side of the chair; a footed cane is placed slightly to the front and to the side of the right armrest and a standard cane is hooked over the front portion of the armrest.

The patient moves toward the front of the chair seat, positions the feet parallel or anteroposterior and flat on the floor, and places the right hand on the armrest.

To rise, the patient leans the trunk forward and pushes strongly with the right upper and lower extremities; the left extremities assist if able.

The patient grasps the cane with the right hand and establishes balance before ambulating.

Return to Sitting

The patient approaches the chair and turns toward the chair, leading with the right upper extremities, until the right side is nearest the chair.

The footed cane is placed in front and to the side of the right armrest or a standard cane is hooked over the armrest.

The right armrest is grasped with the right hand and the patient continues to turn until the back is toward the chair seat.

The right upper and lower extremities are used primarily to lower the patient into the chair slowly; then the body is positioned back in the chair.

CRUTCHES

For descriptive purposes, assume the patient is NWB on the left lower extremity (LLE).

Rise to Stand

The patient moves toward the front of the chair seat and places the right foot approximately 6 to 8 inches forward.

The handpieces of both crutches are grasped in the left hand and the crutches are positioned vertically slightly in front and to the side of the chair; the right hand holds the armrest.

To rise, the patient leans the trunk forward and pushes with both hands and right lower extremity (RLE).

The patient establishes balance and uses the right hand to place one crutch in the right axilla; the remaining crutch is placed in the left axilla.

The crutches are positioned to form a tripod before ambulating.

Return to Sitting

The patient approaches the chair forward and turns, leading with the right extremities, until the back is toward the chair.

The patient steps back until the edge of the chair seat contacts the RLE.

The crutches are removed, one at a time, from the axillae; the handpieces are grasped with the left hand; and the crutches are positioned to the side and vertically.

The right hand is positioned on the arm rest and, using the upper extremities and RLE, the patient lowers into and then moves back in the chair.

WALKER

For descriptive purposes, assume the patient has generalized weakness in the lower extremities.

Rise to Stand

The walker is positioned directly in front of the chair and close enough to be within the patient's reach to rise to stand.

The patient moves toward the front of the chair seat; positions the feet parallel or anteroposterior and flat on the floor; and places the hands on the front portion of armrests.

To rise, the patient leans the trunk forward and pushes with both hands and lower extremities.

When standing, one hand at a time reaches to grasp the handpieces on the walker and establishes balance before ambulating.

Return to Sitting

The patient approaches the chair forward and turns toward the chair, leading with the stronger extremities, until the back is toward the chair.

The patient steps back until the front edge of the chair seat contacts one or both lower extremities.

The patient reaches, one hand at a time, to grasp each armrest and lowers the body into the chair slowly using the upper and lower extremities; then moves back in the chair.

Note: For each of these activities, the patient should be instructed to elevate the foot plates or swing the front rigging, position the caster wheels forward, and lock the wheelchair before standing.

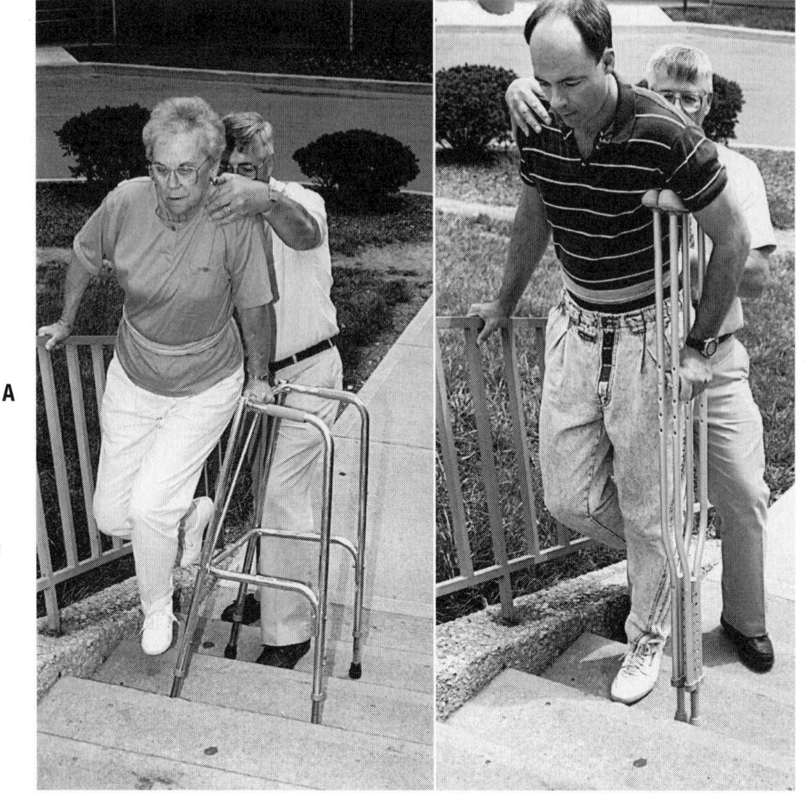

Fig. 9-30 Guarding position for ascending stairs, three-point pattern.

PROCEDURE 9-8

Guarding Techniques for Stairs, Curbs, and Ramps

GENERAL CONSIDERATIONS

The size, stature, weight, and strength of the patient and the caregiver may affect how the techniques presented are applied; some modifications may be necessary, and in some situations, two persons may be required.

The techniques presented for use on stairs are appropriate for use with curbs and ramps.

Regardless of the technique used to guard a patient on stairs, you must prevent the person from falling down multiple steps or forcing you to fall. Therefore you must do the following:

- Maintain a wide stance with your feet; do not place both feet on the same step; use one hand to grasp the safety belt.
- Properly position yourself to maximally protect yourself and the patient.
- Anticipate the actions you will perform in case balance is lost when ascending or descending the stairs.

ASCENDING STAIRS: GUARDING THE PATIENT FROM BEHIND

Position yourself behind and to one side of the patient.

- If a handrail is used, position yourself to the side opposite it.
- If a handrail is not used, position yourself to the side at which the greatest danger or potential for injury exists should the patient's balance be disturbed.
- *Note:* Many caregivers prefer to be positioned to the patient's weakest side or the side of the least functional extremity.

Grasp the safety belt with one hand; be prepared to use your other hand to control the trunk or grasp the handrail when it is available.

Place your outside foot on the step the patient stands; place your other foot on the step below.

PROCEDURE 9-8

Guarding Techniques for Stairs, Curbs, and Ramps—cont'd

Balance Lost Forward

Pull back on the safety belt; use your other hand to pull back on the trunk or to grasp the handrail.

Assist the patient to regain balanced position.

If the patient is unable to regain balance, help lower the person to the steps or move the body toward the handrail.

Balance Lost Backward

Turn your body sideward toward the patient; maintain a wide stance with your feet.

Use one hand to press forward against the pelvis or trunk; use your other hand to grasp the handrail.

Assist the patient to regain a balanced position or help lower the person to the steps or move the body toward the handrail.

Balance Lost to One Side, Toward You

Use one hand or your shoulder to press against the trunk; use your other hand to grasp the handrail.

Assist the patient to regain a balanced position or help lower the person to the steps or move the body toward the handrail.

Balance Lost to One Side, Away from You

Use the safety belt to pull the patient toward you; use your other hand to control the trunk or to grasp the handrail.

Assist the patient to regain a balanced position or help lower the person to the steps or move the body toward the handrail.

DESCENDING: GUARDING THE PATIENT FROM THE FRONT

Follow general considerations listed previously in this Procedure.

Place your outside foot on the step onto which the patient will step; place your other foot on the step below.

Balance Lost Forward

- Move in front of the patient, but maintain a wide stance.
- Use your free hand to press back against the chest or to grasp the handrail; instruct the person to look up and straighten the trunk or to release the aid(s) and grasp the handrail.
- Assist the patient to regain a balanced position or sit on a step.

Balance Lost Backward

- Pull forward on the safety belt; use your other hand to grasp the handrail.
- Assist the patient to regain a balanced position or sit on a step.

Balance Lost to One Side, Toward You

- Use one hand or your shoulder to press against the side of the chest to move the person away from you; one hand grasps the safety belt.
- Assist the patient to regain a balanced position or assist to sit on a step or instruct the person to release the aid(s) and grasp the handrail.

Balance Lost to One Side, Away from You

- Pull on the safety belt to move the patient toward you; use your other hand to grasp the handrail.
- Assist the patient to regain a balanced position or assist to sit on a step or instruct the person to release the aid(s) and grasp the handrail.

DESCENDING: GUARDING THE PATIENT FROM BEHIND

Follow general considerations listed previously in this Procedure.

Place one foot on the step on which the patient stands; place the other foot on the step below.

Balance Lost Forward

- Pull back on the safety belt; use your other hand to control the trunk or to grasp the handrail; maintain a wide stance with your feet.
- Assist the patient to regain a balanced position or assist to sit on a step or instruct the person to release the aid(s) and grasp the handrail.

Balance Lost Backward

- Move so you are somewhat behind the patient; press forward at the pelvis; use your other hand to control the trunk or grasp the handrail; maintain a wide stance with your feet.
- Assist the patient to regain a balanced position or assist to sit on a step or instruct the person to release the aid(s) and grasp the handrail.

Balance Lost to One Side, Toward You

- Use your body to support the patient and to prevent the person from falling to the side.
- Assist the patient to regain a balanced position or assist to sit on a step or instruct the person to release the aid(s) and grasp the handrail.

Balance Lost to One Side, Away from You

- Pull on the safety belt to move the patient toward you; use your other hand to control the trunk or to grasp the handrail.
- Assist the patient to regain a balanced position or assist to sit on a step or instruct the patient to release the aid(s) and grasp the handrail.

Caution: When you pull on the safety belt, you must not pull too quickly or use excessive force. You should attempt to correct the movement of the patient by using a firm, smooth pull on the belt. If you pull with excessive force, you may cause further disturbance of the patient's balance. It is recommended you practice with an unimpaired individual, who can simulate various loss-of-balance movements, to help you develop a sense of the control needed when you use a safety belt.

stride so that the upper foot is on the step the patient is standing on and the lower foot is on the step below the step to which the patient will step (Fig. 9-31). This requires the person to span two steps, which may not be possible for women who wear skirts or for the person with a short stride. *Caution:* Do not stand with your feet parallel to each other and on the same step directly below and in front or to the side of the patient. This position will be unstable if the patient falls forward because it does not provide a wide anteroposterior BOS.

Grasp the safety belt with one hand and the handrail, if one is available, with the opposite hand. Step down one step with each foot after the patient has descended one step; repeat the process to descend all the steps. Teach the patient to stop and gain balance on each step before progressing to the next step. Do not allow the patient to develop momentum when descending the stairs. A too-rapid descent is apt to lead to imbalance and increases the possibility of a fall. (*Note:* If there is no handrail, grasp the safety belt with one hand and position your other hand above and anterior to, lightly touching the patient's shoulder. If your hand does touch the anterior shoulder, it must not restrain the patient's forward movement or cause the patient to alter normal balance.)

Alternative Method. Stand behind and to the side of the patient in the area where there is the least protection. Use an anterioposterior stance with your outside foot on the step on which the patient is standing and your inside foot one step above the step on which the patient is standing (Fig. 9-32).

Grasp the safety belt with one hand and the handrail, if one is available, with your opposite hand. Descend one step with each foot after the patient has descended one step. Teach the patient to stop and gain normal balance on each step before progressing to the next step.

(*Note:* Either of these techniques can provide safety for the patient. Most patients have a greater sense of security when someone is in front of them when they descend stairs. If you are behind the patient and balance is lost forward, you can provide security by gently pulling back on the safety belt and the patient's shoulder; if necessary, seat the person on the stair. You must avoid allowing the patient to pull you forward if a serious loss of balance occurs.)

Ascending a Curb Stand behind and slightly to one side of the patient in an anteroposterior stance. Grasp the safety belt with one hand and position the other hand above and anterior to the patient's shoulder (Fig. 9-33). The patient steps up onto the curb, then you step up onto the curb.

Descending a Curb. Stand in front of and slightly to one side of the patient in an anteroposterior stance. Place your outside foot on the curb and your inside foot on the surface onto which the patient will step.

Grasp the safety belt with one hand and position your other hand anterior to the patient's shoulder or mid-chest. Move back as the patient steps down, then reposition yourself behind the patient if he or she continues to ambulate.

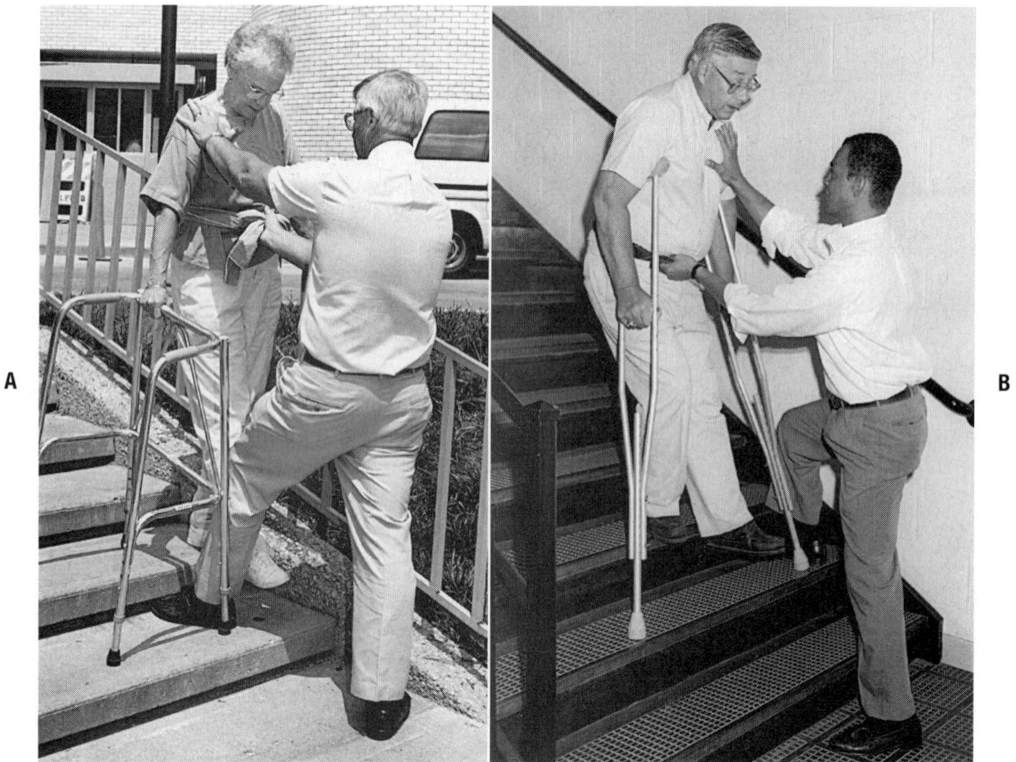

Fig. 9-31 Guarding position for descending stairs, three-point pattern.

An alternative is to stand behind the patient in an anteroposterior stance and with your outside foot at the edge of the curb. Grasp the safety belt with one hand and position your other hand anterior to the patient's shoulder (Fig. 9-34). The patient steps down, then you step down. (*Note:*

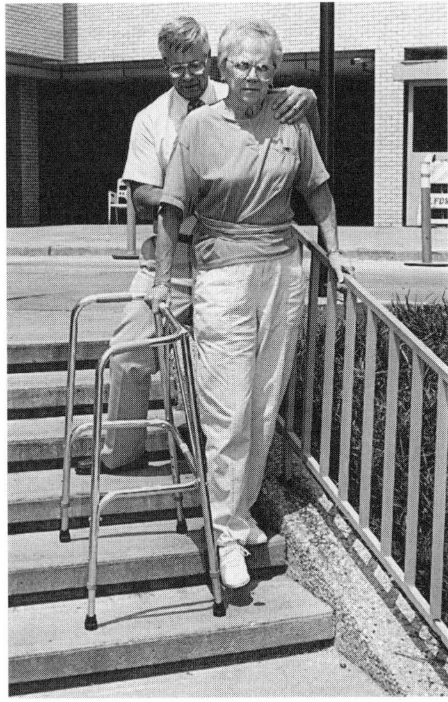

Fig. 9-32 Guarding position for descending stairs (alternative method).

As explained previously, either technique can provide safety for the patient provided you are aware of and alert to the risks involved with each technique.)

Ascending and Descending a Ramp or Incline Stand behind the patient when ascending the ramp, using the techniques previously described regarding the positioning of your feet and hands. You may position yourself behind or in front of the patient when descending the ramp. However, regardless of the position you select, use the techniques previously presented regarding the position of your feet and hands.

Actions If the Patient Loses Balance or Falls

You must be alert and ready to act quickly should the patient lose his or her balance. Your protective reactions must be so well developed that you are able to react automatically to prevent or minimize injury. Proper guarding techniques must be practiced after you understand the rationale and basis for them. In many instances it will not be necessary or desirable to maintain the patient upright. Assisting the patient to the floor or onto a firm object is an accepted procedure, providing proper techniques are used and injury to the patient is minimized. Your primary responsibility is to provide a safe environment and treatment and to protect the patient from injury to the best of your ability.

Level-Ground Ambulation If the patient loses balance forward in a trunk-flexed position, restrain the patient by firmly holding the safety belt; push forward against the pelvis and pull back on the shoulder or anterior chest. Then assist

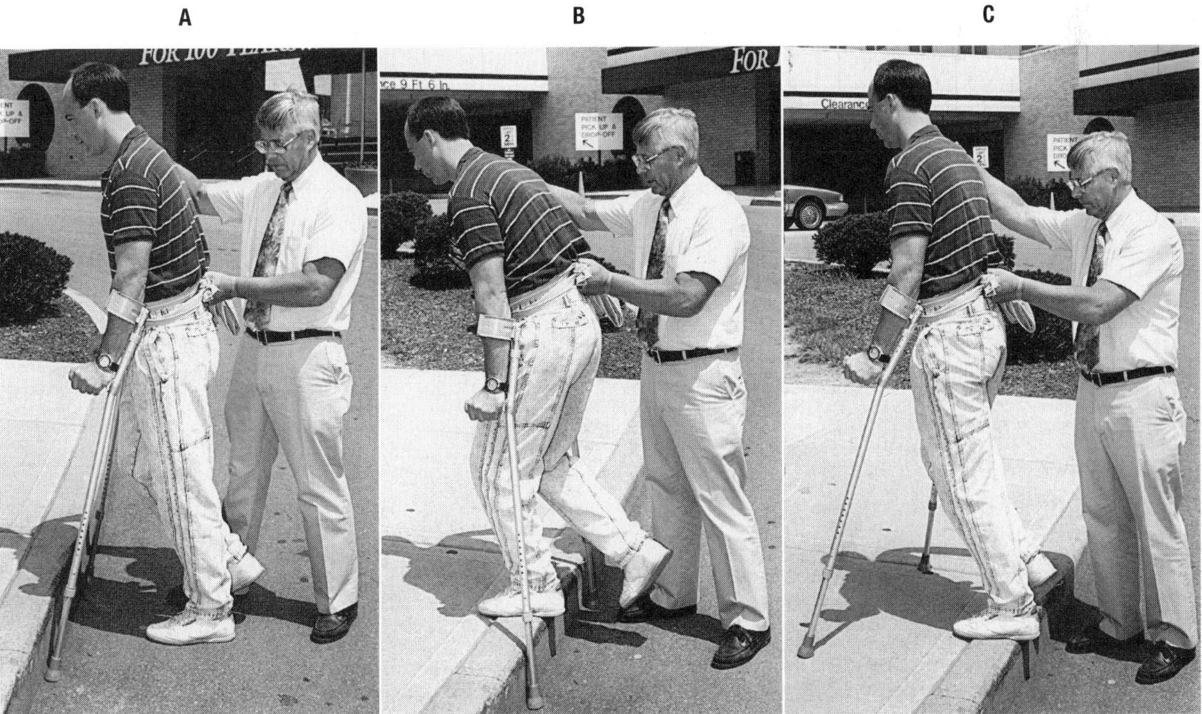

Fig. 9-33 Guarding position for ascending a curb, three-point pattern.

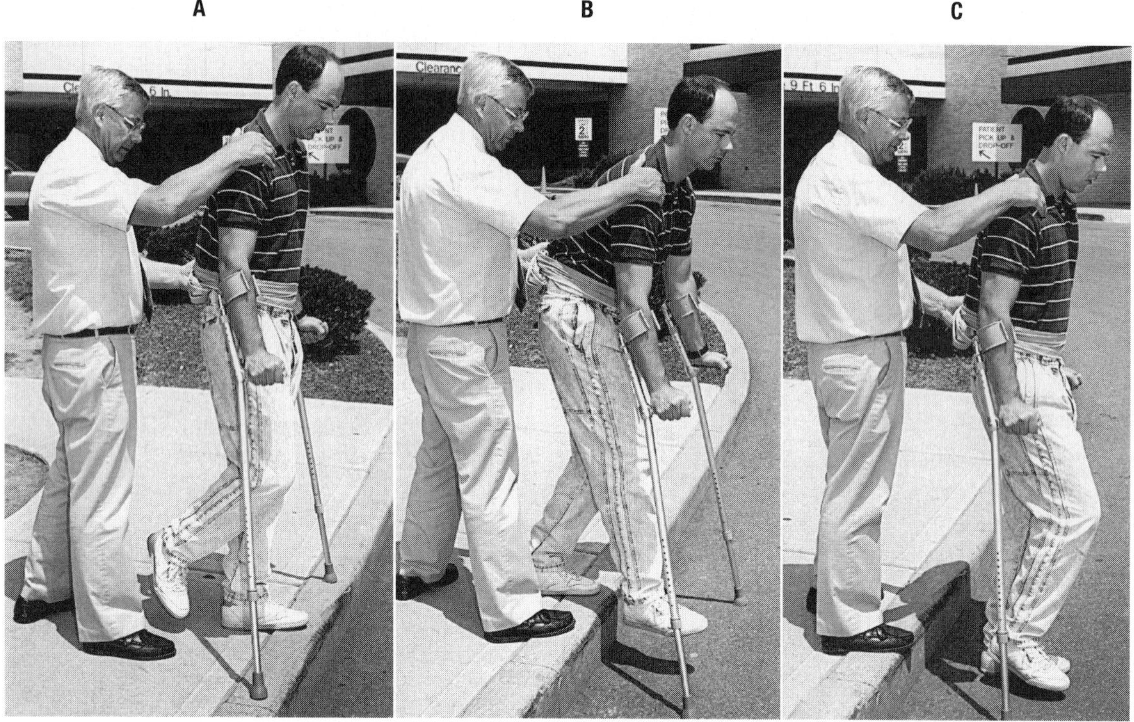

Fig. 9-34 Guarding position for descending a curb, three-point pattern.

the patient to regain balance and to stand erect, providing it has been determined that the patient did not sustain any serious injury. In some instances it will be helpful to allow the patient to lean against you briefly. If the patient loses balance backward, rotate your body so one side is turned toward the patient's back and your anteroposterior stance is widened. Push forward on the patient's pelvis and allow the person to lean against your body. Then assist the patient to regain balance and stand erect.

If the patient falls forward, beyond the point where standing cannot be maintained, instruct the person to quickly release or remove the crutches and reach for the floor. Retard the forward motion by pulling back gently, but firmly, on the safety belt and the patient's shoulder, but do not prevent the patient from reaching the floor (Fig. 9-35, *A*). Step forward with your outside foot as the patient is moving toward the floor and gently retard the descent (Fig. 9-35, *B*). Instruct the patient to cushion the fall by bending the elbows as the hands contact the floor and to lower the body to the floor (Fig. 9-35, *C*). It may be helpful to instruct the person to turn the head to one side to avoid injuring the face (Fig. 9-35, *D*).

If the patient falls backward, beyond the point where standing cannot be maintained, rotate your body so it is turned toward the patient's back and widen your anteroposterior stance. Instruct the patient to release or remove the crutches and allow the person to briefly lean against your body or to sit on your thigh. It may be necessary to lower the patient onto the floor to a sitting position using the safety belt and proper body mechanics (Fig. 9-36) (see Procedure 9-4).

Stairs

Ascending Stairs. When you are positioned behind the patient and balance is lost forward, restrain the person by gently and firmly pulling on the safety belt and the shoulder or hold firmly to the handrail and the safety belt and pull gently and firmly on the safety belt. Move closer to the patient and maintain your anteroposterior stance as you assist the person to regain balance and stand erect. If you are unable to maintain the patient standing, instruct the person to release the crutches and reach for the handrail. Lower the patient to the stair using the safety belt or maneuver the patient toward the wall of the stairway.

If the patient loses balance backward, maintain your anteroposterior stance and press forward against the upper trunk or pelvis as you hold onto the handrail. Assist the patient to regain balance and to stand erect. If you are unable to maintain the patient standing, instruct the patient to release the crutches and grasp the handrail or lean forward. Allow the patient to lean against your body or sit on your thigh or maneuver the patient toward the wall of the stairway. Regardless of which technique you use, you must prevent the patient from falling backward and causing both persons to fall down the stairs.

Descending Stairs. When you are positioned in front of the patient and balance is lost forward, restrain the person

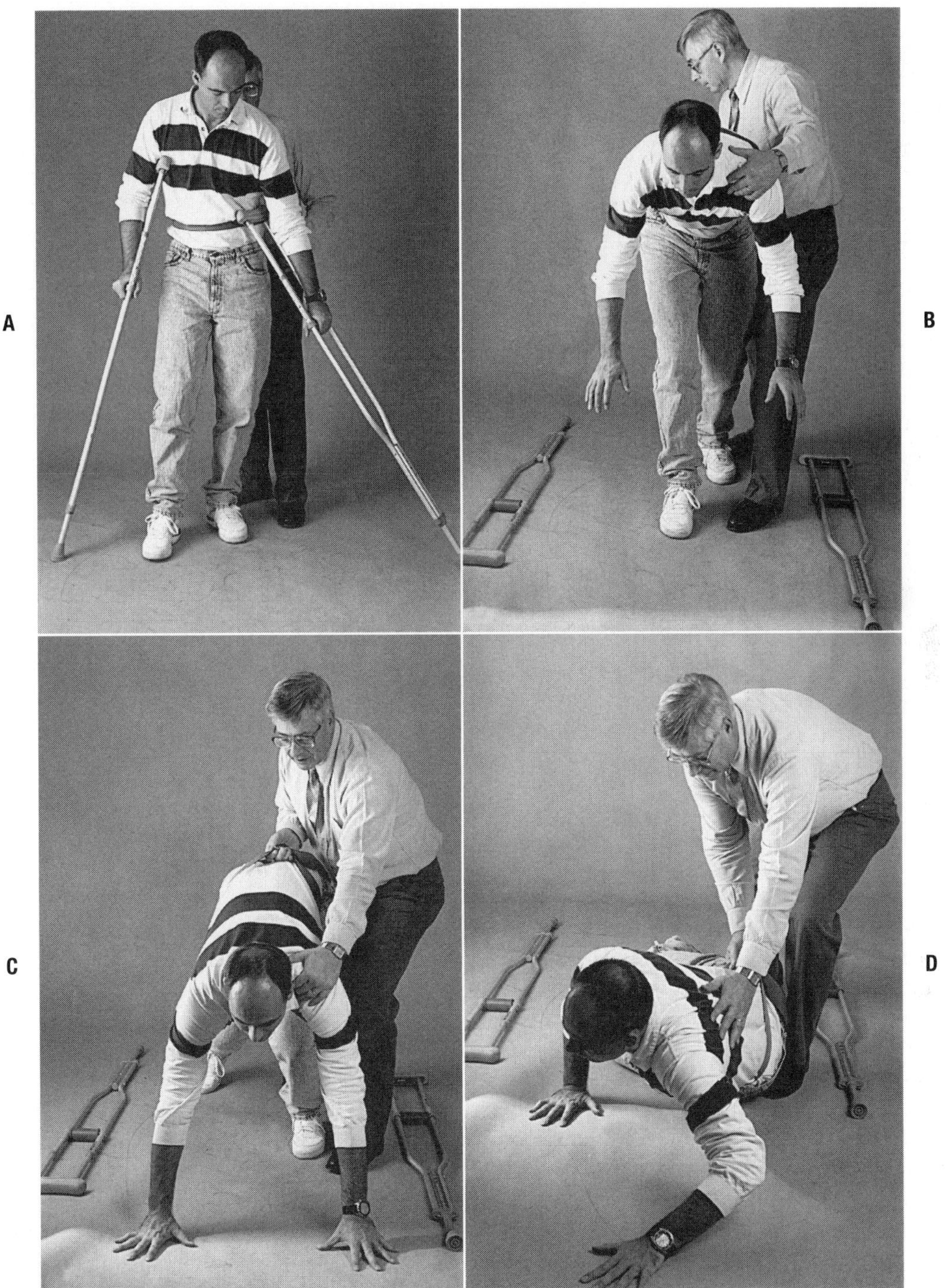

Fig. 9-35 Guarding position for a forward fall.

by gently, but firmly, pushing on the shoulder or chest and gently, but firmly, pulling on the safety belt. You may prefer to hold firmly to the handrail and the safety belt and move your body toward the patient's chest. Assist the patient to regain balance and to stand erect. If you are unable to maintain the patient standing, instruct the patient to release the crutches and grasp the handrail or push on the pelvis or chest while grasping the handrail to maneuver the person toward the wall of the stairway. Regardless of which technique you use, you must prevent the patient from falling forward and causing both persons to fall down the stairs.

If the patient loses balance backward, restrain the patient by pulling forward with one hand on the safety belt and one hand grasping the handrail. Move closer to the person while maintaining your anteroposterior stance. Assist the patient

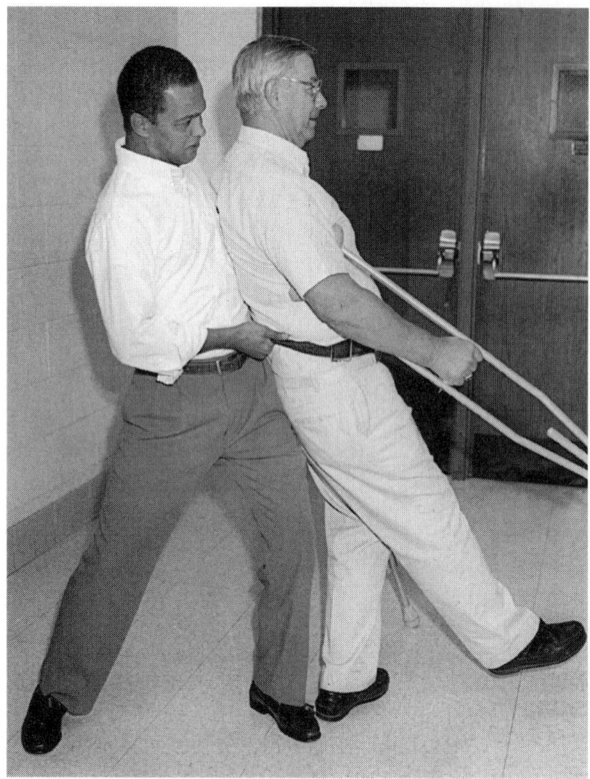

Fig. 9-36 Guarding a person when balance is lost backward.

to regain balance and to stand erect. If you are unable to maintain the patient standing, instruct the patient to release the crutches and grasp the handrail or instruct and assist the patient to sit on a step.

When you are positioned behind the patient and balance is lost forward, restrain the person by pulling back on the safety belt while you hold the handrail or by pulling back on the safety belt and on the anterior shoulder. The patient may briefly lean backward against you to regain balance and to stand erect. If you are unable to maintain the patient standing, instruct the patient to release the crutches and grasp the handrail, or pull back on the safety belt and instruct the patient to sit on a step. Regardless of which technique you use, you must prevent the patient from falling forward and causing both persons to fall down the stairs.

If the patient loses balance backward, restrain the patient with gentle, but firm, forward pressure against the pelvis and upper thorax or hold the handrail and prevent the patient from falling backward with your body. Assist the patient to regain balance and to stand erect. If you are unable to maintain the patient standing, instruct the patient to release the crutches and grasp the handrail or instruct and assist to sit on the step.

These same techniques can be used for both curbs and inclines (see Procedure 9-8).

AMBULATION FUNCTIONAL ACTIVITIES

These components of ambulation with an aid are frequently overlooked during the ambulation training program. If a patient is to be fully independent, it is important to teach the person to move backward and sideward, to turn to the left and to the right, and to perform a 180-degree arc. These movements are necessary because they are components of basic, functional ambulation activities. The patient will need to move backward to be able to sit or to move away from a door that opens toward him or her. A sideward movement is required in narrow spaces (such as the area between two rows of seats in a theater or a narrow hallway or doorway). Turning is required to change direction of movement or for positioning before sitting or performing other activities that require a change of direction. You should not assume that each patient would be able to perform these activities without being taught. Failure to teach the patient these activities may result in decreased independence or an increased risk of injury for the patient.

Backward Movement

Four-Point Pattern Instruct the patient to move one ambulation aid backward and then to step back with the opposite lower extremity; then move the other ambulation aid backward and steps back with the opposite lower extremity. Continue to repeat the pattern as necessary.

Two-Point Pattern Instruct the patient to simultaneously move one ambulation aid and the opposite lower extremity backward and then move the opposite aid and lower extremity backward simultaneously. Continue to repeat the pattern as necessary.

Three-Point Pattern Instruct the patient to start with the crutch tips lateral to, but even with, the toes of the shoes. Then step back approximately 6 inches and reposition the crutches. Continue to repeat the pattern as necessary.

An alternative, advanced technique is to instruct the patient to place the crutches approximately 6 inches behind the heels to form a reverse tripod. Then step back through the crutches to create a forward tripod. The crutches are repositioned and the pattern is repeated as necessary.

The first technique is a more stable method because the crutches remain in front of the patient to preserve the forward tripod position. The second pattern should be used only with patients who have excellent balance and coordination.

Three-One–Point Pattern Instruct the patient to step back with the stronger or less affected lower extremity while maintaining the crutches in front of or even with the weaker or more affected lower extremity. Then the patient steps back with the crutches and the weaker or more affected lower extremity to place them in line with the normal foot. Continue to repeat the pattern as necessary.

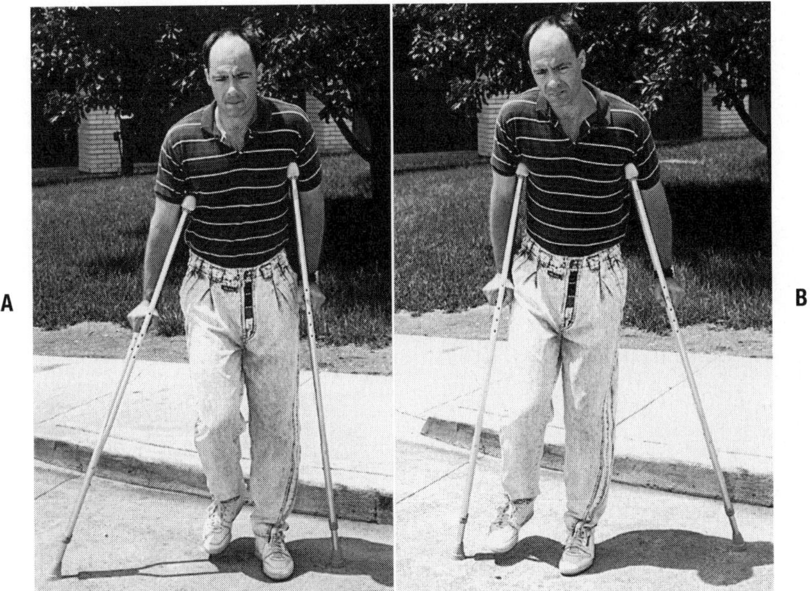

Fig. 9-37 Sideward movement to the patient's right.

An alternative, advanced technique is to instruct the patient to simultaneously move the crutches and the weaker or more affected lower extremity backward; then the patient steps backward with the normal lower extremity until it is behind the other foot and crutches. Continue to repeat the pattern as necessary.

Sideward Movement

To move to the right, instruct the patient to position the left ambulation aid next to the outside of the left foot and the right aid approximately 6 to 8 inches away from the right foot. The patient steps to the right and repositions the aids to sidestep again (Fig. 9-37).

For the four-point, two-point, and three-one–point patterns, instruct the patient to position the aids as described previously to sidestep with the right foot and then with the left foot. Reposition the aid and repeat the pattern as necessary.

For the three-point pattern, instruct the patient to position the crutches as described previously and then support the body weight on the hands and sidestep to the right. Reposition the crutches and repeat the pattern as necessary.

The patient is instructed to reverse the process to sidestep to the left.

Turning Movement

The patient should be taught to turn to the left and to the right regardless of which extremities are weakest or most affected. However, the weaker or more affected lower extremity will require more protection or support when the turn is performed and care must be taken if the patient pivots on that lower extremity. It is suggested the patient learn to pivot on the stronger lower extremity regardless of which lower extremity is weaker, regardless of the direction of the turn, and regardless of the type of gait pattern used. The ambulation aid should be used to protect the weaker or more affected lower extremity and to provide stability similar to the way the ambulation aids are used during level-ground ambulation (Fig. 9-38). For example, the patient who uses bilateral ambulation aids or a walker to protect the RLE can be taught to turn to the right by initially shifting weight onto the LLE. The aid and the RLE are moved slightly forward and toward the right as the patient pivots toward the right on the LLE. This pattern is repeated until the turn has been completed. The aid is moved in the direction of the turn to provide support and stability by maintaining the patient's COG and vertical gravity line over the BOS. To turn to the left, the aid and RLE are moved forward and to the left as the patient pivots on the LLE.

If the patient is unable to bear weight or pivot on the LLE, the person can be taught to pivot on the RLE while elevating the LLE from the floor and moving the aid to the left.

It will be more difficult for the patient to turn (pivot) when standing on a carpeted surface. It may be necessary to teach the person to lift the weight-bearing foot from the carpet to initiate the turn or pivot, while supporting weight on the aid and on the weaker lower extremity, if it is possible to bear weight and pivot on the weaker extremity.

Encourage each patient to use caution when turning. This is particularly important for the elderly, poorly coordinated, or mentally confused patient. *Caution:* Turning by pivoting on a lower extremity on which a total hip replacement has been recently performed is *absolutely contraindicated*. The

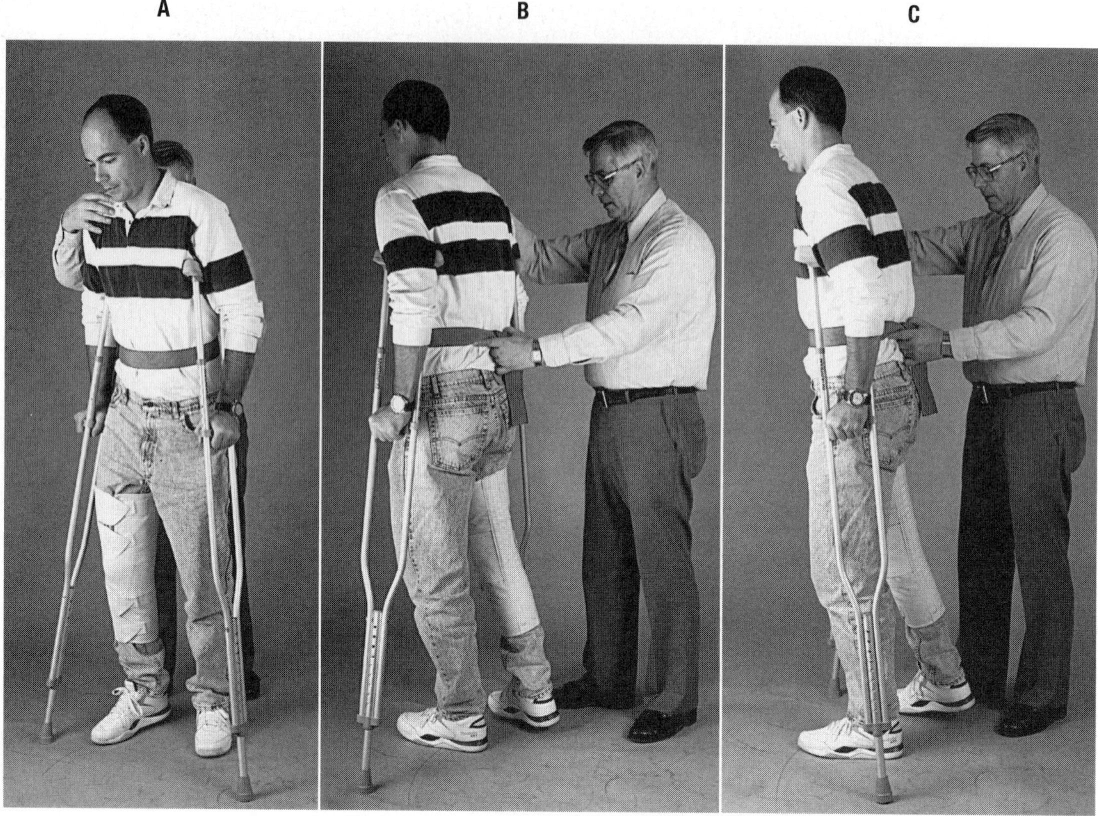

Fig. 9-38 Guarding position for turning movement.

patient who has undergone a hip replacement must learn to pivot while bearing weight on the nonsurgical lower extremity and must avoid rotation of the pelvis or hip while bearing weight on the surgically affected lower extremity.

Curbs and Stairs

Two approaches are used to ascend and descend multiple steps (stairs): (1) with the use of a handrail (banister), and (2) without it. It is usually desirable to initiate stair activities with the patient using a handrail to provide maximum stability and a sense of security. However, most patients should be taught to manage stairs without using a handrail because there are likely to be instances when a handrail will not be available.

When a handrail is used, teach the patient to ascend and descend with the handrail on both the left and the right side of the stairs because handrails may be located on both sides of the stairs or on only one side of the stairs in the patient's environment. For example, most stairs leading to a basement or to the second floor of a residence will have only one handrail, which could be located on either the left or right side of the stairs. If there is only one handrail and it is located on the right wall of stairs leading from the first to the second floor, it will be on the patient's right when ascending the stairs, but on the left when descending. Therefore it is important to have the patient ascend and descend stairs using a handrail on either side of the stairs to ensure independence. The patient may develop a preference if two handrails are available. Right-handed patients may prefer to use a handrail on the right because they can use their dominant (stronger) upper extremity on the handrail. Similarly, left-handed patients would probably prefer to use a handrail on the left. In most stair patterns in the United States, the right side of the stairway is used for ascending and descending, so teaching the patient to use the right handrail will prepare the person for that pattern.

The patient who has only one functional upper extremity and who requires a handrail for support may experience difficulty using a unilateral handrail, depending on its location and on whether the stairs are ascended or descended. A patient with a nonfunctional left upper extremity and a limited functional LLE, but who has functional right upper and lower extremities, can be used as an example. Suppose the home has a handrail on the left wall of the stairs leading from the second floor to the first floor. To descend the stairs, the patient must be taught to reach across the body with the right upper extremity and grasp the handrail as the person steps down first with the LLE and then steps down to the

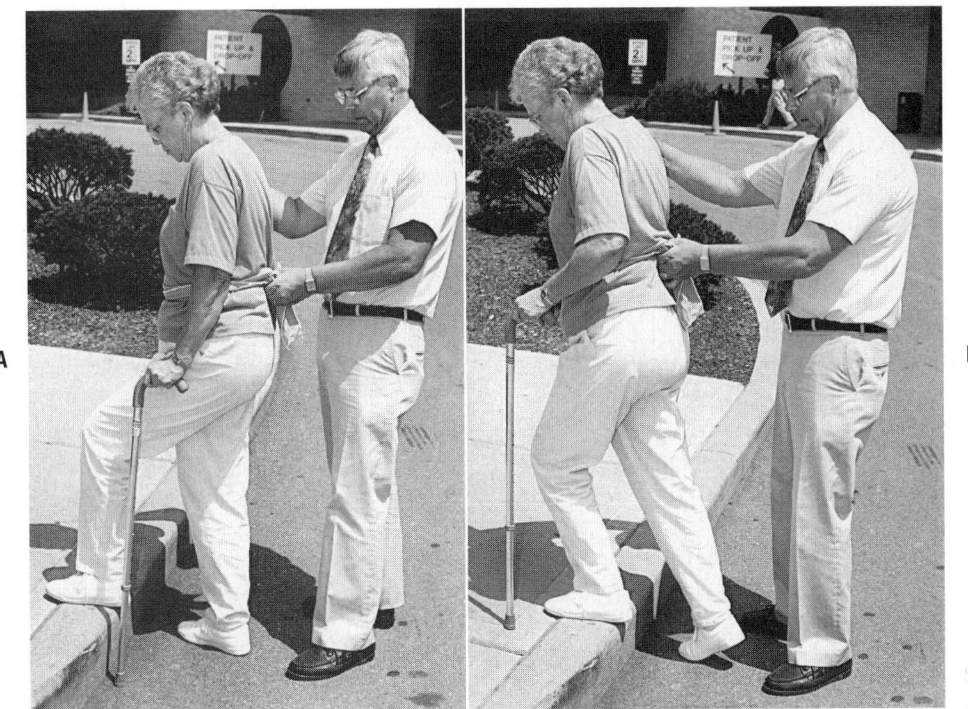

Fig. 9-39 Guarding position for ascending a curb with a unilateral cane.

same step with the RLE. An alternative method is to have the patient descend the stairs backward so the right upper extremity will be next to the handrail. If this method is used, the patient steps down with the LLE and then steps onto the same step with the RLE. To ascend the stairs, the handrail will be on the patient's right side and the right upper extremity can be used in the conventional manner. The patient steps up with the RLE and then steps onto the same step with the LLE.

Now suppose the handrail is on the right side of the stairs. To descend the stairs, the patient uses the right upper extremity to grasp the handrail, steps down with the LLE, and then steps to the same step with the RLE. However, to ascend the stairs, the patient must be taught to face the handrail, grasp it with the right upper extremity, step up with the RLE first, and then step up onto the same step with the LLE.

These examples demonstrate the need to interrelate information about the patient and the anticipated environment as you plan and progress through the training program.

Portable, temporary curbs or stairs can be used initially, but actual curbs and stairs should also be available for instruction and practice. Demonstrate the pattern to the patient and reassure the patient you will provide protection. The patient should not be challenged by a complete flight of stairs (approximately 10 to 12 steps) until a series of three to five steps or a single curb have been practiced. Patients who are NWB on one lower extremity and who have a cast or an orthosis that limits the movements of the lower extremity must be guarded more carefully. You must be certain the patient has sufficient strength, balance, coordination, and endurance to perform curb and stair climbing. The patient who lacks these physical qualities may find it necessary to ascend and descend stairs by sitting and advancing one step at a time using the upper extremities and one or both lower extremities. This method is usually the least desirable and should be used only when the patient is unable to use the other methods described.

Ascending a Curb

Bilateral Canes. The patient places the stronger or less affected lower extremity onto the curb, then elevates the body using the lower extremity while simultaneously raising the weaker or more affected lower extremity and both canes onto the curb. An alternative technique is to have the patient place the canes onto the step, step up with the strongest lower extremity, then raise the weakest lower extremity onto the curb. *Note:* This method decreases the amount of assistance available from the canes because the angles of the shoulders, elbows, and wrists are changed.

Unilateral Cane. Instruct the patient to place the stronger or less affected lower extremity onto the curb, then elevate the body onto the curb using the strongest lower extremity while simultaneously raising the weaker or more affected lower extremity and cane onto the curb (Fig. 9-39). An alternative technique is to have the patient place the cane onto the curb simultaneously with the strongest lower extremity, then raise the weakest lower extremity onto the curb (Fig. 9-40).

Bilateral Crutches

Three-One–Point Pattern. Instruct the patient to place the stronger or less affected lower extremity onto the curb. The patient elevates the body, using the strongest lower extremity, and simultaneously raises the crutches and the weaker or more affected lower extremity onto the curb.

Three-Point Pattern. Instruct the patient to place the weight-bearing lower extremity onto the curb with the affected lower extremity held in extension at the hip and knee and in external rotation at the hip or with the knee flexed. The patient elevates the body using the strongest lower extremity and simultaneously raises the crutches onto the curb and brings the opposite lower extremity forward (see Fig. 9-33).

Standard Walker. If the curb is low (4 inches or less), instruct the patient to place the walker onto the curb, place the stronger or less affected lower extremity onto the curb, and elevate the body onto the curb using the upper and lower extremities while simultaneously raising the weaker or more affected lower extremity onto the curb (Fig. 9-41). If the curb is a standard height (6 to 8 inches), instruct the patient to turn so the back is toward the curb and the walker is in front of the body. The patient places the stronger or less affected lower extremity onto the curb and elevates the body onto the curb while simultaneously lifting the walker and other lower extremity onto the curb. Then the patient backs away from the edge of the curb before turning to move forward. Some patients may be able to ascend the curb forward using the first method described, but this may be difficult because the walker will be too high for proper use of the upper extremities. The patient should try both methods to determine which is most efficient and safe.

Descending a Curb

Bilateral Canes. Instruct the patient to simultaneously place the weaker or more affected lower extremity and both canes down onto the surface below the curb while slightly flexing the stronger or less affected hip and knee. This latter action will help to lower the patient's COG as the canes are lowered. The patient lowers the body with the strongest lower extremity and steps down with that extremity after the canes and the opposite lower extremity have been placed on the lower surface.

Unilateral Cane. Instruct the patient to simultaneously step down with the weaker or more affected lower extremity and cane while flexing the stronger or less affected lower extremity slightly (Fig. 9-42, *A*). The patient lowers the body with the strongest lower extremity and steps down with that extremity after the cane and opposite lower extremity have been placed on the lower surface (Fig. 9-42, *B*).

Bilateral Crutches

Three-One–Point Pattern. The same procedure described previously for bilateral canes should be taught.

Three-Point Pattern. Instruct the patient to place the crutches down onto the lower surface by slightly flexing the

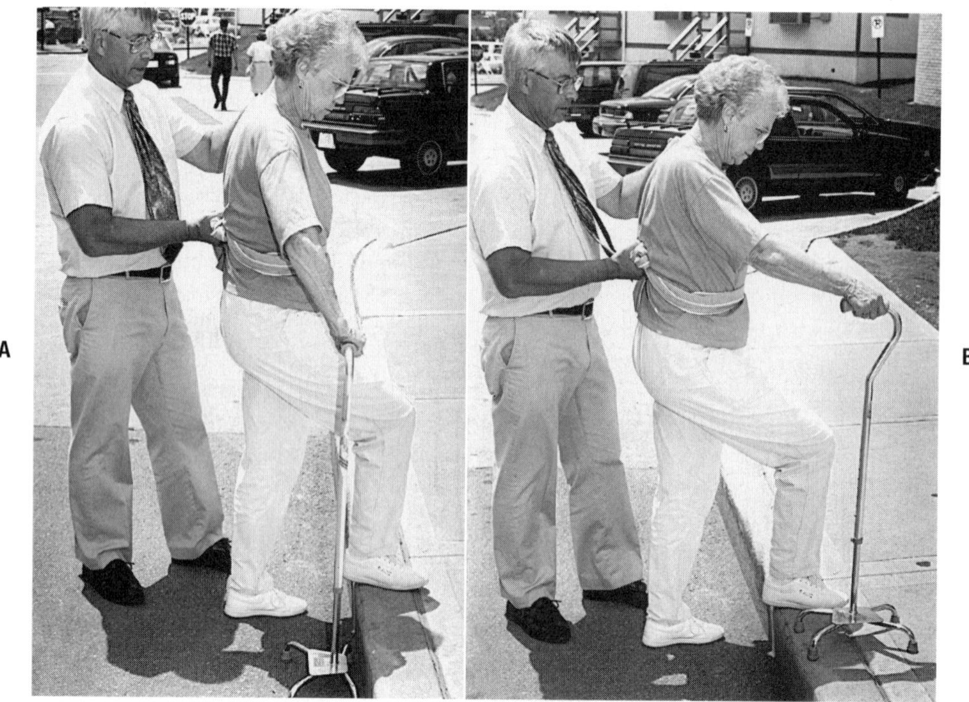

Fig. 9-40 Guarding position for ascending a curb with a unilateral four-footed cane.

strongest hip and knee. The weaker or more affected lower extremity is positioned in front of the patient and over the edge of the curb. The patient steps down using the strongest lower extremity after the crutches are resting on the lower surface.

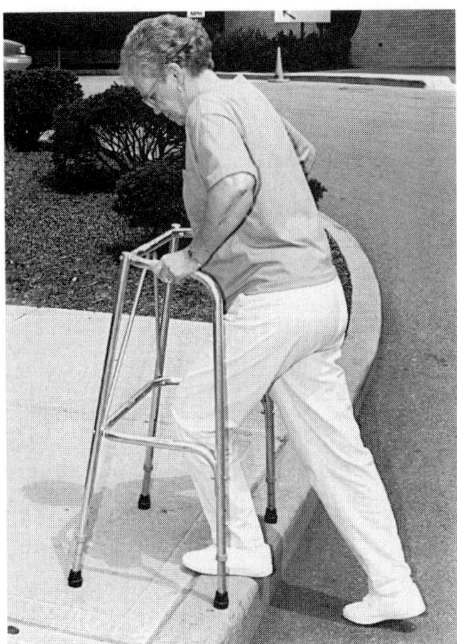

Fig. 9-41 Patient ascending a curb with a walker.

Standard Walker. Instruct the patient to move to the edge of the curb and place the walker down onto the lower surface while flexing the strongest hip and knee slightly (Fig. 9-43, *A*). The weaker or more affected lower extremity is positioned in front of the patient and over the edge of the curb. The patient moves the weaker or more affected lower extremity forward while lowering the body with the stronger or less affected lower extremity and the upper extremities and then steps down with the strongest lower extremity (Fig. 9-43, *B*).

When the patient descends a curb or stairs, it is important to teach the person to flex the hip and knee of the supporting lower extremity as the ambulation aid is being placed onto the step below the step on which the patient stands. This technique is especially necessary for the patient using bilateral axillary crutches because it improves the patient's balance and stability. For example, if the patient does not flex the hip and knee to lower the body, the distance between the top of the axillary rest and the axilla will increase greatly when the crutches are placed down on the next step and the stability of the crutches will be reduced significantly. If only the trunk is inclined forward, the COG will shift forward and the vertical gravity line may not remain within the BOS. In addition, the tendency for the axillary crutches to slip forward or backward is increased when the distance between the axillary rest and the axilla is excessive; this will further reduce the patient's stability. Do not

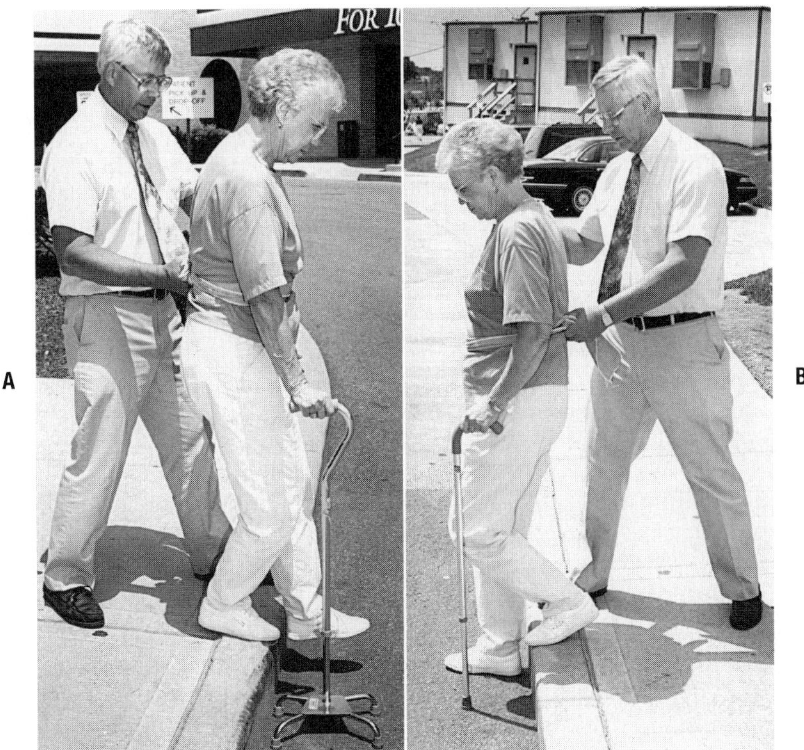

Fig. 9-42 Patient descending a curb with a unilateral cane.

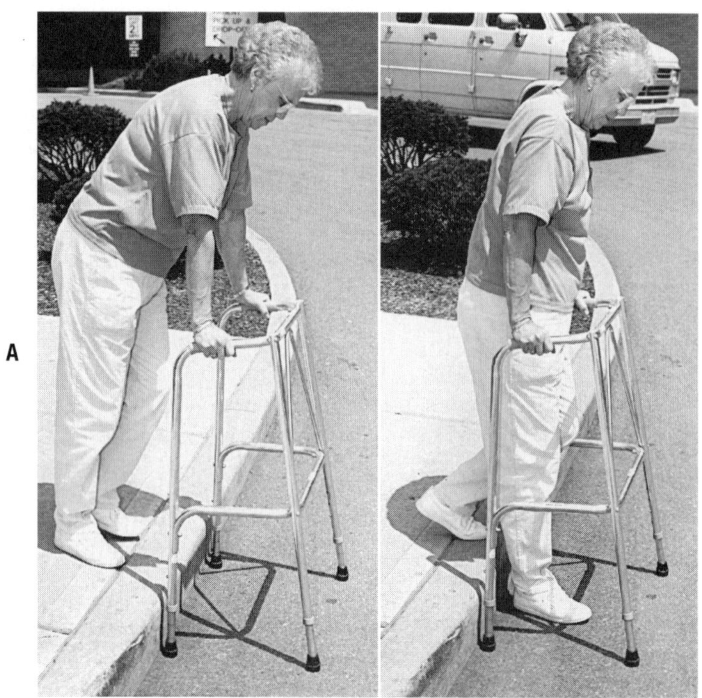

Fig. 9-43 Patient descending a curb with a walker.

overlook teaching this simple technique during the training program; the patient's safety will be improved when it is used (Procedure 9-9).

The same sequences described for the curb can be repeated to ascend and descend stairs. However, the patient should be taught initially to use a handrail when ascending or descending stairs to increase stability and safety. As has been noted previously, the patient should learn to use a handrail on the right and left to ascend and descend the stairs, regardless of which lower extremity is the weaker or more affected, because it may be necessary to use a handrail on either the left or right. In addition, it is important to teach the patient to ascend and descend stairs without using a handrail to enhance independence. Refer to Procedure 9-9 for specific instructions.

Modifications of the patterns used for curbs may be necessary for stairs without handrails and can be used for any ascending or descending activity.

Ascending and Descending Stairs Using a Handrail

Bilateral Canes. The patient may be instructed to hold both canes in one hand and use the other hand on the handrail. An alternative method is to hold a cane in each hand, grasp the handrail and one cane simultaneously, and use the other cane as described for a curb. The cane held simultaneously with the handrail is held parallel to the direction of the handrail. The lower extremities are used in the same way as described for a curb.

Unilateral Cane. The patient may be instructed to hold the cane and the handrail simultaneously or to hang the cane on the forearm farthest from the handrail, on the belt, or in a pocket and use the strong hand to grasp the handrail or grasp the handrail with one hand and use the cane in the other hand as described for ascending and descending a curb. The lower extremities are used in the same way as described for ascending and descending a curb.

Bilateral Axillary Crutches. Instruct the patient to place both crutches under the axilla farthest from the handrail and hold the handpieces, then grasp the handrail with the hand nearest to the handrail (see Fig. 9-30, *B*).

An alternative method is to have the patient place one crutch under the axilla farthest from the handrail and to hold the other crutch perpendicular to the crutch in the axilla, using the hand that grasps the crutch handpiece; the hand without the crutch grasps the handrail (Fig. 9-44).

A third method is to have the patient place one crutch under the axilla farthest from the handrail and hold the other crutch parallel with the handrail with the hand that grasps the handrail. The patient should try each of these methods to determine which is the most functional. The lower extremities are used in the same way as described for ascending and descending a curb. (*Note:* The person who uses forearm crutches can also be taught to use these techniques.)

Standard Walker. *Caution:* These techniques are suggested only for the patient who has good balance, trunk control, and extremity strength. They should be performed only

PROCEDURE 9-9

Independent Ascending and Descending of Stairs with Assistive Aids

For descriptive purposes, assume the RLE is the affected or weaker lower extremity when a single cane is used and when NWB and PWB crutch patterns are used.

Caution: Whenever a fixed handrail is available, the person should use it for security and stability.

CANE

Ascending Pattern

The patient faces the stairs and steps up one step with the LLE.

The LLE is used to elevate the body as the RLE and cane ascend simultaneously onto the same step.

The patient establishes balance before ascending to the next step and then repeats the previous activities.

Descending Pattern

The patient steps down one step with the RLE and cane simultaneously and uses the LLE to lower the body.

The LLE descends and balance is established with both feet on the same step. These activities are repeated for the next step.

CRUTCHES: NONWEIGHT BEARING

Ascending Pattern

The patient faces and stands close to the stairs and uses the crutches for balance and support and steps up with the LLE.

The LLE is used to elevate the body as the crutches are lifted onto the same step. The patient extends and externally rotates the RLE so the toes will not strike or become caught under the front edge of the stair tread.

Balance is established before ascending to the next step and these activities are repeated to ascend the next step.

Descending Pattern

The patient stands with the LLE and crutches positioned toward the front portion of the stair tread; the RLE is held forward of the front edge of the stair tread so the heel will clear.

The patient balances on the LLE and lowers the body by partially flexing the left hip and knee; the crutches are placed toward the front portion of the stair tread on the step below.

The patient uses the crutches for balance and support to step down with the LLE.

The person establishes balance and then repeats these activities to descend to the next step.

CRUTCHES: PARTIAL WEIGHT BEARING

Ascending Pattern

The patient faces and stands close to the stairs and uses the crutches and RLE (PWB) for balance and support to step up with the LLE.

The LLE is used to elevate the body; step up with the RLE and lift the crutches simultaneously onto the same step.

Balance is established before ascending to the next step.

Descending Pattern

The patient stands with the feet and crutches positioned toward the front portion of the stair tread.

The patient balances on the LLE and lowers the body by partially flexing the left hip and knee, then lowers the RLE and crutches simultaneously to the front portion of the stair tread on the step below.

The crutches and RLE (PWB) are used for balance and support to step down with the LLE onto the same step.

Balance is established before descending to the next step.

Note: These same patterns can be used for ascending and descending a curb or other type of single elevation. When two-point and four-point patterns are used, the patient ascends the stairs leading with the stronger lower extremity followed by the other lower extremity and then the assistive devices are lifted simultaneously or alternately. To descend the stairs, the assistive aids are lowered to the step below simultaneously or alternately and then the patient steps down with the weaker lower extremity first, followed by the stronger lower extremity. If there is no strength difference between the lower extremities, either lower extremity may be used as the lead extremity.

when a handrail is available and when all of the feet of the walker fit on the stair treads when the walker is positioned along the patient's side. You may prefer to teach these as techniques to be used for emergency situations rather than as routine techniques.

Ascending. Instruct the patient to face the stairs and to position the walker along the side farthest from the handrail with the closed side of the walker next to the body. The front feet of the walker are placed one step above the step on which the patient stands; the rear feet remain on the step on which the patient stands (Fig. 9-45).

The patient grasps the handrail and the front handgrip or the midpoint of the horizontal bar of the walker. The patient steps up with the stronger or less affected lower extremity, elevates the body with the upper and lower extremities, and then steps up with or lifts the weaker lower extremity. The walker is advanced up one step by the patient and the procedure is repeated. The final step at the top of the stair is

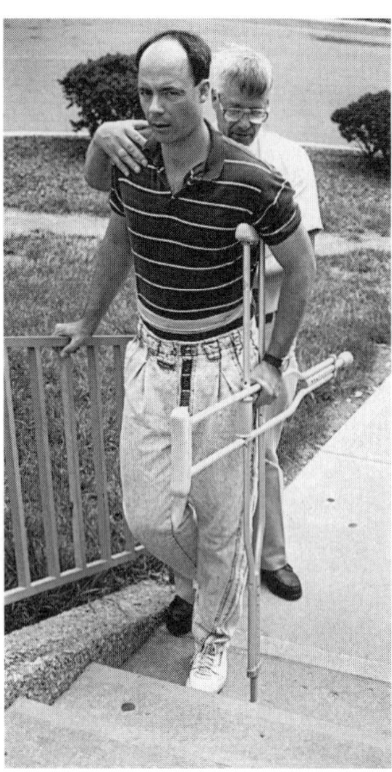

Fig. 9-44 Patient ascending stairs with bilateral axillary crutches (alternative method).

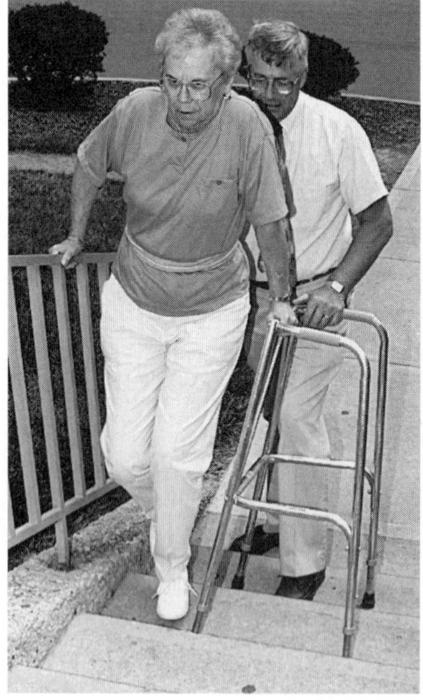

Fig. 9-45 Patient ascending stairs with a walker.

performed by placing the walker on the upper surface and using it for support as the patient steps up.

Descending. Instruct the patient to face the stairs and to position the walker along the side farthest from the handrail with the closed side of the walker next to the body. The front feet of the walker are placed one step below the step on which the patient stands and the rear feet remain on the step on which the patient is standing (Fig. 9-46).

The patient grasps the handrail and the rear handgrip or the midpoint of the horizontal bar of the walker. The weaker or more affected lower extremity is lowered by slightly flexing the hip and knee of the strongest lower extremity, then the body is lowered using the upper and lower extremities, and the person steps down with the strongest lower extremity. The walker is advanced down one step and the procedure is repeated. The patient descends the final step using the same method described to step from a curb.

Ascending and Descending Stairs Using Axillary Crutches *Caution:* These procedures are suggested for the patient who has good balance, trunk control, and strength in both upper extremities and one lower extremity (Figs. 9-47 and 9-48). The pattern for ascending and descending stairs is described in Procedure 9-9.

Patients with Casts or Knee Immobilizers

Below-Knee Cast. To ascend stairs or a curb, the patient has several options. Each method is designed to protect the foot and lower leg immobilized by the cast, to maintain balance, and to promote safety and stability for the patient.

Instruct the patient to extend the hip and flex the knee to 90 degrees, keeping the knee at 90 degrees, so the toes will clear the curb or the stair lip or *riser*. As an alternative, instruct the patient to extend the hip and knee and externally rotate the hip (see Fig. 9-47) or to flex the hip and knee to 90 degrees so the toes will clear the curb or the stair lip or riser. The last method does not provide as much protection to the foot and cast as the other two methods and is not recommended.

The method selected for each patient will depend on the patient's strength, balance, coordination, and, in some instances, personal preference. The patient should try each of these methods to determine which one is the most efficient.

To descend stairs or a curb, there are several options. First, the patient can flex the hip and knee to 90 degrees so the heel clears the stair tread and then position the lower leg in front of the body when stepping down, or the patient can partially flex the hip and maintain the knee in extension so the heel clears the stair tread (see Fig. 9-48, *A*). Do not teach the patient to flex the knee to 90 degrees with the hip extended because the toes are apt to contact the curb surface or stair tread when stepping down (see Fig. 9-48, *B*).

Full-Length Cast or Knee Immobilizer. To ascend stairs or a curb, the patient should extend and externally rotate the hip so the toes clear the stair lip or riser or the front of the curb when stepping up. The immobilized extremity will trail the body as the patient steps up.

To descend stairs or a curb, instruct the patient to partially flex the hip so the heel clears the stair tread or curb. The immobilized lower extremity remains in front of the patient and leads the body when stepping down.

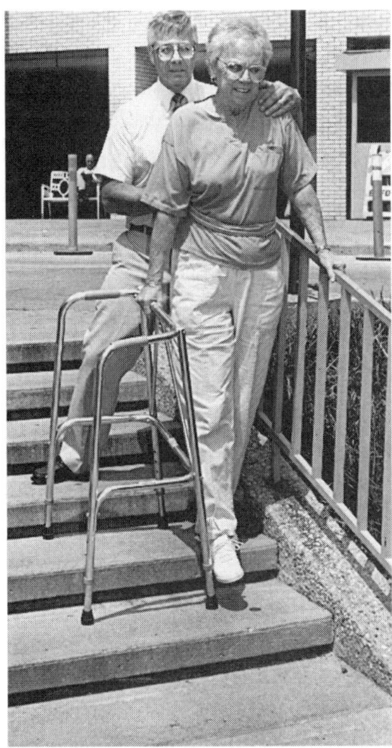

Fig. 9-46 Patient descending stairs with a walker.

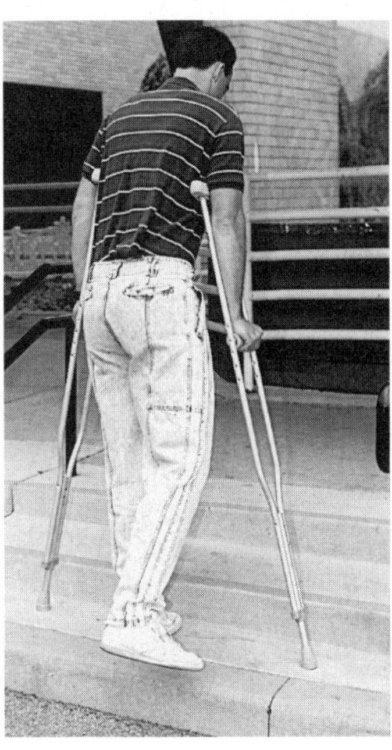

Fig. 9-47 Patient independently ascending stairs using bilateral axillary crutches, three-point pattern.

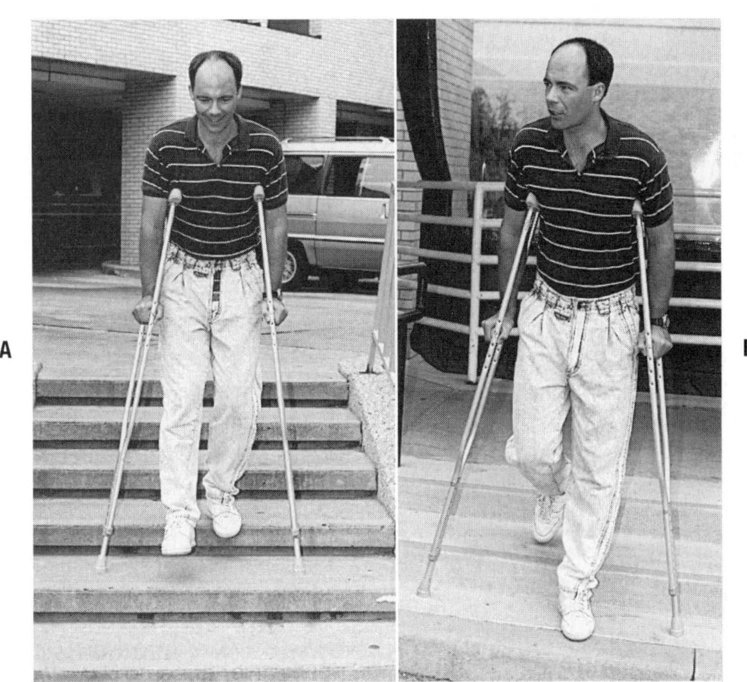

Fig. 9-48 **A,** Proper way to descend stairs independently using crutches, three-point pattern. **B,** Improper way.

Doors

Patients who use ambulation aids should be taught how to manage opening and closing various types of doors. The patient should be familiar with several techniques to control doors with and without self-closing devices (automatic door closers). It is likely that the patient will prefer to use only one of these techniques, but independence will be enhanced if more than one method is learned and mastered.

Self-Closing Door If the door opens away from the patient, the door is approached at an angle so the person faces the side of the door that will open (that is, back to the hinges) (Fig. 9-49, *A*). Instruct the patient to remain close to the door and the doorknob, latch, or crash bar; use one hand to open the door; and shift the body weight onto the opposite crutch and lower extremity, if weight bearing is permitted on that extremity (Fig. 9-49, *B*). The door is opened with a quick push, and the patient returns the hand from the doorknob or crash bar to the crutch. The crutch nearest to the door is moved so the crutch tip engages the floor and the bottom of the door and serves as a doorstop. The door can be opened wider by repeating this procedure as the patient moves through the doorway.

The patient moves through the doorway by pushing against the door to open it farther and by repositioning the crutch tip to keep the door open. The person must be certain the final step through the doorway will place the body beyond the closing arc of the door. (*Note:* If the door has a crash bar, the patient should open the door by pushing on the crash bar near to where it is attached to the door close to the door latch; this will give the patient the greatest advantage to open the door with the least expenditure of energy. A crutch tip can be used to keep the door open or with the back to the door; the body can be used to keep the door open while moving sideward [Fig. 9-49, C].)

Some patients may prefer to place both crutches under the axilla farthest from the crash bar, holding them with the corresponding hand while grasping the crash bar with the hand nearest to the crash bar. The person may use the crash bar as a support when stepping through the door. The patient must be instructed to push downward rather than outward on the bar while moving through the doorway to avoid opening the door too wide and affecting the BOS. The crutches will need to be repositioned into each axilla to take the last step through the doorway.

If the door opens toward the patient, instruct the patient to approach the opening edge of the door at an angle, facing toward the hinge side of the door (Fig. 9-49, *D*). By being positioned at an angle to the door, the patient will be able to open the door a smaller amount than would be necessary if standing directly in front of it. The patient positions the body close to the door, but slightly outside the area needed to open it. The body weight is shifted onto the crutch handgrip farthest from the doorknob or latch and the hand nearest the doorknob to open the door by quickly pulling on the doorknob and then returning the hand from the doorknob is used to grip the aid (Fig. 9-49, *E*). The crutch nearest to the open edge of the door is moved so the crutch tip engages the floor and the bottom of the door to serve as a doorstop (Fig. 9-49, *F*). If necessary, the door can be opened wider before the patient moves through the doorway. The patient moves through the doorway by pushing against the door and repositioning the crutch tip against the bottom of the door (Fig. 9-49, G). The person must be certain the final step through the doorway will place the body beyond the door frame and the closing of the door.

The same procedures can be used for forearm crutches, canes, or a walker.

Standard Doors Instruct the patient to use the same positions and techniques previously described for a door that opens away from or toward the person. However, the patient will need to open the door only wide enough for the crutches, canes, or walker and the patient to move through the doorway. The door does not need to be opened to its full width if the patient is taught to move through the doorway at an angle. The crutch or cane tip or the walker feet are not required to restrain the door. The patient will need to turn to close the door, then move sideward or backward after the door has been closed to resume the gait pattern and direction. When the door opens toward the patient, it may be necessary to back up while opening the door, especially if the door cannot be approached at an angle toward or facing the opening edge of the door.

Ascending or Descending Ramps, Inclines, or Hills Instruct the patient to ascend a ramp, incline, or hill using techniques similar to those used to ascend a curb or stairs. Teach the patient to advance the aid and the stronger or less affected lower extremity before advancing the weaker or more affected lower extremity; a shorter stride may be necessary (Fig. 9-50). With a full-length cast or knee *immobilizer,* the patient will need to extend and externally rotate the hip to clear the foot when ascending the ramp, incline, or hill and will need to flex the hip when descending. With a below-knee cast, that extremity should be extended at the hip and flexed at the knee when ascending. On a steep incline or hill, the patient may need to "zigzag" by moving diagonally when ascending.

The patient is instructed to descend a ramp, incline, or hill using techniques similar to those used to descend a curb or stairs, but the stride and placement of the ambulation aid(s) should be shortened (Fig. 9-51). Instruct the patient to advance the weaker or more affected lower extremity and ambulation aid before advancing the stronger or less affected lower extremity using a short stride. With a full-length cast or knee immobilizer, the patient will need to partially flex the hip to clear the foot and thus the immobilized extremity will lead the movement. With a below-knee cast, the hip and knee should be partially flexed, with the foot positioned

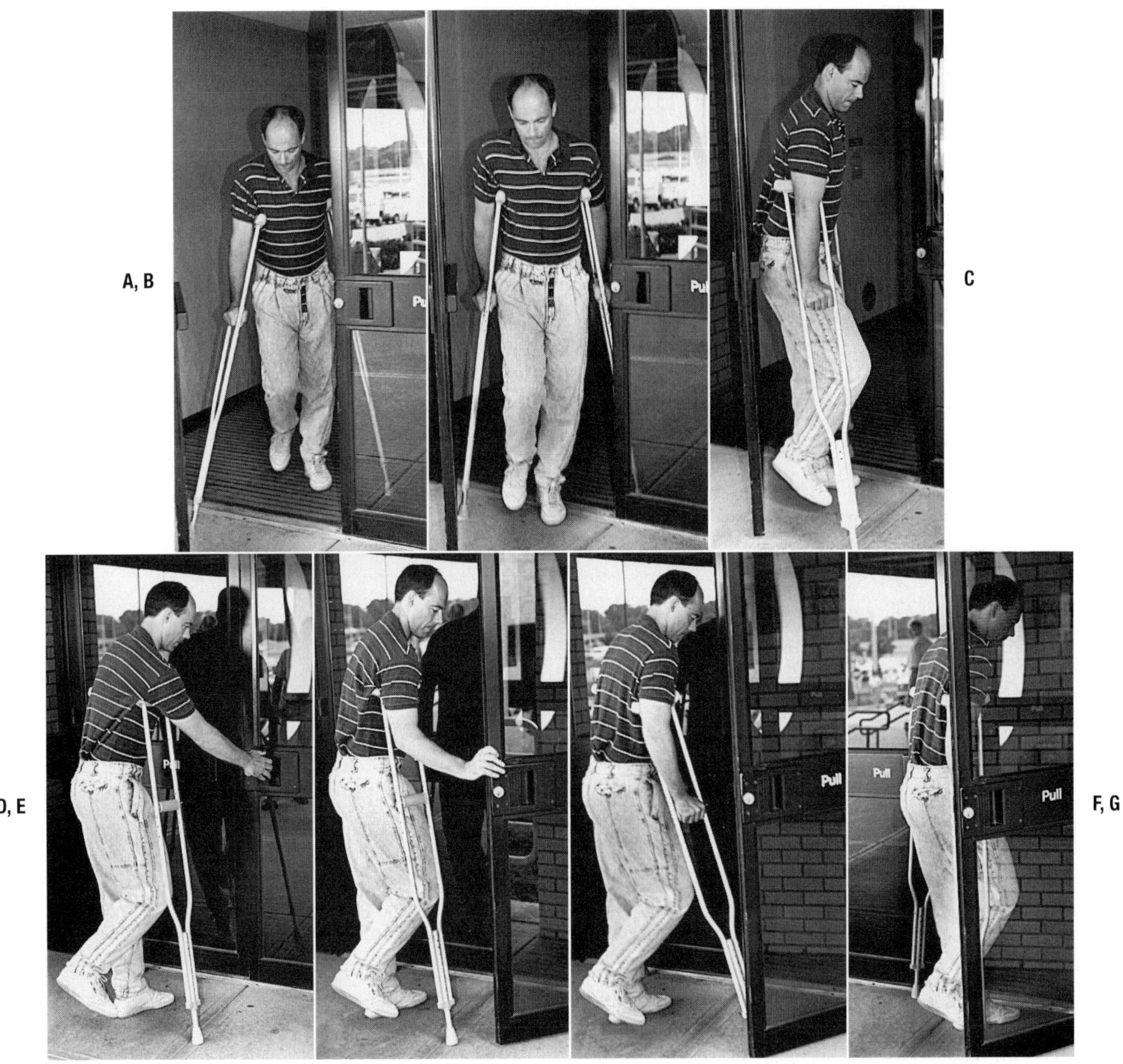

Fig. 9-49 **A** through **C,** Use of bilateral axillary crutches to negotiate a self-closing door that opens away from the patient. **D** through **G,** Use of bilateral axillary crutches to negotiate a self-closing door that opens toward the patient.

in front of the body to clear the foot; alternatively, the hip should be partially flexed and the knee extended to clear the foot. The affected lower extremity should not be allowed to trail the body. On a steep incline or hill, the patient may need to zigzag by moving diagonally when descending.

Elevator Access The patient should be taught to enter and leave the elevator in a forward position whenever possible. The ambulation aid or the patient's hand or arm can be used to activate the device that automatically prevents the door from closing, but the patient will need to determine the type of device used (such as photoelectric beam, pressure bar, or rubber-covered flange on the edge of the door). The patient should be taught to observe the area where the floor of the elevator and the floor of the corridor meet. There may be a space between the two surfaces, and the tip of the crutch, cane, or walker must not be placed in that space. Furthermore, when some elevator cars stop, their floor may not be level with the corridor floor; the patient should be alert for this potential hazard. After the patient is in the elevator, it will be necessary to turn around to face forward in preparation to exit the car and to use the control panel.

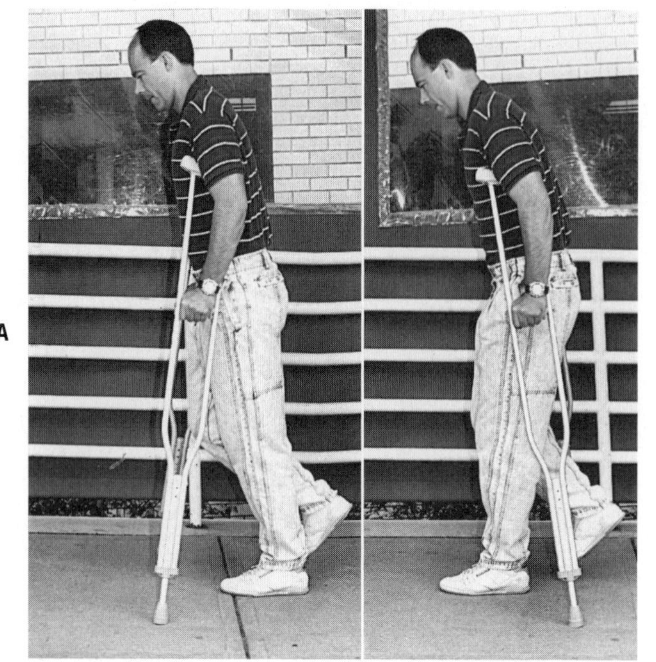

Fig. 9-50 Patient ascending a ramp with bilateral axillary crutches, three-point pattern.

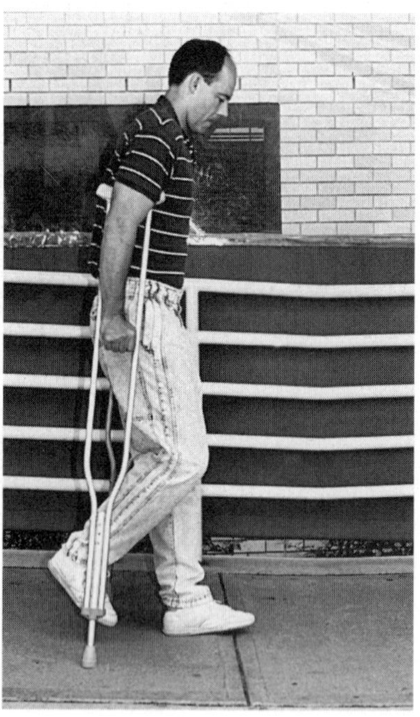

Fig. 9-51 Patient descending a ramp with bilateral axillary crutches, three-point pattern.

PROCEDURE 9-10

Standing Transfers into an Automobile

INDEPENDENT TRANSFER WITH CRUTCHES

Instruct the patient to approach the passenger door at an angle; position yourself to guard by standing behind and to one side.

The patient reaches to open the door, opens it, and shifts the crutches into the hand farthest from the car.

The free hand is positioned on a solid surface of the car (that is, roof, back of the seat, dashboard, door frame) and the patient pivots so the body is toward the car seat.

The body is lowered onto the car seat using the upper extremities and functional lower extremity.

The patient pivots and places the lower extremities into the car; the crutches are placed in the car; the car door is closed and the seat restraints are applied.

Note: For many persons, the transfer will be performed more easily if the car seat is positioned back as far as possible. This position will make it easier to place the lower extremities and crutches in the car.

Automobile Access Frequently, the patient will find it more convenient to enter and leave the car from the passenger side to avoid interference from the steering wheel. An automobile with two doors is usually easier for the patient to enter and exit because the door is wider, providing more space in which to sit, and the access to the rear seat area is more convenient for storage of the aid (Procedure 9-10).

To enter the car, instruct the patient to approach the car door at an angle so it opens away from the body (Fig. 9-52, *A* through *C*); open it only as far as necessary to have access to the seat. The patient pivots the body to face away from the car interior and places both crutches in one hand; the other hand can be placed on the back of the seat or on the dash or on the door with the window rolled down (Fig. 9-52, *D*).

A, B

C

D, E

F

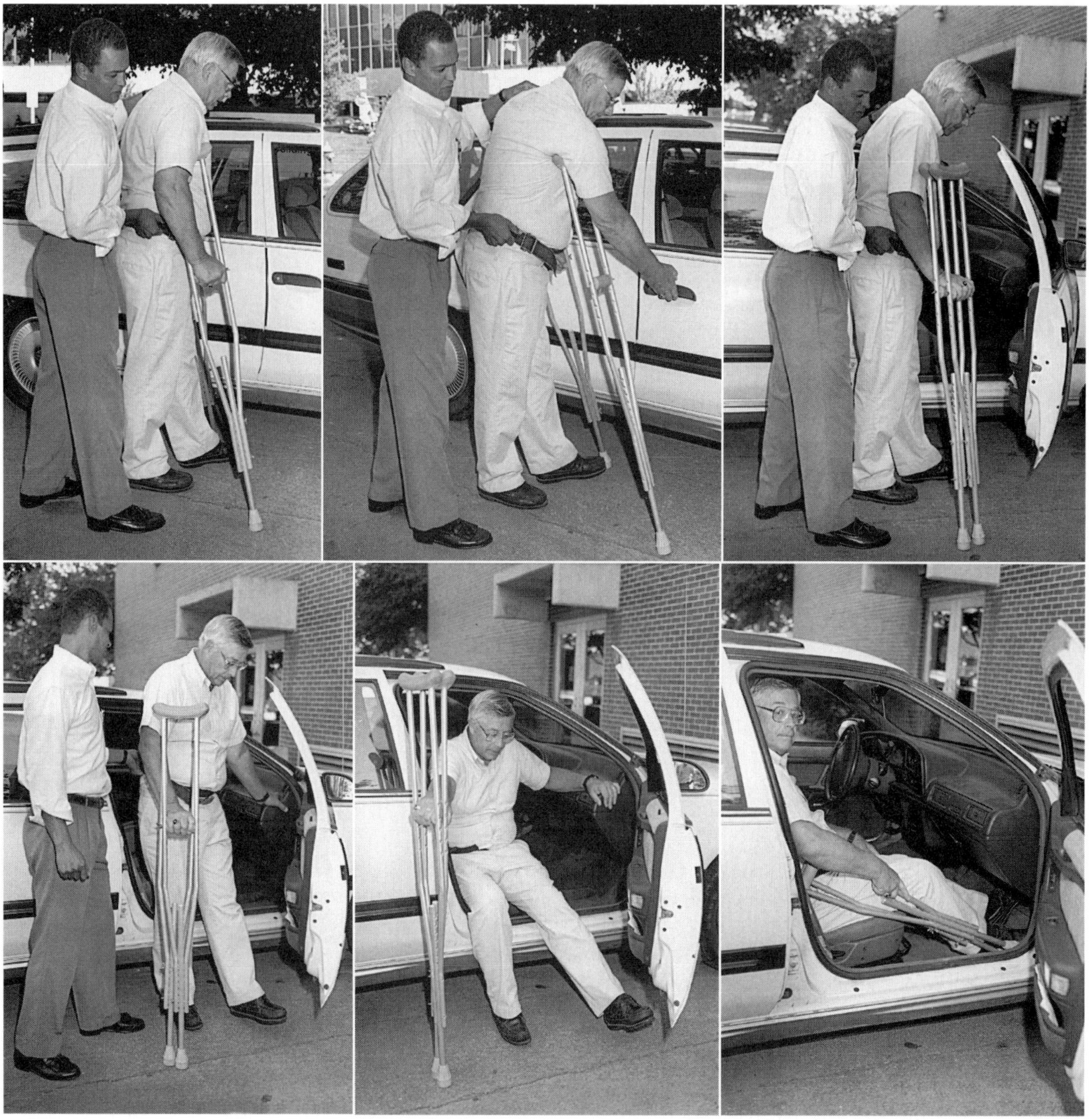

Fig. 9-52 Transfer from crutches into a motor vehicle: **A,** The person approaches the passenger door at an angle. **B,** He reaches for the door latch. **C,** The door is opened and crutches are placed in one hand. **D,** The person pivots and places the free hand on the dash. **E,** He lowers his body onto the car seat using the upper extremities and uninvolved lower extremity. **F,** The lower extremities and crutches are placed in the car.

The person lowers onto the seat and places the lower extremities and ambulation aid(s) into the car (Fig. 9-52, *E* and *F*). The patient will need to slide across the seat if entered on the passenger side and is to drive. The patient with a full-length cast or knee immobilizer may be more comfortable in the back seat because the extremity can be placed on the seat. To drive an automobile with an automatic transmission with the RLE immobilized, it can be placed on the front seat or on the floor on the passenger side of the car, or the seat can be adjusted to its most rearward position to provide more space between the front seat and the foot controls. The patient with a full-length cast or knee immobilizer on the LLE will have difficulty driving the vehicle because it will be difficult to position the LLE and still have access to the steering wheel and to the foot controls. *Caution:* A person with an immobilized lower extremity should not attempt to drive an automobile with a standard transmission.

To leave the car, instruct the person to open the car door, obtain the ambulation aid, and adjust the body so the lower extremities are placed outside the car. The patient grasps both crutches in one hand and places the other hand on the back of the seat, on the dash, or on the door frame with the window rolled down. The patient uses the upper and lower extremities to push to stand, positions the crutches in each axilla, and steps away from the car. It may be necessary for the patient to turn to close the door and then to move backward before resuming the gait pattern and direction of travel.

Transferring to the Floor from Crutches

There may be instances when a patient desires to sit on the floor or ground. Several methods can be taught to the patient to allow movement from standing to sitting on the floor. This activity is not to be confused with a protective fall; this is an activity the patient controls and performs independently.

If the patient is NWB on one lower extremity and uses bilateral axillary crutches, both crutches are dropped to the floor and balance is maintained briefly on the strongest lower extremity; then reach forward toward the floor with the upper extremities while flexing the stronger lower extremity and extending and externally rotating the hip of the most affected lower extremity. The patient lowers the body using the strongest lower extremity until the hands contact the floor. The person can kneel on the strongest knee or turn the hips and sit on the hip of the strongest lower extremity to complete the activity. Another method would be to instruct the patient to drop both crutches and reach backward toward the floor with the upper extremities, flex the hip of the weaker or more affected lower extremity and slide the heel forward on the floor, then flex the hip and knee of the strongest lower extremity. The patient lowers the body using the strongest lower extremity until the hands contact the floor and then sits on the floor to complete the activity. Alternatively, instruct the patient to shift both crutches to the hand on the side of the weaker or more affected lower extremity and grasp both handpieces (Fig. 9-53, *A*). The hip of the most affected lower extremity is flexed and slides that heel forward on the floor. The body is lowered using the strongest lower extremity and the hand holding the crutches while reaching toward the floor with the opposite upper extremity (Fig. 9-53, *B* and *C*). The person sits on the floor to complete the activity (Fig. 9-53, *D*).

(*Note:* The patient can be taught all of these techniques or only one of them depending on the amount of strength, coordination, balance, flexibility, and personal preference. The same techniques can be used for the patient who is able to partially bear weight on one lower extremity and fully bear weight on the other lower extremity.)

Rising from the Floor to Standing

If the patient is NWB on one lower extremity and uses bilateral axillary crutches, instruct the person to turn so the hands and the foot of the strongest lower extremity are on the floor and to assume a half-kneeling position with that one lower extremity. The hip of the weaker or more affected lower extremity is extended and externally rotated. The crutches are positioned within easy reach and the patient pushes to stand using the strongest lower extremity and the upper extremities. The patient picks up the crutches with one hand and grasps the handpieces while still in a semistanding position. The trunk is straightened, the person stands erect, and positions the crutches in each axilla to complete the activity. Alternatively, the patient turns so the hands and the foot of the strongest lower extremity are on the floor to assume a half-kneeling position, with the hip of the weaker or more affected lower extremity extended and externally rotated (Fig. 9-54, *A*). The crutches are held vertically by the handpieces with the hand on the side of the weaker or more affected lower extremity (Fig. 9-54, *B*). The patient pushes to stand using the strongest lower extremity and the hand on the crutch handpieces (Fig. 9-54, *C* and *D*); after standing, the crutches are positioned into each axilla (see Fig. 9-53, *A*). In a third technique, the patient sits on the floor and flexes the strongest hip and knee so the foot is flat on the floor. The weaker or more affected lower extremity is maintained in front of the body. The patient holds both crutches by the handpieces, using the hand on the same side as the weaker or more affected lower extremity *or* the crutches may be placed between the thighs with both hands grasping the crutch handpieces. The patient pushes to stand using the strongest lower extremity and the upper extremities holding the crutches; after standing, the crutches are positioned into each axilla.

Similar methods or techniques can be used for patients who use ambulation aids other than axillary crutches. In some instances, the patient may prefer to use a firm object (such as a table, chair, sofa, tree trunk, bench, or railing) for support and stability to move to the floor or return to standing. However, the patient will be more independent when it is possible to perform these activities without the use of a firm object because such an object may not be available or accessible. Special needs or techniques may need to be resolved by problem solving with the patient. There are some risks to patient safety associated with this activity, so you must use caution and guard the patient and use a safety belt when these techniques are practiced.

Falling Techniques

Backward The patient should be taught to control the body if a backward fall occurs. Instruct the patient to release the crutches (or other aid) and flex the trunk and head while reaching forward. The force of the fall is absorbed by the buttocks and the patient's head is protected.

It is not recommended the patient be taught to reach backward with the upper extremities for protection. When this method is used, the head will tend to move backward and it is more likely to strike the floor or ground. This method can also produce strains or sprains of the shoulders or elbows and fractures of the wrists. *Caution:* If this activity is demonstrated or practiced, floor mats should be used to prevent injury (Fig. 9-55) (Procedure 9-11).

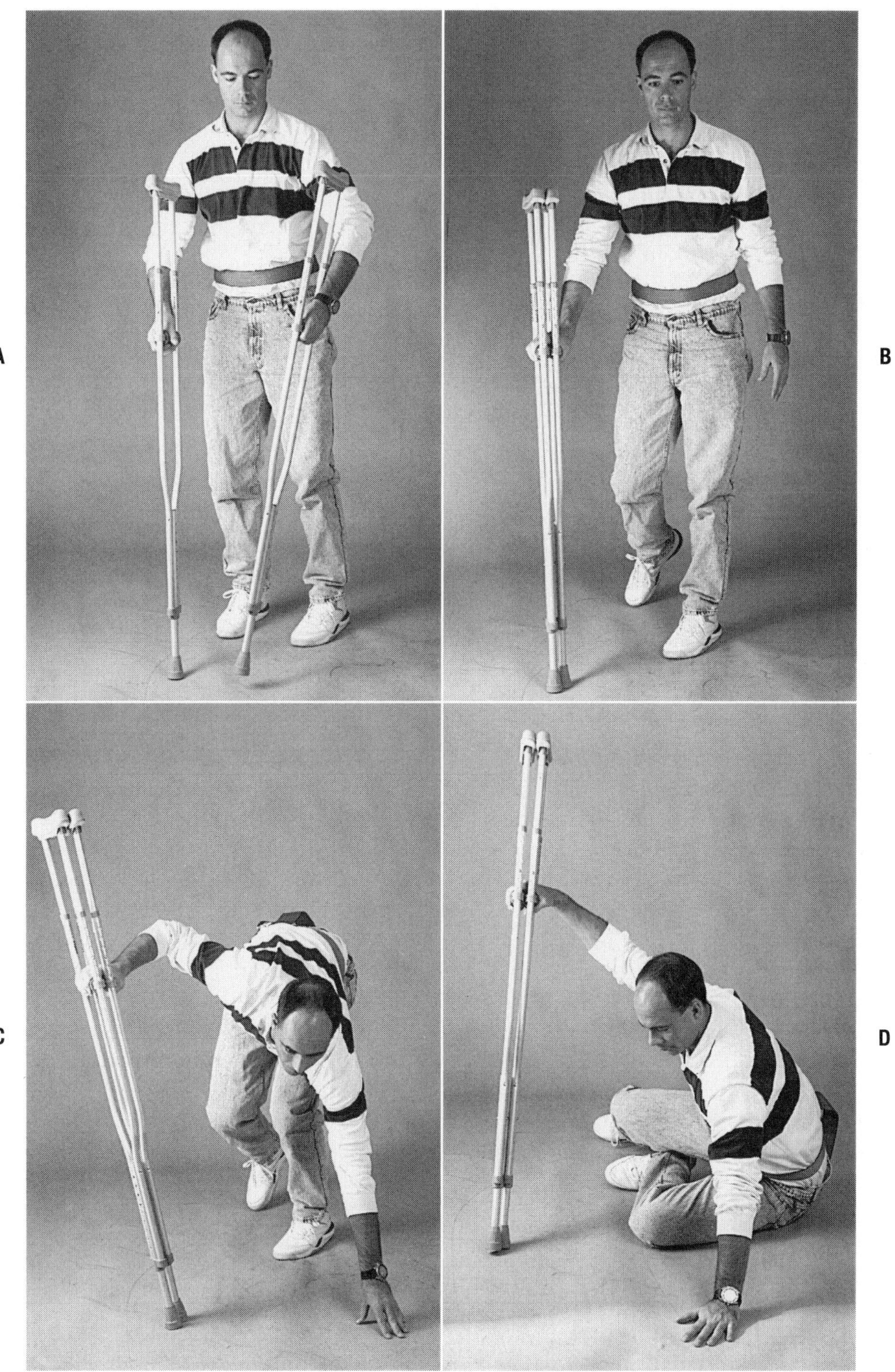

Fig. 9-53 Patient transferring to the floor from crutches.

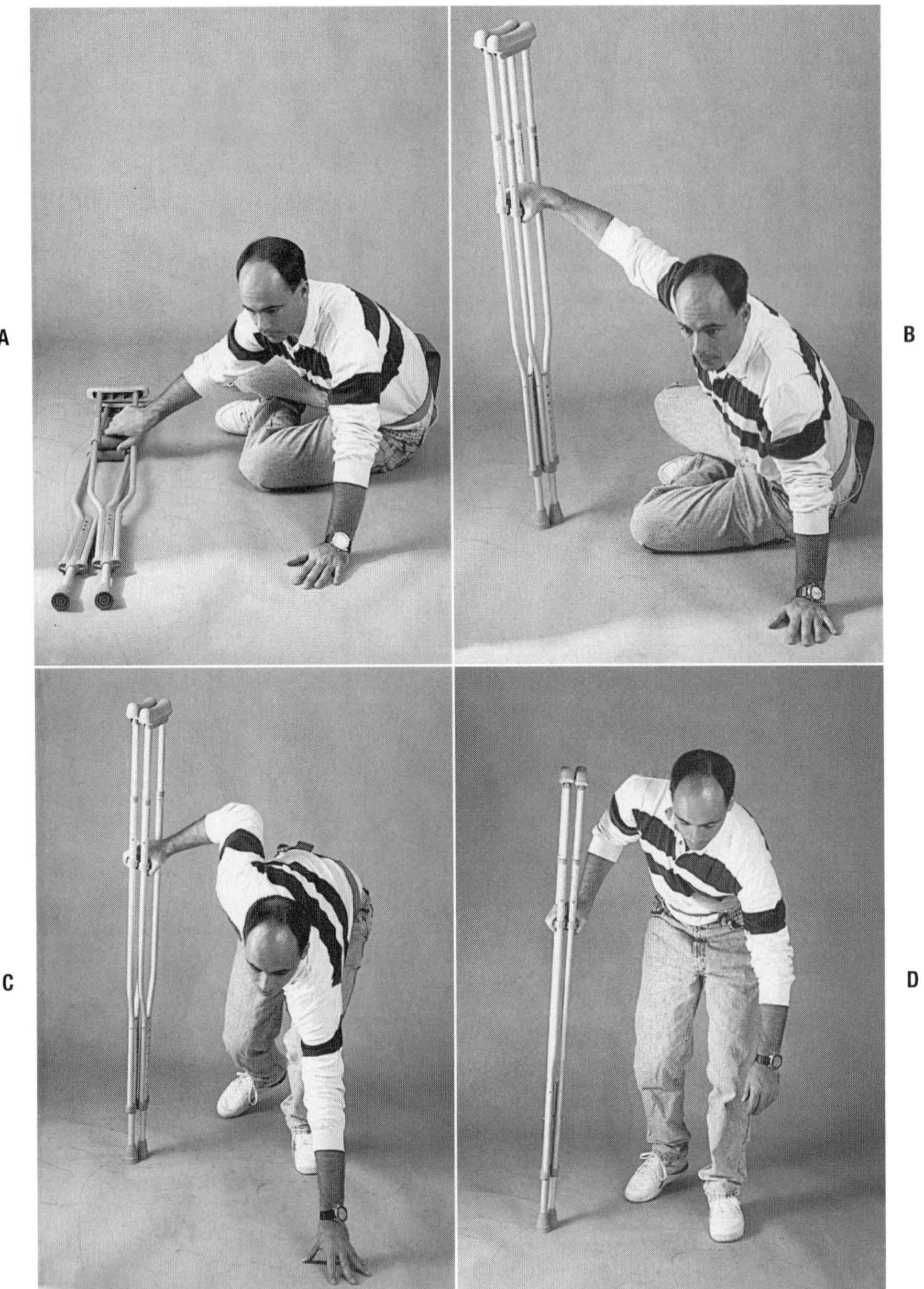

Fig. 9-54 Patient rising from the floor to a standing position using crutches.

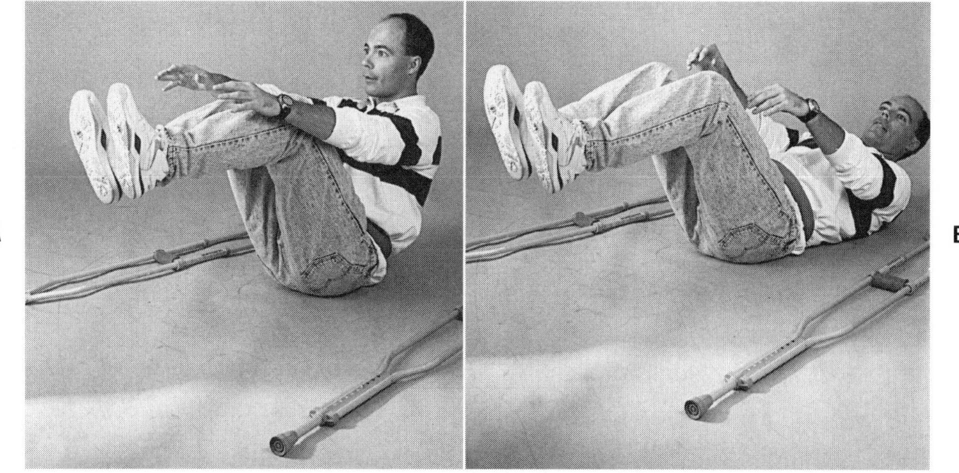

Fig. 9-55 Technique for teaching a patient how to fall backward using crutches.

PROCEDURE 9-11

Protective Fall When Using Crutches

These procedures should be described and demonstrated by the caregiver before the patient attempts them; when the activity is practiced, the patient must be guarded closely and protective mats should be placed on the floor to prevent injury.

FORWARD FALL

The patient releases the crutches and quickly flips them to the side; the crutches must not fall to the floor in front of the body.

The patient reaches forward with both upper extremities and turns the head to one side.

When the hands contact the floor, the elbows are bent to absorb some of the force of the fall.

The body is lowered to the floor and the crutches are gathered in preparation for standing using one of the techniques presented in this chapter if no serious injury has occurred.

BACKWARD FALL

The patient releases the crutches and quickly flips them to the side; the crutches must not fall to the floor behind the body.

The patient tucks the chin toward the chest and reaches *forward* with both upper extremities.

A semiflexed trunk position is maintained so the buttocks will contact the floor first.

The crutches are gathered in preparation for standing using one of the techniques presented in this chapter if no serious injury has occurred.

Forward The patient should be taught to release the crutches, so they fall to each side, and reach toward the floor with the upper extremities. The person should "break" the fall with the upper extremities and lower the body to the floor. Turning the face to one side may reduce facial injuries (see Fig. 9-35).

SUMMARY

Ambulation with an aid or aids can be a potentially hazardous or dangerous activity for a patient. Therefore it is important to emphasize specific precautions to the patient and family to promote safety.

All ambulation aids should be inspected and evaluated frequently for damage or disrepair. Nuts, adjustment buttons, tips, and handgrips must be secure and properly tightened or applied before using the aid for ambulation. The patient should be instructed to examine the equipment periodically and maintain it properly. The family and the patient should be instructed to maintain the environment of the home so it will be free of hazards that could lead to patient injury. For example, small area (throw) rugs should be removed; extension cords should not lie on the floor in an area where people will walk; linoleum or tile floors should not be waxed or highly polished; smooth floor surfaces should be dry and any fluids spilled on them removed immediately; wall or grab bars should be attached to the wall studs, not to the wall board or plaster; one or two handrails may need to be added to stairs; and furniture should be arranged to provide adequate space for the patient to maneuver. Safety information can be provided in written form, and you should document your activities and the patient's performance according to the policies of the facility or agency with which you are employed or associated (Box 9-5).

Each patient must be instructed in the proper gait pattern and how to perform selected functional activities before initiating ambulation or attempting each functional activity. You must guide, encourage, and correct the patient until the person is proficient and competent to perform the gait pattern safely. In addition, you must guard and protect the patient throughout the training sessions by using proper positioning and the safety belt. Demonstrations are helpful and usually necessary as part of the teaching-learning cycle. The family may need to be instructed how to protect or manage the patient at home.

The patient should be reminded to bear the body weight on the hands rather than on the axillary bar of the axillary

Box 9-5 Precautions for Ambulation in the Home

Remove small rugs or mats that are likely to slip or slide (such as area or throw rugs); be extremely cautious when using a bathmat.
Avoid waxing floors or use a "nonskid" wax.
Immediately wipe fluids from noncarpeted floors.
Check ambulation aids frequently for cracks, loose nuts, or worn tips; clean dust and dirt on tips weekly.
Remove items stored on stair steps; be certain stair handrails are secure and strong.
Position furniture in each room to provide a 36-inch-wide unobstructed pathway when possible.
Provide safety (grab) bars for the toilet, shower, and bathtub; be certain they are attached to wall studs or floor.

crutch to avoid possible injury to nerves and circulatory vessels located in the floor of the axilla. The axillary bar must not be used as the primary weight-bearing surface during ambulation or when the patient is standing. Finally, inform the patient and the family how to contact you for advice or assistance after the patient has returned home. This information should be provided in writing and should include your business telephone number and the hours you are available.

self-study ACTIVITIES

- Describe the patient characteristics and abilities necessary to perform the following gait patterns: two-point, four-point, three-point, three-one–point, and modified two-point or four-point.
- Discuss the factors you would consider when selecting each of the following ambulation aids: canes, axillary crutches, platform crutches, forearm crutches, walker, and parallel bars.
- Outline the assessment or evaluation techniques or procedures you would perform before initiating a gait pattern that required ambulation aids or equipment. Provide a rationale for the selection of the techniques.
- Explain how you would initially measure and confirm the fit of each ambulation aid; state the important principles related to the proper fit of the device.
- Explain how you would instruct a patient to use a unilateral ambulation aid and provide a rationale for your instructions.
- Describe how you would guard a patient ambulating on a level surface or on stairs and when moving from sitting to standing and from standing to sitting.
- Describe how you would *monitor* a patient's response to ambulation activities and how you would use the findings to plan the patient's treatment.

problem SOLVING

1. Your patient with a full-length, NWB cast on the LLE uses bilateral axillary crutches and is to be discharged tomorrow. He tells you that he must enter and leave his workplace through a door that has a strong self-closing device. He must pull the door to enter and push it to exit; there is no crash bar and there is a threshold to cross. How would you instruct him to enter and leave the building safely?
2. A 14-year-old girl with a below-knee PWB cast on the RLE must learn to ascend and descend steps so that she can get to her bedroom at home and classrooms at schools. The only handrail at either location is to her right as she ascends the stairs. What instructions or directions will you give her to make this activity safe and effective?

CHAPTER 10

Special Equipment and Patient Care Environments

objectives

After studying this chapter, the reader will be able to:

- Describe the use of the equipment used for special patient needs.
- Describe the precautions necessary when treating a patient using the equipment.
- Understand and apply appropriate measures to resolve a patient emergency.
- Define acronyms used to describe special patient care units (CCU, ER, ICU, MICU, NICU, OHRU, PACU, SICU).
- Describe treatments that could be performed with a patient in a special care unit or who uses special support equipment or systems.

key terms

Alveolus A small hollow; one of the thin-walled chambers of the lungs (pulmonary alveoli) surrounded by networks of capillaries through whose walls exchange of carbon dioxide and oxygen takes place.

Arrhythmia Variation from the normal rhythm, especially of the heartbeat.

Arterial monitoring line (A line) A catheter inserted into an artery and attached to an electronic monitoring system to directly measure arterial blood pressure.

Catheter A rubber, plastic, metal, or glass tube used to remove or inject fluids into a person.

Comminuted Broken or crushed into small pieces.

Cyanosis A bluish discoloration of the skin and mucous membranes caused by excessive concentration of reduced hemoglobin in the blood.

Dialysis The diffusion of solute molecules through a semipermeable membrane passing from the side of higher concentration to the side of lower concentration; a method sometimes used in cases of defective renal function to remove elements from the blood that are normally excreted in the urine (hemodialysis).

Electrocardiogram (ECG or EKG) A graphic record of the heart's electrical action derived by amplification of the minutely small electrical impulses normally generated by the heart.

Endotracheal tube (ETT) A hollow tube, approximately 10 inches long, with an inflatable cuff near one end that is inserted and positioned in the trachea. After the tube has been positioned, the cuff is inflated to maintain the tube's position so the patient can breathe through the tube.

Fistula Any abnormal, tubelike passage within body tissue, usually between two internal organs or leading from an internal organ to the body surface.

Fowler's position A position in which the head of the patient's bed is raised 18 to 20 inches above level with the knees flexed.

Gastrointestinal Pertaining to the stomach and intestines.

Hyperventilation Abnormally prolonged and deep breathing.

Hypoxemia Deficient oxygenation of the blood.

Infusion The slow therapeutic introduction of fluid other than blood into a vein.

Infusion pump (IMED, IVAC) An electronic device designed to automatically control the flow and rate of intravenous fluids into a patient.

Intravenous Administration of fluids into a vein through the use of a steel needle or plastic catheter.

Intravenous therapy The introduction of a fluid into a person's vein; nutrients or medications may be supplied intravenously.

key terms—cont'd

Mediastinum The mass of tissues and organs separating the sternum in front and the vertebral column behind, containing the heart and its large vessels, trachea, esophagus, thymus, lymph nodes, and other structures and tissues.
Micturition Voiding of urine.
Monitor An apparatus designed to observe, report, and measure a given condition or phenomenon such as blood pressure, heart rate, or respiration rate.
Myocardial infarction (MI) Necrosis of the cells of an area of the heart muscle resulting from oxygen deprivation caused by obstruction of the blood supply.
Nasogastric (NG) tube A plastic tube usually inserted into a nostril and ending in the stomach. It can be used to remove fluid or gas from the stomach, monitor the digestive function of the stomach, administer medications or nutrients, or obtain specimens of the stomach contents.
Oximeter A photoelectric device that measures oxygen saturation of the blood.
Patent Open, unobstructed, or not closed.
Pneumothorax Accumulation of air or gas in the pleural cavity resulting in collapse of the lung on the affected side.
Respirator See *ventilator.*
Shunt A passage or anastomosis between two natural vessels, especially between blood vessels.
Suprapubic Above the pubis.
Swan-Ganz catheter A long intravenous tube inserted into a vein (usually the basilic or subclavian vein) and terminating in the pulmonary artery. A monitor attached to the catheter measures the pulmonary artery pressure and the pulmonary capillary wedge pressure; it permits evaluation of cardiac function.
Tachypnea Very rapid respirations.
Tract A longitudinal assemblage of tissues or organs—especially a bundle of nerve fibers having a common origin, function, and termination—or several anatomic structures arranged in a series and serving a common function.
Traction The exertion of a pulling or distracting force to maintain a proper position of bone ends or joints to facilitate the healing process.
Trendelenburg's position A position in which the patient lies supine with the head lower than the rest of the body.
Turning frame An apparatus that allows a patient's position to be changed from supine to prone, and vice versa, by one person by maintaining the patient's position between two frames of the apparatus; the patient may be turned horizontally or vertically depending on the apparatus used.
Ventilator A mechanical apparatus designed to intermittently or continuously assist or control pulmonary ventilation (breathing); also referred to as a *respirator.*
Wedge pressure Intravascular pressure measured by a catheter inserted into the pulmonary artery (Swan-Ganz catheter) to permit indirect measurement of mean left atrial pressure.

INTRODUCTION

Many patients who occupy hospital beds are acutely ill and require extensive nursing care. The equipment and technology available to treat and monitor these patients have improved dramatically during the past several years. Life-supporting or life-sustaining equipment is commonplace. Patients who probably would not have survived life-threatening trauma or illness several years ago are surviving now because of advances in medical treatment and equipment. Requests for treatment of these seriously ill patients by various members of the rehabilitation team have increased, in part because medical and nursing personnel have recognized the advantages of the early application of rehabilitation techniques for these patients. Consequently, the occupational therapist, physical therapist, respiratory therapist, and other caregivers have become integral members of this medical management team. Many of these very ill patients are initially managed in specialized nursing units listed in Box 10-1.

The initial exposure to the equipment and devices used in these units can overwhelm, intimidate, or create apprehension in an inexperienced, uninformed practitioner. In this

Box 10-1 Specialized Patient Care Units

CCU: Coronary (cardiac) care unit or critical care unit
ER: Emergency room
ICU: Intensive care unit or intermediate care unit
MICU: Medical intensive care unit
NICU: Neurologic (neuro) intensive care unit
OHRU: Open heart recovery unit
PACU: Postanesthesia care unit
SICU: Surgical intensive care unit

text, descriptions of some of the equipment and devices used frequently to treat the seriously involved patient are presented to assist the caregiver to become better prepared to treat these patients in a specialized environment. However, the caregiver should be oriented specifically to the equipment and treatment protocols in each employment setting before providing patient care. Also, information should be provided to the caregiver in preparation to react and to know from whom assistance can be obtained if a patient emergency occurs.

ORIENTATION TO THE SPECIAL INTENSIVE CARE UNIT

A typical patient cubicle in an intensive care unit (ICU) is apt to have several types of equipment to monitor the patient's physiologic state, ventilate, provide *intravenous therapy*, deliver oxygen, and remove fluids from the patient (that is, suction). The patient may have *intravenous* (IV) lines, an *arterial monitoring line (A line)*, drainage tubes, oxygen, or leads going from the patient to a *monitor* of vital signs, and may also be receiving respiratory support from a *ventilator (respirator)*. After you have reviewed the medical record, take a few minutes to observe the unit and the patient before you initiate any treatment. Some patients will be alert, others may be comatose or unresponsive, and most patients in specialized care units will be acutely ill or seriously traumatized.

If you are unfamiliar with the equipment applied to the patient, obtain assistance from a nurse in the unit or participate in a program designed to prepare you to treat patients who are in the unit (Figs. 10-1 and 10-2). When the patient is acutely ill, it will be necessary to reduce the intensity of the treatment compared with the intensity you might use

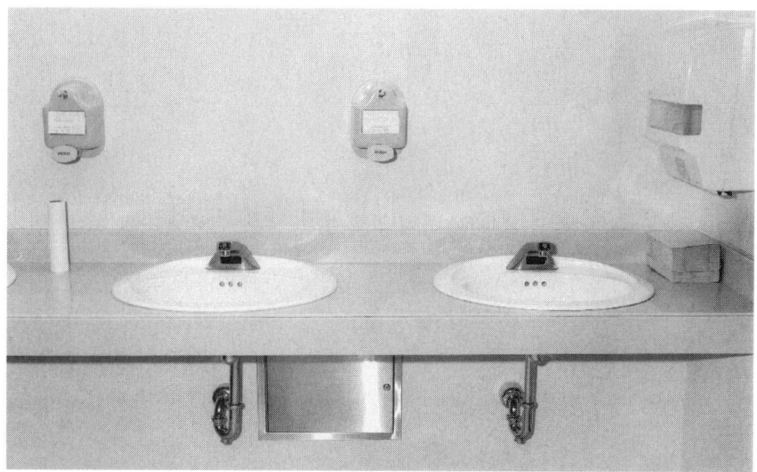

Fig. 10-1 Handwashing area at the entrance to the intensive care unit for use by visitors before entering and when leaving the unit; water flow is activated when the hands are placed beneath the faucet spout.

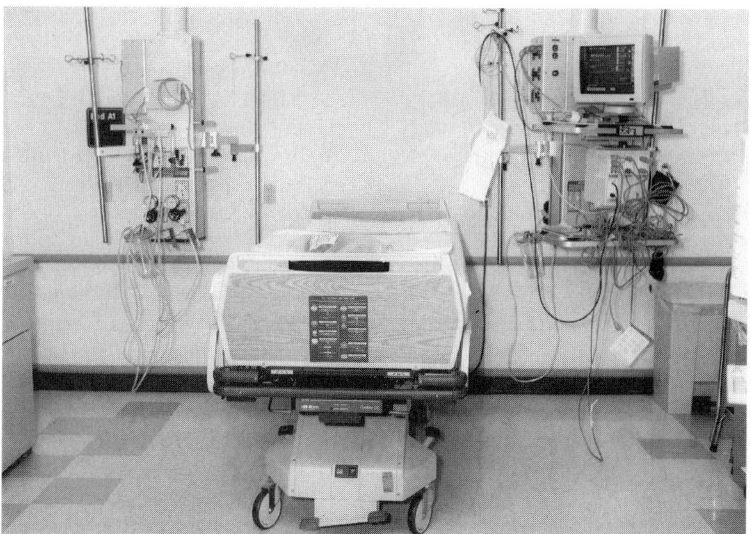

Fig. 10-2 Typical intensive care unit patient unit or cubicle prepared for patient use.

with less ill patients. Shorter treatment sessions, fewer exercise repetitions, and less demand for active participation by the patient may be necessary. Careful and continuous monitoring of the patient's response to treatment will be required. You can accomplish this through observation of and communication with the patient, awareness of vital signs, and a comparison of the current responses with previous responses to the treatment. It is recommended you discuss the patient's current condition with one of the nursing personnel before treatment because a patient's condition may fluctuate from hour to hour or from day to day and you may not be able to rely on information obtained at your previous visit (Procedures 10-1 and 10-2).

The caregiver who treats patients in an ICU is apt to find that the roles in that environment will be very similar to the roles required to treat patients whose conditions are less acute or life threatening. The general, overall goals of treatment for patients in the ICU will be to minimize or prevent the adverse effects of inactivity and immobility and assist each person to become functionally independent.

Caregivers should be aware there are several aspects of care and intervention to be considered when they treat patients in the ICU. One aspect is to prevent the development of contractures through the use of passive and active exercise, proper positioning, and body alignment. In addition, the use of exercise and physical activity will be important to improve the general condition of the patient. Bed mobility training will be necessary because it is a precursor to transfer and ambulation activities that are requisites for functional independence. Passive and active exercise help stimulate the sensory system; therefore sensory awareness and coordination may be enhanced through exercise. Some patients may have respiratory difficulties and they may need to be taught how to breathe more efficiently during their recovery, even when a respiratory aid is being used. Patients with respiratory deficits or who have experienced thoracic or abdominal surgery may need to be instructed how to cough effectively. For some patients, wound care and management will be required and the prevention of pressure ulcers will be particularly important for all caregivers. Protective garments may need to be worn by the caregiver and compliance with the methods used to prevent the transmission of pathogens and

PROCEDURE 10-1

Treating a Patient in an Intensive Care Unit

Review the patient's medical record before each treatment session, even when multiple sessions occur during the same day.

Request information about the patient's current status (such as physical activity level, mental capacity, or alertness) from nursing personnel.

Wash your hands and apply protective garments as necessary.

Observe the equipment or devices used to monitor the patient for current information about the physiologic status.

Observe the type and location of the equipment or devices being used by the patient (such as ventilator, IV line, oxygen, urinary catheter, supplemental nutrition, suction).

Identify the location of all tubes, monitor lead connections, IV line connections and insertion sites, and patient-controlled analgesia; maintain all tubes and leads free of occlusion and tension.

Evaluate or determine the patient's present physical and mental status before initiating treatment.

Observe the patient and monitoring devices frequently; determine the response to the treatment; identify significant change in the condition or physiologic status.

Notify nursing personnel of significant change in the patient's condition or physiologic status; document and record your activities and observations as necessary.

PROCEDURE 10-2

Precautions to Use in the Intensive Care Unit

Avoid occlusion or excessive tension on all tubes, monitor leads, suction units, supplemental nutrition items, and oxygen service.

Observe and assess the patient before, during, and after treatment; determine the objective and subjective response to the treatment.

Modify or cease treatment if the patient exhibits abnormal, unexpected, or undesired response(s) to the treatment (such as changes in vital signs, breathing pattern, indication of increased pain, reduced mental awareness or alertness).

Request assistance from nursing or respiratory service personnel if you identify changes in the function or performance of the patient support systems (such as IV line, monitors, ventilation, supplemental nutrition, or drainage devices).

Note the appearance and odor of visible wounds and wound or urine drainage; observe the general appearance of the patient.

Request assistance, as necessary, to adjust or move equipment or reposition the patient.

At the conclusion of the treatment:

- Be certain the patient is properly positioned.
- Elevate or replace side rails on the bed, if indicated.
- Position the bedside table so it is accessible to the patient.
- Position other personal items so they are accessible.
- Inform the patient of the location of the "nurse call" device; position it so it is accessible.

cross contamination of other patients may be required. Finally, assisting the patient to cope with, adjust to, or overcome painful stimuli may be accomplished through selected exercise techniques, the use of pain-relieving electrotherapy equipment, or by being a compassionate caregiver.

TYPES OF BEDS

The standard manually operated and electrically operated beds are the two most common beds used in a hospital. These beds provide support, access to care, and the ability to alter the patient's position for most patients. However, the acutely ill or traumatized patient frequently requires special features not available on the standard hospital bed (Fig. 10-3).

If the caregiver finds the patient's position to be inappropriate for treatment, several options are available: reschedule the treatment when the patient is positioned more appropriately, temporarily reposition the patient to permit treatment, or treat the patient as much as possible without changing position. If the patient's original position is changed, the caregiver should follow the nursing policies and procedures regarding repositioning the patient. It may be necessary to request the nurse to reposition the patient or readjust the position of the bed, or it may be necessary to have a nurse present when position changes are made by the caregiver. Usually the caregiver should return the patient to the original position at the conclusion of the treatment session and adhere to any time schedule related to patient positioning. For example, a patient may need to follow a turning schedule and may be limited in the amount of time allowed to remain in one position. Therefore the caregiver should be aware of and comply with any special schedule the patient is expected to follow.

Standard Adjustable Bed

Most hospital beds can be adjusted using electrical controls. The controls may be located at the head or foot or on the side rail of the bed or attached to a special cord so the patient can operate them independently. The controls should be marked according to their function and may be operated by using the hand or foot. The bed can be raised and lowered in relation to the floor as a total unit or the upper and lower components can be adjusted separately or together. On most beds, the lower portion is hinged so it can be adjusted to provide knee flexion, which in turn causes hip flexion. On some beds, the lower component will become flexed whenever the upper component is raised. This action creates hip and knee flexion, which is more comfortable for the patient and tends to prevent sliding down in the bed. When the upper portion is raised slightly, the patient's position is referred to as *Fowler's position*. Sometimes when the bed is adjusted with the upper portion raised and the lower portion flexed, the bed is considered to be "gatched."

Most beds have some type of side rails or protective devices. Some rails are lifted upward until the locking mechanism is engaged, whereas other types are adjusted by moving them toward the upper portion of the bed until the locking mechanism is engaged. When a side rail is used for patient security, it is important to be certain the rail is locked securely before you leave the patient. Also, check to be certain the side rail has not compressed or stretched any IV, *catheter*, or other tubing. Adjust the bed into the position that will allow you the best access to the patient and enable you to use proper body mechanics. The prolonged use of bed rails can be a form of patient restraint that may not be permitted legally. If they are used, it should be determined that

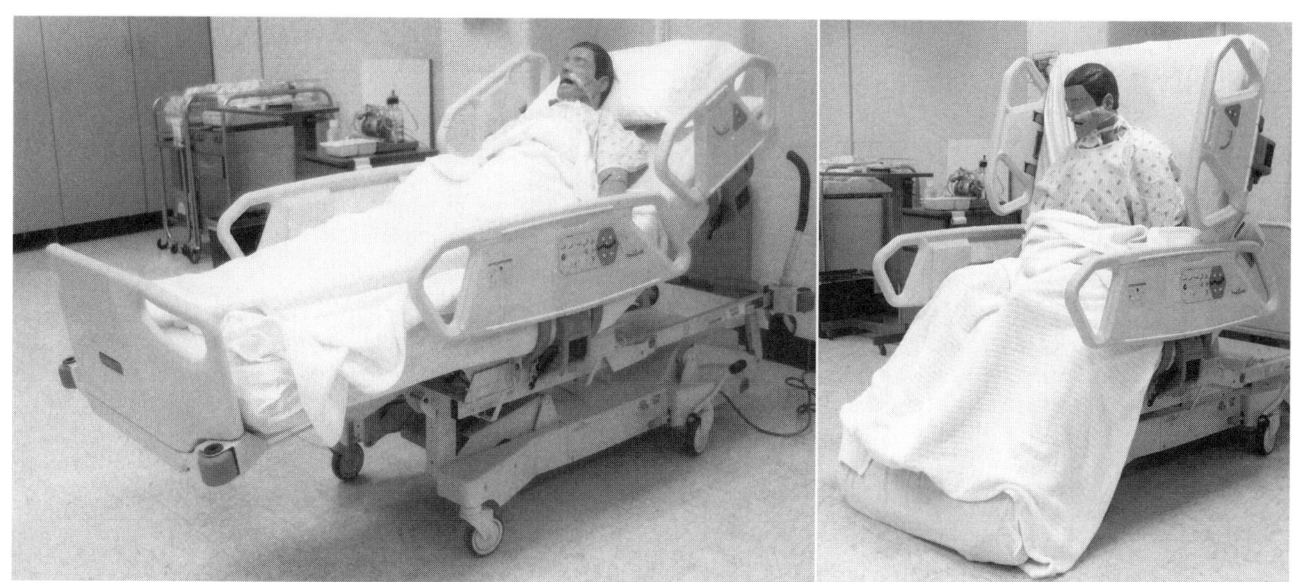

Fig. 10-3 Specialized adjustable bed; allows patient to stand when elevated completely.

patient safety is endangered when they are not in place. Be certain to return the patient to the original, required, or preferred position at the conclusion of the treatment.

The patient will probably have a device that is either located on the side rail or attached to a long electrical cord that is used to contact nursing personnel from the bed. At the conclusion of treatment, the caregiver should be certain the patient has access to the device and is aware of its location or position. This device may be referred to as a "call button."

Turning Frame (Stryker Wedge Frame)

A *turning frame* has an anterior and a posterior frame, each of which has a canvas cover. It has a support base that allows elevation of the head or foot ends of the frames or of the entire bed. A pivot joint allows the patient to be turned in a horizontal plane from a prone to a supine position or from a supine to a prone position by one person. A similar device is the Foster frame.

A turning frame is indicated when skeletal stability and alignment are desired; to permit a patient to be turned horizontally from prone to supine or from supine to prone; when continuous maintenance of skeletal cervical *traction*, such as Crutchfield or a similar type of skeletal traction, is desired; and when a patient must be immobilized after a spinal fracture and safe and efficient change of position from supine to prone, or vice versa, must be performed.

This equipment has several advantages. It allows access to the patient for a variety of therapeutic interventions and nursing care; it allows one person to safely and easily turn the patient from supine to prone, and vice versa; and it allows the patient to be wheeled or transported from one location to another without being removed from the frame. Furthermore, the unit can be elevated or lowered as a unit to several heights or positions and the height of the head or foot of the frame can be changed independently. The patient can be positioned in *Trendelenburg's position* when supine or prone. The unit requires relatively little space, even to turn the patient, and it allows cervical traction to be applied and maintained even when the patient is turned.

The equipment does have several disadvantages. The patient can be positioned only supine or prone and patients who weigh more than 200 pounds or who are more than approximately 6 feet tall will be difficult to position on the frames. Most of the patients who exceed these limits will not be able to tolerate this device for extended periods. Patients are at risk of developing skin problems as a result of shear and pressure forces related to being positioned only prone or supine and contractures may develop unless appropriate exercise and positioning techniques are used. *Note:* The development of new equipment and other technologic advances in patient care have reduced the need for this piece of equipment in most hospitals in the United States and it is rarely used.

Air-Fluidized Support Bed (Clinitron)

The air-fluidized bed is a rectangular or ovoid bed that contains 1600 pounds of silicone-coated glass beads called microspheres. Heated, pressurized air flows through the beads to suspend a polyester cover that supports the patient. When set in motion, the microspheres develop the properties associated with fluids. The patient feels as if he or she is floating on a warm waterbed. Contact pressure of the patient's body against the polyester sheet is approximately 11 to 15 mm Hg.

This equipment is indicated for patients who have several infected lesions or require skin protection and whose position cannot be altered easily (such as persons with burns or spinal cord injury); patients with extensive pressure ulcers or at risk of developing deterioration of the skin (such as obese persons); patients with recent, extensive skin grafts; or patients who require prolonged immobilization (Fig. 10-4).

This piece of equipment has several advantages. It reduces the need for the application of topical medications and dressings by establishing a microclimate environment favorable for the healing process. The temperature of the air in the bed can be controlled according to the needs of the patient. There is reduced pressure on the skin and pressure sores are less likely to develop because of the lowered pressure. Friction or shear forces to the body are reduced significantly or eliminated and the patient can lie on the lesions or wounds for brief periods. When the unit is turned off, the polyester cover becomes a firm surface, which may be beneficial for certain therapeutic interventions or nursing care.

The unit has several disadvantages. The polyester cover (filter sheet) can be damaged (punctured) easily by a sharp object and if the filter sheet is punctured, the microspheres will be expelled. Air flowing across the patient's skin may cause body fluids to evaporate more rapidly than normal

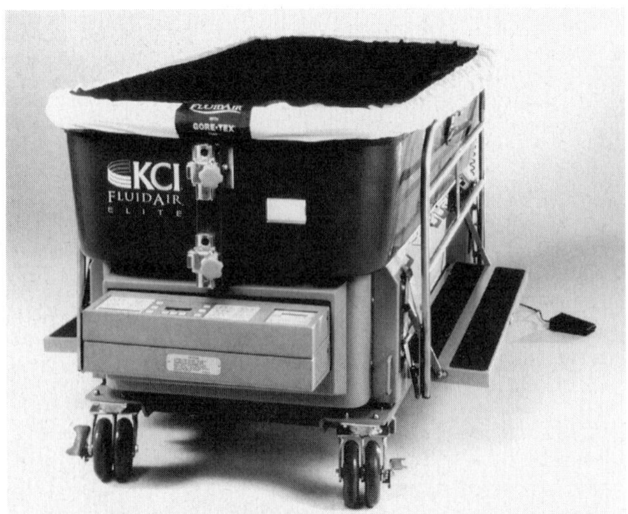

Fig. 10-4 Air fluidization bed. (Photograph courtesy of Kinetic Concepts Incorporated [KCI].)

and it may be necessary to have the patient ingest small amounts of extra fluids to compensate for the fluid loss. A patient may require frequent position changes because of the tendency for fluid to pool in the lobes of the lungs and obese or tall patients are apt to be uncomfortable on this bed. The height of the bed from the floor will probably be fixed, so it may be difficult to provide care or to transfer the patient. A draw sheet can be used to assist in positioning the patient and a two-person sliding transfer from the bed to a stretcher can be performed with the unit turned off. Finally, this is a very expensive piece of equipment.

Posttrauma Mobility Beds (Keane, Roto-Rest)

Posttrauma mobility beds are designed to maintain a seriously injured patient in a stable position and maintain proper postural alignment through the use of adjustable bolsters. The bed oscillates from side to side, in a cradle-like motion, to reduce the amount of prolonged pressure on the patient's skin.

These beds are indicated for patients with restricted respiratory function, patients with advanced or multiple pressure ulcers, or patients who require stabilization and skeletal alignment after extensive trauma or as a result of severe neurologic deficits.

These beds have several advantages. The constant side-to-side motion assists in improving upper respiratory *tract* function and reduces the need to turn the patient to relieve pressure or prevent the development of pressure ulcers. The friction and shear forces associated with turning the patient are eliminated and the constant motion of the bed may provide some environmental stimulation for neurologically impaired patients. Urinary stasis is reduced and bowel function is improved as a result of the constant motion of these beds (Fig. 10-5).

Several disadvantages have also been reported. Some patients may experience signs or symptoms of motion sickness, such as vertigo or nausea, and some patients may feel isolated from the environment as a result of a decrease in their visual orientation. Exercises and other forms of patient care may be restricted because of the bolsters and alignment supports, although some beds have ports or hatches for better access. Finally, sufficient space must be available to allow the bed to oscillate without interference from other objects. The bolsters and alignment supports must be maintained in position to provide proper stabilization and alignment. This is especially necessary for adequate support to the thorax.

Low Air Loss Therapy Bed

The low air loss bed has several segmented and separated air bladders that allow the limited escape of air. The amount of air pressure in each bladder is individually controlled for each patient based on the size, weight, and shape of each patient, and the bed may be adjusted to several different positions (Figs. 10-6 and 10-7).

This bed is indicated for patients who require prolonged immobilization; patients who are at high risk of developing pressure ulcers or who have existing ulcers; patients whose condition requires frequent elevation of the trunk to promote proper respiratory function; and obese patients.

This bed has several advantages. It can be adjusted to accommodate the need to change the patient's position to hip and knee flexion, sitting, or a semirecumbent position. The

A

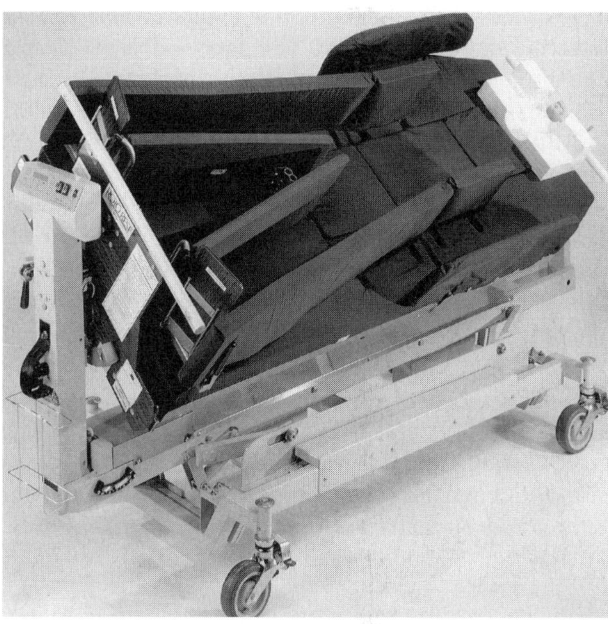

B

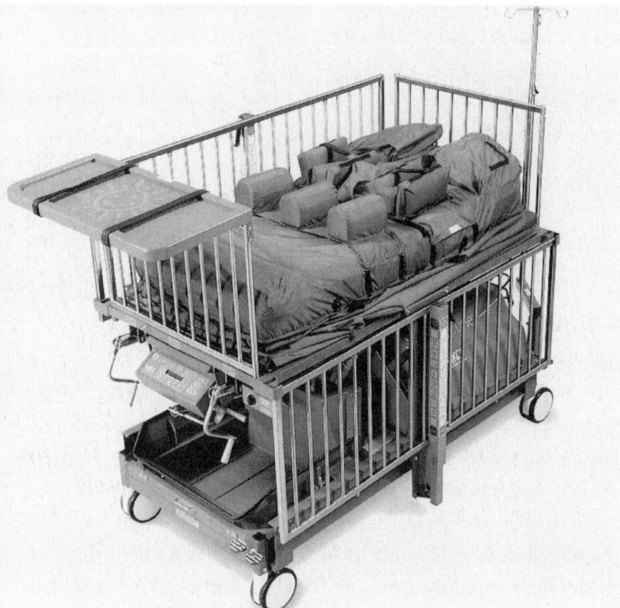

Fig. 10-5 **A,** Roto-Rest bed. (Photograph courtesy of Kinetic Concepts Incorporated [KCI].) **B,** Pediatric bed.

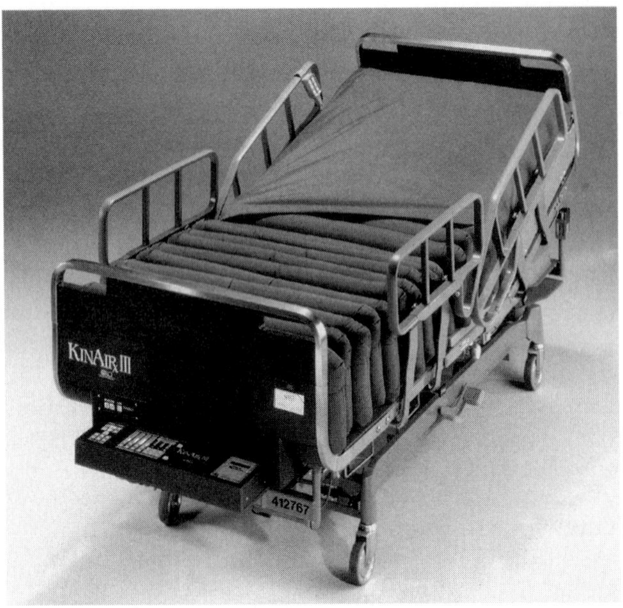

Fig. 10-6 Air suspension bed with individual air bladders. (Photograph courtesy of Kinetic Concepts Incorporated [KCI].)

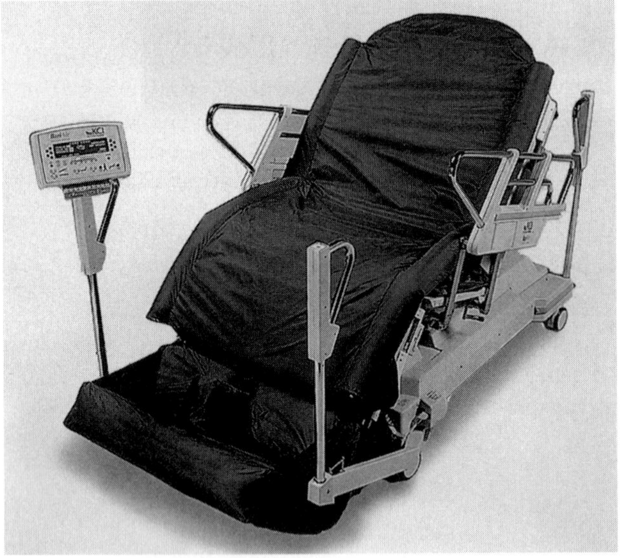

Fig. 10-7 Air suspension bed for a heavy patient (300 to 850 lb). (Photograph courtesy of Kinetic Concepts Incorporated [KCI].)

patient's position can be altered through the use of electronically operated controls. The patient's weight is measured by sensors in the bed and the air bladders are inflated or deflated automatically to distribute the patient's weight.

Several disadvantages have also been reported. The air bladders can be punctured or torn by sharp objects and frequent alterations in the patient's position must be performed to prevent pressure ulcers. (*Note:* To be able to transfer a patient, you should lock the wheels, elevate the patient's trunk approximately 20 to 30 degrees, deflate the seat section, perform the transfer, and turn off the seat deflation control to reinflate the seat.)

The surfaces of the three beds described in this section may not be rigid enough to allow effective performance of the chest compressions required for cardiopulmonary resuscitation (CPR). Therefore a flat rigid wooden or plastic device must be placed beneath the patient to provide a firm solid surface before the initiation of CPR or the person may need to be transferred to the floor. It will be easier to transfer the person when he or she is supine and is first placed on a firm support.

LIFE SUPPORT AND MONITORING EQUIPMENT

Mechanical Ventilators

Most ventilators, also known as respirators, currently use positive pressure to move or propel gas or air into the patient's lungs. The purpose of a ventilator is to maintain adequate and appropriate air exchange when normal respiration is inhibited or cannot be actively performed by the patient. A ventilator may be indicated for diseases or conditions that affect the patient's neurologic or musculoskeletal control of respiration or that interfere with the exchange of gases in the lungs. A ventilator may be used when the patient experiences apnea or when the potential for respiratory distress or failure exists.

An example of respiratory distress that may develop is acute respiratory distress syndrome (ARDS); a similar syndrome affects infants. This syndrome is potentially life threatening and its existence must be recognized soon after it affects the patient so immediate steps can be initiated to counteract the syndrome. Some of the possible causes of ARDS are systemic shock, diffuse respiratory infection, and systemic response to sepsis or extensive trauma. Clinical signs and symptoms include dyspnea, *tachypnea*, *cyanosis*, and *hypoxemia*. The caregiver who treats a patient with ARDS or the infant syndrome must monitor the patient's response to activity and observe the monitoring equipment frequently to be certain the vital signs and arterial blood gases (ABGs) remain within acceptable ranges or limits. The person with ARDS will have a restricted respiratory capacity and will receive respiratory assistance from a ventilator. The person is likely to be intolerant of active exercise, especially resistive exercise, in the early stages of recovery and complete recovery from ARDS may require several weeks. The syndrome is life threatening because it can cause the failure of one or more major organs such as the kidneys; therefore early detection of the syndrome and aggressive treatment are extremely important.

Types of Ventilators

Volume-Cycled Ventilators Volume-cycled ventilators are used primarily for patients who require long-term support. A predetermined volume of gas ("air"), dependent on

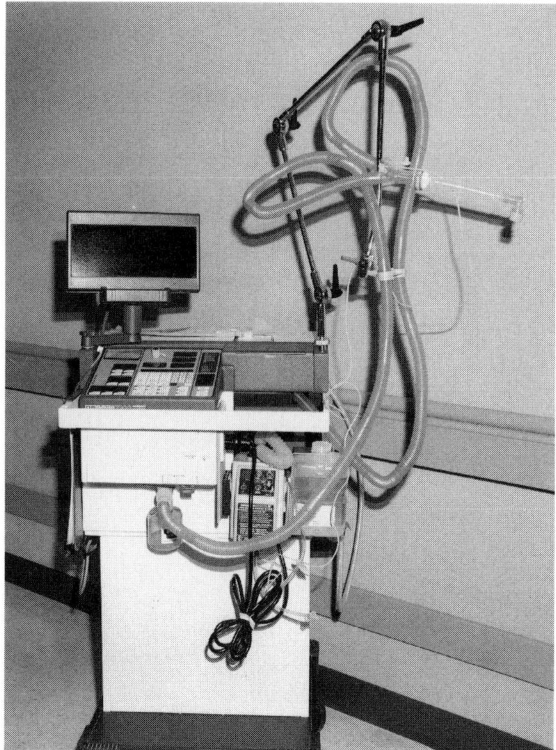

Fig. 10-8 Ventilator with computer functions.

the patient's needs, is delivered during the inspiratory phase of respiration, but the expiratory phase remains passive (Fig. 10-8). This type of equipment is indicated when long-term ventilation assistance is needed, for the patient with severe chronic obstructive pulmonary disease (COPD), after thoracic surgery, and for disorders of the central nervous system and musculoskeletal disorders that affect the respiratory system, such as a cervical spinal cord injury, brain injury, amyotrophic lateral sclerosis, or poliomyelitis.

Pressure-Cycled Ventilators Pressure-cycled ventilators deliver a predetermined established maximum pressure of gas during respiration and the inspiratory phase ends when that level is reached. The expiratory phase remains a passive phase. The flow rate may vary from one respiration cycle to the next.

This device is indicated when only short-term ventilation is needed in the form of intermittent positive-pressure breathing (IPPB) and for selected patients with neuromuscular or musculoskeletal distress.

Negative Pressure Device Negative pressure ventilation is rarely used currently in the management of patients with respiratory problems. The primary types are the tank respirator ("iron lung") and the chest respirator ("turtle shell"). These devices create a negative pressure in the patient's chest so the environmental air pressure exceeds the internal thoracic pressure. Because of this pressure imbalance, air enters the patient's lungs passively to provide inspiration. These devices were used primarily for persons with poliomyelitis.

Box 10-2 Modes of Ventilation

Assist mode: The patient must develop or cause a negative pressure to "trigger" the ventilator to provide assistance to deliver gas, such as oxygen and air, to the patient.

Continuous positive airway pressure (CPAP) mode: This mode superimposes the use of PEEP (refer to the description below) on the patient's spontaneous breathing pattern. It is particularly useful to assist a patient to become weaned from the ventilator or to help maximize the gas exchange capabilities for an immobile, inactive patient.

Control mode: The inspiration phase of respiration begins at timed intervals based on the patient's need for gas.

Assisted control mode: This mode is a combination of the previous two modes.

Intermittent mandatory ventilation (IMV) mode: The patient's ventilation cycle is established so ventilation occurs a minimum number of times per minute. This is the mode that is frequently used to begin to wean the patient from the ventilator and to develop an independent respiration pattern.

Synchronized IMV mode: This mode allows the ventilation cycle to be coordinated with the patient's own breathing cycle.

Positive end-expiratory pressure (PEEP) mode: This mode allows oxygen to be induced into the patient's lungs by maintaining positive pressure at the end of expiration, which increases the alveolar surface area able to absorb the gas induced by the ventilator and leads to maximal alveolar ventilation. The PEEP helps to expand and maintain the *alveoli,* which would normally close at the end of expiration, *patent.*

Modes of Ventilation

Several modes by which patients can be ventilated are described in Box 10-2.

Airway Placement Usually, the gas delivered by the ventilator will be induced into the patient through a tube in one of several possible airways. The tube is referred to as an *endotracheal tube (ETT)* and when it is in place, the patient is considered to be intubated. The possible locations for an ETT are in the oral pharyngeal, nasal pharyngeal, oral esophageal, nasal endotracheal, or oral endotracheal airway. Other means of insertion of the tube include tracheostomy and laryngostomy. Each of these artificial airways provides a clear airway through the patient's nasal, oral, or other passageways to the lungs. The ETT allows suction of the bronchial tree, but insertion of the ETT will restrict the patient from talking. When the ETT is removed, the patient will probably complain of throat discomfort and the voice is apt to be distorted for a short period. The caregiver must avoid disturbing or accidentally disconnecting the tube of the ventilator from the ETT and bending, kinking, or occluding the connector tubing. You should be certain the tubing is not obstructed by the weight of one of the patient's extremities or trapped under the bed rail.

The patient who uses a ventilator can participate in various types of exercise and other bedside activities, including sitting and ambulation. The patient must be informed of the activity and the caregiver must be certain the tubing is sufficiently long to allow the physical activity to be performed. Because the patient will have difficulty communicating orally, questions should be asked that can be answered with head nods or other nonverbal means. The patient's response to the activity must be monitored closely by the caregiver and undue stress to the patient should be avoided. A patient using a ventilator probably will not tolerate exercise as well as other patients, so you should be cautious during treatment. You should monitor the patient's vital signs and be alert for signs of respiratory distress such as a change in the respiration pattern, syncope, or cyanosis.

The ventilator has an auditory and visual alarm that will be activated by various stimuli such as a disconnected tube, coughing by the patient, movement of the tubing, or a change in the respiratory pattern or needs of the patient. During orientation to the special care unit, the caregiver should be instructed how to determine the cause of the alarm and how to return the system to normal function. If this educational program is not provided, the caregiver should know how to obtain assistance from a nurse or respiratory therapist in the unit. The caregiver should be alert for signs or symptoms of respiratory or cardiopulmonary distress exhibited by the patient, such as dyspnea, tachycardia, *arrhythmia*, or *hyperventilation*.

The caregiver should become familiar with the various types of ventilators and modes of ventilation before beginning treatment on any patient. This can be accomplished through one or more inservice orientation programs.

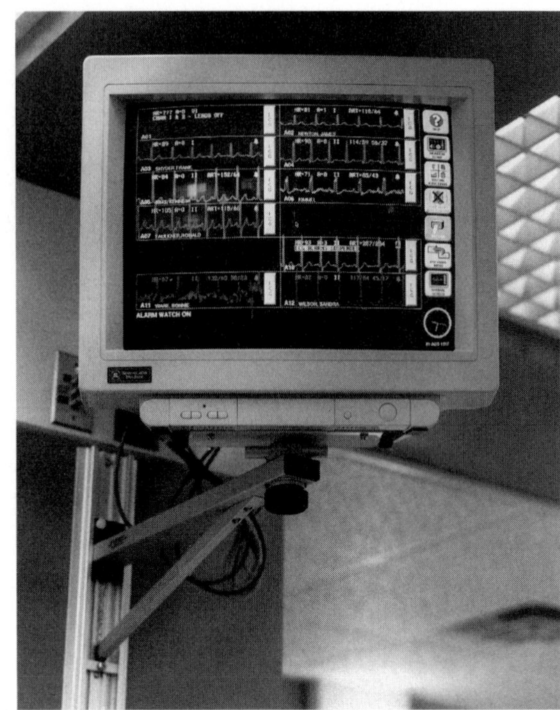

Fig. 10-9 Patient monitor located in nurses' unit in intensive care unit; several patients can be monitored simultaneously.

Monitors

The patient who requires special care may have the physiologic status monitored by various pieces of equipment. Common monitoring parameters include cardiac-vital signs, ABGs, intracranial pressure (ICP), pulmonary artery pressure (PAP), central venous pressure (CVP), and arterial pressure (A line) monitoring equipment. Exercise can be performed by patients who are being monitored, provided care is taken to avoid disruption of the equipment. Many of these units have an auditory and visual signal that may be activated by a change in the patient's condition, a change in the function of the equipment, or a change in the patient's position. In some instances it will be necessary for a nurse to evaluate and correct the cause of the alarm, but in other instances, the caregiver may be able to correct the cause safely. For example, cease exercise and allow the patient to rest until the physiologic state returns to an acceptable level.

The caregiver should recognize the patient's condition is most likely to be unstable and caution should be used to avoid causing stress for the patient. Orientation to the purpose and function of the monitoring equipment and devices is recommended for persons who will treat the patient. *Caution:* Be certain you understand which parameters the various channels on the monitor are measuring or reporting at a given time and which channels are active. The channels can be changed to monitor different parameters at different times or they can be deactivated. Therefore it is important that the caregiver knows which of the patient's physiologic responses are being monitored when treatment is being provided.

Vital Signs Monitor The patients' monitor may display current values of any of the following: blood pressure, respiration rate, temperature, blood gases, or cardiac patterns (Fig. 10-9). A portable unit can be used when a permanent, fixed monitor is not available (Fig. 10-10). Acceptable or safe parameters or ranges for the three physiologic indicators can be set in the unit. An alarm is activated when the upper or lower limits of the ranges are exceeded or when the unit malfunctions. A graphic and a digital display of the values are apparent on the monitor screen so that the caregiver can observe the effects of the exercise and the patient's responses to activity.

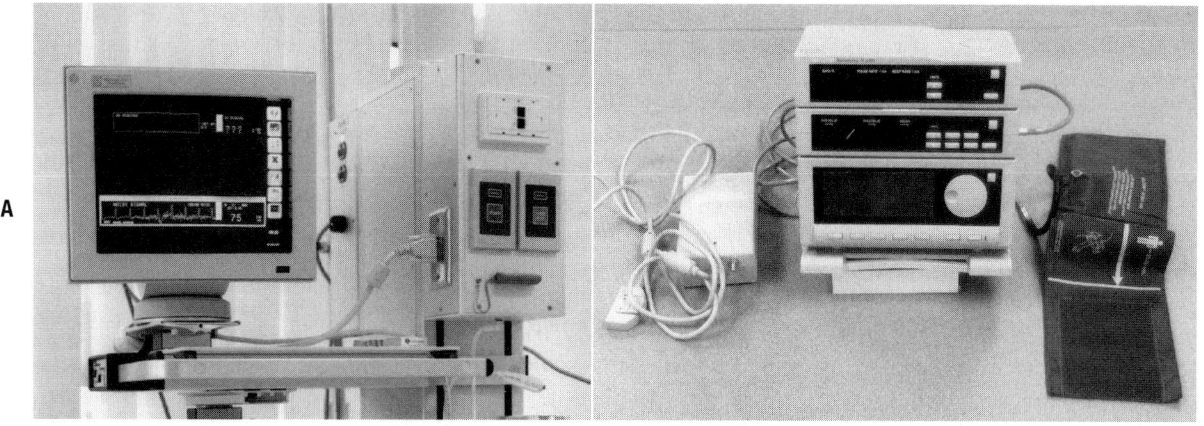

Fig. 10-10 **A,** Patient monitor located in the patient's unit; heart rate, temperature, respiration rate, *electrocardiogram* patterns, and blood gases can be displayed separately or simultaneously. **B,** Portable monitor.

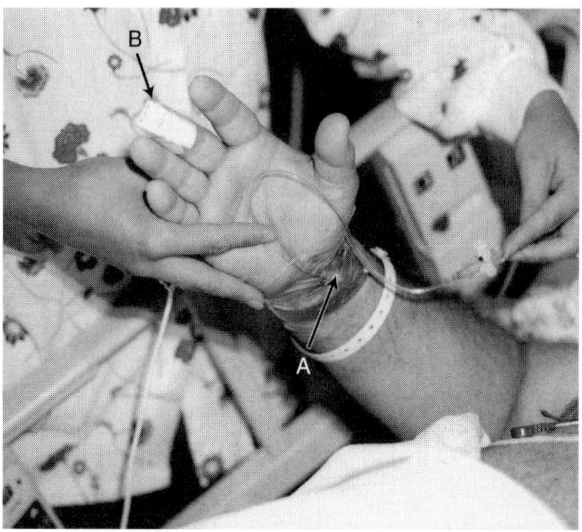

Fig. 10-11 This person has an *A* arterial line inserted at the wrist with *B* an oximeter on the middle finger.

Oximeter This photoelectric device is used to measure the oxygen saturation (SaO_2) of the patient's blood by recording the different modulations of a transmitted beam of light affected by reduced hemoglobin (Hgb) and oxyhemoglobin. Usually, the *oximeter* will be positioned on or attached to a patient's finger or ear and it will measure and report the pulse rate and the percentage of oxygen saturation of the Hgb (blood) (Fig. 10-11).

Pulmonary Artery Catheter (Swan-Ganz Catheter) The *Swan-Ganz catheter* is a long, plastic, IV tube that can be inserted into the internal jugular or the femoral vein, guided into the basilic or subclavian vein, and then passed into the pulmonary artery. This catheter is used to provide accurate and continuous measurements of PAP and will detect even very subtle changes in the patient's cardiovascular system, including responses to medications, stress, and exercise.

This device is indicated when measurements of right atrial pressure, PAP, and pulmonary capillary *wedge pressure* (PCWP) are desired. Readings are performed frequently; the monitor screen will show a rolling waveform and a digital reading of the various values will appear. Normal values are right atrial pressure, 0 to 4 mm Hg; PAP, 20 to 30 mm Hg systolic and 10 to 15 mm Hg diastolic; PCWP, 4 to 12 mm Hg.

Exercise can be performed with the pulmonary artery catheter (PAC) in place, but it may be necessary to limit the exercise because of the location of the catheter's insertion. For example, if the catheter is inserted into the subclavian vein, shoulder flexion should be avoided and shoulder motions restricted. Similar restrictions in hip flexion and abduction exist for a femoral vein insertion. Some complications associated with this catheter are pulmonary artery vascular damage, damage to intracardial structures, cardiac dysrhythmias, endocarditis, and sepsis (infection).

Intracranial Pressure Monitor The ICP monitor measures the pressure exerted against the skull by brain tissue, blood, or cerebrospinal fluid (CSF). It is used for patients who have experienced a closed head injury, a cerebral hemorrhage, a brain tumor, or an overproduction of CSF. Normal ICP pressure is 4 to 15 mm Hg, but a fluctuation of as much as 20 mm Hg can occur from a variety of routine activities.

This device is used to monitor ICP easily, to quantitate the degree of abnormal pressure, to properly initiate treatment, and to evaluate the results of treatment. Some of the complications associated with this device are sepsis, hemorrhage, and seizures.

Types of Intracranial Pressure Monitoring Devices

Ventricular Catheter. The ventricular catheter is inserted into a lateral ventricle of the brain through a hole drilled in the skull. This is a highly accurate method to monitor the ICP and it allows withdrawal of CSF.

Subarachnoid Screw. A screw is inserted into the subarachnoid space through a small hole drilled in the skull.

This device permits accurate measurement of the ICP, but it does not permit withdrawal of CSF.

Epidural Sensor. A sensor plate can be placed in the epidural space, but this has proved to be a relatively inaccurate measurement device and has poor reliability; therefore this device is rarely used.

Minimal physical activities can be performed when these devices are in place, but activities that would cause a rapid increase in ICP, such as isometric exercises and the Valsalva maneuver, should be avoided. The patient should be positioned to avoid neck flexion, hip flexion greater than 90 degrees, and lying in a prone position. The patient's head should not be lowered more than 15 degrees below horizontal. As with other devices that use plastic tubing, care must be taken to avoid disruption, disconnection, or occlusion of the tube.

Central Venous Pressure Catheter The CVP catheter is a plastic IV tube used to measure pressures in the right atrium or the superior vena cava. It measures the pressure associated with the filling of the right ventricle (that is, the diastolic pressure). Such measurement is imprecise and may be misleading regarding the function of the right ventricle. Precautions similar to those expressed previously for other catheters also apply when a CVP line is in place. Potential complications are similar to those listed for the PAC.

Arterial Line (A Line) The A line is a catheter that is inserted into an artery, typically the radial, dorsal pedal, axillary, brachial, or femoral artery. The A line is used to continuously measure blood pressure or to obtain blood samples without repeated needle punctures and it usually provides accurate measurements. Potential complications include sepsis, hemorrhage, development of a *fistula* or aneurysm, ischemia, or arterial necrosis.

Exercise can be performed with an A line in place, providing the precautions described previously, especially those related to disruption of the catheter, disturbance of the inserted needle, occlusion of the line, or disconnection of the line from the inserted cannula, are followed (see Fig 10-11).

Indwelling Right Atrial Catheter (Hickman) The right atrial catheter is inserted through the cephalic or internal jugular vein and passes through the superior vena cava to near the tip of the right atrium. This device allows administration of medications, removal of blood for testing, and measurement of CVP. When a central line catheter is used for "hyperalimentation" or total parental nutrition (TPN), it will usually be positioned into the superior vena cava for the delivery of the nutritional solution. The central line can be used with patients who will receive a bone marrow transplant, who have cancer, or who have experienced severe trauma. Some potential complications associated with this device are sepsis and blood clots.

Exercise should be performed with care and precautions similar to those described previously for other catheters should be followed (Fig. 10-12).

Reference Laboratory Values

Reference laboratory values are important because they provide baseline values with which a patient's laboratory findings can be compared. Depending on the diagnosis, physical

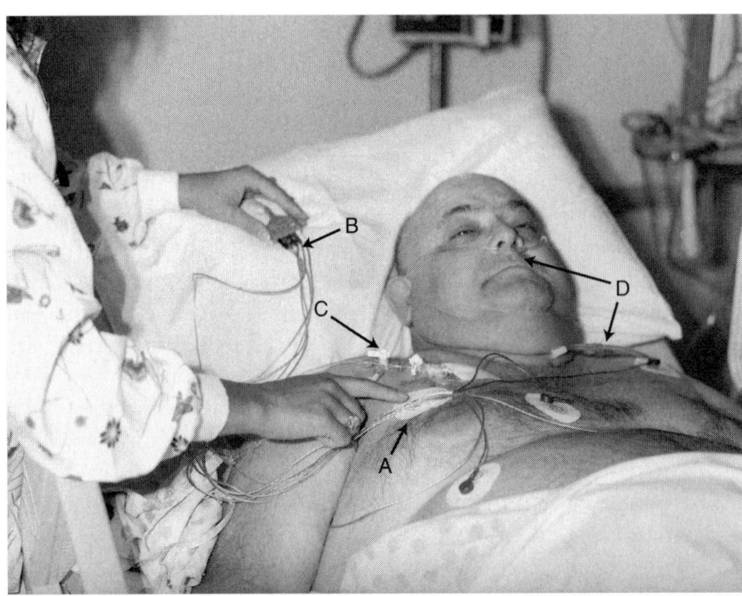

Fig. 10-12 *A,* The nurse is pointing to one monitor lead. *B,* She holds the lead connection to the monitor. *C,* Immediately above her finger is a central line. *D,* Note the nasal cannula for supplemental oxygen.

and mental condition, and institutional or physician guidelines or protocols, the approach to care and treatment will be adjusted for each individual. Persons with the same or similar diagnosis may require very different approaches to care because of differences in their physical responses to the disease, trauma, or condition that they have experienced.

Cardiac status can be determined by examination of the cardiac enzyme levels in the blood after an acute *myocardial infarction (MI)*. When an MI occurs, intercellular enzymes are released into the person's blood. The enzyme creatine kinase (CK) and especially the enzyme found primarily in cardiac muscle, CK-MB, when they are present in the blood, indicate that an acute MI has occurred. These increased values usually return to normal levels within 2 days after the MI. The caregiver must use caution when treating the individual and should be certain to closely observe the patient's vital signs as they appear on the cardiac monitor. The patient can receive basic care and participate in physical activities providing the vital signs, blood chemistry, ABGs, and physical appearance remain within acceptable ranges. Adverse responses to activity such as chest pain, fatigue, hypotension, or cardiac dysrhythmia are indicators that the treatment may need to be modified, altered, or discontinued.

The ABG analysis provides information about the oxygenation level of the blood. A pulse oximeter, often positioned on a fingertip or an earlobe, is used to measure the pulse rate and the percentage of oxygen saturation in the blood. Refer to Table 10-1 for ABG values and ranges.

During exercise or physical activity, a minimum of 90% saturation should be maintained to avoid hypoxemia and possible respiratory dysfunction. If supplemental oxygen is being provided for the patient, it should remain in place during the treatment. If the oxygen saturation falls below 90% and remains there, the treatment should be discontinued and consideration should be given to altering or modifying the treatment in the future. Changes in the individual's respiration rate or pattern may occur because of a reduced oxygen saturation level during exercise. If hyperventilation occurs, the person may benefit from relaxation techniques such as abdominal-diaphragmatic or pursed-lip breathing. If hypoventilation occurs, the person may benefit from deep-breathing techniques and an upright, trunk-supported position.

Blood chemistry analysis provides information about an individual's red blood cell (RBC) and white blood cell (WBC) count, Hgb, and hematocrit (Hct). The WBC, also known as a leukocyte, is one of the body's defense mechanisms for fighting acute or chronic disease or infection. An increased WBC count may indicate the presence of bacterial infection, leukemia, neoplasm, allergic reaction, inflammation, or tissue necrosis. A decreased WBC count may indicate bone marrow deficiency or infection with human immunodeficiency virus or it may be attributable to radiation or chemotherapy treatments. A person with a decreased WBC count caused by an immunosuppressed condition must be monitored carefully and the caregiver must be certain to perform thorough handwashing, apply protective garments, and follow treatment precautions before treatment to reduce the possibility of cross contamination. Depending on the diagnosis and the individual's physical condition, treatment activities may need to be modified, altered, or discontinued according to the patient's response to the treatments and frequent rest periods may be necessary. Precautions for exercise

Table 10-1 Reference Laboratory Values

Arterial Blood Gases (ABGs)	
ph	7.35-7.45
$Paco_2$	35-45 mm Hg
HCO_2	22-26 mEq/L
Pao_2	80-100 mm Hg
O_2Sat. (Sao_2)	95%-98%

ph = acid-base status: <7.35 = acidosis; >7.45 = alkalosis
$Paco_2$ = Partial pressure of carbon dioxide dissolved in arterial blood; influenced by pulmonary function
HCO_2 = Amount of alkaline substance dissolved in arterial blood; influenced by metabolic changes primarily
Pao_2 = Partial pressure of oxygen dissolved in arterial blood; influenced by pulmonary function
O_2 = Oxyhemoglobin saturation or percentage of oxygen carried by hemoglobin

Selected Blood Chemistry Values	
Red blood cells (RBCs)	$4.6\text{-}6.2 \times 10^{12}$/L (male) $4.2\text{-}5.4 \times 10^{12}$/L (female)
White blood cells (WBCs)	$4.3\text{-}10.8 \times 10^9$/L
Hemoglobin (Hgb)	14-18 g/dl (male) 13-16 g/dl (female)
Hematocrit (Hct)	40-54 ml/dl (male) 37-48 ml/dl (female)
Potassium (K^+)	3.5-5.0 mEq/L
Glucose	70-115 mg/dl
Platelet	$150\text{-}450 \times 10^6$/L
Sodium (Na^+)	135-145 mEg/L
Serum creatinine	0.6-1.5 mg/dl (male) 0.5-1.0 mg/dl (female)
Creatine kinase (CK)—total	25-255 μl/L
CK-MB isoenzyme (heart related)	0-5.9 ml/L
CK-MM isoenzyme (muscle related)	5-70 μl/L

Reference values may vary depending on the method used to obtain them or the source that reports them; many are gender or age dependent. The reference values, also referred to as "normal values," used for this table were obtained from the *Encyclopedia and Dictionary of Medicine, Nursing, and Allied Health, Fifth Edition*, Philadelphia. W.B. Saunders, 1992, except the creatine kinase values. Those values were obtained from Laboratory Values in the Intensive Care Unit, *Acute Care Perspectives*, The Newsletter of Acute Care/Hospital Clinical Practice Section–APTA, Winter, 1995.

Table 10-2 Precautions for Exercise with Low Blood Counts

Count	No Exercise	Light Exercise	Resistive Exercise
Hematocrit	<27%	27%-30%	>30%
Hemoglobin	8 g/dL	8-10 g/dL	>10 g/dL
Platelet	<50,000 mm^3	50,000-70,000 mm^3	>70,000 mm^3
White cells	<500 mm^3 with fever	>500 mm^3	>500 mm^3

activities when abnormal blood values exist are presented in Table 10-2.

Because they are bound to the Hgb contained in the cell, the RBCs transport oxygen to tissue cells throughout the body. Anemia occurs when the RBC count is decreased significantly and polycythemia occurs when the RBC count is increased significantly. A patient with either of these conditions may participate in physical activity providing institutional and physician guidelines or protocols are followed and the response to the activity is monitored frequently and consistently.

The Hct is used to measure the volume percentage of packed RBCs in a sample of whole blood. The Hct is particularly important in the diagnosis of polycythemia or anemia. Persons with anemia will not tolerate vigorous physical activity and their vital signs should be monitored frequently and consistently.

The Hgb is the protein contained in the RBC that transports oxygen in the blood; it is frequently referred to as oxyhemoglobin. Anemia, trauma, surgery, or dietary iron deficiency may cause a decrease in the Hgb. A person with a low Hgb will have a reduced tolerance to physical activity and will require frequent rest periods. Persons whose Hgb is less than 8 g/dL should not receive or participate in treatment requiring physical activity.

The caregiver who provides treatment in an ICU (or coronary care unit [CCU]) should become familiar with the reference values of various laboratory tests to understand the implications for treatment when abnormal values are identified. The level of activity that is appropriate or suitable for a given patient can be established by the caregiver to assist the patient to attain maximal function effectively without jeopardizing recovery (see Table 10-1).

Feeding Devices

It may be necessary to provide nutrition for a patient who is unable to feed independently or who is unable to chew, swallow, or ingest food.

Nasogastric Tube The *nasogastric (NG) tube* is a plastic tube inserted through a nostril that eventually terminates in the patient's stomach. Purposes of the NG tube include: removing fluid or gas from the stomach and *gastrointestinal* (GI) tract, evaluating digestive function and activity in the GI tract, administering medications directly into the GI tract, providing a means to feed the patient, allowing treatment to the upper portion of the GI tract, and obtaining gastric specimens. Some patients will complain of a sore throat or may have an increased gag reflex as a result of the tube. The patient will not be able to eat food or drink fluids through the mouth while the NG tube is in place. Exercise can be performed with the NG tube in place, but movement of the patient's head and neck should be avoided, especially flexion or forward bending.

Gastric Tube The gastric tube (G tube) is a plastic tube that is inserted directly into the stomach through an incision in the patient's abdomen. Many of the purposes described for the NG tube also apply to the G tube.

Exercise can be performed providing the caregiver is aware of the presence of the G tube and avoids removing the tube.

Intravenous Feeding, Total Parenteral Nutrition, and Hyperalimentation Devices Intravenous feeding techniques permit *infusion* of large amounts of nutrients that are needed to promote tissue growth. They are a means to achieve an appropriate metabolic state in patients who are unable to, should not, or refuse to eat.

A catheter is inserted directly into the subclavian vein or sometimes into the jugular or another vein and then passed into the subclavian vein. The catheter may be connected to a semipermanently fixed cannula or sutured at the point of insertion. The caregiver should carefully observe the various connections to be certain they are secure before and after exercise. A disrupted or loose connection may result in the development of an air embolus, which could be life threatening to the patient.

Usually, the system will include an *infusion pump*, which will administer fluids and nutrients at a preselected, constant flow rate. An audible alarm will be activated if the system becomes unbalanced or when the fluid source is empty.

Exercise can be performed providing the caregiver does not disrupt, disconnect, or occlude the tubing and cause undue stress to the infusion site. Motions of the shoulder on the side of the infusion site may be restricted, especially abduction and flexion.

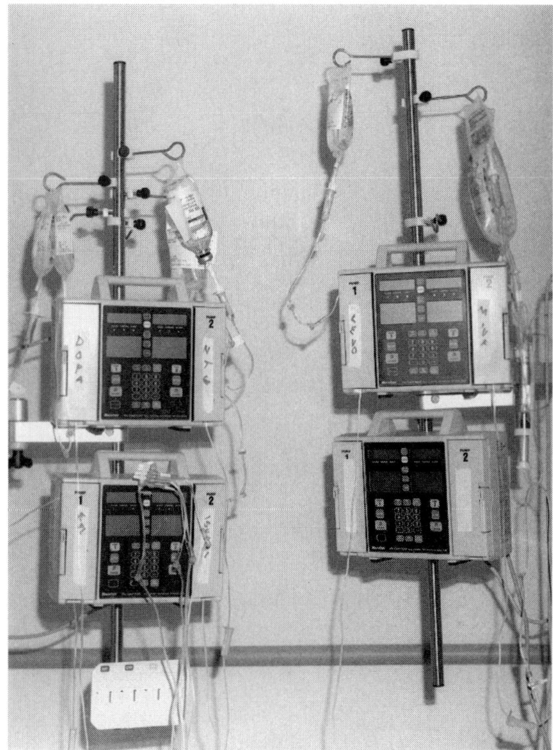

Fig. 10-13 Multiple intravenous line systems with solutions in position for infusion.

Intravenous Infusion Lines Intravenous lines are used to infuse fluids, nutrients, electrolytes, and medications; to obtain venous blood samples; and to insert catheters into the central circulatory system to monitor the physiologic condition of the patient, especially the cardiopulmonary system (Fig. 10-13).

The components of the IV system usually consist of the solution or fluid container, which may be a bottle or plastic bag; a device to measure the number of drops of fluid administered per minute; plastic tubing; a roller clamp to control the rate of the flow of fluid; and a needle to enter the vein. Some IV systems include an infusion pump, which provides a constant, preselected fluid flow rate. Refer to Box 10-3 for a listing of commonly used IV infusion sites.

Most IV insertions are made into superficial veins. Various sizes and types of needles or catheters are used depending on the purpose of the IV therapy, infusion site, need for prolonged therapy, and site availability.

Possible complications associated with the IV administration include infiltration of fluid into the subcutaneous tissue, phlebitis, cellulitis, thrombosis, local hematoma, sepsis, pulmonary thromboembolus, air embolus, or a catheter fragment embolus. The caregiver should use caution to avoid disruption, disconnection, or occlusion of the tubing; stress to the infusion site; and interruption of circulatory flow. The infusion site should remain dry, the needle should remain secure and immobile in the vein, and no restraint should be placed above the infusion site. (For example, avoid applying a blood pressure cuff above the infusion site.) The caregiver should observe the infusion site for signs of infiltration of the fluid into the subcutaneous tissue (such as edema, hyperemia, complaint of site discomfort by the patient, reduced flow of fluid, or infection). Observe the total system to be certain it is functioning properly when you begin and when you end the treatment (Box 10-4).

Exercise can be performed, but disruption, disconnection, occlusion, or overstretching of the tubing must be avoided. If the infusion site is in the antecubital area, the elbow should not be flexed. The patient who ambulates with an IV line in

Box 10-3 Common Intravenous Infusion Sites

Upper extremity: metacarpal and dorsal venous plexus of the hand; basilic, cephalic, and antecubital veins

Lower extremity: dorsal venous plexus and medial, lateral, and marginal veins of the foot; saphenous and femoral veins

Head: superficial scalp veins (often selected for use with infants and the elderly)

Box 10-4 Signs/Symptoms of Intravenous Therapy

INFILTRATION

Cool skin around the site; swelling around the site; swelling of the limb; sluggish flow rate

PHLEBITIS

Pain in limb; erythema; edema with induration; streak formation

THROMBOPHLEBITIS

Painful IV site; erythema; edema with induration; sluggish flow rate

AIR EMBOLISM

Decrease or drop in blood pressure; weak, rapid pulse; cyanosis; loss of consciousness; increase or rise in CVP

INFECTION OF VENIPUNCTURE SITE

Swelling and soreness at the site; foul-smelling discharge

SYSTEMIC INFECTION

Sudden rise in temperature and pulse rate; chills and shaking; changes in blood pressure

ALLERGIC REACTION

Fever; swelling or generalized edema; itching or rash; respiratory distress, especially shortness of breath place should be instructed to grasp the IV line support pole so the infusion site will be at heart level. If the extremity with the infusion site remains in a dependent position, blood flow may be affected, resulting in retrograde flow of blood into the IV line tubing. Similar procedures to maintain the infusion site in proper position should be followed when the patient is treated while in bed, on a treatment table, or platform mat. Activities that require the infusion site to be elevated above the level of the heart for a prolonged period should be avoided so the proper direction of the flow of the IV fluid will be maintained.

Problems related to the IV system that develop as you treat the patient should be made known to nursing personnel. Unless the caregiver has been specifically instructed and trained to adjust, modify, alter, or otherwise correct the IV system, he or she should request a qualified person to correct any problems that develop during the treatment. However, simple procedures such as straightening the tubing or removing an object that is occluding the tubing should be performed by the caregiver.

Urinary Catheters

A urinary catheter can be applied internally (indwelling catheter) or externally. The external urinary catheter is successful only for male patients. A catheter inserted through the urethra and into the bladder is an internal catheter. A condom applied externally to the penis of a male patient with a drainage tube attached to it is an external catheter. No practical, acceptable, or effective external catheter has been developed for female patients.

Urinary catheters are used to remove urine from the bladder so it can drain through plastic tubing into a collection bag (Fig. 10-14), bottle, or urinal. Urinary catheters are used for a patient who has lost voluntary control of *micturition*. This lack of control may be attributable to a spinal cord injury, a disease such as multiple sclerosis, or the physiologic changes associated with old age. Any form of trauma, disease, condition, or disorder that affects the neuromuscular control of the bladder sphincter may necessitate the use of a urinary catheter, including before and following some surgical procedures. The catheter may be used temporarily or for a prolonged period, even for the remainder of the patient's life. Many patients require the use of a catheter and it is not unusual for a caregiver to treat a patient with a catheter. Common complications associated with the use of a catheter are infection of the urinary tract or bladder, development of a urethral fistula, formation of bladder calculi as a result of urinary stasis, and kidney failure. The patient with a spinal cord injury above the T6 cord level may experience autonomic hyperreflexia caused by urine retention. This condition is described in Chapter 12.

Exercises to the lower extremities can be performed by a patient with a catheter provided the caregiver avoids disruption, disconnection, stretching, or occlusion of the drainage tube. You should determine how much free tubing is available before initiating exercise to avoid causing excessive tension on the tubing or the catheter. Urine drains into the collection bag as a result of the effect of gravity; therefore the bag should not be positioned above the level of the bladder for more than a few minutes. The bag should not be placed in the patient's lap when being transported by wheelchair or on the lower abdomen when lying on a wheeled stretcher. Furthermore, the bag and tubing should be positioned and secured to minimize the possibility the bag or the tubing will be pulled or snagged and it should be positioned below the level of the bladder when the patient is being transported. When the patient ambulates, the bag should be positioned and maintained below the level of the bladder, but so it will not interfere with gait or ambulation activities.

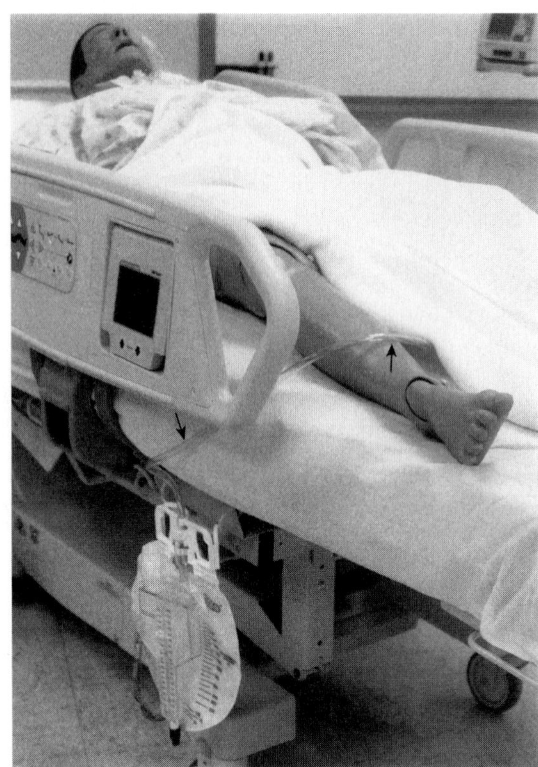

Fig. 10-14 Urinary drainage system with collection bag.

It may be difficult to provide an adequate position to promote drainage when the patient receives hydrotherapy in an immersion tank or sit-in whirlpool. In such cases, the bag can be positioned below the level of the bladder, but the tubing will probably have to be elevated over the edge of the tank or whirlpool before it can be directed downward to the bag. This position of the tubing may prevent urine from draining because it will have to drain upward or against the force of gravity. You should drain any urine in the tubing into the bag before the patient is placed in the water to assist with the future drainage. The bag must not be immersed in the water. At some institutions, treatment protocols may permit clamping of the tubing or catheter before the patient is immersed so the bag can be removed for the length of the treatment. However, the flow of urine should not be occluded for an extended period and should not be occluded frequently to avoid the complications associated with the stasis of urine in the bladder.

The caregiver should observe the color of the urine and be alert for unusual odors associated with it or the urinary system. Foul-smelling urine; cloudy, dark urine; or urine with blood in it (hematuria) should be reported to a physician or nurse. You should also observe the flow and amount of urine in the bag. Any reduced flow or decreased production of urine should be reported. The caregiver should document and verbally report observations of abnormal urine appearance or production promptly so proper treatment can be initiated.

Infection can be a major complication for the person who uses a catheter, particularly if it is an indwelling catheter. All personnel who are involved with the patient should maintain cleanliness when treatment is provided. Precautions must be used when replacing any tubing that has been disengaged from the catheter or the collection bag, when replacing the bag, and when the catheter is inserted into the bladder. Many times it is safer to allow nursing personnel to replace or reconnect the tubing rather than reconnecting it using improper technique. Treatment settings that routinely treat patients with catheters have specific protocols for the care of the tubing and collection bag and the insertion and removal of the catheter. It is important that infection be prevented from developing in the urinary system. Therefore strict adherence to the principles of medical and surgical asepsis is necessary by all personnel.

Foley Catheter The Foley type of indwelling catheter is held in place in the bladder by a small balloon that is inflated with air, water, or sterile saline solution. The catheter has two or three tubes or channels in it. The main channel allows the urine to drain and the other channels are used to inflate the balloon and irrigate the bladder. To remove the catheter, the balloon is deflated, and the catheter is withdrawn.

External Catheter The external catheter (condom) is applied over the shaft of the penis and is held in place by an adhesive applied to the skin or by a padded strap or tape encircling the proximal shaft of the penis. *Caution:* The tape or strap must not be applied too tightly to avoid occlusion of the urethra or the blood supply of the penis.

Suprapubic Catheter Another type of urinary catheter that may be encountered is a *suprapubic* catheter. This catheter is inserted directly into the bladder through incisions in the lower abdomen and the bladder. The catheter may be held in place by adhesive tape, but care should be used to avoid accidental removal.

Oxygen Therapy Systems

Oxygen delivery may be required for a variety of conditions, including after surgery, after MI and other cardiac problems, respiratory diseases, or inadequate lung function. The purpose of oxygen therapy is to provide and maintain an adequate amount of oxygen in the patient's blood in response to the patient's needs when the patient is unable to provide an adequate amount independently. There are several devices or modes that can be used to deliver the oxygen and the selection of the specific device will depend on the patient's condition or illness and functional respiratory capabilities. Regardless of how it is delivered, the oxygen should be humidified to reduce its drying effect on the respiratory mucous membranes.

Modes of Delivery

Nasal Cannula The nasal cannula has two plastic prongs (or points or tips) that are inserted into the patient's nostrils. The points are joined by a plastic connector that rests below the nose and above the patient's upper lip and is secured by tubing positioned above the ears. This mode is used most frequently for patients who require low to moderate concentrations of oxygen (such as patients with COPD).

Oronasal Mask The oronasal mask is a triangular plastic device with small vent holes in it for exhaled air; it covers the patient's nose and mouth. It is used for short periods when moderate concentrations of oxygen are desired, such as to begin to wean a postsurgical patient from long-term therapy, need for higher concentrations of oxygen, or as a temporary approach until a decision is made regarding a permanent form of oxygen delivery.

Nasal Catheter A catheter can be inserted through the nasal passage to the nasopharyngeal junction, which is located just below the level of the soft palate. The uses of this catheter are similar to those described for the nasal cannula.

Tent Occasionally, a tentlike device that encloses the patient's trunk and head may be used, especially if the patient is restless, very young, uncooperative, or extremely ill. The edges of the tent must be sealed to prevent the loss of oxygen; this may require frequent and repeated monitoring of the system by nursing personnel.

Tracheostomy Mask or Catheter Some patients may have a temporary or permanent tracheostomy through which oxygen can be administered by a mask placed over the stoma or by a catheter inserted into the stoma.

In the hospital setting, oxygen is obtained from a wall unit when the patient is in bed or from an oxygen cylinder that accompanies the patient when out of the room. The oxygen in the cylinder, or tank, is compressed or pressurized and there is a regulator on the tank to control the administration of the oxygen to the patient. The rate of flow, in liters per minute, will be determined by a physician and is delivered and maintained by proper adjustment of the regulator valve.

Caution: Oxygen supports combustion, so care must be used to prevent a fire or explosion. Excessive heat, such as a flame, spark, radiator, or even high room temperature, must be avoided. When not in use, the cylinder should be stored in a temperate, dry, and well-ventilated area and should be handled with care to avoid damage to the regulator valve or to the cylinder itself to prevent rapid release of the compressed gas. Cylinders should be transported on a wheeled carrier or on a wheeled pushcart for larger cylinders. Care should be used to avoid dropping or tipping the tank onto the floor to prevent damage to the tank or the control device. When a patient who is receiving oxygen therapy ambulates, the cylinder should accompany the patient in a wheeled carrier or should be carried by another person.

Precautions to be considered when treating the patient who is receiving oxygen include avoiding disruption, disconnection, or occlusion of the tubing; maintaining the prescribed flow rate; and maintaining a free flow of oxygen. In addition, you should be alert for signs or symptoms of respiratory distress exhibited by the patient. If the patient complains of dyspnea or shortness of breath, cramping in the calf muscles, or exhibits cyanosis of the nail beds or lips, the person may be experiencing respiratory or circulatory distress. Exercise or physical activity should cease, the oxygen delivery system should be evaluated for improper function, and qualified personnel may need to be contacted for assistance. The patient may obtain symptomatic relief by standing and partially flexing the trunk, using the upper extremities placed on a firm object for support. Do not place the patient supine; instead, allow the person to lean forward slightly when seated. The patient may rest with the forearms on the thighs, on the chair armrests, or on a firm table to relieve respiratory distress. The prescribed flow rate *must not* be altered when the patient performs exercise. Complications can develop if the patient receives an overdose of oxygen, especially COPD patients, whose usual dose is 2 liters per minute. Careful monitoring of the patient's response to the exercise or activity must be performed to avoid or quickly identify an adverse response and to provide appropriate emergency care.

Chest Drainage Systems

Chest drainage tubes may be used to remove air, blood, purulent matter, or other undesirable material from the patient's chest or pleural cavity. These tubes are inserted through an incision in the chest and may be connected to a mechanical or gravity-based suction system (Fig. 10-15). There are three types of chest tube bottle systems, and these use one, two, or three bottles. The one- and two-bottle systems function by gravity, whereas the three-bottle system and the commercially available disposable systems use a pump to create suction (Fig. 10-16).

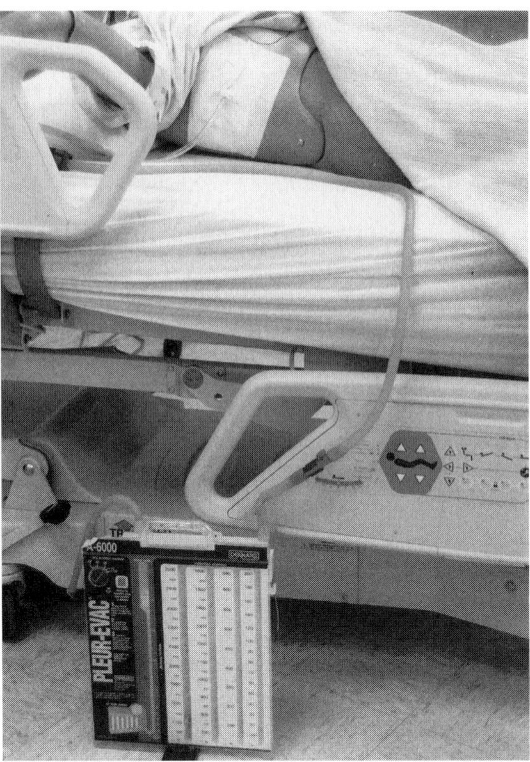

Fig. 10-15 Chest drainage system with collection reservoir.

The chest tubes will be inserted in different locations depending on the type of drainage desired. Tubes that are placed in the anterior or lateral chest wall promote the removal of air (as in treating a *pneumothorax*), tubes placed inferiorly and posteriorly promote the removal of fluids and blood, and a *mediastinal* tube is used to drain blood and fluid, which may be necessary after open chest or heart surgery. The drainage tubes usually will be maintained securely in place with adherent dressings, but care should be used to avoid pulling on them or the connecting tubing. Additional precautions are avoiding disruption of the bottles or containers located on the floor; disconnection or occlusion of the tubing; observing the color of the drainage; observing the system for proper function; and monitoring the patient's response to exercise or activity. For the patient who ambulates, the collection bottles should be kept below the level of the location of the inserted tube.

Ostomy Devices

An ostomy is a surgically produced opening in the abdomen to allow the elimination of feces. More specifically, an enterostomy is the result of a surgical procedure that produces an artificial stoma into the small intestine through an incision in the abdominal wall. Ileostomy and colostomy are

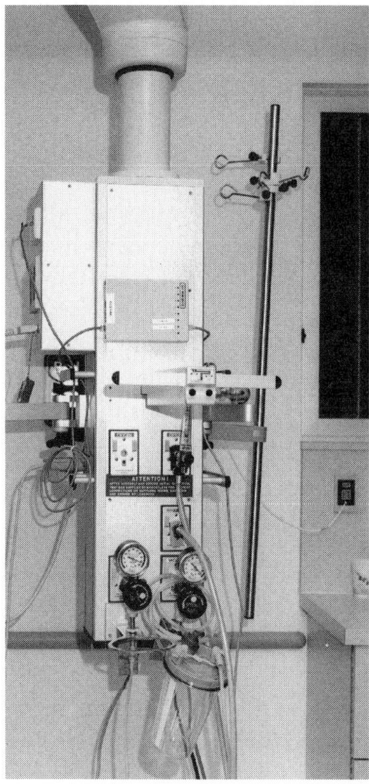

Fig. 10-16 Suction equipment.

types of enterostomy. The stoma is covered with a plastic bag or pouch to collect waste. Most patients will find it necessary to have the collection bag in place at all times, particularly if the waste is more liquid than solid. The location of the ostomy will affect the need for and the extent to which the patient will use the collection bag or pouch.

There are three primary types of collecting devices for the patient with an ostomy; they are designated by the way they are attached to the patient. The bag may be a two-piece pouch that attaches to a skin barrier that adheres to the patient's skin with an adhesive; a one-piece pouch attached to a skin barrier; or an adhesive-backed pouch that adheres to a separate skin barrier. The pouch may be disposable or reusable. Components of the system include an odor-proof plastic pouch, a skin barrier, a filter for gas release, and a means to attach the pouch to the skin barrier or the skin barrier to the skin, such as an adhesive seal or belt tabs.

The caregiver should be aware the patient has an ostomy and excessive stress to the attachment of the pouch should be avoided during treatment. Most patients can be treated with minimal concern for the development of complications or the need to restrict exercise or activity. The patient with a recent ostomy may be sensitive to and concerned about whether the system will function properly. The caregiver should avoid activities that may cause the patient to experience a socially embarrassing event (such as leakage of waste or intestinal gas). Usually, it is desirable to schedule the patient's treatment after the pouch has been emptied or to coordinate it with the patient's bowel habits.

Traction

Traction applied to an extremity can be used to align fracture segments, stretch soft tissue, reduce muscle spasm or contractures, and immobilize the patient. It may be applied to the skin or to a skeletal structure and it may be applied constantly or intermittently. Skin traction must be applied with low weights because of the intolerance of the skin and soft tissue to excessive force. Skeletal traction is applied through a pin or wire inserted into bone to which traction ropes and weights are attached. Skeletal traction is used to position, immobilize, and align fracture segments to promote their proper healing.

Types of Skeletal Traction

Balanced Suspension Traction

Balanced suspension traction is used primarily to treat displaced or *comminuted* femoral fractures. A splint under the femur (Thomas splint) and one under the lower leg (Pearson attachment) are used to balance and suspend the extremity. A pin or wire such as a Kirschner wire or Steinmann pin is inserted through the tibial plateau to provide traction to the distal femoral segment. Because of this arrangement, the traction will remain "balanced" even when the patient moves in bed. Exercises can be performed to the noninjured extremities and ankle movements can be performed on the injured extremity. This type of traction requires prolonged immobilization of the patient, which can lead to secondary complications such as contractures, pressure ulcers, and sepsis. The more recent use of internal or external fixation devices, as described later in this section, has reduced the need for this type of traction and enhanced the functional recovery of the patient.

Skull Traction Skull traction is applied by tongs (such as Crutchfield, Gardner-Wells, Vinke, or Barton tongs) positioned into small holes drilled in the outer layer of the patient's skull. The traction is applied through a rope-weight arrangement and is used for patients with a fracture or dislocation of one or more cervical vertebrae.

Precautions to be aware of when treating the patient who has skull traction are to be certain the traction weights hang freely after the patient has been repositioned; avoid removal or release of any traction weight during treatment, unless prescribed; avoid bumping the weights because doing so will create motion through the rope to the fracture site; and note the condition of the site of the pin. Look for bleeding, skin disruption, drainage, or signs of inflammation at the site of the pin insertion. Any unusual observations should be documented and reported promptly.

A device frequently referred to as a "halo" can be applied to provide traction and stability to the cervical spine. The device is held in place by four pins inserted into the patient's skull and a metal ring that connects the pins to which four vertical uprights are attached. The uprights are anchored to two over-the-shoulder plates, which are connected to a padded vest worn over the upper body. With the "halo" in place, the patient can be mobile and can sit, stand, and perform various activities. Exercise of the extremities can be performed, but care should be used when movement of the shoulder is attempted or when the muscles that attach to the cervical vertebrae are contracted to avoid stress to the fracture site and to the corresponding nerve roots of that area.

External Fixation External fixation is a form of stabilization and traction that uses a variety of frames applied externally to the patient's extremity (such as Haynes, Hoffmann, or Anderson devices). These frames hold pins that have been inserted into the bone fragments of a severe fracture to maintain the fracture in alignment. This form of fixation allows earlier and greater mobility for the patient while providing excellent alignment and stabilization of the fracture segments. Ambulation on both lower extremities and exercise of the noninjured extremities or areas of the body can be performed, though weight bearing on the involved extremity may be contraindicated or limited. This form of fixation is particularly beneficial for a comminuted, an extensive open, or an infected open fracture or when bone grafts are involved. Be careful to avoid excess stress to the exposed frame and pins and observe the insertion sites for evidence of adverse reactions to the pins (such as infection or bone deterioration). *Note:* Care must be taken when the patient uses ambulation aids so the external apparatus is not struck or does not interfere with the ambulation pattern.

Internal Fixation This method of treatment uses hardware applied internally to or within bone to maintain its alignment and stability after fracture reduction. The hardware can include transfixation screws, bone plates, wires, nails, and intramedullary rods. The technique usually provides a shorter period of immobilization, a stable fracture site, maintenance of local circulation, and more rapid return to functional activities.

Depending on the location and type of fracture, the hardware used to fixate the fracture, and the patient's general condition, the treatment procedures selected will vary. Early active or passive mobilization of the joints proximal and distal to the fracture should be initiated. Isometric exercise of the muscles that cross the fracture and that are immobilized (as in a cast) can be done to maintain muscle tone, local circulation, and muscle awareness. Active and active resistive exercise for the muscles and joints of the noninvolved extremities should be performed to maintain or improve range of motion and strength.

Ambulation after fracture in a lower extremity can usually be performed within a few days after the fracture has been reduced and fixated. The amount or type of weight bearing depends on the location of the fracture, the type of fixation device, the general condition of the patient, and the desires of the surgeon.

Caution may be necessary to protect the fracture site and soft-tissue incision, if a surgical open reduction was performed, until healing occurs. The open reduction of the fracture has the potential for wound infection, which is a disadvantage of this procedure. In addition, the complication of the development of a venous embolus may occur after a femoral fracture. If the embolus is transported to the pulmonary artery, a life-threatening condition exists.

Patient-Controlled Analgesia

The patient-controlled analgesia (PCA) system allows the patient to self-administer a small predetermined dose of pain medication intravenously on demand, as frequently as every 6 minutes. A reservoir of the medication is connected by tubing to an IV line and to a small control module or pump, which the patient wears on the wrist. When medication is desired, the patient presses a button on the control module; the medication moves to a small area in the control module and then passes through tubing into the IV line. The unit will not deliver more medication than the premeasured dose each time the patient activates the button. In addition, the patient cannot receive the medication more frequently than a predetermined period (for example, every 6 minutes). The number of requests the patient has made and the number of doses the unit has delivered are recorded by the unit and are available for review. This device should not interfere with the patient's exercise program or other activities. However, the precautions outlined for IV lines should be followed.

Dialysis Treatment

Dialysis is used for patients who experience acute or end-stage renal disease (ESRD). The single leading cause of ESRD is type 2 diabetes, followed by high blood pressure, glomerulonephritis, and cystic kidney. The objectives of dialysis are to prevent infection, restore the normal level of fluids and electrolytes, control the acid-base balance, remove waste and toxic materials, and assist in or replace normal kidney function.

An important issue for dialysis patients is regular access to removal of waste products from the body. There are two types of generally accepted methods of artificial kidney treatment: hemodialysis and peritoneal dialysis. The majority of dialysis patients receive hemodialysis, which may be provided through a prosthetic *shunt* or an arteriovenous fistula. Blood is pumped out of the patient's body to the dialyzer, which cleanses the blood of wastes, and the cleaned blood is returned to the body from the machine through connecting tubing. Dialysis in this method is usually performed for 2- to

4-hour periods, or longer, and is done at least three times per week. Advantages of this method are that trained professionals are with the patient during the procedure and there is minimal disruption of lifestyle between treatments.

In peritoneal dialysis, the inside lining of the abdomen acts as a natural filter. Wastes are taken out by means of the cleansing fluid, dialysate, which is washed in and out of the body in cycles. The dialysate solution is delivered into and removed from the abdomen through a catheter, which has been surgically implanted in the abdominal wall. This method of dialysis is repeated several times a day or can be done automatically by a machine (cycler) during the night. Advantages of this method are the patient can do the treatment alone and at the times and place desired.

Exercise and activity can be performed safely, but excessive activity involving the area of the shunt and application of any occlusive item, such as a blood pressure cuff, or restraint to the upper arm of the extremity containing the shunt, should be avoided. Care should be taken to avoid pulling on the peritoneal tube or the tubing attached to it and to avoid occluding the drainage tubing.

SUMMARY

It may be necessary to treat a patient who is very ill or whose condition requires highly specialized care or the use of a variety of devices and equipment to maintain life. These patients should be treated with caution and frequent monitoring. A patient who uses any of the devices, systems, or procedures described in this chapter should be evaluated whenever treatment is provided and the response to treatment should be documented at the conclusion of each treatment session. Any complications or problems encountered or any deviations from the expected treatment results should be noted. Serious or unusual adverse patient responses to treatment should be discussed directly with an appropriate person such as a physician or nurse. Remember that many of these patients are acutely ill and probably will not tolerate exercise or physical activity as easily as less ill patients would. You are encouraged to proceed carefully by maintaining the program within the functional and physiologic capacities of each patient.

self-study ACTIVITIES

- Describe how you might alter or modify your treatment plan and program to accommodate the types of patient conditions presented in this chapter.
- Explain the immediate and long-term actions you would perform if the patient exhibited adverse responses to the treatment received.
- Define the following: IV line, SICU, CCU, PACU, A line, NG tube, skeletal traction, external fixation, TPN or hyperalimentation, and ventilator. (Select other acronyms or terms and define them also.)
- Outline the components you believe should be included in a program designed to orient or familiarize a therapist with the equipment, environment, and patient therapy devices that are apt to be encountered in an ICU.

problem SOLVING

1. You are treating a patient in an ICU who is on a ventilator. The treatment includes active assistive exercises to the extremities. During one of the treatment sessions, the alarm on the ventilator sounds. What are your immediate actions at this time and what would you do if the patient exhibited signs of respiratory distress?
2. You have been asked to give instructions for ambulation to a 45-year-old patient with a comminuted fracture of the right lower extremity. He has an external fixation device and is apprehensive about ascending and descending stairs. What instructions or directions would you give him in teaching this necessary activity?

CHAPTER 11

Basic Wound Care and Specialized Interventions

objectives *After studying this chapter, the reader will be able to:*

- Describe and demonstrate how to establish and maintain a sterile field.
- Describe the functions of a dressing and a bandage.
- Describe and demonstrate the proper application and removal of a dressing.
- Describe and demonstrate the proper application and removal of a bandage that covers a dressing.
- Assess and stage a pressure ulcer.
- Describe four tests to assess peripheral venous and arterial circulation.
- Describe and demonstrate girth measurement.
- Describe a treatment approach for lymphedema.
- Describe the principles and function of compression garments and how to measure the extremities for a garment.
- Describe the functions of chest physical therapy and demonstrate postural drainage positions.

key terms

Autolysis The disintegration of cells or tissues by the enzymes of the body or cellular components in wound fluid.

Chest physical therapy Gravity-assisted bronchial drainage with techniques for secretion removal and breathing techniques.

Debridement The removal of devitalized tissues from or adjacent to a traumatic or infected lesion to expose healthy tissue.

Epithelialization Healing by the growth of epithelium over a denuded surface.

Erythema Redness of the skin caused by congestion of the capillaries in the lower layers of the skin.

Eschar A dry scab; devitalized tissue.

Exudate A fluid with a high composition of protein and cellular debris that has escaped from blood vessels and is deposited in tissues or on tissue surfaces.

Granulation Any granular material on the surface of a tissue, membrane, or organ.

Induration The quality of being hard; abnormal firmness of tissue with a definite margin.

Lymphedema A functional overload of the lymphatic system in which lymph volume exceeds transport capabilities resulting in obstructed lymph flow.

Maceration The softening of a solid or tissue by soaking.

Necrosis The morphologic changes indicative of cell death.

Slough A mass of dead tissue in, or cast out from, living tissue; pronounced *sluf.*

Sterile Free from any microorganisms; *aseptic.*

Ulcer A local defect or excavation of the surface of an organ or tissue produced by sloughing of necrotic inflammatory tissue.

INTRODUCTION

The care and management of a wound is an important aspect of patient treatment with which a caregiver may be involved. The ability of the caregiver to establish and maintain a sterile or clean environment during the application of a dressing and the ability to avoid contamination of the wound, other persons, equipment, or treatment areas is of paramount importance. The application of the principles and techniques of proper hand washing and the use of protective garments (see Chapter 2) are necessary activities for the caregiver when treating a wound. A wound that is contaminated or is caused by pressure to the tissue overlying a bony prominence requires consistent and persistent care to enhance the healing process. The judicious application of protective positioning (see Chapter 5), nursing procedures, topical or systemic medications, appropriate nutrition and hydration supplements, and skin care are critical components of wound care.

The caregiver must be able to recognize the type of wound, the phase of healing it represents, and the factors that affect wound healing. Each wound should be assessed to determine its size, depth, and appearance so subsequent assessments can be compared with the initial findings. The procedures to assess, classify, and stage a wound are presented later in this chapter.

Information about establishing a sterile field and the application of a sterile dressing and its covering (that is, secondary) bandage to protect the wound from contamination and application of a topical medication are described. The caregiver must remember that prevention of wound contamination and prevention of cross-infection of others are critical elements of wound care.

Girth measurement is an important process, when performed over time, to provide objective evidence of either edema or atrophy in a limb. These measurements also provide evidence of treatment success for a variety of disorders. Serial measurements and techniques are discussed in this chapter, as is volumetric measurement of the hand and foot.

Edema occurs when venous or lymphatic vessels or both are impaired; we will focus primarily on *lymphedema*. When impairment is so great that the lymphatic fluid exceeds the lymphatic transport capacity, the result is an abnormal collection of high protein fluid in the interstitial spaces. Lymphedema can be primary (congenital, usually found in the lower extremities) or secondary (caused by surgical removal of lymph nodes; by tumor invasion of the lymph nodes; injury or infection to the lymph drainage system; or radiation therapy, which can damage the lymph channels). Lymphedema can be found in any part of the body, but is most often limited to the extremities.

Patients who have experienced an axillary or groin dissection should be informed that secondary lymphedema is a possibility and should be provided instruction about preventive measures because this is a lifelong, chronic condition. Fortunately, effective treatment for both primary and secondary lymphedema is available from caregivers with specialized education. Treatment methods of complete (or complex) decongestive therapy (CDT), which includes manual lymph drainage (MLD), lymphedema care and precautions, compression pump, compression bandages or garments, and therapeutic exercises, are discussed. Two measurement techniques for upper and lower extremity compression garments are also included in this chapter.

Chest physical therapy (CPT), also known as cardiopulmonary physical therapy, is an important part of care for those patients with respiratory disease (such as chronic obstructive pulmonary disease [COPD], cystic fibrosis, pneumonia, asthma, carcinoma of the lung) or those who have experienced surgery or injury (for example, cardiac or thoracic surgery, lung operations, or fractured ribs). The caregiver should be aware of specific methods of chest care used in a particular setting. In some facilities, a physical therapist will be responsible for all aspects of CPT, including postural drainage, percussion and vibration, and airway clearance (such as suctioning and cough techniques). In other settings, respiratory therapy or nursing, or both, will have defined interventions for the respiratory-involved patient. Suctioning techniques through the nose, mouth, or endotracheal tube are not presented in this text. However, examination and evaluation techniques and the treatment methods of postural drainage and secretion removal and goals for the patient who receives CPT are described.

THE STERILE FIELD

As the term indicates, a *sterile* field is designed to maintain the sterility of objects contained within the field, such as dressings or bandages, and to prevent contamination of the objects, which in turn could contaminate the patient. The sterile field is a form of surgical asepsis designed to keep the area free from pathogens. Usually a nonabsorbent, sterile towel or the outer cover or wrapping of a package that contains sterile supplies is used as the base for the sterile field. Once the field has been established, additional sterile objects can be added to the field cautiously.

It is important to know and to apply the four rules of asepsis when you establish the field and when you use items that are part of the field:

- Know which items are sterile.
- Know which items are not sterile.
- Separate sterile items from nonsterile items.
- If a sterile item becomes contaminated, the situation must be remedied immediately.

Contamination occurs any time a sterile item physically contacts a nonsterile item. Often the remedy is to discard the contaminated item and it may also be necessary to reestablish the sterile field.

Only items that have been specifically sterilized or packaged and identified as sterile until the package is opened can be considered sterile. If an item has been autoclaved, be certain that black lines appear on the tape used to seal the package. These black lines indicate that the item has been sterilized or can be considered sterile. The outer packages of prepackaged sterile items should be checked to be certain that the items in the package were labeled as sterile when packaged and that they are still sterile (that is, the outer package is completely sealed and dry) (Fig. 11-1).

Once the field has been established (that is, set up), care must be taken to maintain sterile conditions in the area and avoid contamination of the field. Guidelines for maintaining the sterile field are presented in Box 11-1. In general, if you remember and follow the four rules of asepsis, contamination of the field will be avoided. If you have any question as to whether an item is sterile, consider it contaminated and do not use it. If the object has come in contact with other objects that were considered sterile, all of the items should be discarded and only new items known to be sterile should be used.

It is imperative to maintain the sterile field once it has been established. The level of care provided by the caregiver when a sterile technique is required may affect the healing process and possibly the patient's life. Procedures designed to protect the patient and the caregiver and to prevent wound contamination must be followed diligently and consistently.

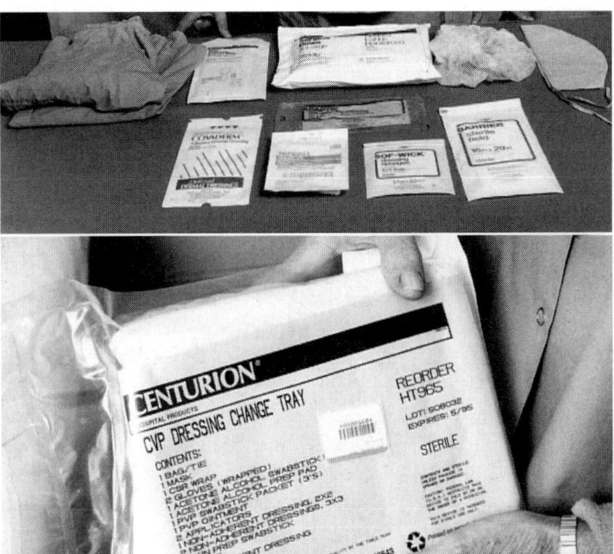

Fig. 11-1 Sterile packaging.

Box 11-1 Guidelines for Maintaining a Sterile Field

Do not talk, sneeze, cough, or reach across a sterile field. The air currents or moisture droplets from your nose or mouth can convey pathogens onto the field.

Do not turn your back to the field because contamination of the objects in the field can occur when you are not able to observe the field.

Do not allow a nonsterile object to come in contact with a sterile object and do not allow a sterile object to come in contact with an unsterile object.

Do not leave the field unattended, even if it is covered with a sterile towel or other sterile item. In your absence the field can become contaminated.

A 1-inch border at the edges of the field is considered to be unsterile. Avoid placing any sterile item within 1 inch of the outer edge of the field and do not touch this area with sterile gloves or other sterile objects.

When you wear sterile protective clothing, the portions that are considered sterile, until they come into contact with an unsterile object or environment, are the gloves, the front of the gown above waist level, and both sleeves of the gown. The remainder of the gown is considered to be unsterile.

Remember: Any liquid is affected by gravity. Therefore when forceps or other items that have been stored in a liquid disinfectant are used, they should be handled so the tip or end that has been in the disinfectant is held downward. If the tip or end of the object is held upward, the fluid will flow to a nonsterile area on the object. Then, when the tip or end is held downward again, the fluid will flow from the nonsterile area back to the sterile area, thereby contaminating the object.

The base and the area surrounding the field should be void of moisture because moisture is apt to contain microorganisms and can penetrate the field by direct contact, absorption, or the wicking property of any of the materials on the field. Moisture is considered to be a source of contamination, so the field must remain dry. If the base of the field or any of the sterile materials on the field become wet, they should be considered contaminated.

To reduce or avoid movement over the field, position the items on the field in the order they will be used so the items that are to be used first are nearest you.

The area below the surface of the sterile field, which will usually be tabletop height or waist height, is considered unsterile. Any item that falls to or is located below waist or tabletop level should be considered contaminated.

General cleanliness of the treatment area, including the furniture, floor, walls, and lavatories, should be maintained to reduce the proliferation or deposition of microorganisms. Hand-washing techniques and practices described previously should be used when a sterile field is required.

Box 11-2 Basic Goals of Wound Care and Management

- Protect the wound and surrounding tissue from additional trauma.
- Reduce strain on the tissues near the wound.
- Protect the tissue in the area of the wound from mechanical stress or movement.
- Reduce the number of pathogenic microorganisms in and around the wound.
- Expedite the healing process.
- Decrease or reduce the formation of scar tissue.

WOUND MANAGEMENT

Dressings and bandages are important items associated with the care and management of wounds and the caregiver must apply the concept of the prevention of wound infection. The basic goals of wound care are listed in Box 11-2. Three phases of wound healing are described in the literature: (1) the inflammatory, (2) proliferative, and (3) remodeling (maturation) phases.

The inflammatory process initiates wound healing. Its function is to limit tissue damage, remove injured or damaged cells, and repair the injured tissue. It is the body's initial local defense response to injury or trauma and it begins immediately after injury or trauma.

The inflammatory process consists of at least three stages: (1) vascular, (2) *exudate*, and (3) reparative stages. During the acute phase of healing, the vascular stage is characterized by hyperemia because of a change in cellular filtration pressures and an increase in the permeability of cells. These factors usually produce local edema, warmth, *erythema*, and discomfort, which are the cardinal signs and symptoms of inflammation.

The exudate stage can have any of several appearances: serous (blister), purulent (pus), fibrinous (clotting), or hemorrhagic (bleeding). In this stage, a fluid passes through the walls of vessels into adjacent tissues or spaces to help deposit fibrins and leukocytes, which are necessary to initiate wound healing.

During the reparative stage, damaged cells are replaced, and true wound healing begins. Damaged cells are removed through phagocytosis, which is accomplished by polymorphonuclear cells and monocytes.

The proliferative phase overlaps the inflammatory phase and *granulation*, *epithelialization*, and contraction of the wound site occur. The fibroblastic cells proliferate and collagen tissue develops to initiate scar formation. According to one theory of healing, the fibroblasts and capillary buds develop at the edges of the wound and gradually advance toward the center of the wound. A bed of granulation tissue forms gradually over the surface of the wound and the epithelial margins begin to migrate toward the center of the wound on top of this granulation bed. This process leads to contraction of the wound and eventually to formation of a scar.

The remodeling phase overlaps the proliferative phase and is characterized by the organization of the collagen tissue into a more definitive and finite pattern. Another factor associated with this phase is the increase in tensile strength of the tissue that covers the wound (that is, scar tissue). Because the wound heals from the edges toward the center of the wound, it is important to use care when removing a dressing from the wound. The dressing should be removed gently and from the edges first to avoid disrupting the healing process, particularly if there is an exudate associated with the wound that adheres to the dressing.

Wounds heal by first (primary) or second (secondary) intention. First-intention healing occurs in wounds whose edges are closely related or whose edges have been approximated by sutures, staples, or other similar means. These wounds tend to heal with less likelihood of infection, in a shorter period, and with less scar formation. This is the preferred and most effective method of healing.

Second-intention healing occurs in wounds with large surface areas, with distracted edges, or in which a large amount of tissue has been lost. These types of wounds heal by the gradual filling of the wound with granulation material. These wounds may become infected more easily, usually require an extended healing time, and are apt to exhibit excessive scar formation. When possible, these wounds are transformed into wounds that are better able to heal by the use of skin grafts, skin flaps, or other similar surgical techniques.

Several factors can affect wound healing either favorably or unfavorably. Infection or the presence of high numbers of pathogens in the wound or its surrounding tissue will delay or complicate the healing process. The size, extent, distances between the edges, location, and type of wound can all affect healing. A large, deep, irregularly shaped wound usually requires additional time to heal, as does a wound that is located where there is limited or impaired circulation (such as the shin) (Box 11-3).

The nutritional status of the person is also an important factor. A person with poor nutritional status will experience more difficulty and require a longer healing time. A wound in an elderly patient may not heal as rapidly as a similar wound in a younger adult because of differences in circulation and metabolic responses to the wound. Some medications may aid or enhance wound healing, whereas other medications may delay the healing process. The patient who has a chronic illness or who is generally debilitated probably will exhibit a delay in the healing of the wound.

Wound Classification

A wound can be classified as an abrasion, a puncture, a laceration, a burn, an incision, or an ulceration. An abrasion is a wound caused by rubbing or scraping the skin or mucous membrane. A skinned elbow or knee and a floor or carpet burn are examples of an abrasion. A puncture is a wound

Box 11-3 Factors That Affect Wound Healing

Depending on the presence or absence of the following factors, a positive or negative effect or influence on the healing of the wound may occur.

EXTRINSIC FACTORS

- Pressure applied to soft tissue that overlies a bony prominence
- Shear force applied to the skin, especially to the heels and sacrum
- Maceration of the skin caused by body waste, perspiration, or skin-to-skin contact (that is, skinfolds)
- Infection
- Reduced activity leading to prolonged immobility

INTRINSIC FACTORS

- General health of the patient
- Condition of the skin
- Body build and composition
- Nutritional status
- Hydration status
- Distance between the edges of the wound
- Location of the wound
- Adequacy of blood flow to the wound

Adapted from Morey S: *Pressure Ulcer/Wound Care*. Presented at Ohio Physical Therapy Association Annual Conference, April 17, 1997. Columbus, OH.

caused by a pointed object or instrument. Wounds from nails, pinpoints, or bullets are examples of a puncture wound. A laceration is a wound produced by the tearing of body tissue. A blow from a blunt object or an injury caused by a machine is likely to be a laceration.

A burn is caused when the skin contacts dry heat (fire), moist heat (steam), chemicals, electricity, or radiation. Burns are classified according to their depth and size. A burn may be described as superficial, partial thickness, deep partial thickness, or full thickness. When the upper layer of the epidermis is affected, the wound is superficial; when the lower layers of the epidermis are involved, the wound is a partial-thickness wound; and when the dermis is affected, the wound becomes a full-thickness wound.

An incision is a cut or wound made by a sharp instrument such as a scalpel. An ulceration is the result of an excavation of the surface of an organ or tissue, which is produced by the *sloughing* (that is, falling away) of necrotic inflammatory tissue. Skin ulcers are often located on the distal lower extremities, especially in the area of the malleoli. A pressure ulcer may develop in the tissue that covers a bony prominence (such as the sacrum, calcaneus, greater trochanter) when relief of pressure at the site does not occur.)

The preceding information is limited in its scope and comprehensiveness, but it provides a basic description of the process of wound healing and its relationship to wound management. The reader should refer to other sources listed in the Bibliography for additional information about the wound-healing process.

Box 11-4 Primary Risk Factors Associated with Pressure Ulcers

Pressure to tissue overlying bony prominences, especially the sacrum, heels, greater trochanters, and ischial tuberosities.
Shear and friction forces applied to the skin.
Inadequate or improper nutrition, including appropriate and adequate fluid intake.
Insensitive body areas, especially those insensitive to pressure.
Persistent incontinence, which leads to skin irritation, maceration, or breakdown.
Metabolic or systemic disorders or diseases, especially diabetes.
Persistent use of tobacco products.

Pressure Ulcers

A pressure ulcer, incorrectly referred to as a decubitus ulcer, pressure sore, or bedsore, is one type of wound that can complicate the care of many patients. Although a pressure ulcer may be prevented through an aggressive treatment plan of ongoing skin care, frequent changes in the patient's position, proper and adequate nutrition, and the relief of or reduction in pressure to the soft tissue that overlies bony prominences, there is no assurance that these activities will prevent the development of one or more pressure ulcers. The patient's age, body condition and composition, and disease state; the presence of circulation or metabolic disorders; and the mobility capability of the patient are factors that contribute to the risk of pressure ulcers. Therefore each caregiver who treats the patient must be involved with the prevention of pressure ulcers (Box 11-4).

Causes A pressure ulcer is a wound that develops as a result of two primary factors: (1) pressure to soft tissue that exceeds the normal capillary pressure of the local circulation and (2) shear force to superficial skin. The soft tissue located over a bony prominence, especially the greater trochanter, sacrum, calcaneus, malleolus, and ischial tuberosity, are sites where a pressure ulcer is most likely to occur. In those areas, the capillaries that transport oxygen and nutrients to and remove waste products from the tissue become compressed between the underlying bone and the external pressure source. (*Note:* Table 5-1 presents the locations at which pressure ulcers are most likely to develop depending on the patient's position.) When the capillaries are compressed for a period, they become occluded, ischemia occurs, and the potential for tissue *necrosis* exists. If necrosis does occur, tissue is destroyed, and a partial- or full-thickness wound will be evident.

Contributing factors in the development of a pressure ulcer are a shear force or friction applied to the patient's skin, which may occur during position changes, transfers, or exercise activities. A shear force created by the caregiver's hand or the bed linen may produce friction to the skin, which causes increased surface heat and erosion of the epidermis. The combination of prolonged pressure and episodes of shear force applied to the same area of the body causes trauma to the capillaries, skin, and underlying soft tissue and a pressure ulcer can develop (see Box 11-3).

Patient Assessment Each patient who is admitted to a health care facility or treated at home should be assessed to determine the potential risk to develop a pressure ulcer. In addition, the person's functional abilities such as bed mobility, activity level, wheelchair or ambulatory mobility, feeding, chewing and swallowing capability, and transfer performance should be determined. Information about previous and current medical history, level of mental competence, nutritional status, skin condition, general physical condition, and psychosocial factors are other components of the initial assessment. Identification of specific risk factors should be one of the major outcomes of the initial assessment and examination.

Risk Factors Some of the risk factors related to the development of a pressure ulcer are presented in Box 11-4. A risk assessment at the time of admission of a patient to any health care facility or when the person is treated at home by a health care practitioner is a standard of care recommended by several agencies or regulatory bodies, including the Agency for Health Care Policy and Research (AHCPR); National Pressure Ulcer Advisory Panel (NPUAP); Omnibus Budget Reconciliation Act (OBRA); Association for the Advancement of Wound Care (AAWC); and the Wound, Ostomy, Continence Nurses Society (WOCN). The patient who is at risk to develop pressure ulcers should be identified at admission, the risk factors should be documented, and a prevention program should be initiated promptly. Every person who has contact with the patient, such as housekeeping personnel, family members, aides, and technicians, in addition to primary caregivers, should be considered members of the prevention team. These individuals are able to observe the patient several times during the day; therefore observations, comments, or suggestions from nonprimary caregivers can be helpful to the primary caregivers. Prevention should be a responsibility shared by multiple individuals.

Preventive Interventions Relief of pressure to the soft tissue that overlies a bony prominence is the primary method of pressure ulcer prevention. Relief of the pressure can be accomplished by elevating the area from the pressure source (such as use of a pillow beneath the calf to elevate the heel slightly from the mattress when the person is supine), by changing the patient's position frequently so an area is not in prolonged contact with a source of pressure (that is, use of a turning or positioning schedule to relieve weight bearing on a specific bony prominence), or by positioning the patient so an area is not in contact with a source of pressure (that is, position the patient in a partial side-lying position with the use of pillows or foam wedges so the person does not rest directly on the lowermost greater trochanter) and to separate bony prominences. If the patient is able to independently alter position, instruction on how and when to do so should be provided (that is, perform pushups or lean to one side and then to the other while seated in a wheelchair; lift the pelvis from the mattress using the lower extremities when supine; use a trapeze to elevate the upper body from the mattress when supine). These activities should be performed several times per hour.

Pressure reduction is another preventive method by which the amount of pressure to an area is decreased, but not fully relieved. Air-fluidized, low-air-loss, eggcrate foam, closed cell foam mattress overlays or oscillating beds; air or water mattresses; seat cushions (*Caution:* Do not use the ring, "donut" type of cushion because the rim of the cushion will create pressure, which is apt to occlude capillaries and deprive the local tissue of a proper blood supply and flow); bony joint protectors (that is, heel or elbow guards); and wound protection dressings are examples of pressure reduction aids or approaches. Shear force and friction can be reduced if a draw sheet is used to position or transfer a patient; double socks are used to protect the heels; the head of the bed is elevated to the lowest level of comfort and function for the patient (that is, at approximately 30 degrees of elevation; the patient will tend to slide down over the bed linen, creating shear to the sacrum and scapulae); the patient is instructed to avoid rubbing the heels or elbows on the bed linen when lying supine; and the patient is not dragged across the bed linen when turned, positioned, or transferred (Box 11-5).

Skin Care Frequent inspection of and attention to care of a patient's skin, particularly for the patient who is incontinent, are important preventive activities. Prompt cleansing of the skin; maintenance of dry, clean skin of the perineum, buttocks, and upper thighs; and the use of topical agents to provide a moisture barrier or moisturize dry skin may be necessary for many patients. In addition, the use of lubricants, protective dressings (that is, films, hydrocolloids, hydrogels), and paddings should help minimize shear and friction. *Caution:* Massage of the tissue that overlies a bony prominence should be avoided because it may traumatize the local capillaries, which are apt to be fragile and susceptible to injury.

Caregivers whose treatment requires handling of the extremities, especially the upper extremities, should be aware of the possibility of causing a skin tear when treating elderly patients because their skin tends to be fragile. A skin tear should be assessed and measured before treatment. The area should be cleaned gently with normal saline solution, and the wound edges should be dried by patting the area with gauze. Small pieces of detached epithelium that appear to be traumatized can be debrided by a qualified caregiver and skin that appears to be viable and nontraumatized should be repositioned gently over the wound. A nonadherent dressing should be applied and covered with a protective bandage.

Box 11-5 Guidelines for Pressure Ulcer Intervention and Management

Provide pressure relief or reduction to the body areas susceptible to ulcer development.
Develop and follow a schedule to alter patient position as one method to accomplish the previous guideline.
Determine the nutritional and fluid intake needs of the patient; establish an appropriate diet and feeding schedule to meet the needs.
Initiate mobility activities for the patient that are possible, safe, and appropriate; include bed, wheelchair, and ambulation activities. Shear forces must be avoided.
Perform debridement of necrotic tissue, as necessary, to promote healing.
Perform wound and skin cleansing as necessary; avoid the use of toxic agents, including many types of soaps, hydrogen peroxide, and povidone-iodine (Betadine).
Perform consistent and thorough perineal care, especially when the patient is incontinent.
Rinse the ulcer with a sterile saline solution with an appropriate pressure at the time of dressing changes.
Develop and follow a schedule to observe, evaluate, remove, and apply dressings that is appropriate for the patient and personnel involved.
Provide education to all caregivers involved with the patient's care, including the patient's family members; include information on prevention, care, and management.
Plan and follow a program designed to prevent the development of pressure ulcers, especially for persons who demonstrate a high risk of developing pressure ulcers.

All caregivers should avoid activities or procedures that intensify the established risk factors for a given patient. Prolonged, excessive pressure over time to areas of bony prominences and shear and friction forces must be avoided during exercise, transfers, mobility activities, and turning or positioning of the patient. Straps used to attach splints or orthoses must not be applied too tightly and footwear must fit properly to avoid friction or blister development. The caregiver must be aware of the potential for injury or damage to the patient's skin and must adjust the treatment program to avoid trauma to it (Table 11-1).

Wound Classification and Staging A pressure ulcer should be assessed and classified according to its stage or level of tissue destruction. The stage designation also provides a diagnosis of the amount or type of tissue insult and injury that has occurred. If the epidermis and a portion of the dermis are involved, the wound is considered to be a partial-thickness wound, and the ulcer is considered to be superficial. When the entire dermis and underlying fascia, muscle tendon, or bone are involved, the wound is considered to be a full-thickness wound, and the ulcer is considered to be deep (Fig. 11-2). Box 11-6 lists and describes the four stages associated with a pressure ulcer. These stages can be described as being progressive: Stage I becomes Stage II and Stage II becomes Stage III; however, the stages cannot be described regressively. That is, as a Stage III ulcer heals, it does not revert to Stage II. Instead, as a Stage III wound heals, it continues to be classified as Stage III, but the percentage of the wound that has healed is reported or a measurement and description of the open area of the wound are used to indicate the improvement or healing of the wound. A wound cannot be staged if its depth cannot be measured or visualized; therefore a wound covered with *eschar*, or necrotic tissue, cannot be staged until the wound surface is exposed through *debridement* of the eschar.

Table 11-1 Goals of Wound Management Dependent on Wound Stage and Appearance

Stage	Appearance	Goals
I	Erythema that does not blanch when pressure is intact	Remove, relieve pressure, keep area clean; avoid friction and shear forces.
II, III	Granulation/nondraining	Maintain moist wound bed; protect surrounding tissue; observe for infection.
II, III	Granulation/draining	Maintain moist wound bed; protect surrounding tissue; observe for infection; absorb exudate.
IV	Necrotic/nondraining	Maintain moist wound bed; protect surrounding tissue; observe for infection; soften and remove eschar, necrotic tissue.
IV	Necrotic/draining	Maintain moist wound bed; protect surrounding tissue; observe for infection; absorb exudate.
II, III, IV	Infected wound	Protect the surrounding tissue; absorb exudate, and contain infection.

Adapted with permission from Kendall K, Porter C, Carroll C, Lamare RNC, Tilley JG: Evolution of Sacred Heart Hospital's wound assessment sheet. In *Acute Care Perspectives*, Newsletter of the Acute Care/Hospital Clinical Practice Section, Alexandria, VA: American Physical Therapy Association, Summer 1995, p. 8.

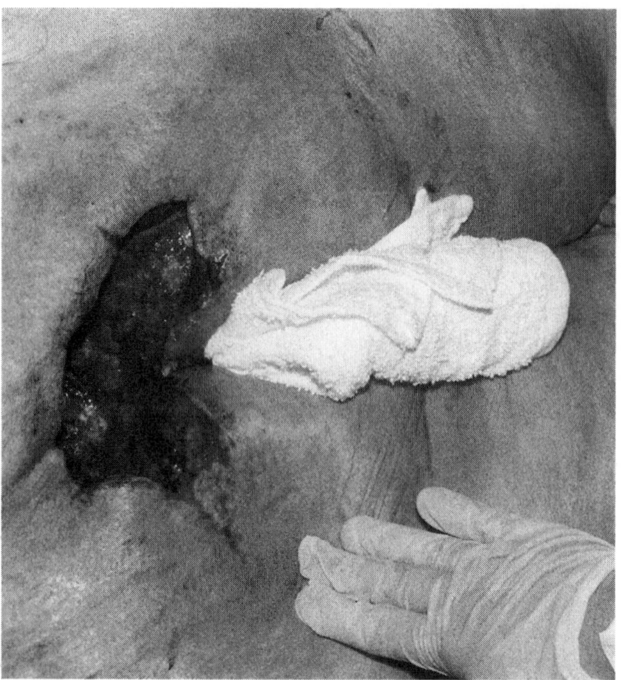

Fig. 11-2 Sacral pressure ulcer; stage III.

Box 11-7 Pressure Ulcer Assessment Factors

Identify the wound stage.
Measure the wound size.
Measure the wound depth.
Observe and describe the tissue at the wound edges.
Examine the wound for areas of tunneling or undermining; measure the length or depth.
Observe and describe the characteristics of any exudate (viscosity, amount, color).
Observe and describe the characteristics of any necrotic tissue (color, adherence, texture, consistency, amount).
Describe any wound odor.
Observe and describe the characteristics of the surrounding skin (dry, macerated, color, texture, blistered, edematous, firm, soft).
Observe and describe characteristics of wound healing:
- Granulation
- Epithelialization
- Budding
- Wound contraction

Adapted with permission from Kennedy KL: *Wound Caring*. Copyright © 1997 Professional Education Systems, Inc. (800-647-8079). No further reproduction may be made without consent from the publisher.

Box 11-6 Staging a Pressure Ulcer 

Stage I: Erythema is present, the skin is intact, and the erythema does not blanch when pressure is applied.
Stage II: Skin loss occurs, which may affect only the epidermis or may penetrate into the dermis, but not through it; the wound bed is free of necrotic tissue and usually appears moist and pink. Classified as a partial-thickness wound.
Stage III: Tissue loss that includes the epidermal and dermal skin layers with penetration into the subcutaneous tissue; some necrotic tissue may be present; tunneling or undermining may occur; an exudate may be observed; and the wound may be infected. Classified as a full-thickness wound.
Stage IV: Destruction of deep tissue such as fascia, joint tissue, and bone may be affected; necrotic tissue is likely to be present; tunneling or undermining may occur; an exudate may be observed; and the wound may be infected.
Partial thickness indicates that the epidermis and upper portion of the dermis are involved, but the wound does not reach the subcutaneous tissue; the wound is considered to be superficial. Full thickness indicates that the epidermis and entire dermis and subcutaneous tissues are involved; fascia, joint tissue, and bone may be affected; the wound is considered to be deep.

Adapted with permission from Kennedy KL: *Wound Caring*. Copyright ©1997 Professional Education Systems, Inc. (800-647-8079). No further reproduction may be made without consent from the publisher.

Wound Assessment Several methods or parameters can be used to assess many characteristics of the wound; examples are provided in Box 11-7. The size is determined by measuring the longest and widest portions of the wound. The measurements are stated in centimeters, and a disposable, plastic overlay can be used to measure the wound. The overlay should be positioned on the wound so its top is directed toward the patient's head and the measurements are made based on the configuration of the face of a clock. Length measurements are made along a line from 12 o'clock (head) to 6 o'clock (foot) and width measurements are made from 9 o'clock (left) to 3 o'clock (right).

The depth is measured by inserting a sterile cotton-tipped swab vertically into the wound until it contacts the bottom or floor of the wound. The caregiver uses a finger or thumbnail to indicate where the upper portion of the shaft of the swab exits the wound; the distance from the end of the swab to the mark on the shaft indicates the depth. The swab and plastic overlay must be discarded in a proper container immediately after each is used for a patient. A swab can be used to determine the amount of undermining of the edge of the wound or tunneling of the wound into surrounding soft tissue. A technique similar to the one described for measuring the depth can be used to measure undermining and tunneling by inserting the swab horizontally. Probing of these areas should be performed gently and cautiously because it will not be possible to observe the tissue that the swab contacts. The caregiver should wear clean, nonsterile gloves when performing these measurements.

Table 11-2 **Dressing Choices and Preferred Uses**

	Type of Dressing						
Stage or Condition	**TF**	**HC**	**HyG**	**AL**	**WD**	**WW**	**PS**
I	X	X					
II	X	X	X			X	
III		X	X	X		X	X
IV				X		X	X
Necrotic/draining				X	X	X	
Necrotic/nondraining			X		X	X	
Noninfected	X	X	X	X	X	X	
Infected				X	X	X	

In *Acute Care Perspectives*, Newsletter of the Acute Care/Hospital Clinical Practice Section, Alexandria, VA: American Physical Therapy Association, Summer 1995, p. 8.
TF = transparent film, HC = hydrocolloid, HyG = hydrogel, AL = alginate, WD = wet to dry, WW = wet to wet, and PS = packing strip.

Another assessment component is to observe and describe the color patterns or necrotic tissue of the wound and to estimate their percentage of content in the wound. Red color is indicative of the process of granulation, yellow or grayish-brown is the color of slough, and eschar will appear black. Epithelial tissue will appear to be pink and shiny and indicates that coverage of the wound by new skin is occurring. Photographs taken periodically can be used to document the condition of the wound and the surrounding tissue (skin).

Wound Care Usually, nursing personnel will be the primary caregivers responsible for the care of a pressure ulcer; however, other caregivers are involved with various aspects of wound management and care. The basic elements of wound care include debridement of necrotic tissue, wound cleaning, wound dressing, and the possible use of adjunctive therapies or interventions.

Debridement The removal of necrotic tissue from the wound allows the wound to heal more effectively. Debridement can be performed with sharp instruments (that is, scalpel, scissors), mechanically, chemically, or with *autolysis*. Sharp debridement is the most rapid method and a scalpel or scissors are used to remove thick adherent eschar and other devitalized tissue. Depending on state statutes, practice acts, and the policies and procedures of the facility, a variety of persons who have the appropriate training may legally perform sharp debridement. Mechanical debridement can be performed through pressure irrigation, the removal of dressings, hydrotherapy, electrical stimulation, a combination of hydrotherapy and ultrasonography, and the use of dextronomers. The use of enzymes to debride is another method, in which enzymes are applied to the wound, or the patient's self-produced enzymes are the active agent; this is known as autolysis, or autolytic debridement. Enzymatic debridement tends to be more effective for small areas of necrosis or when the patient is unable to tolerate other methods. Nutritional support may be necessary to promote improvement in skin condition to increase the development of subcutaneous tissue and improve or maintain the patient's metabolism. Some patients may require supplemental enteral or parenteral feedings to ensure that sufficient nutrient levels are attained.

Dressings Care of the wound usually requires the selection and application of one or more types of dressings. The purposes of the dressing are to protect the wound, assist the healing process, reduce infection or contamination of the wound, and remove exudates and toxic waste when the dressing is removed. Tables 11-2 and 11-3 present information about the selection and effects of several types of dressings. Dressings that prohibit observation of the wound may need to be removed more frequently than dressings that permit observation. Some dressings cause *maceration* of the surrounding skin and a moisture barrier may need to be applied when those dressings are used. Dressings should be removed carefully to avoid trauma to the wound surface or surrounding tissue. The wound and its surrounding skin should be observed and assessed each time a dressing is removed and documentation should be made of noticeable changes from previous observations.

Summary Pressure ulcers are caused by pressure to the soft tissue that overlies a bony prominence. When the tissue is trapped between the bony prominence and a source of external pressure, the capillaries in the tissue are occluded, leading to local ischemia and tissue necrosis. Contributing factors are shear force and friction applied to the skin. Many risk factors predispose the patient to the development of a pressure ulcer; therefore every patient, on admission to a health care facility or who is treated at home, should be assessed for these risk factors. If one or more risk factors are identified, a specific, aggressive prevention program should be initiated. Integral components of such a program are

Table 11-3 Product Selection Based on Wounds Severity

Dressing	Value/Effects
Transparent film (Bioclusive, Tegaderm, OpSite)	Dressing of choice for stages I and II wounds with blister formation over bony prominences; resists shear; may be applied to heels prophylactically; self-adherent and allows wound to be observed; may be used for autolytic debridement. Do not use on draining or infected wounds.
Hydrocolloid (Duoderm, Restore [paste or granules])	Dressing of choice for stages II and III wounds with minimal drainage; provides moist wound bed; absorbs small amount of drainage; self-adherent and provides cushioning over bony prominence. Do not use on infected wounds; medications cannot be used under the dressing.
Hydrogel (Vigilon, ClearSite, NuGel)	Recommended for stages II and III wounds with dressing covering the gel; moist wound bed is maintained; recommended for use on skin tear, cover with rolled absorbent material (Kling); may cause maceration of surrounding healthy tissue; does not protect wound from external soiling.
Wet to wet	Safe choice for unstaged wounds; use on stage II partial-thickness wounds and stages II and IV wounds; dressing will need to be changed every 8 hours to maintain moist wound base; should moisten dressing with saline solution before removal if dressing is dry to prevent bleeding and disruption of granulation bed; moisture barrier must be used on surrounding tissue to prevent maceration.
Wet to dry	Use on stages II and IV wounds for debridement; slough and necrotic tissue adhere to dressing and are removed with dressing.
Calcium alginates (CaAl) (Kaltostate, Algosteril)	Use to absorb heavy drainage but will require a secondary dressing to cover the CaAl; may be used on infected wounds.

Adapted with permission from Kendall K et al: Evolution of Sacred Heart Hospital's wound assessment sheet. In *Acute Care Perpspectives*, Newsletter of the Acute Care/Hospital Clinical Practice Section, Alexandria, VA: American Physical Therapy Association, Summer 1995, p. 8.

Box 11-8 Pressure Ulcer Documentation Guidelines

Describe the site or location of the ulcer.
Identify the stage of the ulcer based on the classification system of the NPUAP.
Measure and report the size of the total surface area of the ulcer.
Measure and report the depth of the ulcer.
Determine the evidence or extent of ulcer tunnels or undermined areas; report tissue destruction underlying intact skin along the margins of the ulcer; measure the width and length.
Estimate and describe the percentage of color (black, red, yellow) and the percentage of the ulcer covered with new skin; describe the composition of the ulcer (such as granulation and epithelialized tissue).
Estimate and describe the type and amount of exudate (such as viscosity, color, consistency).
Describe the odor associated with the ulcer after it has been rinsed with sterile saline solution.
Observe for and report whether edema or induration exists in the tissue surrounding the periphery of the ulcer.
Observe for and report whether signs of inflammation are present in the tissue surrounding the ulcer; measure and report the area in which signs appear.
Observe and describe the condition of the skin surrounding the ulcer (such as dry, moist, loose, taut, warm, discolored).

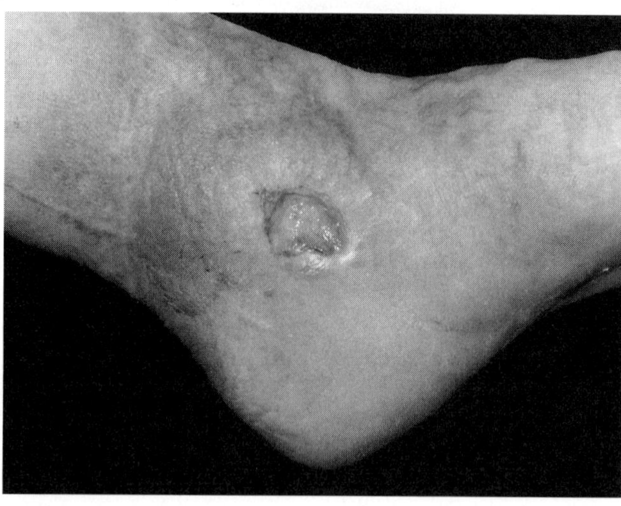

Fig. 11-3 Stasis ulcer; stage III (healing). Located at left medial malleolus.

proper skin care, pressure relief or reduction, proper positioning, and frequent position changes.

If a pressure ulcer occurs, it should be classified and described accurately and objectively so appropriate documentation can be made (Box 11-8). Wound care such as debridement, the use of dressings, and proper nutrition are important aspects of treatment. An interdisciplinary care

Box 11-9 Peripheral Venous and Arterial Circulation Tests

VENOUS SUFFICIENCY TESTS

Percussion Test

Used to assess the function of the values of the saphenous vein.

With the patient standing, the caregiver palpates a proximal segment of the saphenous vein with the fingers of one hand; then uses the fingers of the other hand to tap (percuss) a distal segment of the vein.

A fluid movement will be sensed by the fingers on the proximal segment during percussion if the valves are not functioning properly.

Both lower extremities can be tested and the results are compared.

Deep Vein Thrombophlebitis Test

Used to assess the possible presence of a thrombus.

The caregiver grasps and squeezes the patient's calf while passively forcing the foot into dorsiflexion. If the patient complains of pain in the calf, a positive response is reported; this is known as a positive Homans' sign.

Another method is to apply a blood pressure cuff around the patient's calf and to inflate it gradually; a patient with an acute condition would not tolerate an inflation pressure higher than 40 mm Hg; once the pain threshold has been reached, do not further inflate the cuff; test the noninvolved lower extremity first if only one extremity is suspected of having a deep vein thrombosis.

ARTERIAL SUFFICIENCY TESTS

Rubor of Dependency Test

Used to evaluate the arterial circulation by observing skin color changes that occur with the lower extremity elevated and level.

When the patient is supine, observe and record the color of the plantar surface of the foot (normal = pinkish); elevate the lower extremity approximately 45 to 60 degrees for 1 minute (abnormal = rapid loss of color).

Return the extremity to level; observe and record the color of the plantar surface (normal = rapid pink flush; abnormal = 30 seconds or longer for color to appear; color will be bright red).

Venous Filling Time Test

Used to determine the length of time required for superficial veins to refill, after they have been emptied, as a result of arterial flow through the capillaries into the veins (*Note:* Patient must have a normal venous system).

The patient is supine and the lower extremities are elevated 45 to 60 degrees for 1 minute; then the legs are dangled over the edge of the bed or table; refilling of the veins is observed and timed (normal = 10 to 15 seconds for refilling).

Claudication

Used to measure the length of time a patient can walk before claudication is experienced.

The patient walks on a level-grade treadmill at 1 mile per hour until claudication occurs; the time elapsed is recorded when calf pain prevents continuation of walking.

The test can be repeated at specified intervals and the time elapsed values can be compared.

Adapted from Morey S: *Pressure Ulcer/Wound Care*. Presented at the Ohio Physical Therapy Associated Annual Conference, April 17, 1997. Columbus, OH; O'Sullivan SB, Schmitz TJ: *Physical Rehabilitation Assessment and Treatment*, 3rd edition. Philadelphia: F.A. Davis, 1994.

team should be established to maximize the care and management of the patient and the wound.

Peripheral Vascular Conditions

Wounds caused by venous or arterial insufficiency or diabetes should be differentiated from a pressure ulcer. In some instances, the location and appearance of the wound will be sufficient to determine the type of wound and its cause. For example, a wound located directly over a bony prominence is suggestive of a pressure ulcer; a wound located in the area of the medial malleolus accompanied with edema and dark, dusky skin discoloration is suggestive of a venous insufficiency wound (Fig. 11-3); and a small wound located near the ankle accompanied by localized edema is suggestive of an arterial insufficiency wound or a wound caused by diabetes.

Several assessment methods or tests are available to evaluate the status of venous and arterial circulation in the lower extremity. Peripheral venous circulation dysfunction can be caused by defective or deficient valves, occlusion of the veins, or limited function of the "calf-pumping" mechanism. Usually, peripheral arterial circulation dysfunction is attributable to some form of occlusion of arteries, which is associated with atherosclerosis. Both circulatory systems may exhibit acute or chronic conditions. Some tests that can be performed to determine the function of the venous and arterial peripheral circulation are presented in Boxes 11-9 and 11-10. Other evaluative procedures are examination of the patient's skin, measurement of the skin temperature, palpation of the pulse at various sites, evaluation of sensation, auscultation of an artery, and measurement of blood pressure. Doppler ultrasonography and air plethysmography may be performed, but they require specific training and special equipment.

Treatment procedures or activities for these types of wounds are beyond the scope of this text. However, the caregiver should be aware of the responsibility to notify the

Box 11-10 General Assessment Activities for Peripheral Vascular Conditions

OBJECTIVE ACTIVITIES

Skin Examination

Observe color and compare with that of opposite extremity.
Observe the condition of the skin (dry, scaly, flexible, firm, loose, adherent, moist, presence of exudate).
Palpate to sense temperature, edema, and general condition.
Observe for absence of hair.
Evaluate superficial sensation; use objects with different textures; apply light pressure; use a monofilament "feeler."

Measure Skin Temperature

Use a thermistor with a probe; measure temperature at various sites or locations along the extremity.
Compare values with those obtained from similar sites or locations on the opposite extremity.

Palpate Pulses

Evaluate all major arterial pulses; refer to techniques and procedures in Chapter 3.
Evaluate the quality and rate.
Compare findings of involved extremity with those of noninvolved extremity.

Auscultation

Use a stethoscope to listen for blood flow in the major arteries of the neck, abdomen, groin, and extremities.
Listen for a swishlike sound, which indicates fluid turbulence known as bruit; a narrow vessel lumen will produce turbulence.

Blood Pressure

Perform measurement on both upper extremities; use a proper size cuff.
Follow the techniques and procedures presented in Chapter 3.

Edema

Observe for and measure edema using palpation, girth, or volumetric measurements.
Compare values obtained from involved extremity with values of noninvolved extremity.
Remeasure periodically to determine whether edema is regressing, progressing, or static.

SUBJECTIVE INFORMATION

Obtain past history of the current condition from the patient or a family member.
Obtain specific information about the current condition or a previous similar or different condition and the effects or result of previous treatments.
Determine personal habits that may affect the condition (that is, eating habits, use of tobacco, reaction to heat or cold, sensory changes).

Adapted from O'Sullivan SB, Schmitz TJ: *Physical Rehabilitation Assessment and Treatment*, 3rd edition. Philadelphia: F.A. Davis, 1994.

patient's physician when one of these conditions is identified. For most patients, prompt medical care and management of any condition that affects the peripheral venous or arterial circulation will be necessary to prevent a serious complication.

Dressings and Bandages

The composition of a dressing and its bandage varies, but in many instances several layers are involved. As an example, a topical medication may be applied directly to the wound, with a nonabsorbent material (such as a Telfa pad) placed over the medication with a second layer consisting of a cotton gauze pad; for large wounds or wounds that exhibit excessive drainage, a third layer of an absorbent material may be used. These three layers make up the dressing.

A fourth layer of a material such as roller gauze and a fifth layer of a material such as an elastic wrap may be used as a bandage. Depending on the purpose of or need for the dressing, the type of wound, and the purpose of or need for the bandage, various layers may be omitted or added. However, you should be able to differentiate the purposes or functions of a dressing and a bandage.

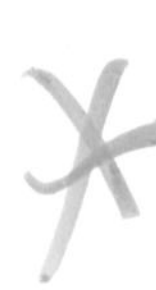

The functions of a dressing are to prevent additional wound contamination, keep microorganisms in the wound from infecting other sites, prevent further injury to the wound, apply pressure to control hemorrhage, absorb wound drainage, and assist in wound healing.

The functions of a bandage are to keep the dressing in place, maintain a barrier between the dressing and the environment, provide external pressure to control swelling, provide support or stability to an area, hold splints in place, and assist the dressing to accomplish its functions.

Removal of a Dressing The caregiver should presume that the wound and dressing are contaminated and therefore should apply nonsterile gloves (that is, use a clean technique) before removing the dressing for self-protection. Once the gloved hand has touched the dressing or the wound, it must not touch any other object, especially the patient or caregiver's skin, the clean (sterile) dressing, or any other object in the area. Once the dressing has been removed, it and the gloves should be discarded in a closed container or nonporous bag. The caregiver should remove the gloves without touching the outside of either glove with any exposed skin as described previously. Immediately after the removal and disposal of the gloves, the caregiver must wash the hands to further reduce the possibility of cross-contamination.

To remove a nonadherent dressing, the bandage may be removed independently of the dressing or with the dressing. If you are unfamiliar with the site and shape of the wound,

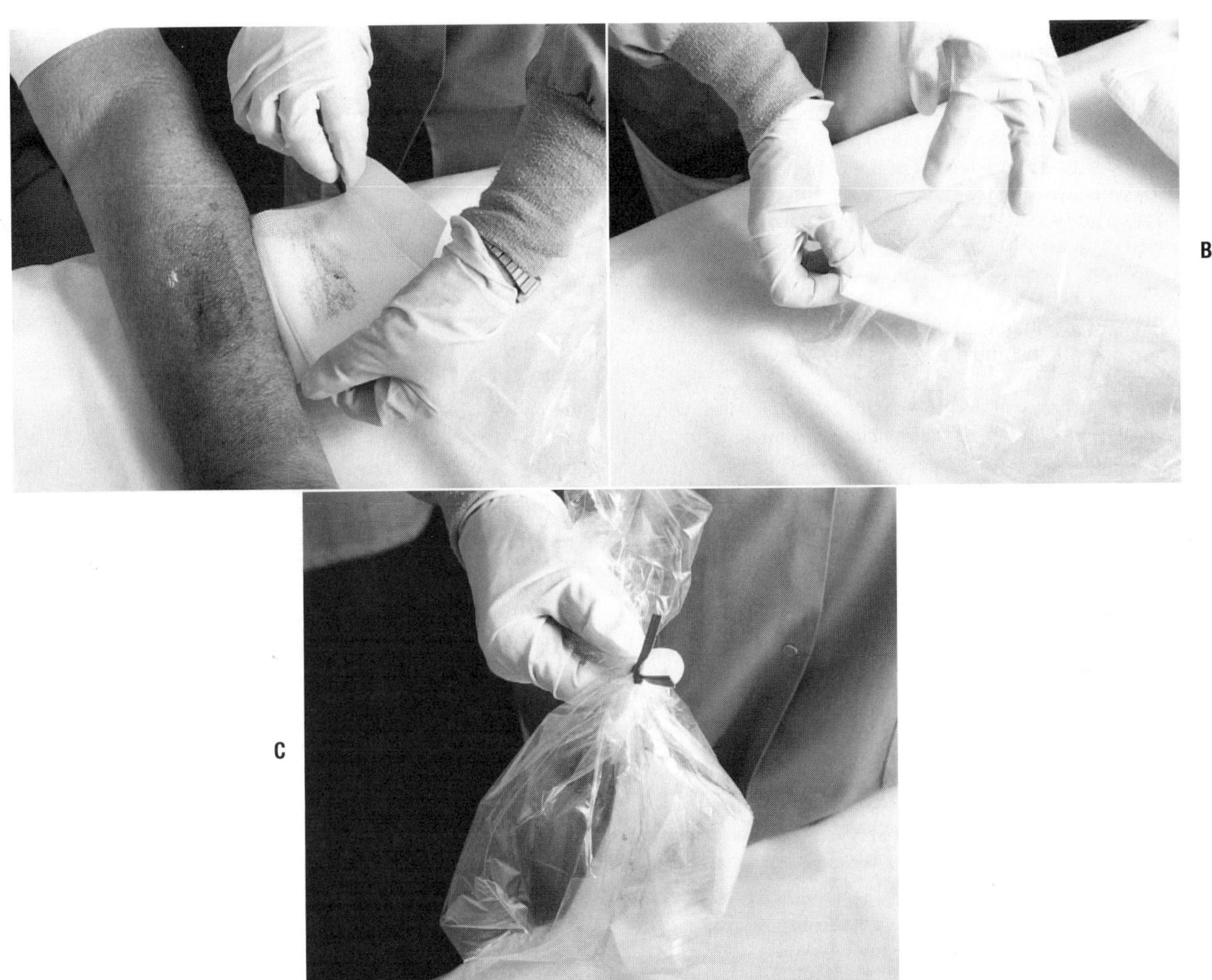

Fig. 11-4 Removal and disposal of a dressing.

request information about it from the patient or other personnel who are familiar with it. The patient may be able to indicate the size and location of the wound on the corresponding extremity or on the caregiver's extremity. Bandage scissors are used to cut through the various layers of the bandage. The blunt tip of the scissors is placed under the edge of the material so it is next to the patient's skin. The initial cut should be made a safe distance from any edge or from the center of the wound. If you are uncertain where or how to cut the dressing, attempt to unwrap or remove the bandage without using scissors to expose the dressing; then carefully remove the dressing layers. As you remove the bandage and dressing materials, mentally note how many layers there are, the materials used, and the sequence of application of the materials. By doing this, you will be prepared to reapply the dressing properly.

The deepest layer of the dressing should be removed by carefully loosening and freeing the dressing from the wound edges and gently pulling it toward the center of the wound; this method disrupts the healing process least. After the dressing has been removed, all dressing materials and your gloves should be discarded in a closed container as described previously and you should wash your hands before you perform any other activity (Fig. 11-4).

When the wound has been exposed, its condition should be evaluated carefully (Box 11-11). Wearing nonsterile gloves, the caregiver should gently and carefully palpate the tissue in the area of the wound to determine the following:

- Temperature of the wound tissue in comparison with the temperature of tissue away from the wound on the same or another extremity
- Tone of the tissue
- Integrity of the wound edges or the area of healing
- Condition of the skin (such as dry, moist, pliable, or tau
- Sensory response or capacity of the tissue

Your observations and findings should be reporte documented using specific and objective terms. A r physician should be notified if you observe advers

Box 11-11 Wound Evaluation

Observe and palpate the condition of the skin surrounding the wound and record your findings.
Observe and record the color of the tissue surrounding the wound.
Observe and record the color and appearance of the wound.
If an exudate is present, note the type and amount.
Determine whether there is an odor; if so, indicate what the odor is and how pervasive it is.
Determine whether there are signs of inflammation or infection.
Determine whether there are signs of pressure or irritation.
Determine whether there is edema or swelling; if so, observe where it is located and in what amount.
State the location and measure the size and depth of the wound.
Determine the type of wound or lesion (such as abrasion, puncture, laceration, burn, incision, ulceration).

or a regression in the healing process or condition of the wound since your previous observation of the wound. Gloves should be worn whenever dressings are changed.

To remove a dressing that adheres to the wound, it may be necessary to soak the bandage and dressing first to reduce disruption of the healing surface of the wound when the dressing is removed. This can be accomplished by soaking the area in a basin, whirlpool, tub, or other similar container. An alternative method is to pour water or a saline solution over the bandage and dressing repeatedly until the hardened exudate has softened. The actual removal of the dressing should be performed as described previously. If a whirlpool is used, the turbine should not be activated until the dressing has been removed from the water. Removal of the dressing material before the turbine is turned on will prevent it from being drawn into the turbine or occluding the drain when the water is released. If edema is associated with the wound, the use of a whirlpool may increase production and decrease removal of excess interstitial fluid (edema) because of the warmth of the water and the dependent position of the extremity when it is immersed.

...plication of a Sterile Dressing After the removal of ...dage and dressing, the wound may require care to en- ...ealing. Before a new dressing can be applied, ...may need to be removed from the surface of ... the process of debridement. Debride- ...ed by gently rubbing the surface of ...se of pulsatile lavage with suc- ...ace of the wound, using a ...el or scissors to excise the ...of the specific methods and ... wound is beyond the scope of this text. Debridement may or may not require the approval of a physician before a caregiver other than a physician can perform it. In many situations, only the physician will be permitted to perform wound debridement. *Note:* Regardless of the method used, the wound should not bleed during or after the debridement process.

A sterile field, with the appropriate wound care materials, should be established and the caregiver should wear sterile, protective clothing appropriate for the patient's condition. If it is necessary to dry the patient's skin before the dressing is applied, a sterile towel should be used. The patient should be positioned to be comfortable and so the wound is accessible (Fig. 11-5, *A* through *C*). *Note:* For some wounds, a clean rather than a sterile technique may be used; facility protocols and policies and procedures should always be followed.

Medications can be applied directly to the wound or to the dressing material and then onto the wound. Medication in a tube or jar should be applied to a cotton swab, gauze pad, or other acceptable applicator and then applied to the wound. The sterile applicator must not contact the unsterile exterior of the tube or jar and care must be used to avoid contaminating the contents of the tube or jar with the applicator once it has contacted the patient (Fig. 11-5, *D* and *E*). Therefore a new swab or gauze pad should be used each time the medication is obtained from the tube or jar.

Select the appropriate dressing material and apply it directly to the medication base over the wound. Be certain you maintain its sterility as it is applied by handling it with sterile gloves or sterile forceps (Fig. 11-5, *F*). Once the initial layer has been applied over the wound, the upper layers of the dressing and the bandage do not need to be applied using sterile technique. Cover the dressing with the appropriate bandage and evaluate the tension, location, and coverage of the bandage. The bandage should have sufficient tension to secure the dressing and control edema, if edema is present or anticipated, but it must not occlude or impede the local circulation. You may have to question the patient about the tension or you can slide a finger under the outer edges of the bandage to determine the tension force.

Some suggestions for the proper application and evaluation of a bandage are listed in Box 11-12. Some indicators of an improperly applied or functioning bandage are the following:

- If the color of the segment distal to the bandage becomes excessively red, blue, or pale, the bandage is usually too tight and is constricting the local circulation.
- If the patient complains of pain, numbness, tingling, or a burning sensation in the segment distal to the bandage, the bandage is usually too tight and is affecting local neural receptors.
- If the exposed distal segment feels cold to the touch when compared with the similar, opposite segment, the bandage is usually too tight proximally and is constricting the flow of arterial blood to the area.

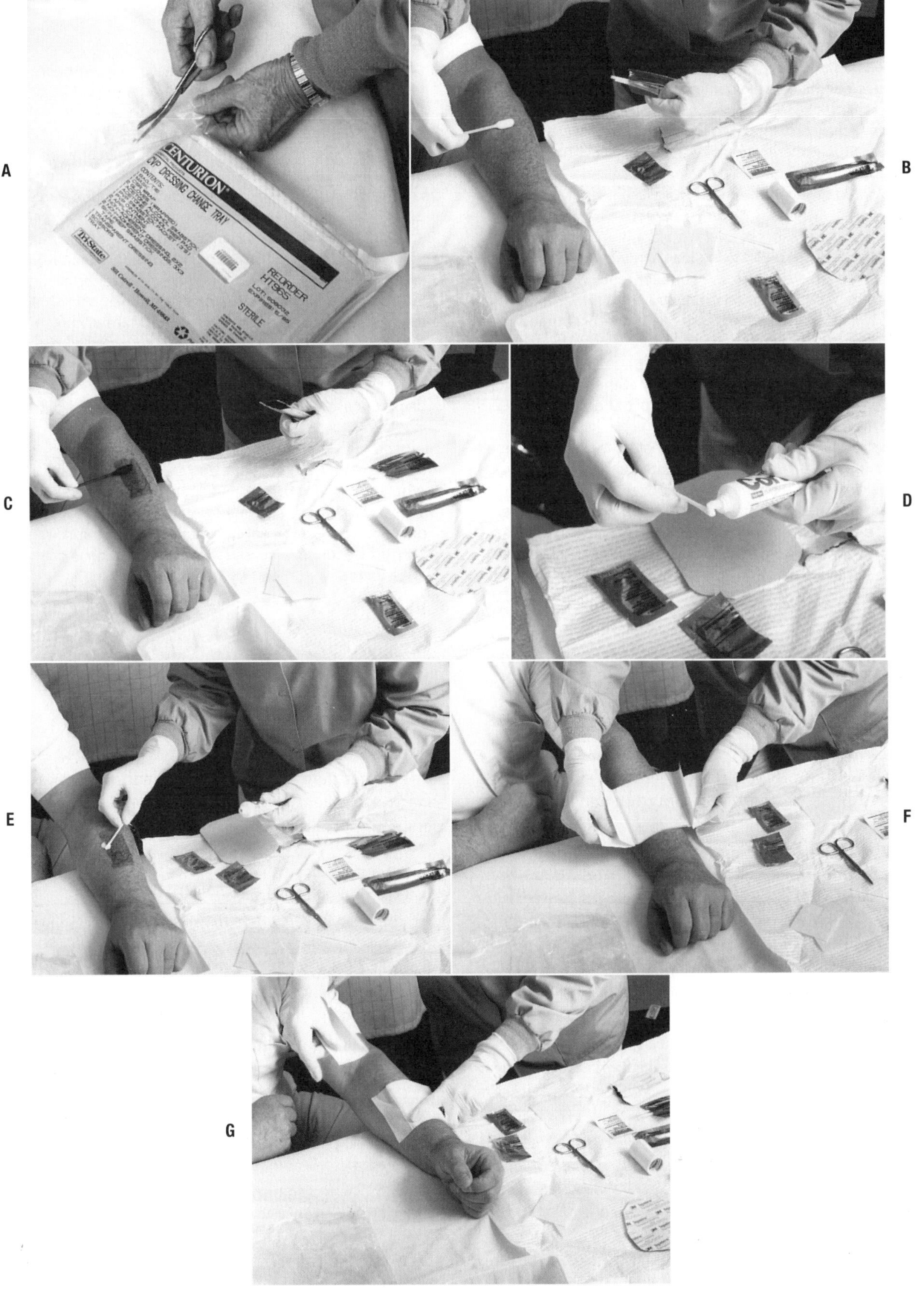

Fig. 11-5 Application of a sterile dressing.

Box 11-12 Guidelines for Applying Bandages

The tension at each turn of the bandage should be equal unless edema is to be controlled. To control edema, the general guideline is to have slightly greater pressure distally than proximally so the edema is passively moved toward the proximal areas of the extremity. This can be accomplished with a low stretch compression bandage providing gradually decreasing pressure from distal to proximal.

Spiral turns are preferred over circular turns because they are less likely to occlude the local circulation.

Each turn should overlap approximately one half of the previous turn to produce pressure and protect the wound.

Avoid wrinkles in the deep layers of the bandage to reduce unnecessary local pressure to the skin caused by the wrinkles.

Bony prominences should be wrapped with caution to avoid excessive pressure; it may be helpful to pad around, but not over, the prominence to reduce pressure to it.

The patient's fingers or toes should not be included in the bandage unless the wound is located on them. They should be visible so they can be observed for signs of excessive pressure such as edema, cyanosis, or temperature change. The patient should be instructed to inform the caregiver if numbness, tingling, or paresthesia develops in the fingers or toes.

Avoid bandaging techniques that cause or create direct contact between two skin surfaces. Use a small gauze or cotton pad between the fingers and toes to separate them. Failure to separate a skin-to-skin contact may lead to skin breakdown because of the effects of the accumulation of moisture and heat.

Do not secure the bandage directly over the wound, over a bony prominence, or where the patient's body weight is apt to rest on the item securing the bandage. If tape is used to secure the bandage, it should not completely encircle the extremity or the segment where the wound is located and it should not be applied to the patient's skin if the bandage will be removed frequently. Safety pins and metal clips must be applied carefully to avoid injury to the patient during and after application. When a safety pin is used, the caregiver should insert a finger under the bandage to elevate it off the patient's skin and avoid puncturing the skin with the pin.

The bandage used to cover a dressing should extend approximately 1 inch above and below the dressing.

The bandage should be removed and reapplied if it turns, slides down or up, becomes wet, or becomes soiled with drainage or if the patient complains of discomfort. Whenever the bandage is removed and the dressing is changed, observe the wound and the surrounding tissue.

- If edema develops in the segment distal to the bandage, the bandage is usually too tight and is constricting the local lymphatic and venous circulation.
- If the bandage changes position, it is usually too loose.

When any of these conditions occurs, the bandage should be removed and reapplied. The patient should be informed of these problems and should become responsible for monitoring the bandage when not being treated or under the direct care of another person. After the bandage has been applied, the caregiver should evaluate the bandage to determine how well it has been applied. The proximally and distally exposed areas of tissue should be observed and palpated; the patient should be questioned about the sensations perceived in the extremity; and the tension of the bandage should be tested. This last activity can be accomplished by simultaneously inserting a finger beneath the deepest layer of the bandage at the proximal and distal edges of the bandage. The pressure should be essentially equal at both sites or slightly greater distally than proximally.

The patient or a family member should be instructed to evaluate the bandage periodically and to remove and reapply it when any of the signs or symptoms of improper application are evident. The length of time the bandage should remain in place; when it should be routinely removed, such as for bathing, for exercise, or if it becomes wet; and how long it can remain removed before it is reapplied should be explained to the patient. You should instruct the patient how to remove and apply the bandage. By observing the patient's performance, you can be more certain the person understands and can perform the procedure. Written instructions may be useful for the patient and the family.

Bandages may be applied and used for purposes other than to cover and protect a dressing. Additional applications and uses and types of bandage materials are presented in Chapter 12.

GIRTH MEASUREMENT

Girth measurement of an extremity to serially measure its circumference is a technique used to evaluate the presence of edema or atrophy. Possible indications for the measurement of the calf or thigh include anterior compartment syndrome, deep venous thrombosis, shin splints or a ruptured gastrocnemius or soleus muscle in the calf, and a ruptured or strained hamstring or quadriceps muscle in the thigh (Fig. 11-6). Indications for upper extremity measurement would include fractures of the humerus, radius, or ulna and severe tennis elbow. Possible causes for atrophy would be postfracture where a cast or splint was necessary for immobilization or from certain muscle disorders such as myotonia dystrophy or amyotrophic lateral sclerosis (ALS). When measuring the upper and lower extremities, measurements should be taken bilaterally for those patients with atrophy or edema in the limb(s) for a base comparison.

A plastic or metal anthropometric measuring tape is recommended for these measurements because these types of

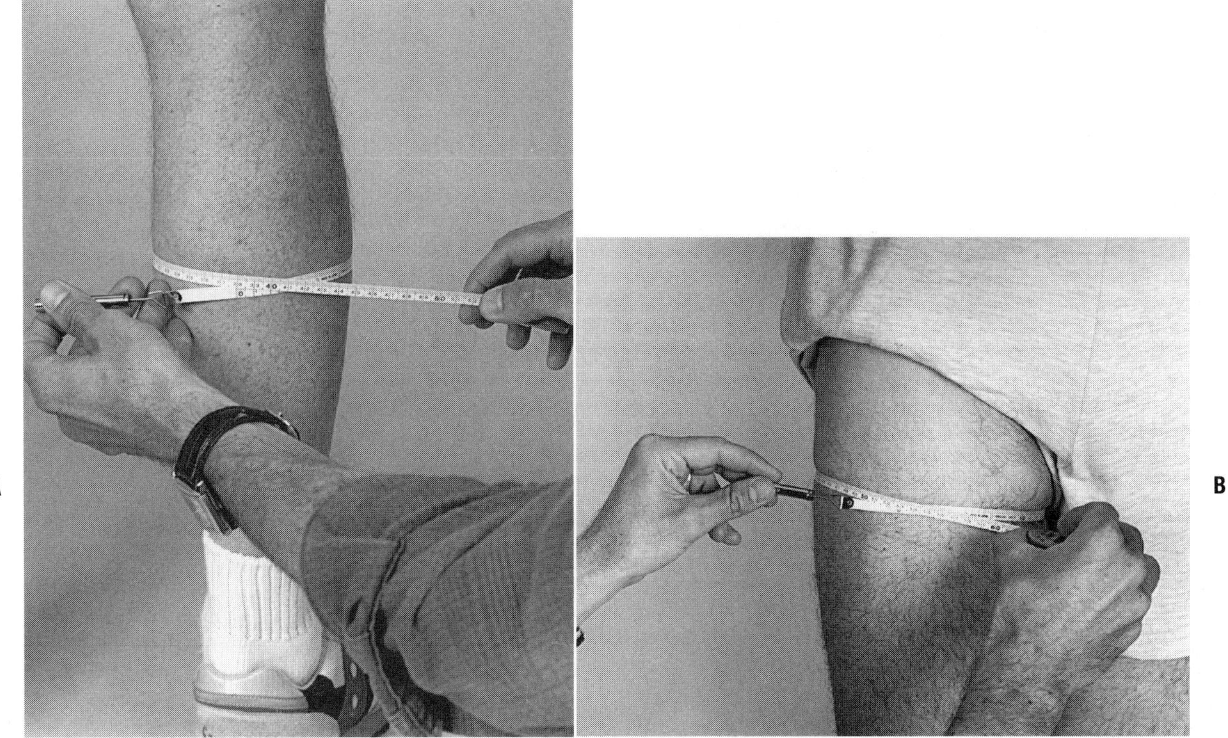

Fig. 11-6 **A,** Girth measurement: calf. **B,** Girth measurement: upper thigh.

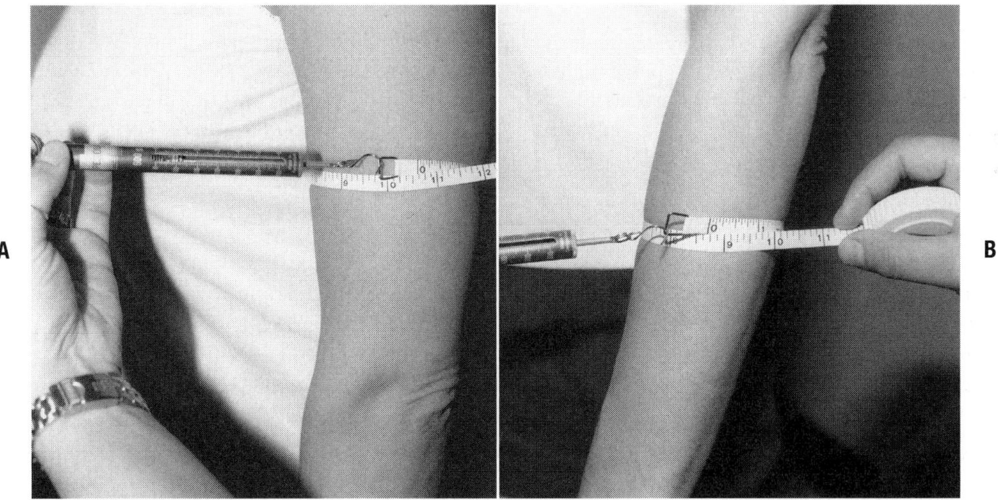

Fig. 11-7 **A,** Girth measurement: upper arm. **B,** Girth measurement: forearm.

tapes will not deteriorate, they are easy to clean, and their calibration marks can be read easily. For lower extremity measurement, the patient should stand on a level surface with feet approximately 6 inches apart, body relaxed. When measuring the upper extremity, expose the extremity in a position of relaxation. Explain the procedure to the patient for either measurement (Fig.11-7). Wrap the anthropometric measuring tape horizontally around the area where the greatest or least amount of girth appears using sufficient pressure to maintain contact with the skin without causing an excessive indentation in the skin. A tension gauge (Fig. 11-8) should be used, if available, when measuring all sites to ensure consistent pressure on the tape. Two measurements to the nearest 0.25 inch should be made at the site and the average of the two is used as the reporting value. A skin-marking pencil can be used to mark the level or location at the base of

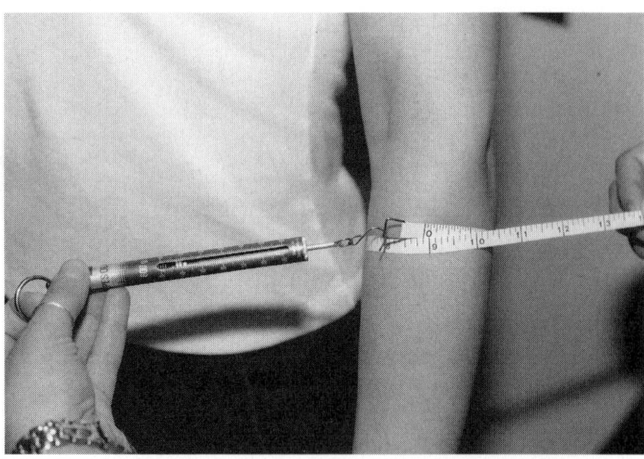

Fig. 11-8 Tension gauge for measuring circumference.

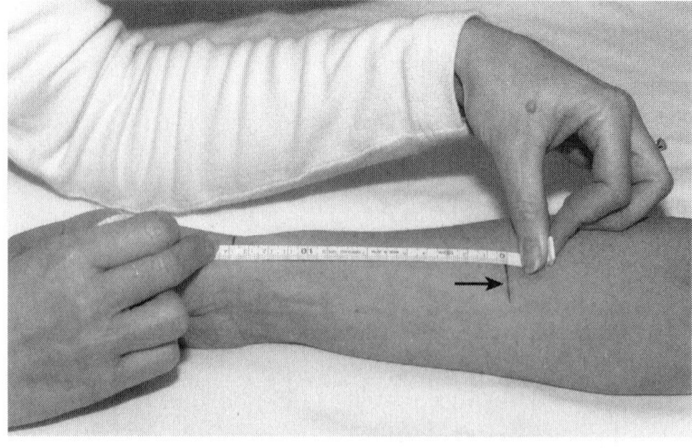

Fig. 11-10 Distance measurement using the base of the radial head as the bony landmark. Note the area at the end of the tape that was marked with a skin pencil.

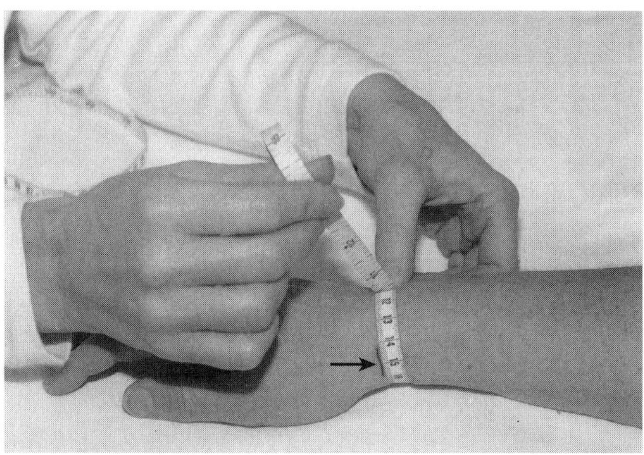

Fig. 11-9 Circumferential measurement of the wrist.

the tape of the circumferential measurement (Fig. 11-9). A measurement, measured in centimeters or inches, should then be taken of the distance from a bony landmark along the extremity to the mark made at the base of the tape to produce a consistent site for future values. Bony landmarks to be considered are the following: the base of the lateral malleolus for the calf; the inferior pole of the patella for the thigh; the tip of the ulnar stylus or the base of the radial head for the forearm (Fig. 11-10); and the olecranon process for the upper arm. Accuracy and reliability of the measurements are enhanced when the same person performs the measurements, a tension gauge is used, the patient is in the same position, measurements are made at the same time of day, and the same tape measure is used. The caregiver should apply the tape horizontally around the extremity with the same tension applied at each measuring session. Serial measurements, performed over a period, will provide objective evidence of the changes in the circumference of the extremity, which indirectly indicates the effect of edema or atrophy in the girth (Procedure 11-1).

Volumetric Measurement

Volumetric displacement, with the use of a volumeter, is a method to measure changes in the distal aspect of an extremity caused by edema or muscle atrophy. The technique is more accurate to use than girth measurements because of the irregular shape of the hand and foot, but it requires some equipment. A volumeter (large enough to immerse a foot and ankle or a hand and wrist) with a spout and a calibrated collection container are necessary. A volumeter with a bar placed near the base is often used for hand/wrist measurement. When using a volumeter with a bar, the person is instructed to immerse the hand so the bar falls between the third and fourth digits (Fig. 11-11).

The volumeter is filled with warm water until it overflows, but it is not ready for use until the water ceases to drip from the spout. The calibrated cylinder is positioned so it will catch the water that overflows when the person immerses the hand or foot into the water-filled volumeter. Instruct the person to immerse the hand or foot slowly and carefully into the water and to remain motionless as the displaced water flows through the spout; the two containers should rest on a firm, level surface. The calibrated container, which is usually a column, collects the expelled water. After the water is collected in the container, it should be placed on a firm, level surface and at a height that allows the caregiver to read the scale at eye level. When a series of measurements are made of the same extremity, conditions such as the water temperature, time of day, equipment, patient position, and evaluator should be replicated at each session to enhance accuracy and reliability of the findings. Differences of several millimeters of water displacement may

PROCEDURE 11-1

Girth Measurements

LOWER EXTREMITY

Expose the extremity; position the patient standing on a level surface so the extremity is relaxed and explain the procedure.

Use a plastic or metal anthropometric measuring tape with well-defined, easily visible calibrations.

Palpate and mark the bony landmark (such as, the lateral malleolus) to be used as the base for the distance measurement site on the extremity; position the free end of the tape on the mark and extend it along the extremity.

Use a skin-marking pencil to mark the site at which the circumferential measurements are to be made (that is, the area of greatest edema or atrophy).

Observe and document the distance measurement value from the bony landmark to the circumferential measurement sites.

For the circumference measurement, apply the tape around the extremity so it contacts the skin firmly and lies flat, but without causing an excessive indentation in the soft tissue; use consistent pressure and a tension gauge, if possible, as you apply the tape.

Record the results for the circumference and the distance from the landmark to the base of the tape; document your activity and identify significant findings.

Measure the contralateral limb for comparison.

UPPER EXTREMITY

Follow the above procedure measuring the distance from a bony landmark (such as the ulnar stylus) to the area where the circumference is to be measured (the area of greatest edema or atrophy); then measure the circumference.

Document both the distance from the landmark and the circumference.

Note: If a tension gauge is used, be sure to mark what tension was used around the circumference to permit more accurate detail of following measurements.

Note: Girth measurements are difficult to perform on irregularly shaped areas such as the hand/wrist and foot/ankle; volumetric measurements are suggested for those areas.

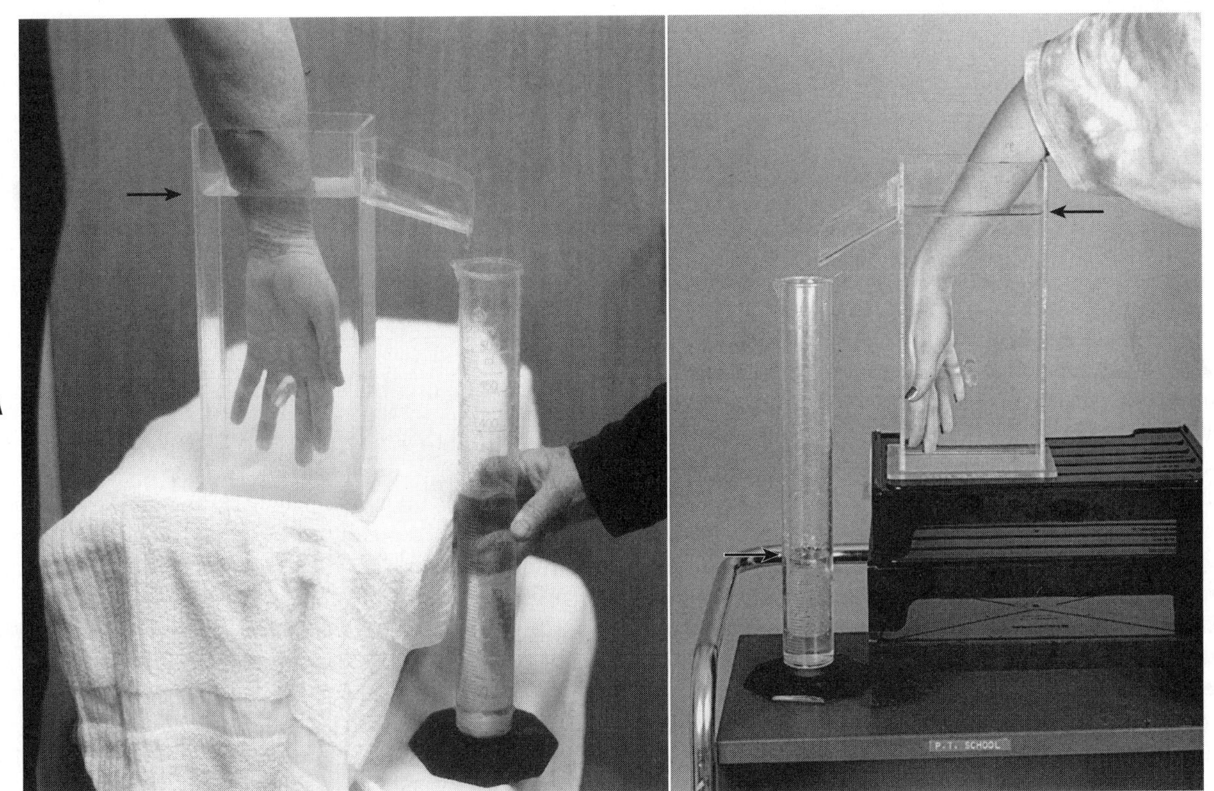

Fig. 11-11 Equipment for volume displacement. **A,** Volumeter showing finger bar. **B,** Volumeter without finger bar. *Note:* Water level is indicated by *arrow.*

PROCEDURE 11-2

Volumetric Measurements

Expose the area to be assessed, seat the patient to assess the foot/ankle, and sit or stand to assess the hand/wrist, inform the patient about the procedure, and obtain the volumeter and a calibrated container.

Fill the volumeter to overflowing with warm water. When water no longer drips from the spout, place the calibrated container beneath the spout, and be certain both containers are on a firm, level surface.

Instruct the patient to slowly and carefully immerse the foot/ankle or hand/wrist, with the hand open and fingers relaxed, into the water until the foot rests on or the fingers touch the bottom of the container. Instruct the patient to leave the part immersed, without movement, until water no longer drips from the spout. *Note:* When using a volumeter with a bar, the person is instructed to immerse the hand so the bar falls between the third and fourth digits.

Remove the calibrated container before the patient lifts the foot or hand from the water so any water that would drip from the part does not drip into the calibrated container. Dry the patient's foot or hand.

Place the calibrated container on a firm, level surface and position yourself to read the scale at eye level.

Record the results, document your activities, and identify significant findings.

Repeat the procedure for the uninvolved extremity for comparison.

occur between a person's left and right hand and between the dominant and nondominant hand. Despite these differences, it will be helpful to measure the displacement of water caused by the unaffected hand or foot to establish a baseline or comparison value for the affected hand or foot. Repetitive measurements can be reviewed and compared to determine the change in volume of the segment being measured (Procedure 11-2).

LYMPHEDEMA

The lymph system is a one-way drainage system designed to rid the tissues of unwanted material and excess fluid. Lymphedema is the result of a functional overload of the lymphatic system in which lymph volume exceeds transport capabilities resulting in obstructed lymph flow, swelling, pain, and susceptibility to infection. Primary lymphedema is a congenital malformation, whereas secondary lymphedema is acquired most commonly after surgical removal of lymph nodes, infection of the lymphatics, radiation therapy for cancer, or trauma. Lymphedema can occur in any body part, but is most often seen in the limbs and it is a chronic condition if left untreated. Although lymphedema is noncurable, there are several indications and contraindications for treatment (Box 11-13) and it can be managed. The CDT—sometimes referred to as Complete/Complex Decongestive Physiotherapy (CDP)—is one treatment protocol (Box 11-14) that can manage this chronic inflammatory condition effectively and minimize associated complications such as repeated infections, cellulitis, lymphangitis, and nonhealing ulcers. The CDT includes MLD, compression bandaging, vasopneumatic compression, patient education about skin care and precautions, compression garment measurement, and remedial exercise. It is a specialized program designed to move fluid from the tissues to promote normal functioning of the lymph system and help alleviate fluid blockage.

The use of MLD as a treatment of lymphedema has become recognized in the United States as an important

Box 11-13 Indications and Contraindications for Lymphedema Treatment

INDICATIONS

Primary lymphedema
Secondary lymphedema
- After trauma, radiation
- After burn
- After obstruction by tumor, scar, inflammation, or parasite

Idiopathic lymphedema
Postoperative edema
Venous ulcer, arterial ulcer
Scar treatment

CONTRAINDICATIONS

Acute infection (patient should be on antibiotics at least 4 days before treatment)
Active cancer
Presence of congestive heart failure
After radiation treatment (requires medical clearance)

Box 11-14 Complete (or Complex) Decongestive Therapy Objectives

1. Enhance lymph drainage through the use of MLD techniques.
2. Control and reduce edema through compression bandaging.
3. Use an intermittent vasopneumatic compression device as an adjunct to MLD.
4. Reduce or eliminate infections through patient education for meticulous skin and nail care.
5. Increase function and enhance lymphatic flow through a gentle, individualized exercise program.
6. Reach a maintenance program of minimal therapy that will preserve the extremity improvements obtained from intense therapeutic intervention, so the patient becomes independent to manage the symptoms.

PROCEDURE 11-3

Instructions for Upper Extremity Lymphedema Bandaging

All bandages start at the wrist; a minimum of three bandages, plus a finger wrap if fingers are involved, will be used for the complete wrap. It is important not to wrap above the elbow with the first two bandages. The third wrap, and fourth if needed, will cross the elbow, but do not return the bandage down across the elbow. Strive to have an even tension, not too tight or too loose, but the bandage should feel firm evenly up the arm when finished. If the hand is not edematous, the finger wrap will not be used. If the wrist appears very small in comparison to the hand and forearm, a strip of foam padding may be used to fill the space before application of the wraps. Start with a finger wrap of 5 cm × 4 m, then a 6 cm × 5 m is applied, followed by an 8 cm × 5 m and a 10 cm × 5m, and if necessary a 12 cm × 5 m.

FINGER WRAP

Prefold in half the 5 cm by 4 in open weave soft cotton bandage, which has a high tensile strength and is available through various manufacturers.

Anchor the white elasticized bandage at the wrist.

Take the bandage to the tip of the thumb (Fig. 11-12, *A*) and wrap around the thumb to its base overlapping by half the width. Anchor again at the wrist and take the bandage to the tip of the index finger, wrap to its base, and anchor at the wrist. Take the bandage to the third fingertip and again wrap to its base ending with a wrist anchor.

Repeat this procedure for the fourth and little fingers, anchoring the final wrap at the wrist. When completed, the palmar surface should be free of bandage (Fig. 11-12, *B*) and the back of the hand should be completely covered as shown in Fig. 11-12, *A*.

6 cm BANDAGE

This short stretch bandage is produced from 100% cotton. It has long-lasting elasticity with strong to firm compression. It provides light resting pressure, but high working pressure. The bandages are permeable to the air and nonirritating to the skin.

Anchor the bandage at the wrist and wrap it around the palm of the hand three to four times to cover the palm and any areas left exposed by the finger wrap (usually at the base of the thumb).

Continue the wrap in a spiral pattern overlapping half of the previous bandage. Wrap to the elbow, but do not cross the elbow.

8 cm BANDAGE

Anchor at the wrist and wrap in a spiral pattern overlapping each spiral by one half. This bandage should cross the elbow and go to the upper arm to approximately the area of the deltoid insertion, but do not return it across the elbow. A square of soft cotton batting should be placed at the antecubital space for comfort before or during application of this third bandage.

10 cm BANDAGE

This bandage and the 12 cm bandage, if necessary, are anchored at the wrist and overlap by one half the previous bandage in a spiral pattern crossing the elbow and ending near the deltoid insertion. These bandages will cover the previous bandages and are used for a large upper extremity.

therapeutic intervention. Dr. Emil Vodder developed the procedure in Cannes, France in the 1930s. It is a superficial massage that differs from therapeutic massage in that it is gentler and is used to encourage fluid drainage from swollen areas by stimulating lymph vessels. Instead of using the kneading motion of massage, MLD involves mild stretching applied to the skin. It is systematically performed to reduce edema to the main lymph nodes in the neck. It increases lymphatic flow, helps break down fibrotic tissue areas, and promotes lymph system collateral development. This manual technique is specifically dependent on the location of the edema, skin tissue and integrity, and the cause of the edema.

Depending on the severity of edema, CDT may need to be performed for a period of 2 to 8 weeks, three to five times per week, before a patient achieves normal or near-normal girth and can be fitted for a compression garment. The MLD is often followed by use of intermittent vasopneumatic compression pumping. When lymph flow is established, a compression pump can be used to further reduce edema and, in conjunction with MLD treatment, can be applied during the control/maintenance phase of treatment. The MLD and compression pumping are followed by compression bandaging of the affected area. Short stretch bandages, with or without the use of foam padding, are used daily to ensure that the appropriate compression is maintained until the limb edema has reached a plateau in reduction. Instructions for lymphedema bandaging are given in Procedure 11-3. The bandages are used to maximally assist compression, for effective increase in lymph system flow, and to prevent reaccumulation of evacuated lymph fluid (see Fig. 11-12). Short stretch bandages are made of extensible elastic material that provides high stability (support), low resting pressure, and high working pressure of the limb. The effectiveness of high working pressure is maximized by muscle and joint activity to pump the fluid proximally. Remedial exercises are performed daily while the extremity is either wrapped or has a properly fitted compression garment applied. While wearing the compression garment(s), patients should perform isometric and active exercises at home that focus on the affected limb(s), such as arm exercises for upper extremities and walking and isometric exercises for lower extremities. All exercise regimens require an individualized approach. Proper assessment of

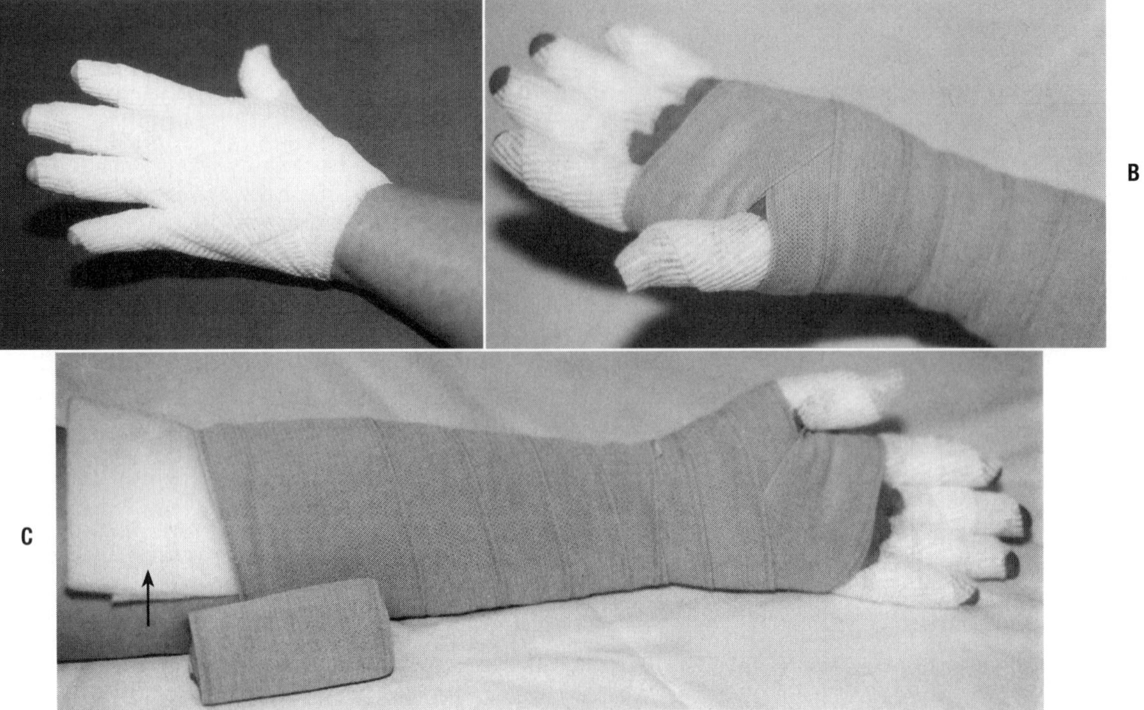

Fig. 11-12 **A,** Initial compression wrap using elasticized gauze. **B,** Short stretch compression bandage; second layer. **C,** Third layer compression bandage with cotton batting, indicated by the arrow, to cushion the antecubital fossa; this bandage ends at the deltoid insertion.

Box 11-15 Precautions for Lymphedema Patients

- Avoid extreme temperatures (hot baths, burns, and travel in extreme hot or cold climates)
- Avoid factors that may cause infection (such as insect bites, manicures, vaccinations, pet scratches, skin punctures and cuts, venography, and lymphography)
- Avoid blunt trauma (lifting heavy objects, tennis or golf, blood pressure cuffs, tight clothing, heavy breast prosthesis, and tight jewelry)
- Avoid use of alcohol and nicotine
- Travel wearing a well-fitting compression garment and elevate limb during flight
- Maintain excellent nutrition (low-salt diet; avoid fried foods)
- Avoid obesity
- Perform meticulous skin and nail care
- Exercise daily
- Treat infections promptly and vigorously
- Seek treatment for even the slightest episode of lymphedema
- Use hypoallergenic soaps and fragrances

patient strength, flexibility, functional limb mobility, and aerobic capacity should be performed before initiating treatment and gradual progression of exercise should be expected. *Caution:* Higher exertion-type exercise may damage the delicate balance of the lymph system and interstitial pressure.

Lymphedema patients have a high risk for developing skin infections because of the decreased flow of high-protein lymph fluid. Precautions are listed in Box 11-15. Meticulous skin and nail care are important to prevent bacterial, viral, and other infections. Because lymphedema weakens the immune system of the affected limb(s), the skin must be kept moist and at an appropriate pH level. A low-pH skin lotion that contains no irritants or perfumes should be applied to the skin and nails daily. Because lymphedema is a lifelong condition, patients must be responsible for meticulous skin care, following precautions, self-massage, applying compression bandages or garments, and performing remedial exercises to ensure that CDT will have long-term success. For this reason, a proficient clinician must educate the patient on all the treatment steps from the first day of treatment.

Lymphedema Certification Although CDT has been used with great success in Europe for years, it has only been recognized as the U.S. standard for lymphedema management within the past decade. Registered nurses, physical therapists, occupational therapists, massage therapists, and other providers from several disciplines offer treatment in the United States. There is a strong self-care aspect to the technique of CDT and lymphedema therapists need to be very proficient. For this reason, the Lymphology Association of North America (LANA) began working on a national CDT certification examination, which became available in 2001.

COMPRESSION GARMENTS

Compression garment uses include control of edema in an extremity, assistance in the return of venous circulation in a lower extremity, and decrease in the formation of extensive scar tissue resulting from a burn. However, our information will be limited to lymphedema. Garments are available in both custom-made and standard prefabricated varieties (Fig. 11-13). Standard garments should not be used for patients whose circumference measurements show extreme deviations when compared to measurement tables; for patients whose length measurements vary greatly from the average; for awkwardly shaped limbs or a deformity; or where a nonstandard compression garment is required. Garments may be obtained in a gradient format in which distal compression is greater than proximal compression. Standard prefabricated garments are less expensive and can be obtained quickly, whereas custom-made garments can take up to 3 weeks to receive. For this reason, most proficient caregivers will measure for a custom-made garment after 7 to 10 days of treatment so the garment will be available at the end of the CDT protocol.

Theoretically compression garments aid in reducing swelling by lessening the amount of edema formed within the involved extremity. The garments are fabricated for an individual patient from a fabric that, because of its elastic properties, produces an external, graduated compression force to the tissues. In addition to their use on the extremities, garments can be fabricated for a patient's head or trunk. These applications would be beneficial to decrease the development of scar tissue for the person who has been burned. A patient's comfort, and therefore compliance, is of importance for the maintenance of progress made during therapy. Therefore the fit is extremely important, as is the material from which the garment is made. The garment can be made from synthetic or cotton fibers; some garments have a soft inner lining.

Disadvantages of these garments are they can be uncomfortable (although more comfortable materials have become available), are laborious to put on (often talc is used on the limb before garment application, but talc should not be used in those patients with known respiratory problems), are unsightly, and typically last no more than 3 to 6 months. Garments should be replaced when they begin to lose their elasticity.

Measurements for a pressure gradient garment for the upper or lower extremity can be performed by using the paper measuring tapes (Figs. 11-14 and 11-15) supplied by a manufacturer or by following the directions on other manufacturers' forms (Fig. 11-16, Procedure 11-4). The paper tapes allow circumferential measurements of the extremity to be made approximately every 1.5 inches from the distal to the proximal aspect of the extremity. Specific landmarks on each extremity are used to properly position the tape before the application of the individual strips that are wrapped around the extremity. Complete instructions and directions, including

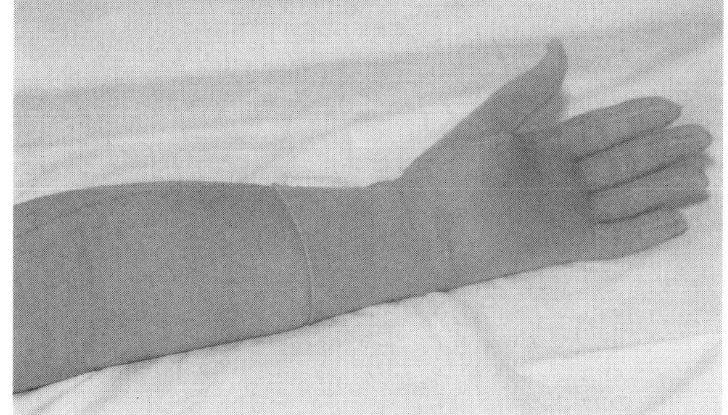

Fig. 11-13 Custom-made compression sleeve with separate glove.

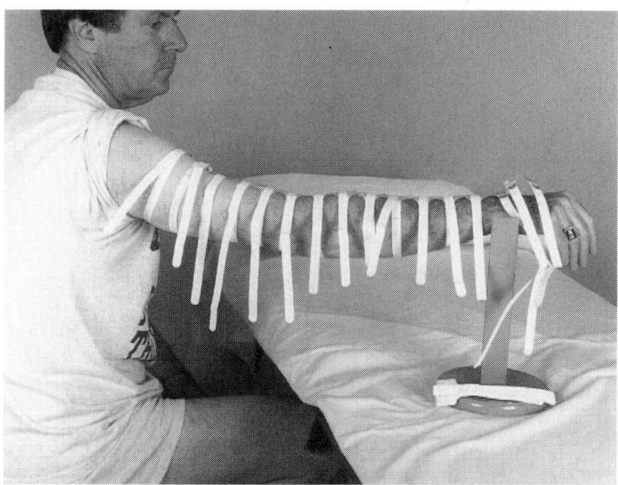

Fig. 11-14 Application of measurement tapes for graduated compression (pressure gradient) garment; upper extremity.

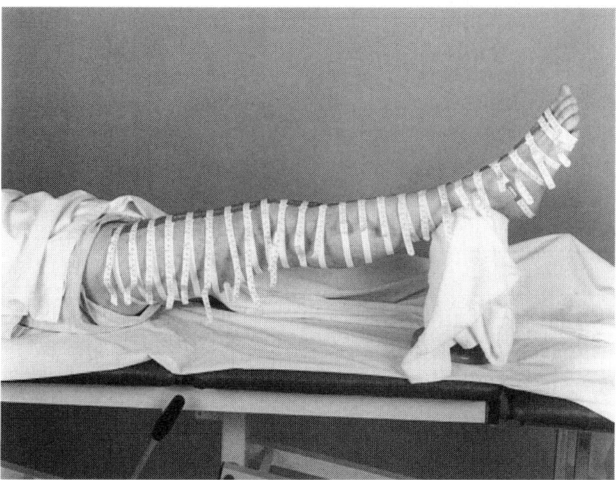

Fig. 11-15 Application of measurement tapes for graduated compression garment; lower extremity.

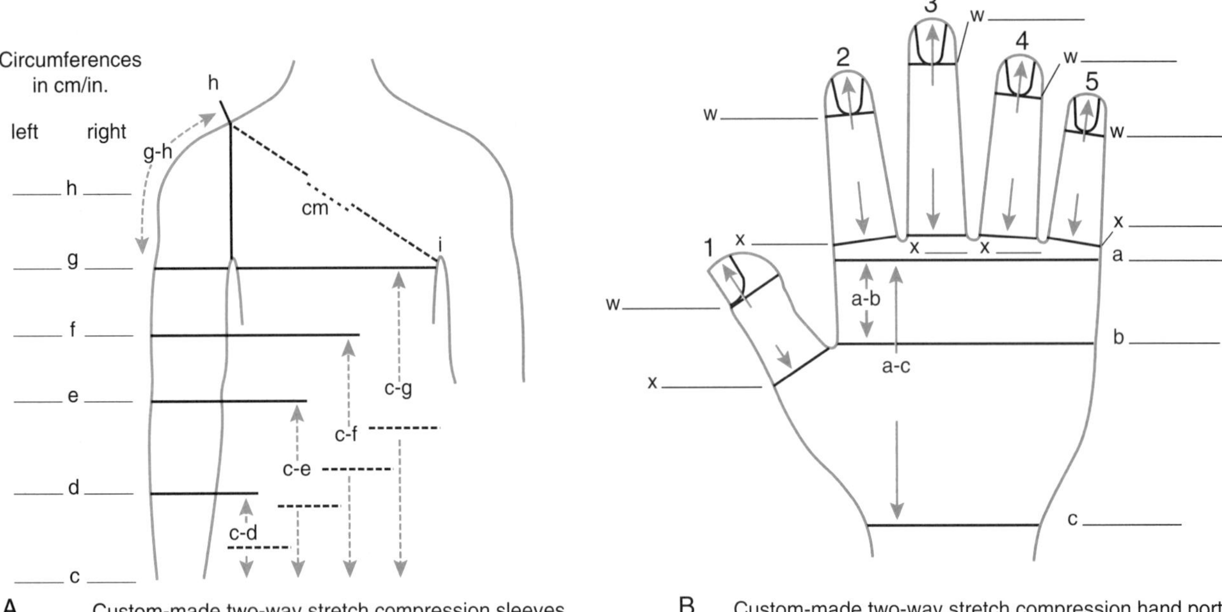

A Custom-made two-way stretch compression sleeves

B Custom-made two-way stretch compression hand portions

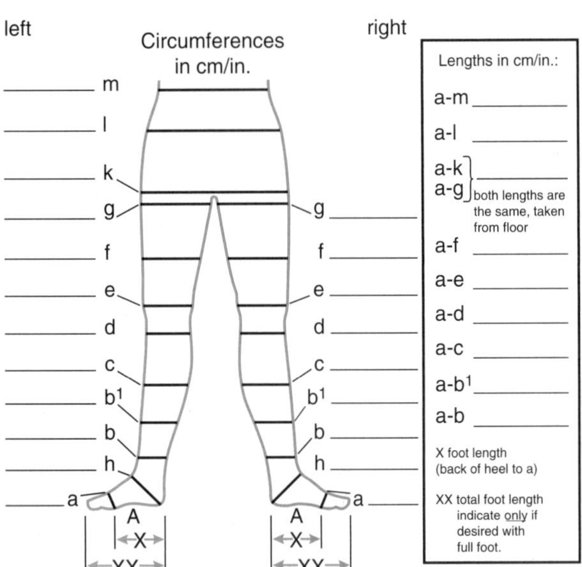

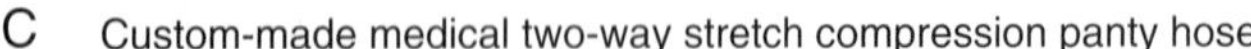

C Custom-made medical two-way stretch compression panty hose

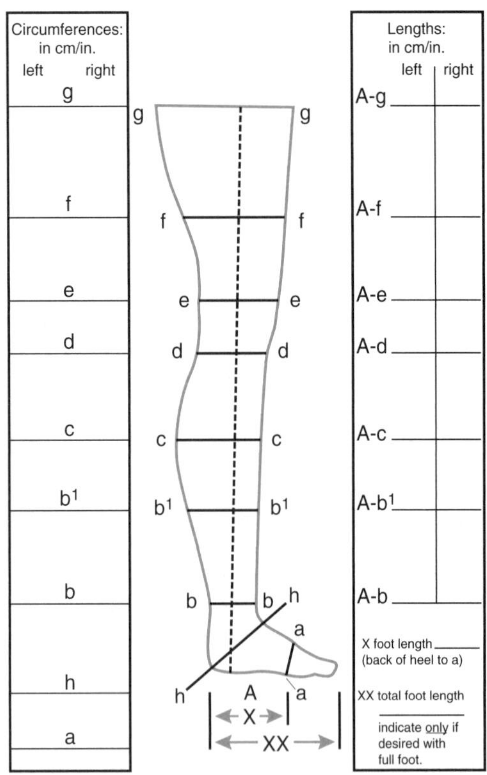

D Custom-made medical two-way stretch compression stockings

Fig. 11-16 Measurements chart for custom-made compression garments; upper and lower extremities. **A,** Two-way stretch compression sleeves. **B,** Two-way stretch compression hand portions. **C,** Two-way stretch compression panty hose. **D,** Two-way stretch compression stockings. (Redrawn with permission from Julius Zorn, Juzo®, 80 Chart Road, Cuyahoga Falls, OH, 2000.)

PROCEDURE 11-4

Measurement of a Pressure Gradient Garment

PAPER TAPE METHOD

Upper Extremity

Explain the procedure and seat the person; support the upper extremity to elevate it; expose the entire upper extremity from the top of the shoulder to the ends of the fingers.

Apply the spine of the measuring tape along the length of the extremity; apply the paper strips at the specified landmarks (elbow, base of the thumb/wrist).

Wrap each individual strip around the extremity; keeping it flat, in close contact with the skin, perpendicular to the spine, and parallel to the strip above and below; do not pull the strip so tight that it causes an indentation in the soft tissue; attach the strip to the spine and follow the manufacturer's instructions for pleating the spine to ensure that the garment's length will be appropriate.

After all the strips are in place, use bandage scissors to cut each strip along the side of the spine that is scalloped (the side that has round indentations); it may be helpful to use cellophane tape to reinforce the attachment of each strip to the spine.

Label the tape with the patient's name; indicate whether it is the left or right extremity; list any specific information or instructions regarding the fabrication; fold the tape and place it in the mailing envelope.

Lower Extremity

Explain the procedure and position the patient supine; support the lower extremity to elevate it from the mattress or mat; expose the lower extremity from the groin to the end of the toes. *Note:* If a leotard ("panty hose")-type garment is to be fabricated, it will be necessary to provide waist and hip measurements.

Apply the spine of the measuring tape along the length of the extremity; apply the paper strips at the specified landmarks (heel/ankle).

Wrap each individual strip around the extremity; follow the same procedure as outlined for upper extremity measurements. *Note:* Extension strips may be added to strips that are not long enough to encircle the extremity; pleats (folds) can be made on the measuring tape to adjust the length of the garment; when edema control is the goal, the extremity should be measured when the least amount of edema is present (that is, measure early in the morning and after CDT if the patient is being treated); many options and modifications are available for the garments (see Figs. 11-14 and 11-15).

MEASURING TAPE METHOD FOR THE UPPER EXTREMITY

Expose the extremity; position the patient so the extremity is relaxed, supported, and elevated from the underlying surface and explain the procedure. If lymphedema is not bilateral, measure the unaffected contralateral extremity to obtain a baseline for comparison. Use a plastic or metal anthropometric measuring tape with well-defined, easily visible calibrations; it will be helpful if the tape can be locked at any length so it will not retract, but can be lengthened.

Use a tension gauge for circumference pressure if available.

To measure each of the circumferences of the extremity, apply the measuring tape around the extremity so it contacts the skin firmly and lies flat, but without causing an excessive indentation in the soft tissue; use consistent pressure as you apply the tape at each mark and apply the tape so each measurement is parallel to the one above and below.

Palpate and mark the ulnar stylus of the wrist to be used as the base for the series of measurement sites on the extremity; take a circumferential measurement at the wrist.

Use a skin-marking pencil to mark the site at which the circumferential measurements of the upper extremity are to be made; the sites should be as equidistant as possible from each other and include the midforearm, elbow, midupper arm, upper arm at the level of the axilla, and, if the sleeve includes the shoulder, measure from the axilla to the tip of the shoulder on the lateral aspect, and from the tip of the shoulder to the opposite axilla (see Fig. 11-16 *A*)

Measure the circumference at each of the sites.

Position the free end of the tape on the ulnar stylus and extend it along the extremity to each of the premarked circumferential sites; document the distances between the ulnar stylus and each circumferential measurement site (see Fig. 11-16).

Document your activity properly on the form provided.

diagrams, are provided with each measuring tape. Other forms of measurement can be accomplished using a plastic-covered cloth tape, an anthropometric tape, or a metal tape (see Fig. 11-7). For the lower extremity, the usual measurement sites are the gluteal fold, upper thigh, lower thigh, knee, calf, distal calf, ankle, instep, and meta-tarsal heads (see Fig. 11-16). Upper extremity measurement sites include the wrist, midforearm, elbow, midupper arm, upper arm at the level of the axilla, and from the axilla to the tip of the shoulder. Should a strap be necessary to secure the upper extremity garment, a measurement from the tip of the shoulder to the opposite axilla must be performed. For brevity, only the explanation for the measuring tape technique of an upper extremity compression garment is explained in Procedure 11-4. If the hand is edematous, it must be measured for a glove or gauntlet (a fingerless glove that may be separate from or that can be attached to an upper extremity sleeve). Hand measurement sites include the circumference of the wrist, midpalm, metacarpal circumference (at the base of the fingers), the base of the thumb and each finger, and the distal interphalangeal joints of the thumb and each finger just below the nails. Distance measurements for the hand include from the wrist to the metacarpal heads, from midpalm to the metacarpal heads, and from the base of the fingers and thumb to either the nail bed for an open-fingered glove or from the base to the tip of the fingers and thumb for a closed-fingered glove (see Fig. 11-16). Two garments should be ordered simultaneously so one garment will be available for use while the other garment is being washed. Use of the two garments alternately will extend the life of each garment. Furthermore, replacement garments should be ordered to be available before the time the current garment has lost its therapeutic value. Instructions about the application, removal, and care of the garment are provided by the manufacturer.

Intermittent Vasopneumatic Compression Devices

Intermittent compression through the use of a vasopneumatic compression pump and sleeve is a method of treatment for chronic or acute edema or swelling and venous insufficiency. A variety of pumps are available. They range in cost from several thousand dollars for more advanced units to several hundred dollars. Pumps range from a single-chambered unit (Fig. 11-17) to up to 12 chambers (cells). Multichambered pumps inflate sequentially from distal to proximal, thereby producing pressure that ascends the extremity, theoretically evacuating the edema with this wave of pressure (Fig. 11-18). Guidelines for pump selection, their number of chambers, the length of time of the pumping session, pumping pressure ranges, and inflation/deflation cycles vary according to the manufacturer.

A trial is recommended for patients to compare pumping devices, if available, before a unit is obtained for home use. Multichambered, sequential pumps are used at relatively low pressures (that is, 40 to 60 mm Hg for the upper extremity and 80 to 90 mm Hg for the lower extremity) and have been advocated as part of a comprehensive lymphedema program. Compression sleeves for the upper and lower extremities are available from most compression pump manufacturers, but some have to be custom-made for particular models. The sleeves are inflated and deflated with the pump (Procedure 11-5). The inflation cycle provides an external compression force to the extremity that assists in removing the edema or

PROCEDURE 11-5

Intermittent Compression Pump

Explain the procedure to the patient and obtain consent, measure the patient's blood pressure, and examine the extremity.

Position and drape the patient according to the diagnosis or condition and extremity involved and apply tubular stockinet and then apply the sleeve to the extremity.

The extremity should be level with or placed above the heart.

Adjust the controls of the unit as necessary (that is, pressure, inflation-to-deflation ratio) and turn on the unit.

Periodically monitor the patient during the treatment session and leave a call device or bell with the patient during treatment.

To conclude the treatment, turn off the unit when the sleeve is deflated. *Note:* If the sleeve is inflated, detach the inflation hose(s) of the unit from the sleeve and deflate it. Remove the sleeve and discard stockinet.

Examine the extremity, measure the circumference (girth) if treating edema, and document your activities and findings.

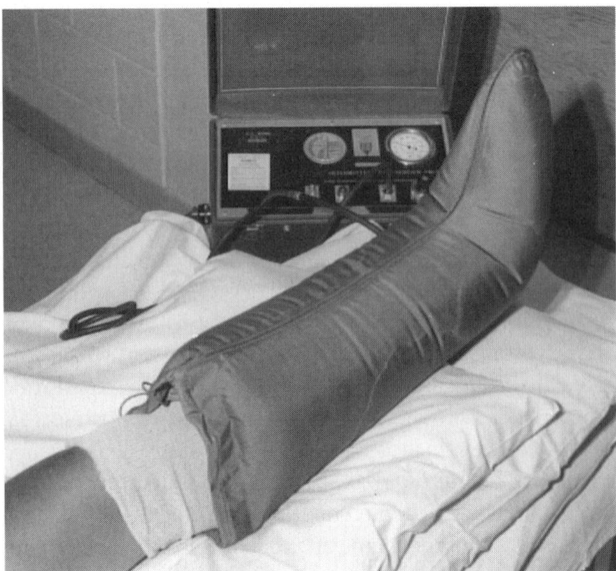

Fig. 11-17 Single-chambered compression pump; lower extremity application.

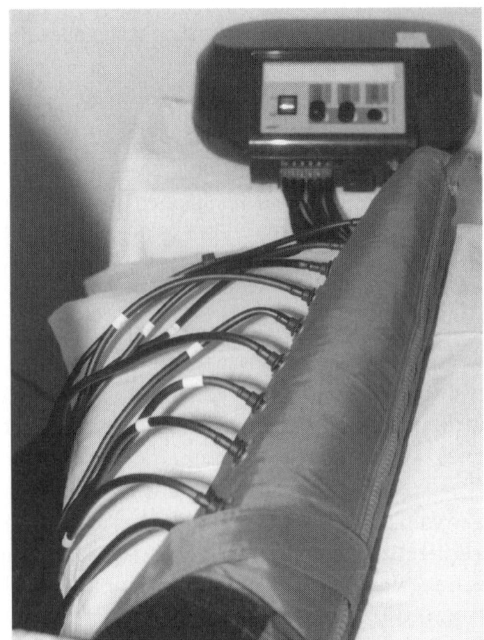

Fig. 11-18 Multichambered, sequential compression pump; upper extremity application.

assists the return of venous blood from the extremity to the heart. (*Caution:* Before using compression to the lower extremity for a venous condition, arterial insufficiency and thrombophlebitis must be ruled out. If arterial insufficiency is present, the inflation phase of the intermittent compression cycle may cause additional occlusion of the arterial circulation and possibly tissue ischemia. If thrombophlebitis is present, the potential exists of causing an embolus to enter the venous system.)

The patient is positioned seated or supine for the upper extremity and supine for the lower extremity, the sleeve is applied, and the extremity is elevated above the level of the heart. (*Note:* Tubular stockinet should be applied to the person's extremity before application of the sleeve to help to maintain cleanliness of the inside of the sleeve.) The amount of pressure in the sleeve and the parameters of the cycle should be established for each patient. Generally, the maximum compression force should be above the patient's systemic diastolic blood pressure, but should not exceed systolic pressure to avoid possible cardiovascular complications. The length of treatment time for compression pumps varies. An example of an extreme protocol would be that the patient is pumped for 2 hours on, 30 minutes off, during waking hours and 6 hours of continuous pumping during the night. The normal length of time for a patient after MLD for lymphedema would be between 30 minutes and 2 hours. A program of intermittent vasopneumatic compression will be advantageous to reduce the edema in an extremity before measurement for a graded compression garment. When this approach is used, the garment can be measured more accurately and will be more likely to control the residual edema. The application of tubular elastic gauze for a finger and hand wrap and low-stretch compression wraps to the extremity after each pumping session will help minimize redevelopment of the edema and should be performed until a permanent graded compression garment is available (see Fig. 11-12).

In addition to mechanical compression, the patient may be instructed to perform active pumping exercises and to elevate the extremity two or three times per hour to assist with edema control. Finger flexion and extension exercises for the upper extremity and active ankle pumping (that is, repetitive dorsiflexion/plantar flexion) for the lower extremity, with the extremity elevated and supported, are two activities that are used frequently.

It is important to observe and converse with the person periodically during each treatment session. Complaints of pain, numbness, tingling, or other forms of paresthesia by the patient may indicate the treatment should be terminated. To conclude a treatment session, the sleeve should be in the deflated mode so the sleeve can be easily removed. If the treatment is terminated with the sleeve inflated, disconnect the hose(s) attached to the control unit from the sleeve. Pressure to the outside of the sleeve will cause it to deflate; when the sleeve has been removed, remove and discard the stockinet. Observe and palpate the extremity and measure the circumference (girth) periodically if lymphedema is the condition being treated. Be observant for skin or circulatory changes that may have occurred as a result of the treatment; document your activities, observations, and measurements as necessary.

These pump units may be rented by or loaned to a person to use at home and the person should be provided with written instructions and directions about use of the unit. Precautions to be followed and a method of communication between the patient and caregiver should be established. In addition, periodic reevaluation of the person's response to or effect of the home treatments should be performed by the caregiver. Contraindications for compression pumps include anticoagulated patients; deep venous thrombosis; and those patients with local cancer or malignancy, severe arterial insufficiency, lymphangitis, cutaneous infection, acute dermatitis, and wet dermatosis. These symptoms may also contraindicate the use of support stockings for vascular conditions.

CHEST PHYSICAL THERAPY

Also called cardiopulmonary physical therapy, CPT is an intervention process concerned with the examination, evaluation, and treatment of patients of all ages with acute and chronic lung conditions. These conditions may be attributable to primary diseases or may be secondary to other medical and surgical conditions. It includes the use of many examination, evaluation, and treatment techniques. The examination and evaluation of a spontaneously breathing and mechanically ventilated patient may include analysis of medical information from the patient's record (chest X-ray, arterial blood gases, history and physical, exercise stress test and tolerance); chest assessment of auscultation, chest wall mobility, palpation, posture analysis, breathing pattern, and chest percussion; evaluation of cough effectiveness and productivity; joint range of motion, muscle testing, observation of noninvasive oxygen monitoring (ear oximetry, transcutaneous oximetry), and identification of respiratory therapy appliances that might enhance CPT; assessment of the stress and tension the patient exhibits; functional evaluation of bed mobility, transfer activities, ambulation on level surfaces and stairs, and need for assistive devices; and observation of mental status and level of acceptance of disease, medical condition, or postoperative status.

Treatment is based on results of the initial and subsequent examination and evaluations. Most of the techniques used fall into the categories of airway clearance (secretion removal), breathing retraining/exercises, and therapeutic exercise. Airway clearance techniques facilitate loosening and removal of secretions from the tracheobronchial tree. Techniques include positioning for gravity drainage (Fig. 11-19); chest percussion, vibration, and shaking; rib springing; cough training, stimulation, and assistance; forced expiratory technique (huff); airway suctioning; and oxygen, bronchodilator, and humidity therapy used in conjunction with CPT treatments. Breathing retraining exercises often include breathing exercises (diaphragmatic, pursed lip, segmental); incentive spirometry (Fig. 11-20); paced breathing techniques;

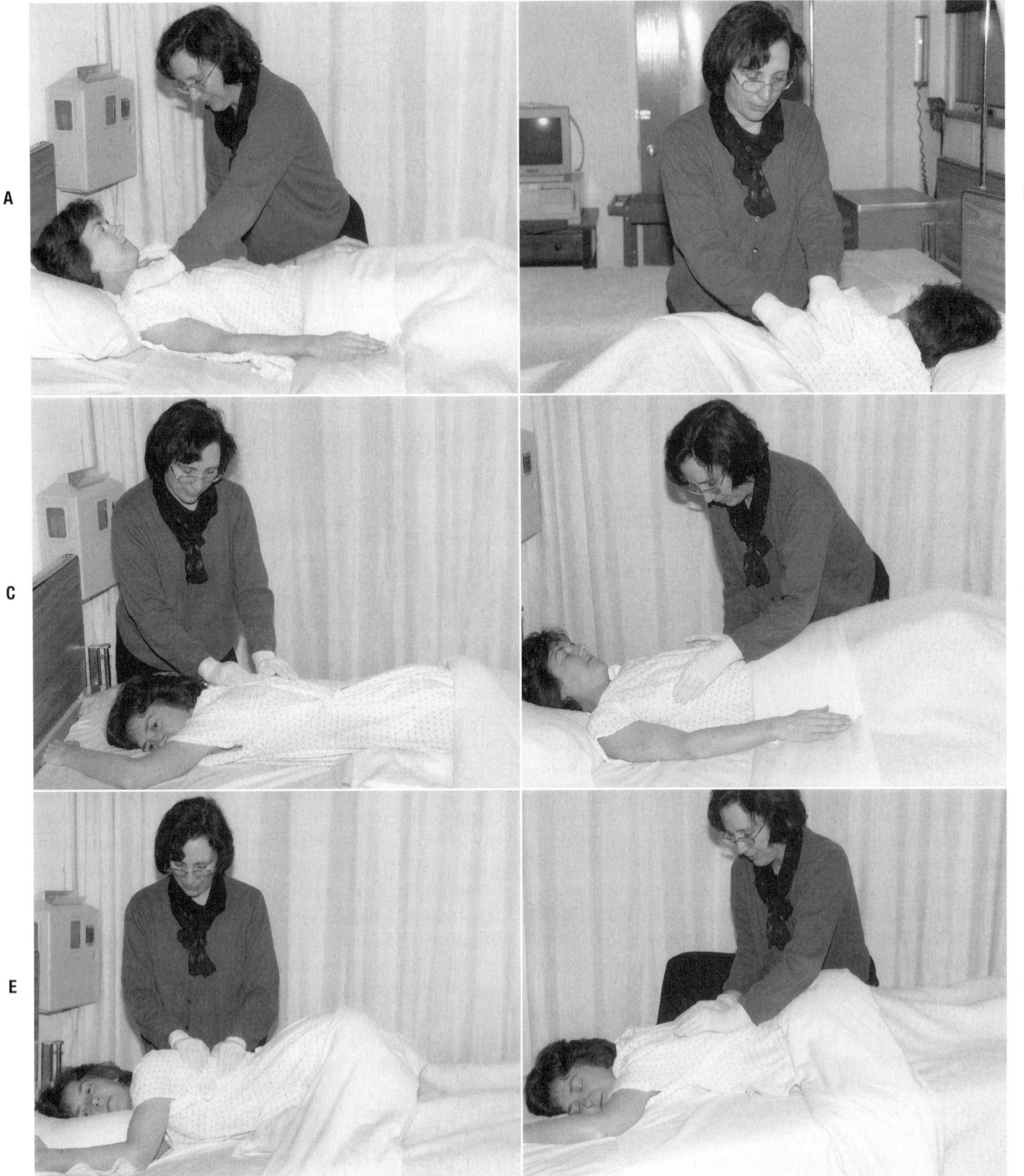

Fig. 11-19 **A,** Postural drainage position for anterior segments, upper lobe. **B,** Postural drainage position for posterior segment, left upper lobe. **C,** Postural drainage position for posterior segment, right upper lobe. **D,** Postural drainage position for anterior basal segments. **E,** Postural drainage position for left lateral basal segment. **F,** Postural drainage position for posterior basal segments.

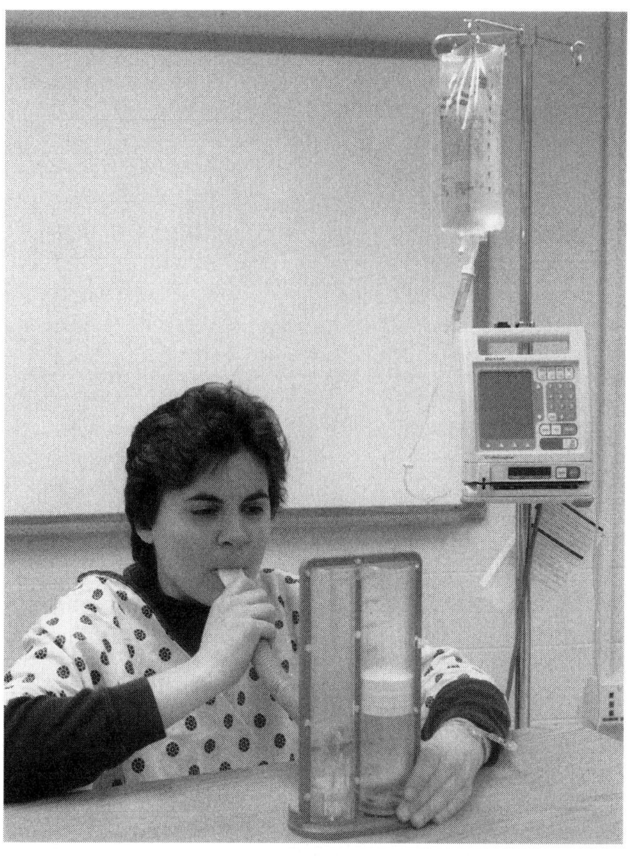

Fig. 11-20 Using an incentive spirometer. Note the IV unit in the background.

glossopharyngeal breathing; sustained maximal inspiration and inspiratory hold techniques; and respiratory muscle strength and endurance exercises. Examples of therapeutic exercise programs with or without oxygen support include relaxation training; posture correction; manual stretching of the thorax; chest mobilization; exercise techniques to improve and maintain range of motion of the chest and shoulders (after thoracotomy); strength and coordination of the trunk and extremities; exercise endurance training; energy conservation techniques (Fig. 11-21); instruction in home care programs; and patient and family education.

Goals of CPT include improvement of airway clearance, ventilation, and exercise tolerance; reduction in the work of breathing; and restoration of the patient to the fullest potential in the inpatient, outpatient, pulmonary rehabilitation, and home care settings. Treatment settings may include medical and cardiac intensive care units, inpatient units, preoperative and postoperative areas, the labor and delivery unit, pediatrics, and the chronic care area. Patients may range in age from the neonate to the very elderly. The CPT home program planning, which assists the patient and family to understand and participate in self-care, promotes optimal pulmonary rehabilitation in the continuum of care.

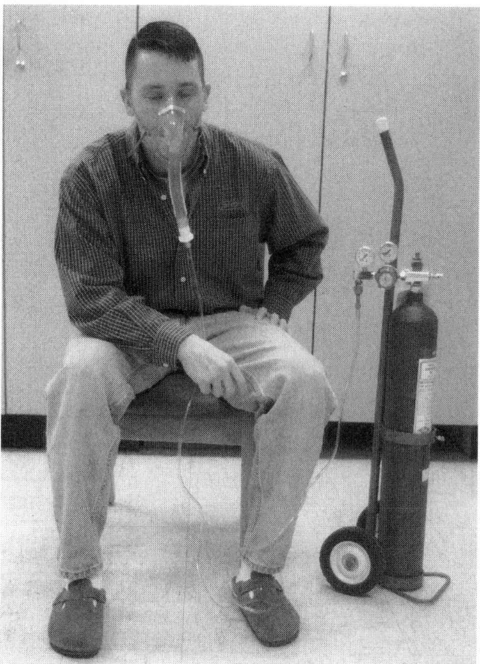

Fig. 11-21 Use of oxygen following exercise. Note the forward trunk position and support by the forearm on the thigh, the oronasal applicator, and portable oxygen cylinder.

Many newer modalities are being clinically tested to be either an adjunct to or a replacement for CPT, especially in the cystic fibrosis population, who need daily CPT. These include, but are not limited to, vests that vibrate the chest wall using pulses of air, airway devices that create waves of pressure through the airway as the patient exhales through the device, high-frequency chest wall compression by an oscillating thoracic cuff, and an intrapulmonary percussive ventilation device.

SUMMARY

Wound care requires the caregiver to comply with many of the principles related to infection control contained in Chapter 2. When the application and removal of dressings and bandages are required for wound care, it may be necessary to develop and maintain a sterile field to protect the dressing materials and to dispose the contaminated materials properly.

For some patients, the prevention of the development of a wound will be an important intervention. This is particularly true for the patient whose condition predisposes the development of a pressure ulcer. Assessment of the risk factors associated with a pressure ulcer and the use of measures to prevent them should be performed for all patients on admission to a health care facility.

The patient with lymphedema should be informed about the risks and preventive measures associated with the condition. Treatment interventions to control edema include the use of specific massage and bandaging techniques, the use of an intermittent compression pump, and the measurement for and eventual application of a pressure garment for the extremity. Girth and volumetric measurements are used to evaluate the size of the extremity after each treatment and provide objective data regarding the results of the interventions used.

A patient who has a respiratory infection or condition that adversely affects respiratory capacity or who is recovering from a surgical procedure affecting the chest or lungs may require chest mobility or lung secretion clearing techniques to improve respiratory status.

self-study ACTIVITIES

- Describe at least five signs or symptoms of an improperly applied bandage and state a corrective action for each.
- Describe at least four instructions or precautions you should give a patient to whom you have applied a bandage.
- List the four rules of asepsis and indicate the importance or significance of each rule.
- Describe and demonstrate how you would evaluate a bandage's tension.
- Describe how you would evaluate a wound at the time a dressing is changed.
- Describe the principles you would use to establish a sterile field.
- Perform girth measurements of an individual's upper and lower extremities.
- Demonstrate how to measure a person for a graded compression garment for the upper extremity.
- Describe six gravity-assisted positions for postural drainage of the lungs.

problem SOLVING

1. You have been asked to give CPT to a patient who has a chest tube in the right lower lobe. What precautions would you take and what postural drainage positions would you avoid?
2. You are treating a patient with a vasopneumatic compression device on the right upper extremity. After 10 minutes, the patient complains of numbness in the right hand. What would you do to alleviate this symptom and what precautions would you take to avoid this situation in the future?
3. You are requested to develop a plan and start a program to prevent the development of pressure ulcers in elderly patients, especially those who have limited mobility. What would you include in your plan and how and with whom would you initiate this program?

CHAPTER 12

Incidents and Emergencies

objectives *After studying this chapter, the reader will be able to:*

- Explain basic, immediate actions to take after selected types of patient injury or acute illnesses.
- Describe precautions to improve safety and reduce patient and employee injury in the treatment setting.
- Differentiate between heat exhaustion and heat stroke through the observation of signs and symptoms and apply appropriate treatment.
- Differentiate between an insulin reaction and acidosis through the observation of signs and symptoms and apply appropriate treatment.
- Differentiate between autonomic hyperreflexia and postural (orthostatic) hypotension through the observation and measurement of various signs and symptoms and apply appropriate treatment.
- Identify the signs and symptoms of choking and apply the Heimlich maneuver.
- Analyze patient care activities and determine the need to modify, reduce, or discontinue treatment.
- Describe at least five ways or means to maintain personal and patient safety.
- Identify factors to maintain a safe treatment environment.

key terms

Acidosis A pathologic condition resulting from the accumulation of acid or depletion of the alkaline reserve in the blood and body tissues; characterized by an increase in hydrogen ion concentration.

Autonomic hyperreflexia (dysreflexia) An uninhibited and exaggerated reflex of the autonomic nervous system as a result of a stimulus.

Cardiac arrest/death The sudden and often unexpected stoppage of effective heart action.

Cardiopulmonary resuscitation (CPR) The reestablishment of heart and lung action as indicated for cardiac arrest.

Convulsion A series of involuntary contractions of the voluntary muscles.

Emergency medical technician (EMT) A person trained to manage the emergency care of sick or injured persons during transport to a hospital or at the scene of injury.

Fracture A break in the continuity of a bone.

Insulin A double-chain protein hormone formed from proinsulin in the beta cells of the pancreatic islets of Langerhans.

Intubation The insertion of a tube, as into the larynx, to maintain an open airway.

Laceration A wound produced by the tearing of body tissue, as distinguished from a cut or an incision.

Orthostatic (postural) hypotension A fall in blood pressure associated with dizziness, syncope, and blurred vision that occurs on standing or when standing motionless in a fixed position.

Seizure A convulsion or attack, as in epilepsy.

Shock Acute peripheral circulatory failure caused by derangement of circulatory control or loss of circulating fluid.

Sternum A plate of bone forming the middle of the anterior wall of the thorax; the breastbone.

Vasoconstriction A decrease in the caliber of blood vessels.

Xiphoid The distal portion of the sternum.

INTRODUCTION

All employees of the patient care area have the responsibility to provide and maintain a safe environment for patient care. In free-standing service units, or in a patient's home, the caregivers and employees should be qualified to provide immediate emergency care. Hospital caregivers and employees should be aware of and follow departmental or institutional policies and procedures regarding emergency situations. In either situation employees should know how to contact and request assistance (such as the use of 911 or local fire, emergency medical, or police telephone numbers and special emergency terms such as "code blue," "code red," and "Captain Thermo"). In addition, you should observe each patient to determine whether the person wears a medical alert bracelet or necklace. These items inform others of special needs or conditions the person may have (such as allergies, implants, pacemakers, diabetes, medication needs).

All caregivers should be informed of their required legal responsibilities and limitations in providing emergency aid, especially as they relate to the "Good Samaritan" statutes of the state in which they work. In some states the employee may be more liable when emergency care is provided by the employee in a hospital or other similar setting where medical equipment or support personnel are available. In most states there is some legal protection for the person who causes additional injury or trauma when emergency care is provided, particularly if the action was a lifesaving or life-sustaining measure. A review of specific professional practice acts and other state statutes may be necessary to determine one's emergency care responsibility in that state.

It should be recognized that the potential for patient and employee injuries becomes greater under certain conditions. Some examples are when there are too few personnel available to manage the patients in the area, too few qualified personnel, excessively busy personnel, personnel who are inattentive to patient needs, poorly maintained or defective pieces of equipment, inadequately trained personnel, and personnel who display careless behavior. The supervisor and all employees should be especially alert when personnel changes occur. Examples of such personnel changes include shift changes, times when some personnel are on vacation or ill and no replacement personnel are provided, during a holiday or weekend when fewer personnel are apt to be used, and when several acutely ill patients are being treated simultaneously.

Some general types of patients that may necessitate closer attention and care by the service unit personnel include elderly patients; debilitated patients; patients with decreased mental competence or cognitive deterioration; patients whose physiologic status has been compromised as a result of extensive burns, a spinal cord injury, a chronic respiratory condition, an acute or chronic cardiac condition, an acute or chronic diabetes; psychologically or emotionally disturbed patients; very young patients; febrile patients; and patients who have been injured or involved in an unusual incident during a previous hospitalization or treatment program.

Caregivers should be aware of and be prepared to respond to an improper referral or prescription by discussing the issue with the referral source before initiating treatment. It may be necessary to delay treatment until the concerns or problems with the referral have been resolved. Precautions or contraindications associated with various treatments should be recognized and applied judiciously to reduce the incidence of injury or trauma to the patient or caregiver. In addition, the caregiver should understand and be aware of the potential problems that may develop in a patient secondary to the primary diagnosis and more care should be used when treating the person with a serious illness or extensive trauma. Supportive personnel should be supervised and guided so they are not requested or expected to perform any treatment activities beyond their education, training, skill, and competence.

Treatment programs or sessions may need to be modified, reduced, or terminated in response to the observed or reported changes in a patient's condition. The patient who convulses without a known cause, experiences incontinence of bowel or bladder without a known cause, loses consciousness without a known cause, or exhibits new or different symptoms from those observed previously should be evaluated carefully before treatment is continued.

The patient who exhibits signs or symptoms of an acute illness or who appears to be experiencing an adverse response to treatment (such as unusual vital signs, vertigo, syncope, nausea, or vomiting) should have the treatment terminated temporarily and should be reevaluated by a physician before being treated again. Nursing and other medical personnel should be apprised of changes in the patient's condition and appropriate documentation must reflect the change.

A mentally competent patient should be informed by the caregiver about the intent, anticipated or desired outcome, and potential risks associated with the planned treatment. All patients should have the opportunity to participate in the process of informed consent, presented in Chapter 1, before receiving treatment and their autonomy regarding deciding whether to receive treatment should be respected. The patient should have the opportunity to ask questions or seek additional information about the treatment. If the treatment is refused, the decision should be accepted and nursing and other medical personnel notified. The caregiver may find it helpful or necessary to confer with a physician, nurse, or other practitioner involved with caring for the patient to assist with the resolution of a dilemma related to a patient's nonconsent. The incident should be documented in the patient's medical record by the caregiver.

Injuries or trauma that may occur to a patient who receives treatment include burns, *lacerations*, muscle strains, ligamentous sprains, heat stress, hematomas, *fractures*, respiratory distress, and cardiovascular distress.

The physical environment in which the patient is treated and the equipment used to treat patients should be maintained to meet the standards established by various agencies. These agencies include the Occupational Safety and Health

Administration (OSHA), Joint Commission on Accreditation of Healthcare Organizations (JCAHO), Department of Public Health (DPH), Commission on Accreditation of Rehabilitation Facilities (CARF), and National Institute of Occupational Safety and Health (NIOSH). The policies and procedures established by the hospital or treatment facility must also be followed.

PRINCIPLES AND CONCEPTS

Health care providers must be aware of the need to maintain a safe environment for treatment. The service unit supervisor or department manager is responsible for developing a safety education and awareness program for all of the employees in the department. Staff meetings and orientation programs regarding environmental, employee, and patient safety should be developed, implemented, and repeated periodically. General guidelines to reduce and avoid patient or employee injury should be included in the unit's policy/procedure or safety manual. Employees should be required to read this material periodically and their comprehension of this material should be evaluated. Failure to provide information and training sessions on safety could create increased organizational or personnel liability and reduce the level of the quality of care.

Written policies and procedures should identify and explain the following:

- Patient scheduling patterns, the least acceptable ratio of personnel to patients, and what is to be done when unacceptable ratios occur.
- The maintenance and monitoring of records such as referrals, patient status documentation (that is, progress reports), treatment protocols, and incident reports.
- Plans for the evacuation and care of patients and the expected function of all personnel at the time of an emergency, such as a fire or disaster.
- First aid or immediate emergency care plans.
- Restriction or access of visitors to the treatment areas.
- Security measures for patient and employee valuables and procedures for items that are lost or found.
- The establishment of equipment inspection, repair, and maintenance records.
- The process and procedures for general infection control and handling of toxic materials (that is, Medical Safety Data Sheets Manual [MSDS]) (see Fig. 1-3).
- The application and use of protective clothing, handling of body fluids, management of patients who are placed in isolation, and changing the dressings of infected wounds.
- Employee job duties, descriptions, and responsibilities.
- Supervisory relationships, lines of communication, a table of organization, the span of control, and the chain of command of the facility and the service area.

The physical environment and equipment should be prepared, inspected, and maintained to ensure the following:

- Proper levels of ventilation, temperature, humidity, light, and noise are provided.
- Routine janitorial and housekeeping services are available and provided.
- Equipment functions according to the manufacturer's standards.
- Structural hazards are minimized or eliminated.
- Equipment is properly attached or fixed to structurally sound and strong areas (that is, it should be attached to wall studs, bolted to the floor, or attached to ceiling joists or rafters).
- Equipment and supplies not in use are stored, line cords and electrical outlets are protected by a built-in ground, and wheels on movable equipment have locks.
- Emergency exits and evacuation routes are clearly marked and displayed for patients, visitors, and employees.
- Emergency equipment (that is, fire extinguishers or hoses, first aid kits, and *intubation* airways) is available, accessible, and ready for use.
- A metabolic cart is available with its components clearly marked and ready to use.
- Floor surfaces are clean and dry, and loose or torn carpeting and other similar hazards (such as line cords on the floor) are eliminated.

Safety related to patient care is the responsibility of the service unit personnel. It is imperative that all personnel understand and comply with safe personal and patient care practices. Regardless of the goal of treatment, the primary responsibility of any practitioner is to "do no harm" to the patient. Employee injuries are frequently associated with activities that require lifting, carrying, pushing, pulling, and reaching. The development, use, and application of proper body mechanics are presented in Chapter 4. It may be helpful to review it for suggestions to prevent injury to yourself and to the patient. You should always be alert to the possibility that patient injury can occur and you should anticipate that unusual events might occur (that is, "expect the unexpected"). The supervisor or department manager has several specific responsibilities, as listed in Box 12-1.

Prevention is an important aspect of patient and employee safety. Care should be taken during an assisted transfer, lifting activities, ambulation activities, and when using equipment. Certain patient conditions, such as wound management, require special attention to avoid infection of the wound and cross-contamination of other persons. Personal cleanliness in the form of proper hand washing before and after each patient's treatment, eating, and toileting is essential for successful infection control. Your personal safety can be maintained best through the use of proper body mechanics, proper personal hygiene, familiarity with the operation of equipment, familiarity with the methods of infection control, and by performing those safety techniques or procedures for which you have been educated or trained.

An injury to a patient can occur even though safety measures are applied diligently and consistently. However, it is less likely to occur when safe practices are used. The primary caregiver of the patient to whom an injury occurs

Box 12-1 Responsibilities of Supervisors

Be certain each employee is qualified and competent for all assigned duties and responsibilities. This will require the supervisor to observe and evaluate each employee's performance at least once a year.

Be certain each employee understands the duties, responsibilities, and expectations of the job. This can be accomplished during the orientation of a new employee and during performance evaluation sessions.

Develop and implement an ongoing safety training and awareness program for unit personnel.

Instruct and teach personnel how to establish appropriate professional interpersonal relations with each patient. Each patient must receive individualized care and should be considered as an entire person rather than as a patient with a specific disability or condition.

Instruct and teach personnel how to obtain informed consent from each patient before initiating or extensively altering treatment.

Instruct personnel to explain all treatment procedures to each patient and to monitor, guide, instruct, or direct the patient during his or her treatment.

Instruct personnel to refer the patient to another caregiver when not skilled or competent to treat the patient.

Instruct personnel to contact the referral source to clarify a referral or prescription that is considered to be inaccurate or incomplete or contains a contraindicated procedure before initiating treatment.

Instruct personnel to clarify any referral or prescription if unsure of its intent or expected outcome before initiating treatment. A verbal referral or prescription should be transferred to written form within 24 hours of its receipt and the written form must be signed by the person who originally provided it.

Be certain personnel report malfunctioning equipment or other forms of breaches of safety and that such situations are corrected promptly.

should follow the steps given in Procedure 12-1. These procedures may vary slightly from facility to facility, but they are necessary to protect the employee, facility, and patient.

Each employee must be aware of the need for the consistent application of preventive measures to maintain a safe environment and the safe care of each patient. The employee's thoughts and behavior should be directed to promote safety for the patient, visitors, other employees, and self. Each employee should be prepared to react to emergency situations quickly, decisively, and calmly. Any emergency or first aid treatment provided by departmental personnel should be performed according to institutional policies and procedures and the training of the employee. Institutional and community agency emergency telephone numbers should be posted by each telephone and employees must use these numbers when assistance is required or desired.

PROCEDURE 12-1

Responses to Patient Injuries

Immediately provide or obtain emergency care for the patient according to established organizational policies and procedures and the competence of the caregiver. Do not leave the patient unattended, but attempt to prevent any further injury and act to stabilize the patient's physiologic status. When it is apparent assistance from trained personnel (such as EMTs, trauma team, CPR team) is needed, they should be contacted before on-the-scene emergency care is initiated to reduce response time. If two or more persons are at the scene, one person should contact the support team while the other begins emergency care.

After the emergency phase is concluded, document the incident with objective and factual information. Indicate the type of emergency care that was given and by whom. List the persons who witnessed or observed the incident, who was notified about the incident, the time the incident occurred, and any events leading up to the incident. Do not confer with the patient or relatives about the incident and do not express information to anyone that would indicate you were negligent or at fault.

Notify your immediate superior, the department supervisor, or the risk manager of the incident.

File the incident report with the appropriate person within the organization; it may be necessary to document the incident in the patient's medical record.

Notify the insurance carrier of the incident; in a large facility, this may be done by the risk manager.

EMERGENCY CARE

Although the role of the caregiver may be to provide immediate first aid, the caregiver should make an effort to obtain immediate assistance from the most qualified individual available, such as a physician, a nurse, an *emergency medical technician (EMT)*, or other medical personnel. In the hospital this may be relatively easy and trained personnel who will react quickly when called are likely to be readily available. However, in the patient's home, an outpatient clinic, a school, an athletic facility, or even an extended care facility, assistance may be difficult to obtain and may require time. Sources of assistance within and external to the setting should be known by the caregiver and the most appropriate source should be contacted promptly. It will require judgment by the caregiver to determine whether assistance should be obtained before or after initiating emergency care or first aid. *Note:* In most situations, it will be best if assistance is requested before initiating emergency care unless the delay of immediate aid is life threatening to the patient. Whatever care has been provided before assistance arrives will have to be explained to the persons who provide additional care. Any objective information about the patient's condition should be provided as well.

BANDAGES

This section presents information about the application and use of bandages when an emergency situation occurs and first aid is necessary. In general, the bandage is used to support or stabilize a segment; to restrict motion of a joint; or to control edema, swelling, or joint effusion when a dressing would not be required. The most common injury that would require the use of a bandage for any of these purposes is a sprain or strain.

Types of Bandage Materials

Materials that are used frequently for a bandage are muslin (unbleached cotton); woven, elastic, porous cotton; rolled gauze; stockinet, which is loosely knit cotton formed into a tube; and adhesive tape (Fig. 12-1). Some of these items will have to be laundered, whereas other items should be discarded after they have been used once. The woven elastic bandage can be used multiple times, but care must be taken when it is washed and dried to preserve its shape and elasticity. It should be washed by hand in lukewarm water, similar to the way a wool sweater would be washed. Excess water should be gently squeezed from the bandage and it should be laid flat on an absorbent towel to dry. Do not hang the bandage from a clothesline because it will stretch because of the weight of the water that remains in its fibers. After it is completely dried, it should be rolled so it will be ready for application. The patient should be given or should purchase several of these bandages so a clean one is available to apply while a previously used one is being laundered and dried. The patient or a family member should be instructed in the proper care of this type of bandage.

Bandages may be named according to their shape, appearance, purpose, design, or material used. Several types of bandages are discussed in the sections that follow. However, a description of the application and use of a bandage, wrap, or strapping with adhesive tape to an area after injury or to prevent an acute injury is beyond the scope of this text, except a tennis elbow wrap or a wrap for a sprained ankle will be presented.

Triangular This bandage is a large piece of cloth cut or formed into a triangle. (For example, a square piece of cloth folded diagonally becomes a triangle.) It is most often used as a temporary sling to support the weight of a patient's upper extremity. When it is used for this purpose, you must be certain the cloth triangle is large enough to contain the patient's forearm and hand. To apply the sling, use the following procedure:

- Flex the elbow of the injured extremity to slightly more than 90 degrees with the palm facing the patient's chest.
- Place the apex of the sling at the elbow and bring the outer end of the sling over the forearm and shoulder of the injured upper extremity (Fig. 12-2, *A*).
- Bring the other end of the sling under the forearm and over the shoulder of the uninjured upper extremity (Fig. 12-2, *B*).

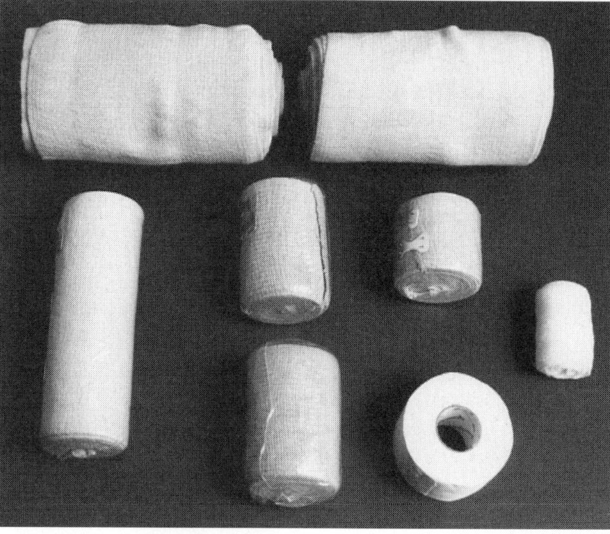

Fig. 12-1 Types of bandages. *Left to right* and *top to bottom,* 6-inch elastic extra long, 6-inch, 4-inch, 3-inch, and 2-inch bandages; adhesive tape; and roller gauze.

- The patient may need to elevate the shoulder of the injured extremity until the sling ends are tied.
- Secure the sling by tying the ends in a square knot positioned to one side of the spinous processes of the patient's neck.
- Have the patient relax the shoulder and be certain the sling trough supports the forearm and hand.
- Pull the free apex end of the sling over the elbow and pin or tape it to the front of the sling.
- Position the patient's hand within the sling and evaluate the height of the hand and forearm, which should be horizontal or elevated slightly above a horizontal position (Fig. 12-2, *C*, and Fig. 12-3).

Cravat A cravat can also be used as a sling, but will not support the patient's upper extremity and the triangular sling.

- To form the cravat, fold a square or rectangular cloth into a series of overlapping layers to the width desired. A belt, necktie, or scarf can be used to form a cravat.
- Loop the cravat over the forearm of the injured upper extremity.
- Tie the two free ends behind and to one side of the patient's neck using a square knot or, if a belt is used, the belt buckle.

Roller Bandage A roller bandage is made of an elastic or a non-elastic material formed in a cylindric roll and fabricated in various widths and lengths. It is used to maintain and protect a dressing, to provide pressure, to maintain a splint, to provide support to a joint, to restrict motion, or to control edema in an extremity.

A B C

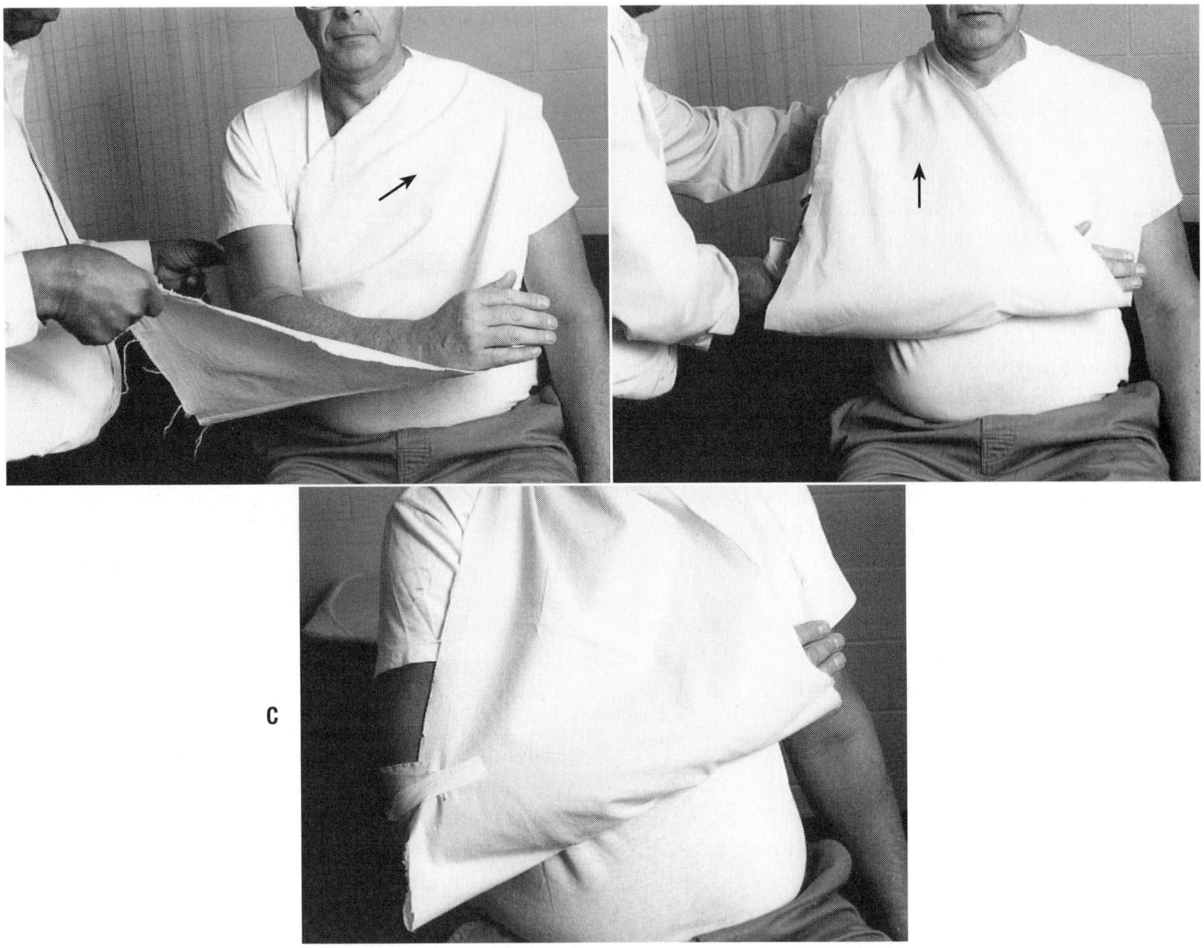

Fig. 12-2 Application of a triangular bandage.

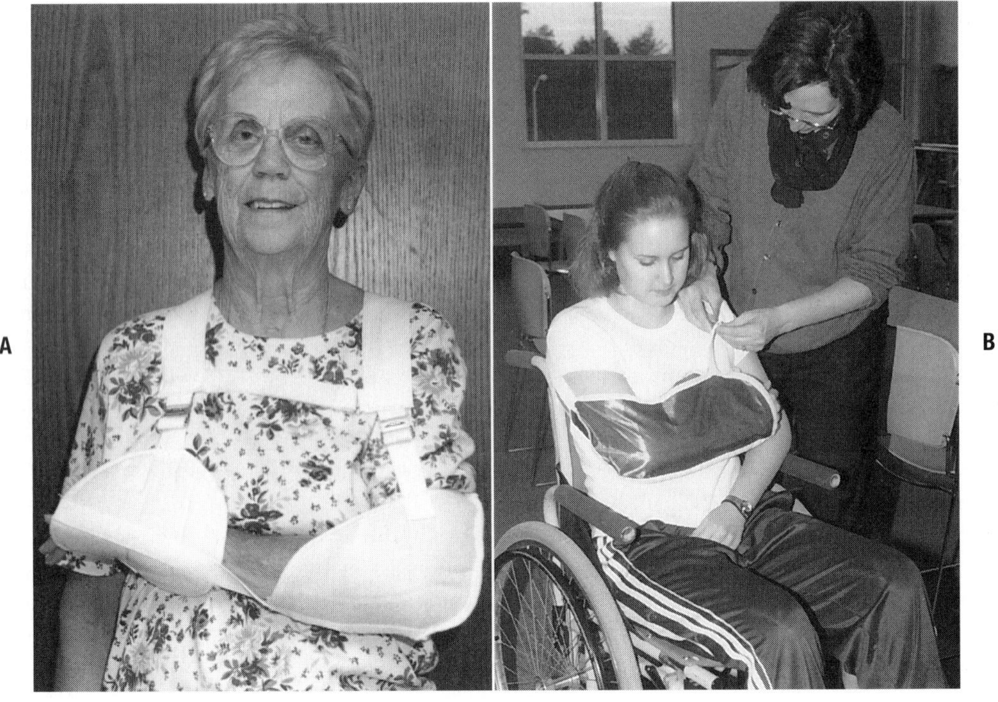

Fig. 12-3 Adjustable slings designed to eliminate pressure to the neck.

Patterns of application are:

Circular. The bandage is applied in a series of overlapping circular turns around a body part to anchor the bandage initially or terminally. It must be applied carefully to avoid occlusion of the local circulation, which could result in decreased blood flow and development of swelling distal to the bandage (Fig. 12-4, *A*).

Spiral. The bandage is applied in a series of overlapping diagonal turns around a body part; these turns may be applied upward or downward. A spiral bandage is less apt to occlude the circulation and will cover a larger area than the circular bandage with the same amount of material (Fig. 12-4, *B*).

Open spiral or oblique. The open spiral is a series of diagonal turns that do not overlap and have an open space between each turn. The bandage begins and terminates with circular anchors and will cover a larger area than the spiral bandage with the same amount of bandage (Fig. 12-4, *C*).

Spiral reverse. The spiral reverse is a series of spiral turns, each of which is folded or reversed on itself midway through each turn. The bandage begins and terminates with circular anchors and is used when the body part or segment being bandaged varies excessively in its shape and circumference (such as forearm or lower leg). The reverse component allows a nonelastic bandage to conform to the change in circumference, so this pattern is usually used with a nonelastic gauze roller bandage (Fig. 12-4, *D* and *E*).

Recurrent. The recurrent pattern is a series of lengthwise layers applied to the anterior-posterior or dorsal-volar surfaces of an extremity or digit. It is used to cover the most distal aspect of a residual limb or the digits. The bandage is anchored with circular turns and may be completed with spiral or figure-of-eight turns (Fig. 12-4, *F* and *G*).

Figure-of-eight. The figure-of-eight is a series of spiral turns applied in alternate directions. The first turn progresses in an inferior-to-superior direction and the second turn progresses in a superior-to-inferior direction. Additional turns follow in the same alternating pattern. This type of bandage can be applied to the foot and ankle, knee, shoulder, hand and wrist, and elbow.

Foot and ankle. Anchor the bandage at the base of the toes and then cross it diagonally over the dorsum of the foot and around the foot (Fig. 12-4, *H*). Bring the bandage diagonally across the anterior ankle, return it to the foot, and repeat the diagonal turns (Fig. 12-4, *I*). Repeat this pattern until the bandage is applied completely. Terminate the bandage with a circular anchor on the lower leg below the belly of the gastrocnemius muscle (Fig. 12-4, *J*). Use a 4-inch bandage for most adults and a smaller width for children.

Hand and wrist. Anchor the bandage at the distal palm, proximal to the metacarpophalangeal (MCP) joints (Fig. 12-4, *K*). Then cross it diagonally through the palm, over the wrist, and diagonally over the dorsum of the hand (Fig. 12-4, *L*). Continue with the figure-of-eight pattern over the hand and wrist. The thumb and fingers are not incorporated in the bandage. Terminate the bandage on the lower forearm with a circular anchor (Fig. 12-4, *M*). Use a 1- or 2-inch bandage for most adults and a 1-inch bandage for children.

Knee. Anchor the bandage slightly below the knee, cross diagonally to the medial or lateral aspect of the knee, and make a circular anchor above the knee (Fig. 12-4, *N*). Return to the lower leg with a diagonal turn and continue with the figure-of-eight pattern until the area is covered (Fig. 12-4, *O*). Terminate the bandage on the thigh with a firm circular anchor (Fig. 12-4, *P*). Use a 4-inch bandage for most adults and a 3-inch bandage for most children.

Elbow. Follow the same pattern as described for the knee, substituting the upper arm and forearm for the thigh and lower leg. Use a 3- or 4-inch bandage for most adults and a 2- or 3-inch bandage for most children.

Spica. A spica bandage incorporates the figure-of-eight pattern, but a large anchor or spica is applied around the pelvis to prevent the distal portion of the bandage from sliding down the extremity to which it is applied. A hip spica is used for a transfemoral amputation or strained groin muscle.

Hip. Anchor the bandage around the patient's thigh, below the level of the injury (Fig. 12-4, *Q*). Wrap the bandage diagonally around the thigh several times using a figure-of-eight or spiral pattern (Fig. 12-4, *R*). Bring the bandage completely around the pelvis, between the iliac crests and the greater trochanters several times and then return the bandage to the thigh (Fig. 12-4, *S*). Complete the bandage with a figure-of-eight or spiral pattern and anchor the bandage on the pelvic spica or on the thigh portion of the bandage. Use a 6-inch bandage for most adults and a 4-inch bandage for most children or small adults. Usually several bandages sewn together or an extremely long bandage are required to accomplish this pattern.

Reminder: It is important to select the proper-width bandage for the size of the area being wrapped. For most adults the following bandage widths are recommended: a 3- or 4-inch bandage for the foot and ankle; a 1- or 2-inch bandage for the hand or wrist; a 2-, 3-, or 4-inch bandage for the elbow; a 3- or 4-inch bandage for the knee; a 6-inch bandage for the thigh; and a 3- or 4-inch bandage for the upper arm. If the bandage is too wide for the area, wrinkles will develop or the bandage will not conform properly to the area. If the bandage is too narrow, it will be insufficient to cover the area or may cause undesired pressure. An elastic bandage is the best type to use for most of these patterns.

Text continued on p. 335

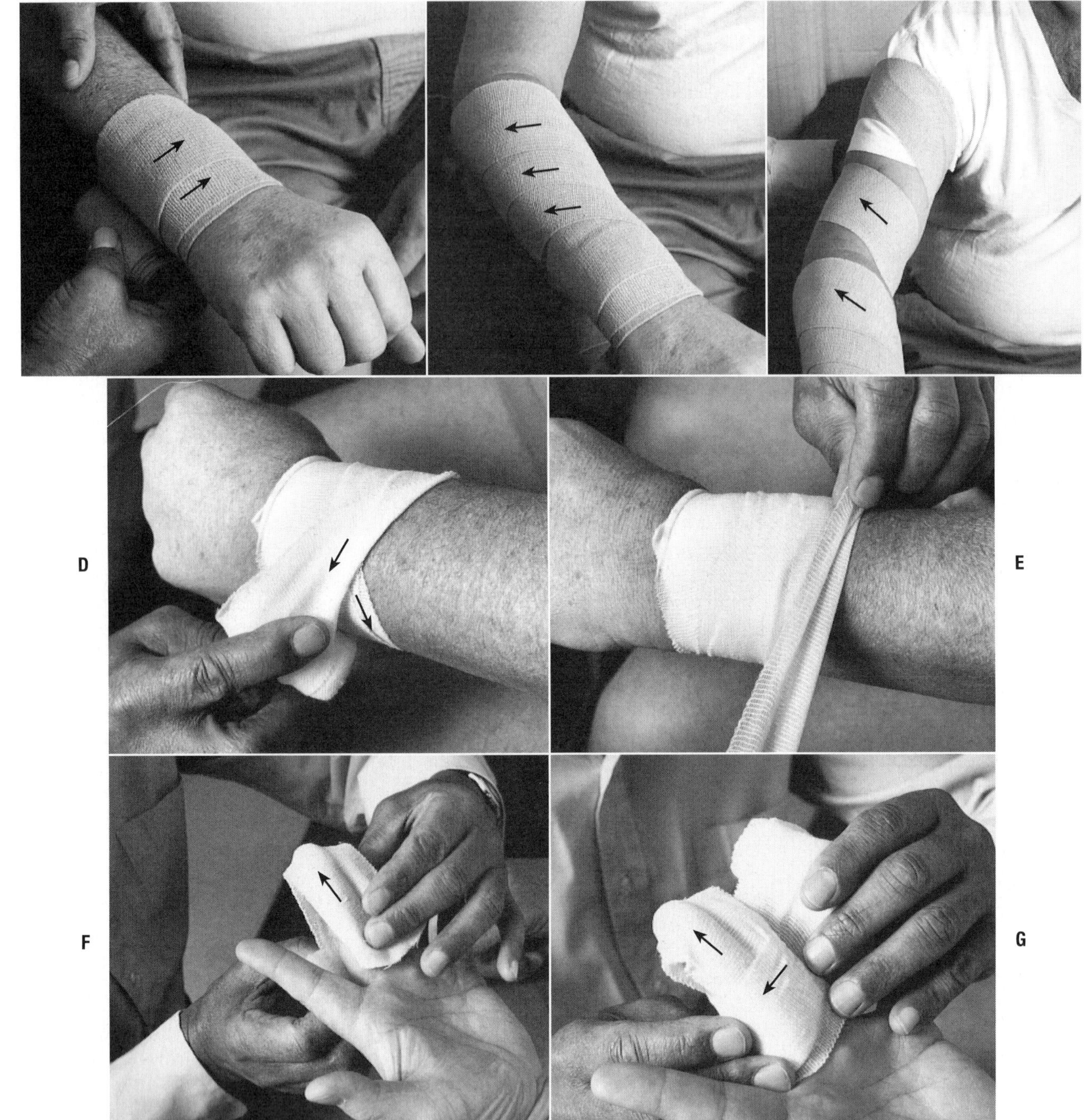

Fig. 12-4 Patterns of application of elastic roller bandage. **A,** Circular. **B,** Spiral. **C,** Open spiral. **D** and **E,** Spiral reverse. **F** and **G,** Recurrent for fingers.

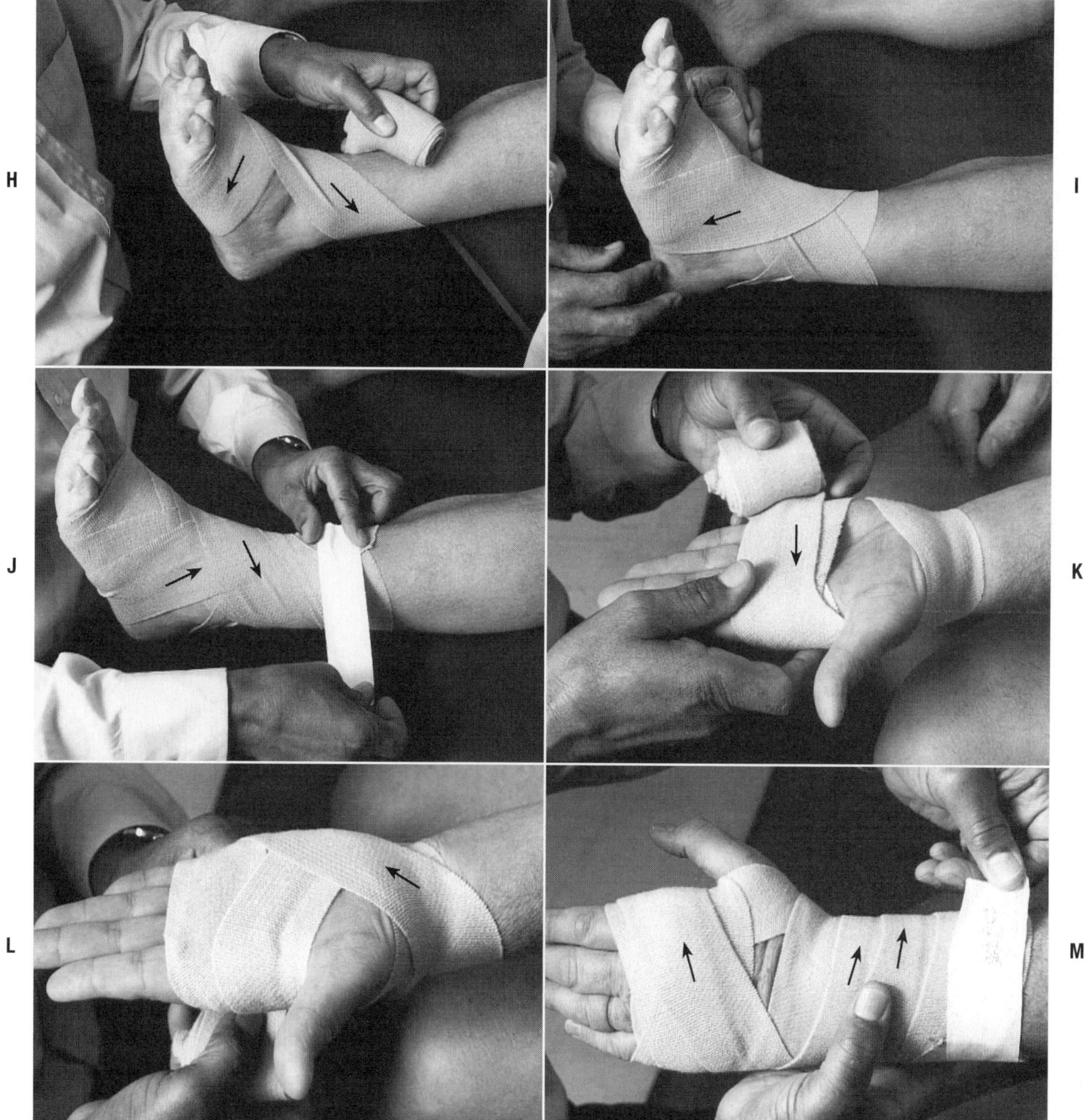

Fig. 12-4, cont'd **H** through **J,** Figure-of-eight for the foot and ankle. **K** through **M,** Figure-of-eight for the hand and wrist.

Continued

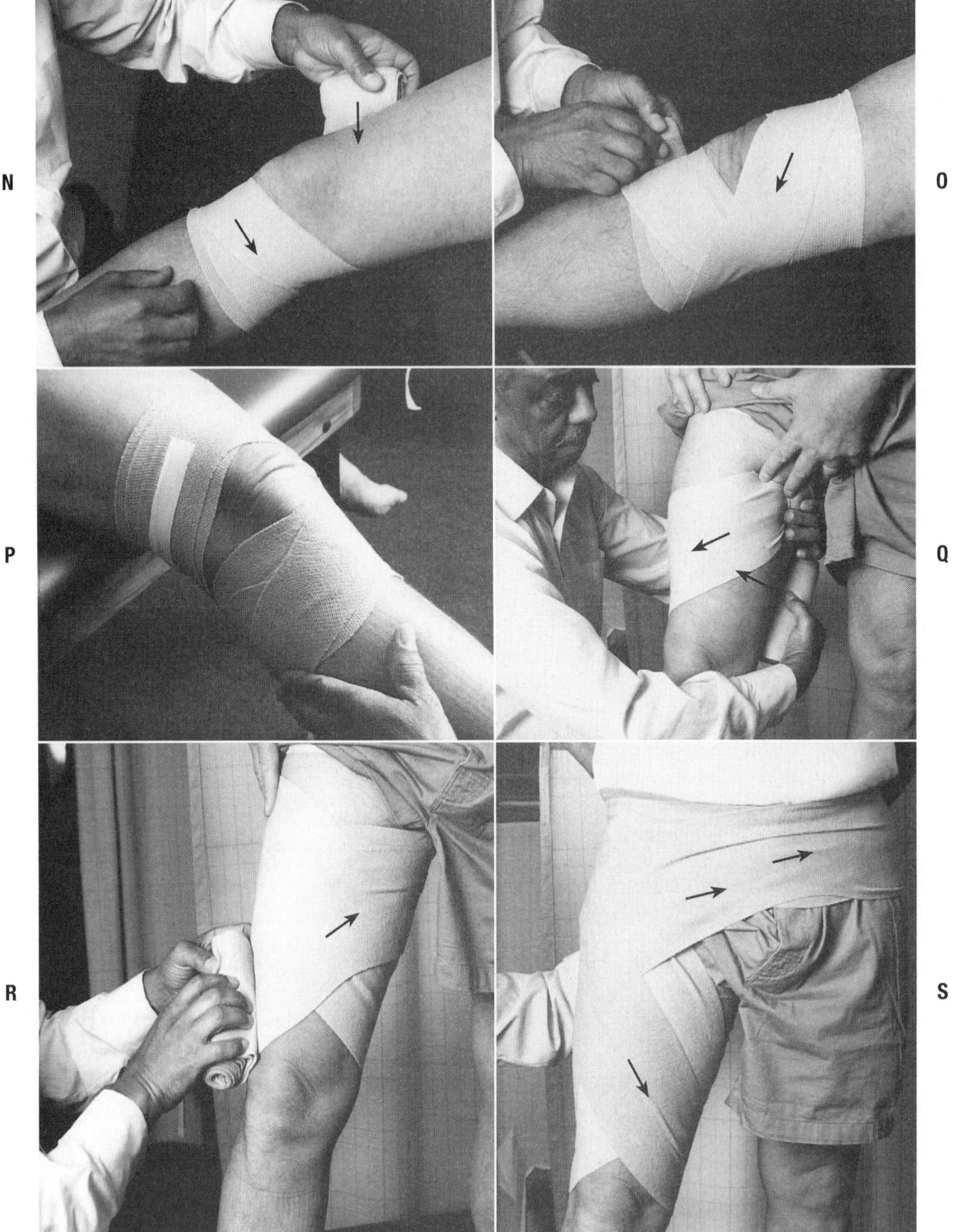

Fig. 12-4, cont'd **N** through **P,** Figure-of-eight for the knee; **Q** through **S,** Spica for hip.

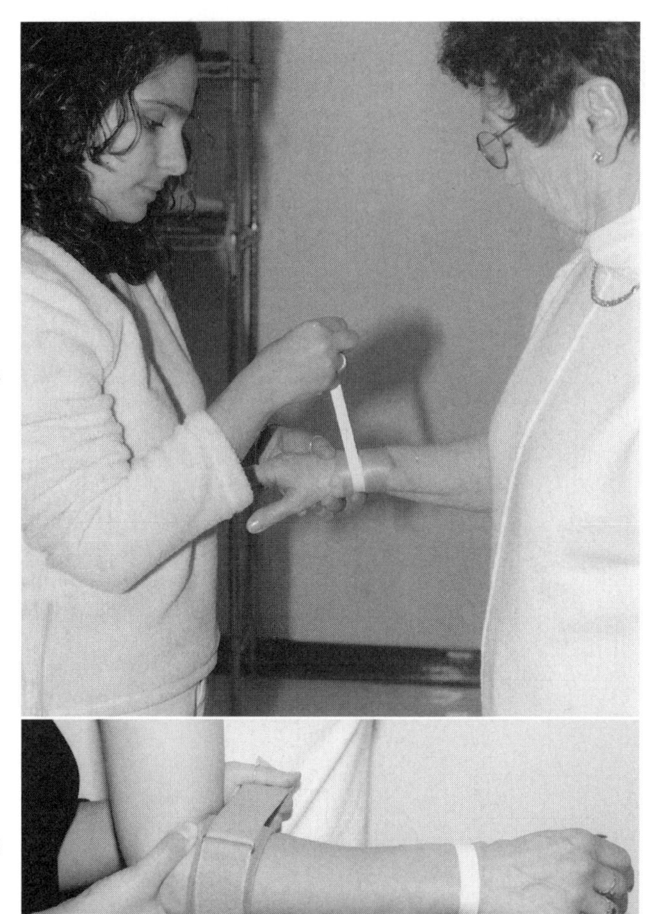

Fig. 12-5 Epicondylitis (tennis elbow) wrap. **A,** Application of underwrap, followed by 0.5-inch-wide adhesive tape. *Note:* The hand should be distracted from the wrist during application. **B,** Tennis elbow strap applied.

Adhesive Tape Bandage Adhesive or athletic tape is used when support or protection to a joint is needed with little or no stretch to the bandage. The usual width of the tape is 1.5 to 2 inches.

Epicondylitis (Tennis Elbow) Wrap. Place an underwrap (a porous polyurethane foam) around the wrist to prevent the tape from adhering to the underlying skin. Distract the wrist by having the patient hold the elbow to the side with elbow bent to 90 degrees and gently pull the wrist and hand away from the forearm. Use athletic tape that is approximately 0.5 to 0.75 inch wide. Place the tape just distal to the radial head and ulnar stylus. Wrap snugly over the dorsum of the wrist followed by "laying on" the tape on the volar surface to avoid compression of blood vessels and the median nerve. Repeat the wrap two or three repetitions and ask the patient to extend and flex the wrist; motion should be limited. When treating for tennis elbow, have the patient wear an adjustable tennis elbow strap approximately 1 to 2 inches distal to the olecranon process (Fig. 12-5).

Ankle Wrap for Sprained Ankle. Following a first- or second-degree ankle sprain, if a commercial splint (elastic or air inflated) is not available, a wrap to prevent further damage to ankle structures and keep them in a protected position can be applied until the sprain has sufficient time to heal. Place an underwrap from the metatarsal heads to approximately 6 inches above the ankle using a spiral and figure-of-eight pattern. Place one or two anchors of the athletic tape just proximal to the fifth metatarsal head and again around the calf just below the head of the gastrocnemius. Start medially on the calf anchor and bring the tape under the calcaneous up to the calf anchor on the lateral side. Repeat with another stirrup anterior or posterior to the previous one. Make sure that pressure is applied on the foot while attaching stirrups to keep the ankle in full dorsiflexion and eversion for a lateral sprain (dorsiflexion and inversion for a medial sprain). Variations of the remainder of the wrap can be done from the addition of heel locks (figure-of-eights around the heels) to using spirals and figure-of-eights around the ankle and up to the calf anchors to complete the wrap. Make sure the wrap is snug, but not so tight it impairs circulation (Fig. 12-6).

Protective Splints or Sleeves Some patients may find it necessary to use a splint or sleeve to immobilize, stabilize,

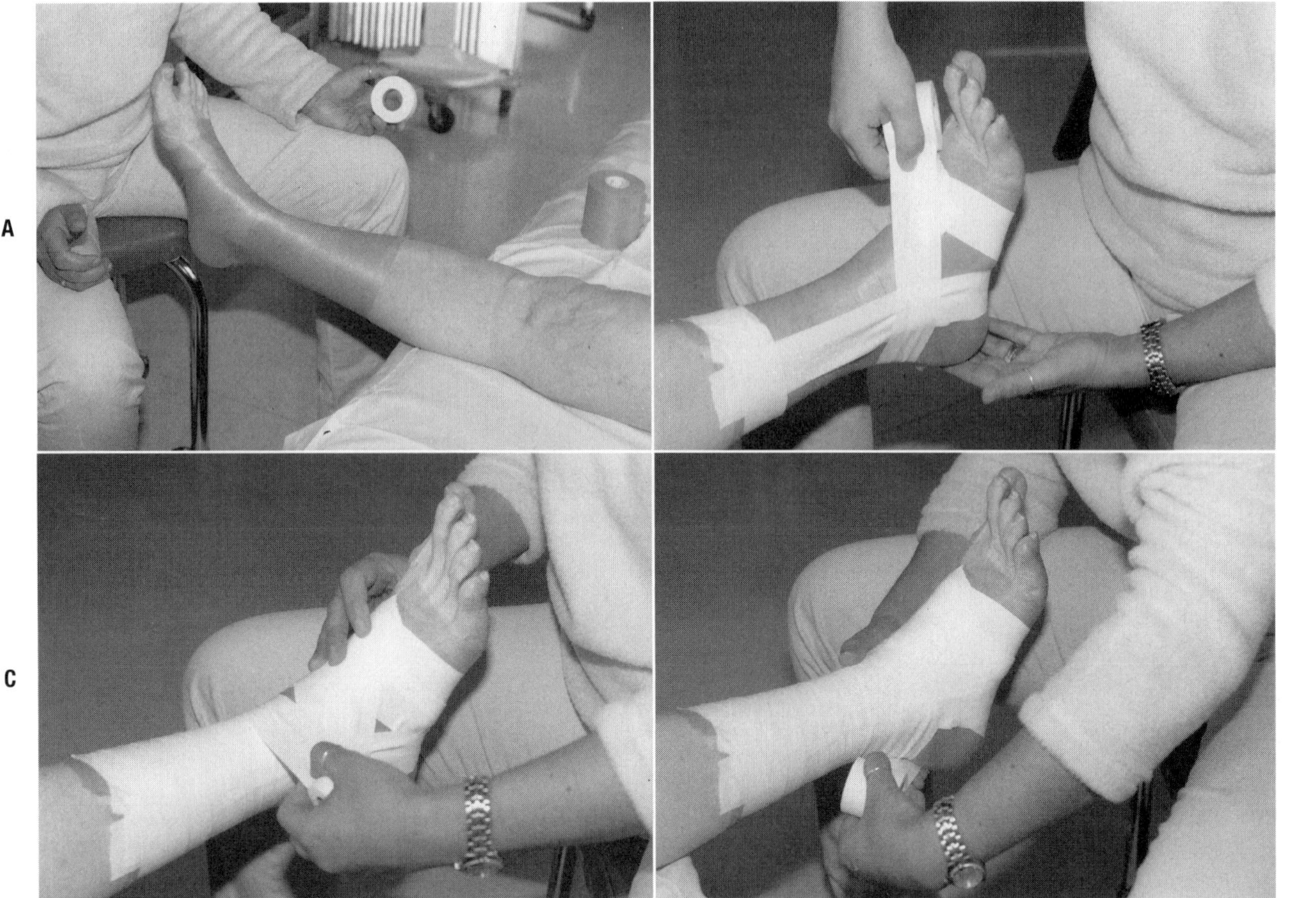

Fig. 12-6 Protective ankle wrap. **A,** Application of underwrap. **B,** Application of a figure-of-eight around the ankle. The two anchors of the stirrups have been applied. *Note:* If the patient is unable to fully dorsiflex the foot, the caregiver should assist by applying pressure into dorsiflexion and eversion or inversion at the ball of the foot while applying the stirrups. **C,** Bandage three fourths completed. **D,** Final figure-of-eight.

and protect a joint or to control edema. The joints affected most frequently are the elbow, wrist, thumb, knee, and ankle. Examples of these devices are presented in Fig. 12-7. Some of these items are available over the counter at a drugstore, pharmacy, sporting goods store, or department store, whereas others must be custom fabricated and fit for the individual. Uses vary from protection during athletic competition, prevention of contractures, or immobilization of a joint during the healing of an injury.

EMERGENCY CARE FOR SPECIFIC CONDITIONS

When an injury or change in the patient's condition requires first aid or emergency care, you should be aware of some of the emergency aid that could be provided. The best way to be prepared to provide emergency care is to participate in an educational program or course provided by a qualified instructor or agency.

Lacerations

The objectives are to prevent contamination of the wound and control the bleeding. Treatment is described in Procedure 12-2.

Shock

The objectives are to identify and reduce or remove the cause when possible and to prevent or reduce the extent of the physiologic state of *shock*. Signs and symptoms of shock include pale, moist, cool skin; shallow and irregular breathing; dilated pupils; a weak, rapid pulse; diaphoresis; dizziness or nausea; and syncope. Treatment is described in Procedure 12-3.

Orthostatic (Postural) Hypotension

Some patients may experience *orthostatic (postural) hypotension*. Usually, this condition is accompanied by signs and symptoms similar to those described for shock. This condition

A

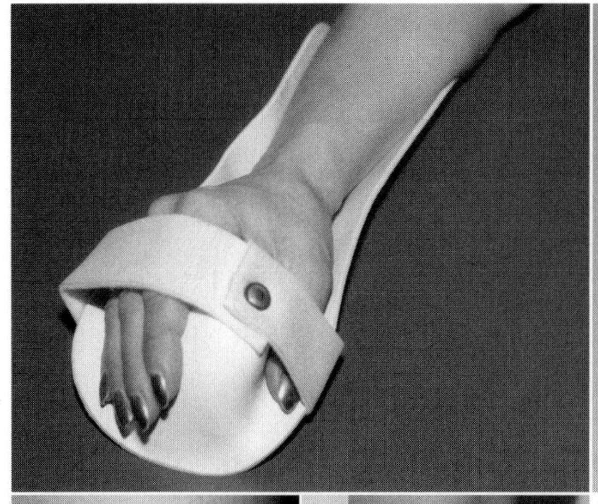

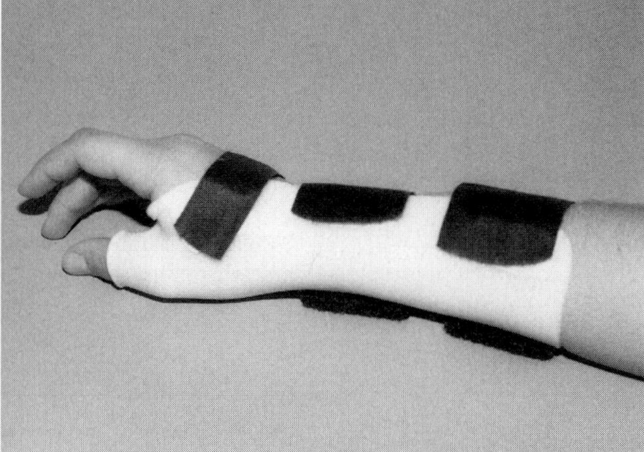

B

C, D

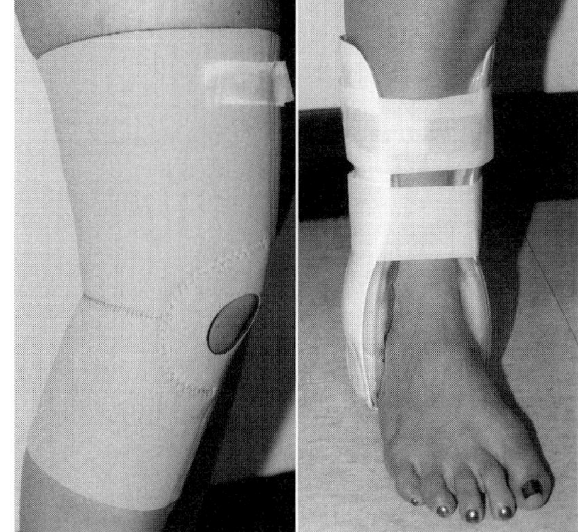

Fig. 12-7 **A,** Positional resting splint. **B,** Immobilization splint for thumb or wrist. **C,** Neoprene knee sleeve. **D,** Air inflated ankle splint.

PROCEDURE 12-2

Treatment of Lacerations

Wash your hands and apply protective gloves; apply a clean or sterile, nonabsorbent towel or similar object to the wound. Continue to wear protective gloves during the treatment of the wound. Obtain additional assistance and contact emergency services personnel as necessary.

Elevate the wound above the level of the heart to reduce blood flow to the area if blood flow is excessive.

In some instances, the wound can be cleansed with an antiseptic or by rinsing it with water.

Place a clean towel or sterile dressing over the wound and apply direct pressure to a bleeding wound.

Encourage the patient to remain quiet and avoid using the extremity.

If there is arterial bleeding (demonstrated by spurting blood), it may be necessary to apply intermittent, direct pressure to the artery above the level of the wound or directly over the wound. This is done most frequently to the brachial and femoral arteries to restrict blood flow to the distal wound site. However, prolonged pressure by the use of a tourniquet should be avoided. The person should be transported to a site where appropriate medical care can be provided unless assistance can be brought to the patient.

PROCEDURE 12-3

Treatment of Shock

Determine the cause of shock (such as excessive bleeding, inability to adjust to moving from a supine to a sitting or standing position, response to excessive heat) and remedy it if possible. Monitor the patient's blood pressure and pulse rate. Obtain additional assistance and contact emergency support personnel as necessary.

Place the person in a supine position with the head slightly lower than the lower extremities. If there are head and chest injuries or if respiration is impaired, it may be necessary to place the person in a supine position, level or with the head and chest elevated slightly. If bleeding is the apparent cause and the wound is visible, attempt to control bleeding as described for a laceration.

A cool compress may be applied to the person's forehead for comfort and a light blanket may be used to prevent loss of body heat.

Have the patient remain quiet and avoid exertion.

After the symptoms have been relieved, gradually return the person to an upright position and monitor to ensure regression of the condition.

Request transportation so the patient can be taken to a facility where proper care and treatment can be provided.

occurs most frequently when the person attempts to stand rapidly from a stooped, kneeling, recumbent, or sitting position. The elderly person, the person who uses antihypertension medication, the person who has a decreased ability to return venous blood from the periphery to the heart (such as the spinal cord-injured person), the person with hypotension, and the person who has been immobilized in a recumbent position for an extended period are most apt to demonstrate orthostatic hypotension. The reduced venous return from the lower extremities results in decreased filling of the left ventricle, which leads to decreased cardiac output and, eventually, decreased cerebral perfusion. As a result, the person experiences dizziness and possibly syncope when rising to stand.

The first aid measures used to resolve hypotension are the same as those listed in Procedure 12-3. Some measures that can be taken to prevent this condition are to wrap the patient's lower extremities, from the feet to the groin, with elastic bandages; apply an abdominal binder or corset; apply elastic hose (half or full length); instruct the patient to perform active ankle dorsiflexion-plantar flexion exercises ("ankle pumps") and alternate knee-to-chest exercises frequently while supine or sitting; allow the person to accommodate to the upright position gradually by slowly elevating the head of the bed to various levels; or use a tilt table to elevate the patient by increments.

In a severe case, it may be necessary to apply a full-body pressurized garment (a G suit) to stabilize the venous circulation. The abdominal binder, elastic lower extremity wraps, elastic hose, and G suit provide external pressure to the veins of the extremities and trunk, which helps return venous blood to the heart and reduces the pooling or collection of venous blood in the lower extremities and abdomen. The active use of the lower extremity muscles will assist in "pumping" or moving the venous blood toward the heart and reduce the pooling of venous blood in the lower extremities. The gradual elevation of the patient from a recumbent to a sitting or standing position assists the vascular system to accommodate physiologically to the changes in position.

Fractures

The objectives are to protect the fracture site and avoid further injury to it, prevent shock, reduce pain, and prevent wound contamination if the bone ends have penetrated the skin. Emergency care should *not* include any attempt to align the fracture segments or "set" the fracture. Treatment is described in Procedure 12-4.

Burns

The objectives are to prevent wound contamination, to relieve or reduce pain, and to prevent shock. Treatment is described in Procedure 12-5.

Convulsions/Seizures

The objectives are to protect the person from injury should a fall or excessive involuntary movements of the extremities occur and to protect the person's modesty or privacy. Treatment is described in Procedure 12-6.

PROCEDURE 12-4

Treatment of Fractures

Obtain information about the injury from the conscious patient (such as its cause, location, the extent of discomfort, and any restriction of motion). Obtain additional assistance and contact emergency services personnel as necessary.

Observe the site of injury or the position of the extremity; examine and evaluate the patient's general appearance and condition. Monitor blood pressure and pulse rate.

Gently palpate the area and surrounding tissue to evaluate swelling or edema and tenderness. Deformity and soft-tissue bruising may indicate a fracture has occurred.

Avoid movement or activity that has the potential to cause additional damage.

Apply support to the site to stabilize it, but do not attempt to align the bone ends. Use a firm object to stabilize the fracture before transporting the patient. A pillow folded around the site, canes or crutches applied on either side of a lower extremity fracture, or a flat piece of wood applied to either side of the fracture site can be used; on small extremities a large magazine can be wrapped around the site.

Cover an open fracture site with a sterile towel or dressing, but do not attempt to reinsert the bone ends beneath the skin.

If a spinal fracture is suspected, use extreme caution when handling the patient. Place the patient on a firm, flat board, and maintain the head and neck in a neutral position. To insert the spinal board, logroll the patient, avoiding forward, backward, or side bending of the spine. At least three persons will be required to roll or lift the patient. Evaluate the level of neurologic sensation and function by asking the patient to move an extremity or report any response to a stimulus applied to the skin. Evaluate the patient for signs of shock, bleeding, and additional injuries. Obtain qualified medical assistance rather than attempting to transport the patient with minimal assistance or without sufficient immobilization. This is a serious injury, and the patient must be handled carefully.

Request transportation so the patient can be taken to a facility where proper care and treatment can be provided.

PROCEDURE 12-5

Treatment of Burns

Remove or eliminate the agent causing the burn or remove the patient from the agent; contact skilled personnel when the burn wounds are extensive or involve the face, hands, perineum, or feet. Obtain additional assistance and contact emergency services personnel as necessary.

Cut away or remove clothing near the site of the burn, but do not attempt to remove clothing that lies over or is part of the wound. Remove jewelry from the patient if edema has not developed and the jewelry can be removed without causing additional trauma.

A clean or sterile dressing or towel can be loosely laid over the wound. In some instances a moist dressing will be more comfortable for the patient. Do not apply any cream, salve, ointment, or similar substance (such as butter or lard) to the wound because this will mask the appearance of the wound and may lead to infection or a delay in healing.

If the wound has been caused by a toxic chemical, use a copious amount of water to wash the wound site to dilute the substance. However, avoid washing the chemical onto an unaffected portion of the skin to prevent causing a burn to that area.

Observe the patient for shock, respiratory distress, and other injuries. Prepare the patient for transportation or transport to a facility that is prepared to manage this type of injury.

PROCEDURE 12-6

Treatment of Seizures

Place the person in a safe location and position; do not attempt to restrain or restrict the convulsions. Obtain additional assistance and contact emergency services personnel as necessary.

Monitor the rate and quality of respiration. There may be a period of tonic contraction of all body muscles, which will cause respiration to cease for up to 50 to 70 seconds. After this has ended, respirations may be slower and deeper than normal for a brief period.

Assist in keeping the patient's airway patent, but do not attempt to open the mouth by placing any object between the teeth. Never place your finger or a wooden or metal object in the patient's mouth, and do not attempt to grasp or position the tongue.

When the convulsions subside, turn the person's head to one side in case vomiting occurs.

Allow the patient to rest after the convulsions cease and protect modesty and privacy. It may be helpful to cover the person with a blanket or screen from view. Some patients' sphincter control may be lost during or at the conclusion of the *seizure,* resulting in the involuntary discharge of bladder or bowel contents.

The patient should be evaluated by a physician to determine the cause of the seizure if the cause is not known.

Choking

The objectives are to restore and maintain a patent airway and normal breathing. Treatment is described in Procedure 12-7.

Heat-Related Illnesses

The objectives are to remove or reduce the cause of the illness and return the individual to a state of normal homeostasis.

The two primary forms of heat-related illness are heat exhaustion and heat stroke (Table 12-1). Of the two, heat exhaustion poses the least threat to life, whereas heat stroke is considered a medical emergency because it can be life threatening. Both illnesses can result from a hot, humid environment; vigorous physical activity; dehydration; and depleted body electrolytes. Persons who are treated with hydrotherapy and persons who participate in vigorous aerobic exercise in a warm, humid environment should be observed periodically for signs or symptoms of heat exhaustion or heat stroke. Heat stroke may follow heat exhaustion if the person is not treated properly when the signs of heat exhaustion appear. Muscle cramps in the legs and abdomen may be the initial indicators of a heat-related illness. Rest, increased fluid intake, and gentle stretching and massage to the affected areas are methods used to relieve these symptoms.

Heat Exhaustion When the signs and symptoms of this condition are observed, it is important to cool the person and counteract the effects of dehydration. Emergency first aid treatment procedures are presented in Procedure 12-8. You may need to treat the person for shock and you should be alert for signs or symptoms of heat stroke. The person should not be given salt tablets by mouth as part of the treatment. The ingestion of excess salt may interfere with the person's ability to readjust the electrolyte balance to a normal state. Fluids containing selected electrolytes can be administered frequently to assist the person to compensate for the loss of electrolytes from excessive exercise.

Heat Stroke This condition is life threatening and its signs and symptoms must be recognized quickly so emergency first aid treatment can be initiated promptly. Emergency first aid treatment procedures are presented in Procedure 12-9. The individual with heat stroke will require care and treatment by qualified medical personnel and must be transported to a medical facility as quickly as possible.

Insulin-Related Illnesses

The objectives are to restore the person to a normal *insulin-glucose* state and to remove, correct, or compensate for the cause of the condition.

It is important to differentiate between the conditions of hypoglycemia (hyperinsulinemia, or an insulin reaction) and

PROCEDURE 12-7

Treatment for Choking

When assisting a *conscious* adult or a child who is more than 1 year old:

- Ask the person if he or she is choking. If the person can speak, cough, or breathe, do not attempt to provide further assistance.
- If the person is unable to speak, cough, or breathe, check the mouth and remove any visible foreign object.
- If the person cannot speak, cough, or breathe, position yourself behind him or her. Clasp your hands over the person's abdomen slightly above the umbilicus but below the diaphragm.
- Use the closed fist of one hand, covered by your other hand, to give three or four abrupt thrusts against the person's abdomen by compressing the abdomen in and up forcefully (Heimlich maneuver; Fig. 12-8). Continue to apply the thrusts until the obstruction becomes dislodged, is relieved, or the person becomes unconscious.
- Obtain advanced medical assistance.

When assisting an *unconscious* adult or child who is more than 8 years old:

- Place the person in a supine position and request help from others to contact advanced medical assistance.
- Open the person's mouth and use your finger to attempt to locate and remove the foreign object (finger sweep).
- Open the airway by tilting the head back and lifting the chin forward and attempt to ventilate using the mouth-to-mouth technique.
- If this approach is unsuccessful in initiating respiration, give 6 to 10 subdiaphragmatic abdominal thrusts using the heel of one hand reinforced by the other hand (Heimlich maneuver).
- If this approach is unsuccessful in initiating respiration, repeat the finger sweep, open the airway, attempt to ventilate, and perform the abdominal thrusts. Be persistent and continue these procedures until the object is removed or advanced medical assistance arrives. (*Note:* Avoid performing a blind finger sweep in children who are younger than 8 years old. Instead, lift the chin to expose the oral cavity and remove a foreign body if you see it).
- After the object has been removed, it may be necessary to initiate CPR techniques to stabilize the person's cardiopulmonary functions.

When assisting a conscious infant (younger than 1 year old):

- Support the head and neck with one hand and place the child in a prone position over your forearm, with the head lower than the trunk and your forearm supported on your thigh.
- Perform four forceful interscapular blows with the heel of your free hand.
- Immediately after applying the blows to the upper back, turn the infant supine with the head lower than the trunk, and perform four thrusts to the lower *sternum* with two fingers.
- Repeat the back blows and sternal thrusts until the object is expelled.

When assisting an *unconscious* infant:

- Place the infant supine and request help from others to contact advanced medical assistance.
- Perform a tongue-jaw lift and remove any foreign object if it is visible.
- Open the airway using the head tilt-chin lift technique described previously and attempt to ventilate the infant.
- Perform four back blows and four sternal thrusts if respiration has not been started.
- If the foreign body has not been removed, repeat the sequence until the foreign object is extracted.
- If the foreign body has been removed and the infant is not breathing, initiate basic CPR techniques (that is, open the airway, use mouth-to-mouth and nose ventilation, and perform chest compressions with two fingers to initiate a heart rate).

Note: All persons who have experienced a choking incident should be examined by a physician as soon as possible. This information is based on the recommendations of the American Heart Association. A pamphlet containing diagrams and this information can be obtained from most affiliate offices of the American Heart Association.

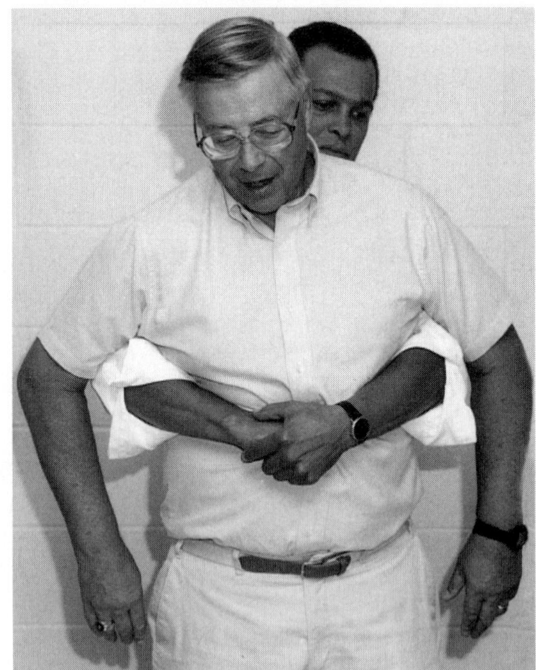

Fig. 12-8 Application of the Heimlich maneuver: hands are positioned above the umbilicus and below the diaphragm and pressure is exerted in and up.

Table 12-1 **Signs and Symptoms of Heat-Related Illnesses**

Observations	Heat Exhaustion	Heat Stroke
Skin	Profuse diaphoresis	Dry; no diaphoresis
Nausea	Present	Present
Headache	Present	Present
Breathing	Shallow, rapid	Labored
Pulse	Weak, rapid	Strong, rapid
Color	Pale	Flushed or changes to gray
Temperature	Normal or slightly elevated	Very elevated (106°-110° F)
Behavior	Exhaustion, collapse	Exhaustion, collapse, convulsions
Consciousness	Unconscious	Unconscious
Eyes	Pupils normal	Pupils contract, then dilate

PROCEDURE 12-8

Treatment for Heat Exhaustion

Place the person in a comfortable position in a shady or covered area or room that is well ventilated. Loosen or remove the person's outer clothing and monitor the vital signs. Obtain additional assistance and contact emergency service personnel as necessary.

Sponge the person's forehead and neck with a cold compress or ice bag. Cool wet towels or sheets can be used to cool the person and water or a solution containing electrolytes may be given by mouth if the person is conscious.

Observe the person for shock or other physiologic changes and treat the symptoms as appropriate. Vomiting, refusal of fluids, or loss of consciousness indicates that the condition is becoming worse.

Request transportation so the person can be taken to a facility where proper care and treatment can be provided if no relief of signs and symptoms occurs within a short time or if further progression of the signs or symptoms occur.

PROCEDURE 12-9

Treatment for Heat Stroke

Place the person in a semireclining position in a shady or well-ventilated covered area or room. Remove the outer clothing and monitor the pulse and respiration rates. Obtain additional assistance and contact emergency services personnel immediately.

Cool the person quickly with large amounts of cool or cold water or apply cold, wet compresses, towels, or sheets to the body. Ice bags can be applied to the wrists, ankles, each groin area, each axilla, and lateral neck areas to cool the large blood vessels.

This is a life-threatening condition and prompt emergency care must be provided; the person should be transported to a medical facility as rapidly as possible.

hyperglycemia *(acidosis)*, as outlined in Table 12-2. An insulin reaction can be caused by too much systemic insulin, too little food intake, or excessive exercise in relation to the metabolic state of the person. Acidosis can be caused by too little systemic insulin, the intake of too much food or improper food (that is, excessive sugar), or insufficient physical activity in relation to the metabolic state of the person; therefore treatment should be scheduled accordingly.

Table 12-2 **Warning Signs and Symptoms of Insulin-Related Illnesses**

Observations	Insulin Reaction	Acidosis
Onset	Sudden	Gradual
Skin	Pale, moist	Flushed, dry
Behavior	Excited, agitated	Drowsy
Breath odor	Normal	Fruity odor
Breathing	Normal to shallow	Deep, labored
Vomiting	Absent	Present
Tongue	Moist	Dry
Hunger	Present	Absent
Thirst	Absent	Present
Glucose in urine	Absent or slight	Large amounts

Insulin Reaction If the person is conscious, provide some form of sugar (such as candy or orange juice). If the person is unconscious, glucose may need to be provided intravenously. The person should rest and all physical activity should be stopped. This condition is not as serious as acidosis, but the person should be given the opportunity to return to a balanced metabolic state as quickly as possible. It may be necessary to counsel the person how to balance food intake and exercise or monitor the blood glucose levels and insulin dosage more carefully.

Acidosis Acidosis can lead to a diabetic coma and death can occur if this state is allowed to persist. It should be considered a medical emergency that requires prompt action, including assistance from qualified personnel. The patient should not be given any form of sugar. Usually an injection of insulin is needed and a nurse or physician should provide care as quickly as possible.

Autonomic Hyperreflexia (Dysreflexia)

The objectives are to determine and remove the noxious stimulus causing the condition and to return the person to a level of normal homeostasis.

Autonomic hyperreflexia occurs in individuals with a relatively recent complete injury to the cervical and upper thoracic portions of the spinal cord down to the T6 cord level. Signs and symptoms include severe hypertension, bradycardia, profuse diaphoresis above the level of the cord lesion, a pounding headache, a general feeling of discomfort, red skin blotches, and piloerection ("goose bumps"). The person may convulse, respiration may become difficult, and may become unconscious.

Various noxious stimuli below the level of the spinal cord lesion (such as bladder distension caused by urine retention, fecal impaction, open pressure ulcers, tight straps from an orthosis or urine retention bag, localized pressure, or exercise) may cause a massive sympathetic system response that cannot be controlled or counteracted by higher centers in the brain because of the location of the spinal cord injury. The result is uncontrolled, widespread peripheral arterial *vasoconstriction*, which causes severe hypertension. This condition should be considered a medical emergency and a physician should be contacted for immediate assistance. Treatment is described in Procedure 12-10.

PROCEDURE 12-10

Treatment of Autonomic Hyperreflexia

Initially place the person in a sitting or semirecumbent position to reduce the hypertension. Do not place the person supine.

If the noxious stimulus can be identified, it should be removed or relieved if possible. A common stimulus is an occluded catheter or a completely filled urine retention bag, which prevents drainage of urine from the bladder.

Monitor the person's vital signs frequently, provide reassurance, and obtain qualified medical assistance.

Be aware that this condition could occur at any time and be prepared to assist the patient.

Cardiac Arrest/Death

The objective is to maintain the cardiopulmonary system at a level sufficient to sustain life until the person can be transported to a medical facility.

All health care practitioners should be trained and certified to perform *cardiopulmonary resuscitation (CPR)*. The information presented in this section is a summary of the CPR techniques developed by the American Heart Association. This group advocates the use of the acronym ABC to identify the three important components of CPR and the sequence in which they should be managed: (A) airway, (B) breathing, and (C) circulation.

Guidelines for CPR recommend that qualified medical assistance be contacted by using the 911 emergency telephone service or by calling a community emergency medical technical support unit (such as an emergency medical service, local fire department, police department, or hospital) *before* the initiation of CPR by an individual. Early contact with a medical assistance team or unit will permit the team to reach the victim as rapidly as possible. If CPR is initiated before contacting more qualified medical assistance personnel, their assistance will be delayed. Therefore when more than one person is available at the scene, one should initiate CPR while another contacts advanced medical assistance immediately (Procedure 12-11).

When a rescuer is alone, an attempt should be made to contact qualified medical assistance before starting CPR unless no reasonable access to a means of contact is possible or it would require extraordinary time. If wireless communication is used (cellular phone, CB radio) the exact location of the victim must be provided so other rescuers can find the site. It should be administered until qualified medical personnel arrive, or until the patient is revived and exhibits the ability to maintain vital signs independently, or until the initial rescuer is unable to continue providing support. Alone, CPR is usually not sufficient to revive or maintain life for a person who experiences a sudden cardiac death ("heart attack"), but it is one link in a chain of events designed to provide the best opportunity for survival. The sequence of the chain of events appears in Box 12-2 and the activities should be performed in the shortest possible time. *Note:* An automatic external defibrillator (AED) may not be available until the EMTs arrive; however, if it is available, it should be used promptly. The AED is programmed by an internal computer that instructs the user how to apply the unit (Fig. 12-9). The AED units have become more accessible to the general public, especially on commercial aircraft and cruise ships; in office buildings, public schools, public service vehicles, and colleges; and at facilities or events where large numbers of persons gather. At some locations, a resuscitation unit (Ambu Bag) may be available to provide respiration for the patient. The caregiver squeezes and releases the flexible canister ("bag") at the rate of normal breathing producing a cycle of inspiration and expiration (Fig. 12-11).

PROCEDURE 12-11

Cardiopulmonary Resuscitation (Adult)

Call 911 or the appropriate medical service before initiating CPR.

Determine the condition of the patient by gently shaking and asking "Are you all right?" or "How do you feel?" If the patient does not respond, place in a supine position on a firm surface. Open the airway by lifting up on the chin and pushing down on the forehead to tilt the head back.

Check for respiration by observing the chest or abdomen for movement, listen for sounds of breathing, and feel for a breath by placing your cheek close to the mouth. If none of these signs are present, the patient is not breathing, and you should initiate breathing techniques.

Pinch the patient's nose closed and maintain the head tilt to open the airway. Place your mouth over the patient's open mouth and form a seal with your lips; perform two full breaths, then evaluate the circulation. Some persons prefer to place a clean cloth over the patient's lips before initiating mouth-to-mouth respirations. If available, a plastic intubation device or mask can be used to decrease the contact between the caregiver's mouth and the patient's mouth and any saliva or vomitus (Fig. 12-10).

Palpate the carotid artery for a pulse. If there is no pulse, you must begin external chest compressions. If an AED is available, it should be used when there is no palpable pulse (see Fig. 12-9).

To initiate chest compressions, kneel next to the patient, place the heel of one hand on the inferior portion of the sternum just proximal to the *xiphoid* process, and place your other hand on top of the first hand. Position your shoulders directly over the patient's sternum, keep your elbows extended, and press down firmly, depressing the sternum approximately 1.5 to 2 inches with each compression. Relax after each compression, but do not remove your hands from the sternum. The relaxation and compression phases should be equal in duration. This can be accomplished by mentally counting "one thousand one," "one thousand two," "one thousand three," and so on, for each phase.

If you perform all CPR procedures without assistance, you should perform 15 chest compressions and then perform 2 breaths. You must compress at the rate of 60 to 100 times per minute, depending on the age of the person. Continue these procedures until qualified assistance arrives or the patient is able to sustain independent respiration and circulation. If you are alone, attempt to gain assistance from other persons by calling loudly for help.

The patient should be transported to a medical facility promptly for additional care and evaluation.

Note: Extreme care must be used to open an airway in a patient who may have experienced a cervical spine injury. In such cases, use the chin lift, but avoid the head tilt. If that technique does not open the airway, the head should be tilted slowly and gently until the airway is patent.

These procedures are appropriate to use for adults and for children 8 years of age and older. A pamphlet or booklet containing diagrams and instructions for CPR techniques can be obtained from most affiliate offices of the American Heart Association.

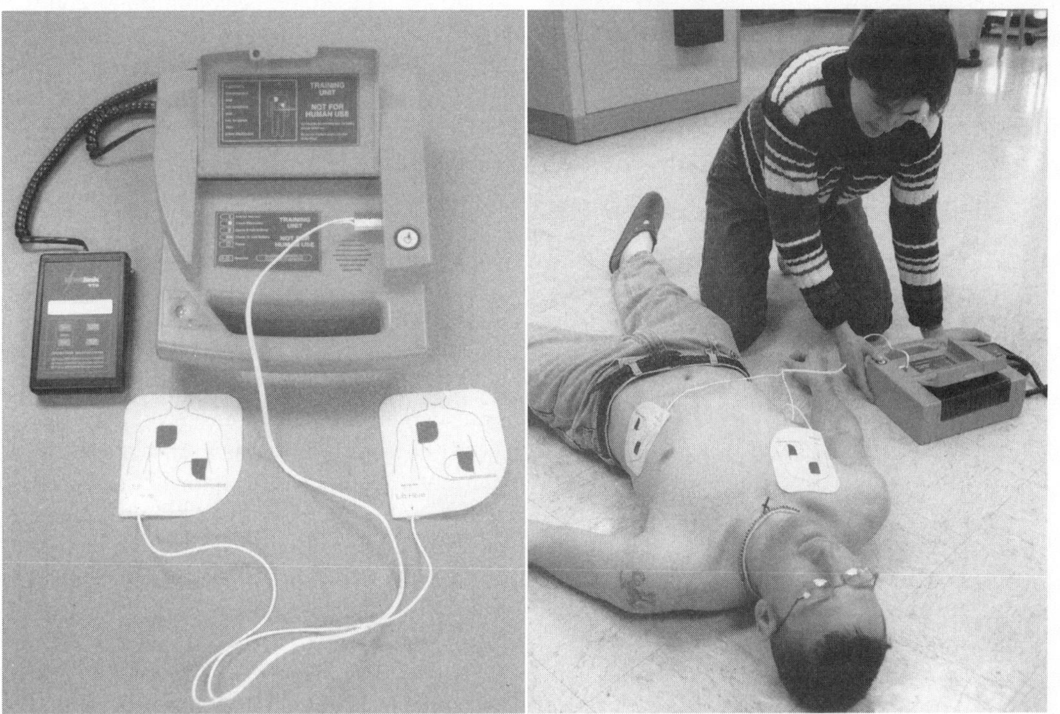

Fig. 12-9 **A,** An AED training unit. **B,** Demonstration of the application of an AED unit.

Box 12-2 Chain of Events to Follow Cardiac Death

Early access and use of 911 or similar emergency contact
Early application of CPR
Early application of an AED
Prompt response by EMTs and transport to a medical facility
Admission to a cardiac care unit

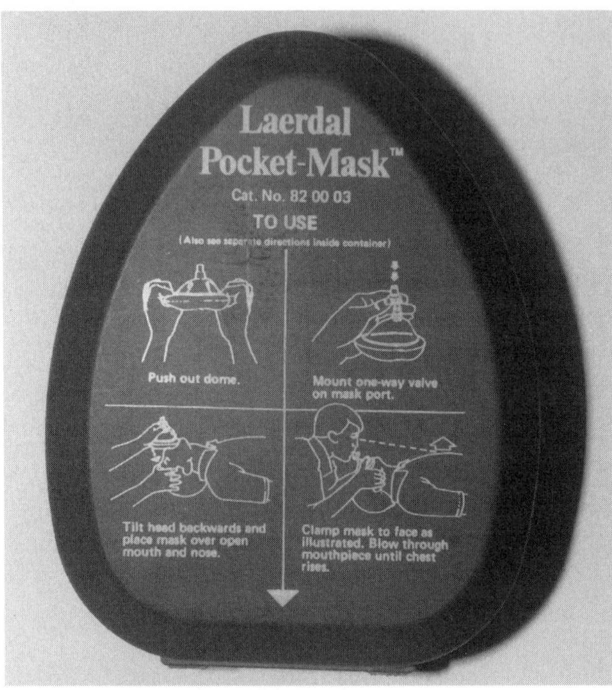

Fig. 12-10 Example of an oronasal mask.

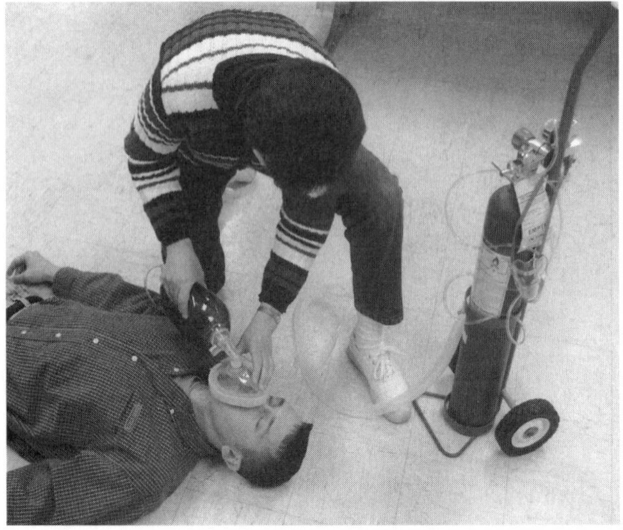

Fig. 12-11 Use of a resuscitation device (Ambu bag).

SUMMARY

The guidelines presented elsewhere in this text regarding the patient care and treatment environment; general patient safety considerations; and the employment of qualified, competent, and properly trained personnel should be reviewed. The patient must be informed of the intent and desired outcome of treatment. The caregiver should be prepared to provide emergency care or obtain assistance if an adverse reaction to the treatment occurs.

Emergency equipment (such as metabolic or crash cart) and supplies should be accessible in the treatment area and the telephone numbers of qualified advanced medical assistance personnel should be posted near all telephones (such as 911, internal emergency numbers or codes ["Doctor Blue," "Doctor Heart," "Captain Thermo"], and other external numbers). Periodic reviews of emergency procedures should be included in staff education programs and CPR retraining of personnel should be performed by qualified instructors at least every 2 years.

Special care and attention should be provided to any patient whose condition has the potential to develop into a more serious problem. For instance, patients who require full-body immersion or who use a therapeutic pool should be provided with fluids before, during, and after treatment to avoid heat exhaustion. The patient injured at or above the T6 cord level should be monitored for noxious stimuli, especially retention of urine to avoid autonomic hyperreflexia. Treatment for patients with diabetes should be scheduled so patients will not be adversely affected by an insulin injection or food intake before receiving treatment. These persons should be counseled to adjust their food or insulin intake according to the type of treatment or amount of physical activity required. The patient with a history of *convulsions* should be reminded to use anticonvulsive medications consistently and according to the prescriptive instructions.

Each patient's vital signs should be monitored frequently, especially patients whose conditions have the potential to lead to an emergency. The Valsalva maneuver should be avoided by requiring the patient to breathe regularly during exercise. A patient who has been recumbent for extended periods or who has a reduced ability to return peripheral venous blood to the heart should be observed and monitored when moving from a recumbent or sitting position to a more upright position. This individual should be given the opportunity to accommodate gradually to an upright position and measures should be used to relieve symptoms of hypotension. The patient should be protected until it is determined the person has accommodated sufficiently to sit or stand safely without experiencing the symptoms of orthostatic hypotension.

Finally, the caregiver should observe each patient for signs or symptoms of an abnormal physiologic response to treatment and should be prepared to act when an emergency occurs.

self-study ACTIVITIES

- Describe your responsibilities, obligations, and actions for a patient who experiences an injury during or as a result of treatment.
- Explain how you would treat a person who has experienced heat stroke, heat exhaustion, an insulin reaction, acidosis, or autonomic hyperreflexia.
- Differentiate the signs and symptoms of heat exhaustion and heat stroke.
- Differentiate the signs and symptoms of orthostatic hypotension and autonomic hyperreflexia.
- Outline what you believe should be included in a safety orientation and prevention program for caregivers in both inpatient and outpatient facilities.
- Describe the activities you would perform to monitor a patient's response to treatment.
- You find it necessary to apply a bandage for each of the conditions listed. For each of the following conditions, state the type of bandage you would select, state the rationale for your selection, and apply a bandage on another person: (1) to control joint effusion/swelling after a recent right ankle sprain; (2) to protect the distal aspects (tips) of the center two fingers of the left hand; and (3) to support the proximal, medial tissue of the left thigh after a recent muscle strain.

problem SOLVING

1. You are in your first special clinical education experience where you assist the athletic trainer at a rural high school in Texas. During the early fall, football practice is in progress and the temperature is 88° F with a relative humidity of 85%. What preparatory actions would you take, what possible medical emergency should you anticipate occurring, and what actions would you perform if an emergency occurred?

1. You are treating an 85-year-old woman with a fractured right femur. She has a long leg cast on her right lower extremity and you are at bedside to get her up and ambulate her with a walker. As she stands, she complains of dizziness and becomes diaphoretic. What is your initial action? What would you do to assist in determining the possible causes for this patient's reaction?

CHAPTER 13

Americans with Disabilities Act: A Review

objectives ***After studying this chapter, the reader will be able to:***

- Explain the purpose of the Americans with Disabilities Act.
- Describe the emphasis of the four primary titles of the act.
- Define the terms associated with the act.
- Discuss the roles a consultant could perform related to the Americans with Disabilities Act.
- Describe the major environmental assessments to be performed for a residence, workplace, and community.
- Describe actions an employer or businessperson can perform to respond to the employment and accessibility requirements of the Americans with Disabilities Act.

INTRODUCTION

Discrimination toward employment and access to workplaces, businesses, and transportation has existed for many years for persons with disabilities. Groups and organizations such as the Equal Employment Commission, President's Committee on Employment of People with Disabilities, National Easter Seal Society, Paralyzed Veterans of America, Multiple Sclerosis Society, Arthritis Foundation, and American Physical Therapy Association have advocated improvement in mobility, access, and employment opportunities for persons with disabilities. Previous federal legislation was designed to protect persons with disabilities from discrimination through the use of certain requirements or incentives. The Civil Rights Act of 1964, Fair Housing and Architectural Barriers Act of 1968 and its amendments in 1988, Section 504 of the Rehabilitation Act of 1973, and Education for all Handicapped Children Act of 1975 are examples of legislation that pertains to persons with disabilities. However, the Americans with Disabilities Act (ADA), which was signed on July 26, 1990, provided enforceable prohibitions and standards that ban discrimination based on disability. The ADA was designed to extend the civil rights for people with disabilities to improve their opportunity for employment by private sector employers; for access to public bus and train service, including AMTRAK; for access to public accommodations and services; and for access to certain types of telecommunications. The ADA is federal antidiscrimination legislation designed to remove employment and access barriers for individuals with disabilities.

The ADA has five titles: Title I, Employment; Title II, Public Service (including public transportation); Title III, Public Accommodations; Title IV, Telecommunications; and Title V, Miscellaneous Provisions. Compliance with most of the regulations and requirements of the ADA was mandated to occur no later than 2 years after the act was signed. At this time, all deadlines for compliance with all regulations have been exceeded and the legislation is in full effect. It is important to understand that the ADA interfaces or is related to other state and federal laws, such as the Family and Medical Leave Act (FMLA), Occupational Safety and Health Act, and workers' compensation laws in effect in each state. Employers, owners, managers, administrators, and persons who are involved with the employment of workers should become familiar with these acts and laws to understand how they may interact with the ADA. Information and assistance with these relationships can be obtained from state and federal departments of labor and local or federal Equal Employment Opportunity Commission (EEOC) offices.

It has been estimated there are approximately 49 million persons of all ages with disabilities in the United States. To date, only approximately 25% of these people are full-time employees.

DEFINITIONS

Individual with a disability: Person who has a physical or mental impairment that substantially limits one or more major life activities. Self-care, walking, speaking, breathing, learning, working, and performance of manual skills are major life activities according to the ADA. The ADA protects an individual if a person has a record of or is regarded as having impairment.

Reasonable accommodation: Making modifications at the job site or workplace that will enable persons with disabilities to easily perform a specific job. Some examples of reasonable accommodations are having a physically accessible workplace, restructuring a job, or adjusting a work schedule or hours of work to meet an individual's needs.

Undue burden: An action necessary to provide a reasonable accommodation that would cause the employer or owner significant difficulty or expense. Several factors are considered to determine whether a hardship would occur for the employer or owner; these factors include the size of the business, number of employees, type of operation of the business, nature and cost of the needed accommodation, and whether the accommodation would have an adverse effect or pose a risk to other employees.

Qualified individual with a disability: A person who can perform the essential functions of a given job or activity, with or without the benefit of reasonable accommodation. In other words, the person must have the knowledge, skills, and mental and physical capabilities to perform the essential elements of a particular job.

Covered entity: An employer, employment agency, labor organization or joint labor management organization, or state and local governments are examples.

Disability: A condition caused by an accident, trauma, genetics, or disease, which may limit a person's mobility, hearing, vision, speech, or mental function; a person may have one or more disabilities.

Handicap: A physical or attitudinal constraint that is imposed on a person, regardless of whether that person has a disability, which places the person at a disadvantage.

Many of the terms in these definitions are not specific and therefore are subject to interpretation. The person with a disability, the employer, an attorney, and state or federal agency personnel may differ in their interpretation of the language contained in the ADA. At the time the act became effective, it was anticipated there would be a great amount of litigation related to the meaning and interpretation of ADA language; however, this has not occurred.

GENERAL ASPECTS OF THE AMERICANS WITH DISABILITIES ACT

It was previously indicated the ADA contains four primary titles, each of which addresses a specific protected category and has separate compliance requirements. Persons in the private sector who own, manage, or lease a business or are employers and who are involved with any type of business, public service, housing, or workplace regulated by Titles I and III should become familiar with the provisions of those titles. All private sector employers who employ 15 or more persons are required to comply with Title I. In addition, because of the requirements of Title III related to accessibility to public accommodations and most commercial facilities, employers and business owners and their agents are affected even if they employ fewer than 15 persons.

Title I prohibits an employer from discriminating against a qualified individual with a disability on the basis of that disability alone. This prohibition affects job application and hiring procedures, opportunities for advancement, compensation and salary matters, and job training activities. An employer could be considered to have discriminated against a qualified person with a disability if the employer does not make reasonable accommodations for the individual or denies employment based on the need to make reasonable accommodations unless the employer can demonstrate that the needed accommodations would cause an undue hardship on the operation of the business (Box 13-1).

When a qualified individual with a disability is hired, the employer is required to make accommodations for a known disability that would enable that employee to achieve the same level of performance and to enjoy benefits equal to those of an average, similarly situated person without a disability. However, the accommodation does not have to ensure equal results or provide exactly the same benefits. The employee must request the accommodation and may suggest an appropriate accommodation. The employer is allowed to review and propose more than one type of accommodation and to select the one that is most appropriate or reasonable without leading to undue hardship, providing it effectively allows the person with a disability to perform the job. Accommodations must be determined based on each individual's needs because the nature and extent of a disabling condition and the requirements of a job will vary. Examples of reasonable accommodations, depending on the disabling condition and job requirements, are adjusting the height or changing the cutout area of a desk, adjusting the height and location of shelves, relocating file cabinets, repositioning telephones and other pieces of office equipment, modifying

Box 13-1 Examples of Workplace Accommodations

- Modification of work schedule
- Modification of job activities or requirements
- Employee reassignment or relocation
- Modifications to the physical plant
- Assistive devices such as teletypewriter (TTY), telephone amplifier, large-print manuals
- Elevation of existing furniture or equipment for wheelchair users
- Accessible restrooms, entrances, hallways, doorways, and parking area

standard office or telecommunications equipment, modifying testing and training activities or procedures, and providing readers or interpreters for persons with a vision or language impairment.

Title III is designed to protect persons with disabilities on the basis of their disability from discrimination related to full and equal access to services, facilities, accommodations, goals, privileges, and advantages of any place of public accommodation by the person who owns, leases, or operates a site, place, or facility classified as public accommodation. Virtually every type of private entity or business whose operation affects commerce is considered to be a public accommodation. Examples of public accommodations are a hotel or motel; restaurant or bar; theater or auditorium; convention center or lecture hall; grocery store, shopping center, or sales or retail establishment; laundromat, gas station, or professional office; public transportation building; museum or library; park or zoo; amusement park; places of education; day care center or senior center; and gymnasium, spa, or bowling alley. For existing facilities and those to be constructed, structural physical barriers must be removed or not included. Title III usually requires removal, modification, or alteration of structural barriers when the changes can be made reasonably and accomplished without significant difficulty or expense. The installation of ramps; widening of doorways; use of door hardware that is more functional than a knob that must be turned; provision of an alternative pathway with a firm surface to buildings, parking areas, or areas within a building; installation of support (grab) bars or rails; increase in space in restrooms to accommodate a wheelchair; creation of accessible parking spaces; use of telephones and water fountains accessible from a wheelchair; and curb cutouts are typical adjustments that can be made to provide greater access for persons with disabilities (Figs. 13-1 and 13-2).

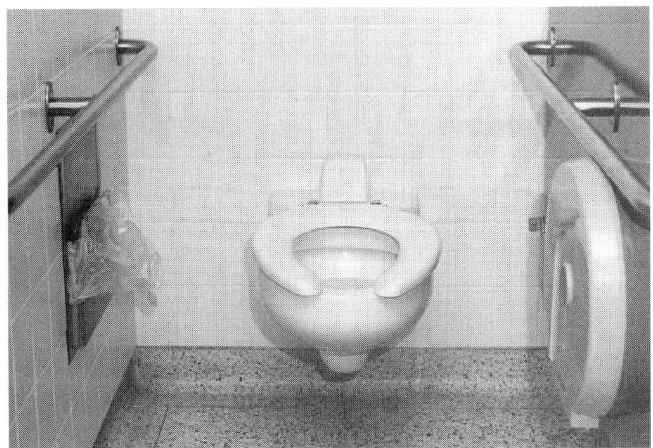

Fig. 13-1 Addition of "grab" rails in a public restroom with a slightly elevated commode.

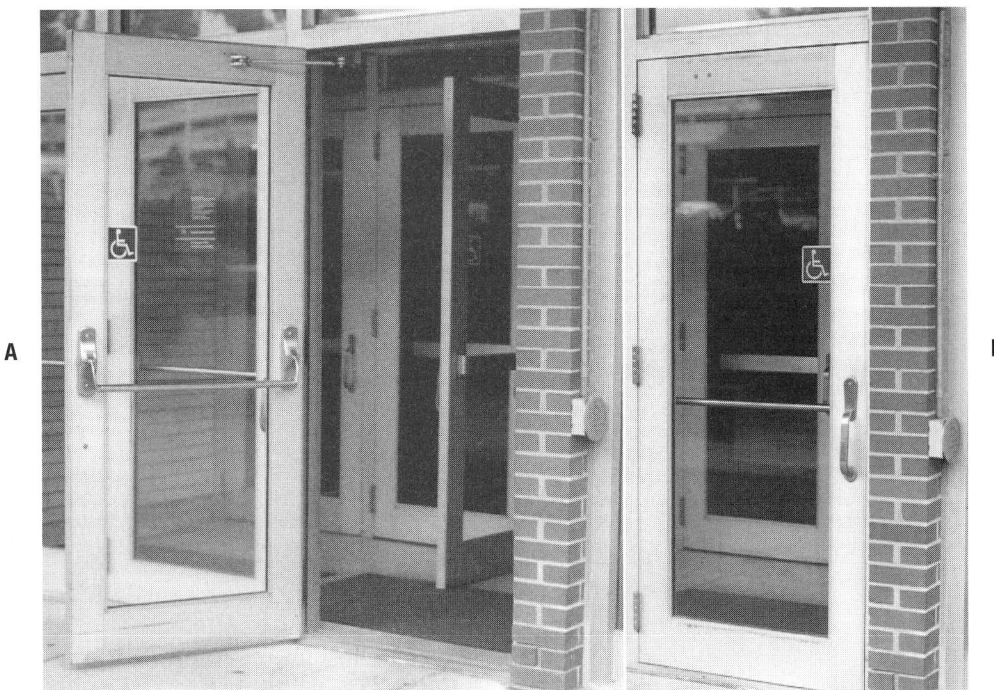

Fig. 13-2 **A,** Pressing the control disk opens the outer and inner doors. *Note:* the threshold of the outer door may be difficult for some persons in wheelchairs to wheel over. **B,** Electrically operated door on a public building; the control disk is located on the brick column; doors close after a preset time period has elapsed.

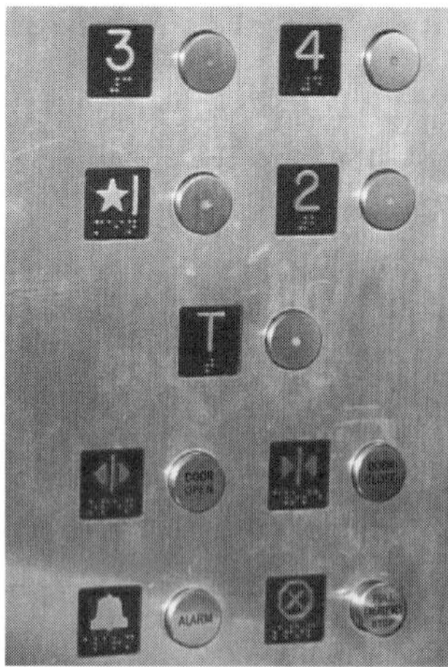

Fig. 13-3 Elevator controls with Braille symbols.

In addition, auxiliary services and aids must be provided to individuals with a vision or hearing impairment (Fig. 13-3). Auxiliary services could be as simple as having the server in a restaurant read the menu selections to persons who are visually impaired or having the server be prepared to use a pad and pencil to communicate with persons who are hearing impaired. An aid that may be required is a telephone or an outlet for a portable device that will serve the needs of persons with hearing impairments, such as a telecommunication display device (TDD). The provisions of Title III do not apply to exempted entities, including private clubs and establishments that are exempt from Title II of the Civil Rights Act of 1964, religious organizations or entities controlled by religious organizations, and entities operated by governments that are exempt from Titles I and II. Figures 13-4 to 13-9 provide examples of Title III requirements or accommodations.

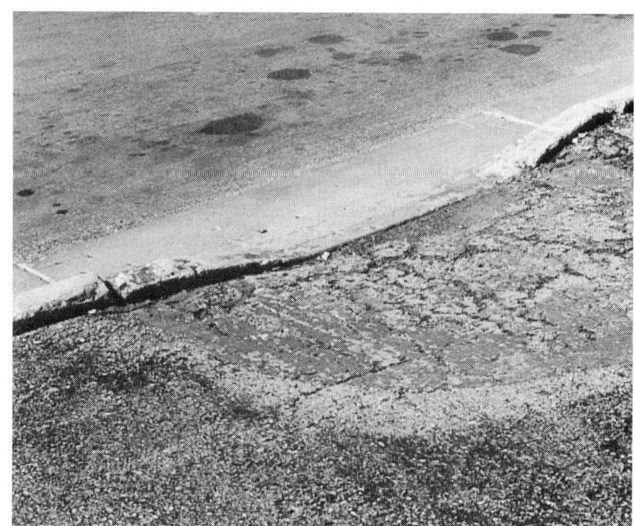
Fig. 13-4 Curb cutout showing uneven surfaces, narrow opening, and lack of crosswalk markings. Unfortunately, some cutouts may not be in good repair or functional for wheelchair access.

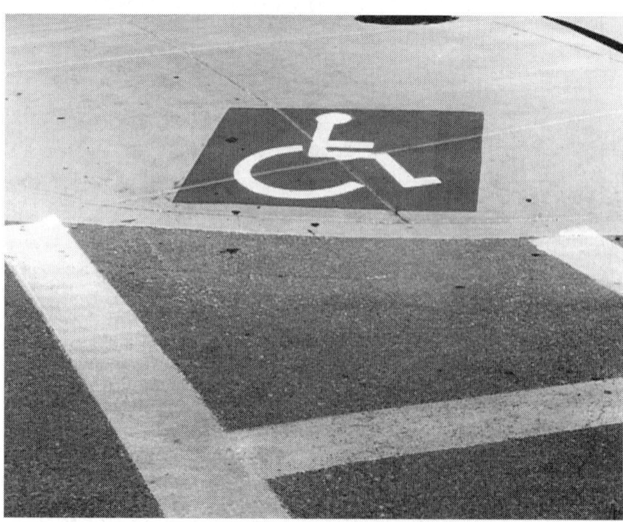
Fig. 13-5 Curb cutout showing smooth, gradual elevation from street level to sidewalk; width of cutout; crosswalk markings; and large turning area on sidewalk in all directions.

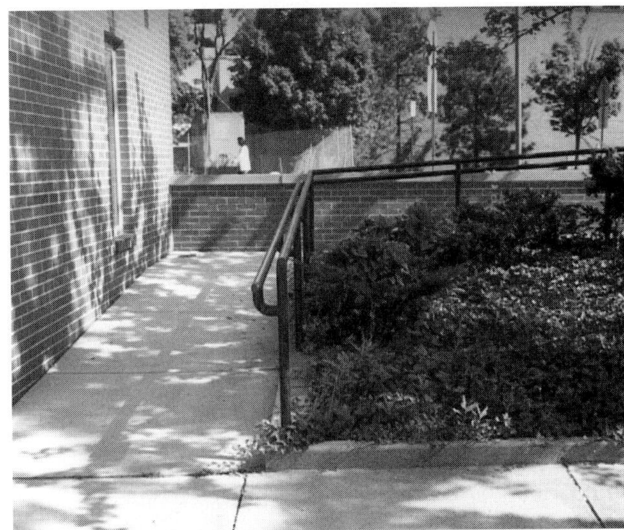

Fig. 13-6 Ramp to public building showing ramp width, even surface, and adequate space to turn wheelchair where direction and slope of ramp change.

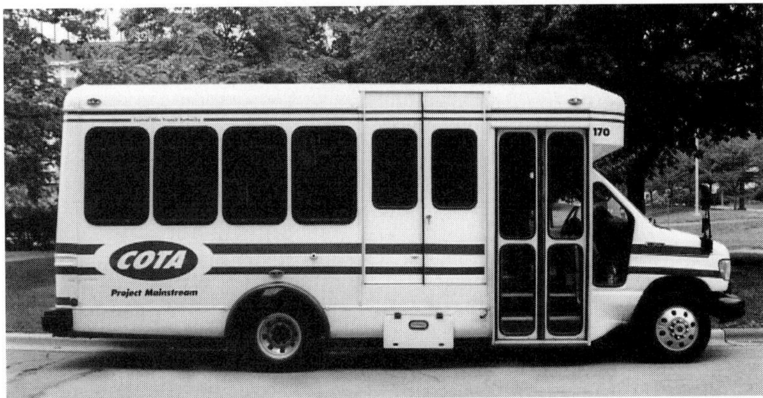

Fig. 13-7 Vehicle used to transport persons from home to another location and return. A lift is used to accommodate wheelchair users and open space with restraints for wheelchairs is available in the vehicle.

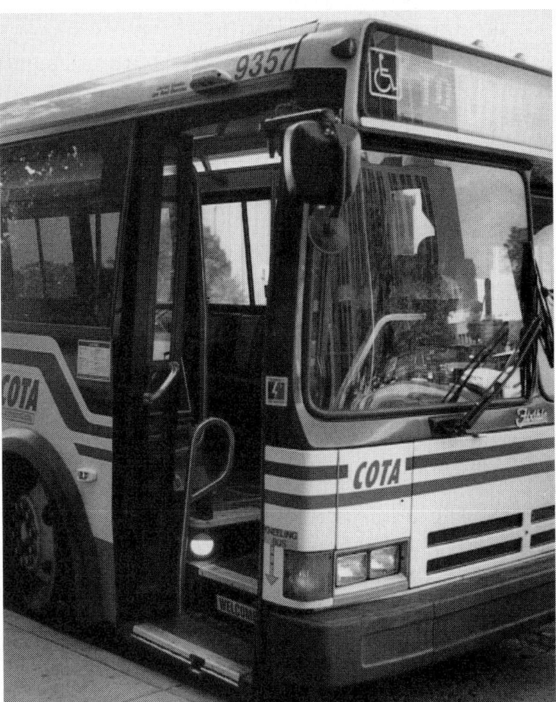

Fig. 13-8 Kneeling bus in lowered position (operated by Central Ohio Transit Authority).

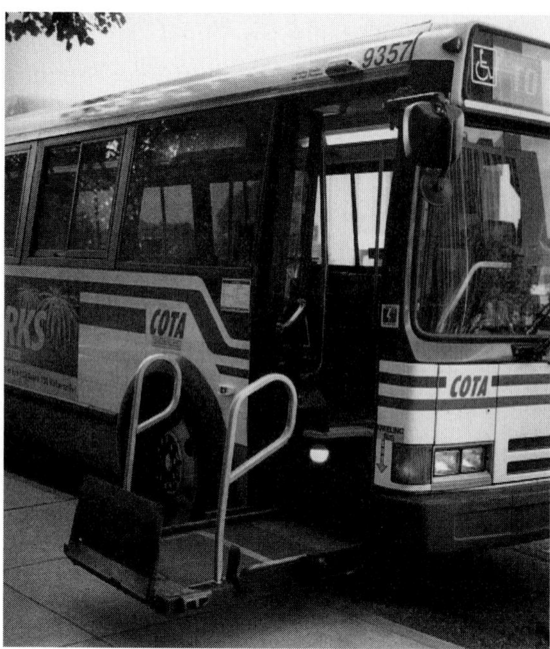

Fig. 13-9 Bus with lift being lowered; vertical panel prevents a wheelchair from rolling off the lift and another panel or bar prevents the chair from rolling toward the bus (not in photograph).

Box 13-2 Suggestions for Employers for Hiring Persons with Disabilities

Learn where to locate and how to recruit people with disabilities.
Learn how to communicate and interact with people who have disabilities.
Be certain that company applications and employment forms do not ask for disability-related information and they are formatted to be accessible to all persons with disabilities.
Prepare written job descriptions that clearly and specifically identify the essential functions of a job.
Be certain that company medical examinations, evaluations, or tests comply with the ADA.
Be prepared to provide reasonable accommodations needed by a qualified applicant to compete for the job.
Treat the individual with a disability with dignity and respect.
Know that persons protected by the ADA include persons with acquired immunodeficiency syndrome, cancer, mental retardation, deaf, blind, learning impaired, or brain injured as a result of trauma.
Train supervisors and other employees about making reasonable accommodations.
Use procedures to maintain and protect medical records as confidential.
Prepare and train all employees to communicate, interact, and work with people with disabilities.

COMPLIANCE AND IMPLEMENTATION OF REGULATIONS

Employers, managers, administrators, and persons with disabilities should become educated about the employment of persons with disabilities. Consultation with human resources personnel, legal counsel, external qualified consultants, current employees with disabilities, and department supervisors is a recommended initial step. Review of the application form, process, and procedures; selection and hiring procedures; and evaluation, advancement, and training opportunities and activities will help to determine the current and necessary level of compliance with Title I. Time should be spent to determine the essential functions of a job; prepare a comprehensive job description written in functional terms; observe the workplace layout and environment; and prepare an on-site job analysis for each job of the business. The physical and mental requirements of the job should be identified and any special skills or abilities that are needed. Specific education and training qualifications and any certification or licensure credentials that are required should be listed. The employer and any agents involved with the hiring process must be aware of restrictions associated with the limits imposed on preemployment inquiries of applicants. During the preoffer or application phase of the employment process, disability-related questions, medical history information, and medical examinations are prohibited by the ADA unless they are specifically job related. An applicant can be asked whether he or she can perform specific essential job functions such as lift and carry objects, stand for prolonged periods, climb a ladder, or use specific pieces of office equipment. When an interview is conducted, the questions asked and the discussion should relate to the information requested on the application and the functional requirements of the job. The interviewer is permitted to ask the applicant about the duties that were performed in a previous job. Questions about any visible physical characteristics of the applicant, present health status, and psychiatric history or previous addiction to drugs are prohibited (Box 13-2).

Medical examinations or evaluations are permitted if they are performed after an offer of employment has been made providing all employees in a specific job category receive the same type of examination. The medical information that is obtained must be placed in a file or separated from the person's personnel file. Preemployment tests for illegal drug use are permitted because such testing is not considered to be part of a medical examination by the ADA. However, employers and their agents should understand that a person who has successfully completed a drug or alcohol abuse rehabilitation program or is enrolled in such a program and is drug free is protected from discrimination by the ADA. When a person with a disability is hired and the disability is made known, the employer should be prepared to address the need for reasonable accommodation to provide a better opportunity for the employee to perform the job as mentioned previously. An ADA catalog has been produced by the National Easter Seals Society that lists videocassettes and audiocassettes, books, and posters that address the ADA and attitude awareness, training, and issues related to employment, transportation, and housing. One item listed in the catalog is *The Workplace Workbook; An Illustrated Guide to Job Accommodations and Assistive Technology* developed by the Dole Foundation and designed as a resource for businesses on accommodating people with disabilities and types of problems that may be caused by inappropriate workspace design.

The employer must consider the requirements for accessibility contained in Title II that are different from the reasonable accommodation requirements of Title I. Consultation with a knowledgeable architect, qualified design professional or health care professional (such as physical therapist, occupational therapist (OT), industrial health specialist), or current employees with disabilities may assist the employer to reach decisions necessary to comply with Title III. Existing facilities classified as public accommodations are required to remove structural architectural barriers where removal is readily achievable. Access into a facility or an establishment for persons with disabilities, freedom of movement, and access to goods and services once inside the facility should be given immediate attention. Suggestions and examples of how this can be accomplished have been presented previously. If the removal of existing architectural barriers is not readily achievable, the facility, establishment, or entity must provide its goods, services, facilities, privileges, advantages, or accommodations through alternative methods if such methods are readily achievable. To comply with these requirements, a business may need to provide a "drive-through" window, offer home deliveries, or provide catalog sales. *Note:* "Readily achievable" is defined as being able to be accomplished easily and performed without difficulty or expense. The categories of the accessibility audit requirements for public accommodations are contained in Box 13-3. Specific requirements, specifications, and guidelines for each of these categories are contained in the *Code of Federal Regulations*, Department of Justice, Civil Rights Division, 28 CFR, Part 36, July 1, 1994 (revised). According to data available from the President's Committee on Employment of People with Disabilities, approximately 80% of the costs to make existing facilities accessible have been less than $1000.00 and 50% of the changes have cost less than $50.00. Extensive remodeling of a facility usually is not required, but creative and innovative ways of thinking are important elements to be used to resolve the majority of accommodation or accessibility problems.

A qualified and knowledgeable health care professional consultant is a valuable resource for an employer. Activities or roles that could be expected of such a consultant are presented in Box 13-4. The employer should review and evaluate the person's credentials, qualifications, and past consultation experiences to determine the level of expertise before contracting for services. The desired and expected outcome or product of the consultation, time frame for the consultation, costs and expenses anticipated, and method of payment for the services should be clearly identified to the satisfaction of the persons involved with the consultation.

The ADA also provides some tax incentives to encourage employers and business owners to comply with the act. The Internal Revenue Service allows a deduction of up to $15,000 per year for expenses associated with the removal of qualified architectural and transportation barriers. In addition, small businesses are eligible to receive a tax credit of up to $5000 for certain costs that are incurred to comply with the ADA. When the two incentives are added, a small

Box 13-3 Accessibility Audit Requirement Categories

Ramps and slopes
Doors and hallways
Signage
Stairs and elevators
Flooring
Obstacles and protrusions
Reach range and clear space
Seating
Equipment (for example, telephones, drinking fountains, controls and receptacles, toilet rooms)
Accessible path and walkway
Parking and loading zone
Alarms, signs, and warnings
Area for emergency refuge

Box 13-4 Activities for an Americans with Disabilities Act Consultant

Educate employers, managers, supervisors, employees, and persons with disabilities about the ADA, particularly Titles I and III.
Perform on-site job analysis; identify essential job functions.
Perform on-site environmental evaluation.
Help develop function-based job descriptions.
Advise on job-related accommodation needs.
Advise on the removal of physical barriers and the improvement of access internally and externally.
Perform physical capacity and functional ability testing of current and prospective employees based on essential job functions.
Help develop policies and procedures related to compliance with the ADA.

business owner could accrue $20,000 in tax incentives in 1 year. As in all tax-related matters, consultation with a tax advisor is recommended to review and assist with the preparation and filing of the appropriate documents.

ASSESSING THE ENVIRONMENT

Introduction

Many persons whose physical abilities have been compromised or reduced because of injury, illness, or disease will need to adapt to their environment, or the environment may need to be modified to permit mobility and function that are safe and energy conserving. Therefore a health care professional may be asked to perform an assessment of the person's current and future environments. The assessment process is related to the concepts and recommendations contained in the ADA, especially when the person's workplace and use of community services and buildings are to be assessed. Three primary environments to be evaluated are the person's residence, place of employment, and the community. Persons who use a wheelchair or ambulation aids for mobility usually encounter environmental barriers that adversely affect their mobility or functional capacity. These persons frequently require accommodations to enable them to gain greater mobility or improved functional capacity. Furthermore, persons with a visual or hearing deficit may also require modifications to their residences, workplaces, and community to enhance their functional abilities.

The application of universal design concepts for the living areas of persons with a handicap or who are elderly should be considered during the environmental assessment process. Wider doors and halls; the use of lever-type doorknobs and faucet handles; relocation of lighting controls and electrical outlets; recessed areas under sinks, cabinets, and work counters; varied heights of countertops; and relocation of cabinets for easier access are some examples of universal design features for the home. The use of these and other similar building accommodations will permit greater accessibility and function for the elderly, persons of differing statures, or the wheelchair user without requiring extensive remodeling or cost. Persons who are building a new home or remodeling an existing one may find it beneficial to incorporate suggestions associated with the universal design approach.

Assessment Process

Several activities are necessary to perform an assessment of the environment, including the following: at least one interview with the patient, family, and employer; at least one site visit to the residence, workplace, and most frequently used community sites; completion of an assessment form or record; and a final written document containing recommendations, diagrams, photographs, or plans of proposed residence and workplace modifications designed to improve mobility, access, or functional abilities. The process may require several interview sessions or site visits and should be performed using interprofessional collaboration. Individuals who may be involved include a physical therapist, an OT, a social worker, a nurse, a public health practitioner, an architect, a contractor, and an employer. When possible, the patient and a family member should be present during at least one site visit. Periodic, short, predischarge home visits by the patient can assist to identify the patient's abilities and limitations and the barriers to mobility and function in the residence. Also, it may be possible to determine what modifications are needed and whether they can be accomplished to sufficiently meet the patient's needs. It may be helpful to perform one visit in the evening or after dark and during inclement weather. Planning for the patient's return to community life must be initiated well in advance of the anticipated date of discharge, especially the assessment process, to permit sufficient time to perform any needed modifications or obtain any needed special equipment for the residence or workplace. Materials and items to be used for the site visits are a tape measure (at least 6 feet long); flashlight; graph paper to plot changes; camera; voice recorder; assessment form; and, in some instances, a laptop computer.

The amount and type of remodeling or structural changes that can be accomplished may depend on factors such as whether the person owns or rents the residence; whether the present structure and grounds can accommodate the remodeling or construction desired; whether the modifications will comply with building code requirements; whether the costs of the modifications are reasonable and affordable; whether a qualified contractor is available; whether the residence is single or multiple level; and what effect the modifications may have on the subsequent sale or rental of the residence. In spite of these factors, fulfilling the needs of the patient is the most important consideration. It should be recognized that not all modifications may be able to be completed at the same time, and priorities may need to be established to complete the entire project. The assessor(s) should identify the modifications necessary to improve the person's mobility or function and provide recommendations how to complete them. This activity should be done through consultation with the person, family members, and employer. Consultation with an architect and contractor is recommended for major remodeling or construction projects. An awareness of the requirements by the health care professional for access and reasonable accommodations in the workplace contained in the ADA will assist in providing meaningful suggestions and recommendations. A variety of environmental assessment forms can be found in the literature or through Internet sources. Many treatment facilities have developed forms that specifically meet their needs and those of the patient-related community environment.

Basic areas or items to be considered during the assessment of a person's residence, workplace, and community are presented in Boxes 13-5 through 13-7.

Box 13-5 Basic Assessment of the Residence

EXTERNAL FEATURES

- Sidewalk/driveway: condition, type of surface
- Garage/carport: attached/detached, size, access
- Approach to entry: steps, porch, landing, illumination
- Entry: door width, threshold
- Access to grounds

INTERNAL FEATURES

- General considerations: door widths, thresholds; hall widths; presence of stairs; location, height, access to electrical outlets/switches; size, space available in rooms; type, access to lighting; location, access to communication units (telephone, computer); location, access to safety devices (smoke/carbon monoxide detectors, circuit breaker panel, surveillance/security controls, emergency exit); location, access to heating/cooling controls; access to/operation of windows; floor surfaces/coverings.
- Living/family room: furniture configuration, ability to reposition; type, access to furniture; location, access to entertainment equipment.
- Kitchen: access; location, layout, and position of sink, counter surfaces, cabinets; location, type, access to appliances and their controls; location of plumbing.
- Bathroom: access to sink, commode, tub/shower, mirror, medicine cabinet; location of plumbing; safety features present or needed (such as grab bars).
- Bedroom: location, height, access to the bed; location, access to other furniture, closet, and clothes.

Box 13-6 Basic Assessment of the Workplace

EXTERNAL FEATURES

- Location, condition, type of surface of parking area
- Location and availability of designated parking spaces
- Approach to entry; steps, illumination, platform
- Entry: door width, size, means of opening/closing, threshold
- Location, type of surface, condition of sidewalk

INTERNAL FEATURES

- Access to work station/office
- Door and hall widths
- Floor surfaces and coverings
- Access to job equipment, supplies, cabinets, desk, work surface, and space
- Access to rest room and its facilities
- Access to eating area and its facilities
- Access to elevator, escalator
- Access to water fountain, refreshment machines

Note: Compliance with requirements for reasonable accommodations stipulated by the ADA should be determined.

Box 13-7 Basic Assessment of the Community

- Location, type, and access to public transportation
- Location, type, and condition of sidewalks and curb cuts
- Location and access to designated parking spaces at restaurants, shopping centers, grocery stores, theaters, banks, and other public buildings
- Entry to buildings: steps, door widths, means of door opening/closing, thresholds
- Access to facilities in public buildings: telephone, rest room, counter surfaces, checkout areas, aisles, emergency exits, water fountain, elevator, escalator

Note: Compliance with requirements for reasonable accommodations stipulated by the ADA should be determined.

SUMMARY

On July 26, 1990, the ADA was signed and most requirements contained in it became effective on July 26, 1992. Each of the four primary titles contains regulations, guidelines, and prohibitions specific to that title. The purpose of the ADA is to prohibit discrimination against persons with disabilities, based on the disability, through comprehensive and enforceable prohibitions. The act was designed to extend the civil rights for people with disabilities in the areas of employment (Title I); access to certain types of public transportation, including AMTRAK and access to government employment, facilities, and services (Title II); access to goods, services, and facilities classified as public accommodations (Title III); and access to auxiliary devices and aids such as telecommunications (Title IV) (Box 13-8).

The ADA is complex legislation that requires careful study before an individual can become reasonably familiar with it. Many terms and concepts are not defined specifically and at times may appear to be ambiguous and subject to interpretation; therefore assistance or consultation with a variety of persons, including an architect, an attorney, an industrial health specialist, or a health care professional, may be necessary to gain information and suggestions about compliance with the act. Many resources are available that provide specific information about the many requirements of the ADA; several of them are located in the Bibliography.

Although most of the requirements of the ADA have been in effect since July 1992, increased education is needed for employers, persons with disabilities, members of many professions, students enrolled in health care education programs, and society in general about the purpose and extent of the ADA. Many health care professionals profess themselves to be advocates for persons with disabilities, but they have not been active in promoting or providing information about

Box 13-8 Summary of Americans with Disabilities Act Titles I through IV

TITLE I: EMPLOYMENT

Employers may not discriminate against an individual with a disability in hiring or promoting if the person is otherwise qualified for the job. Employers will need to provide "reasonable accommodations" to individuals with disabilities, including job restructuring and equipment modification, but they need not provide accommodations that impose an "undue hardship" on business operations. Regulated by the EEOC.

TITLE II: PUBLIC SERVICE

State and local governments may not discriminate against qualified individuals with disabilities. All government facilities, including public transportation and communication, must be accessible. Regulated by the Secretary of Transportation.

TITLE III: PUBLIC ACCOMMODATIONS

Public accommodations operated by private entities such as restaurants, hotels, retail stores, and theaters may not discriminate against individuals with disabilities. Auxiliary aids and services must be provided to individuals with vision or hearing impairments or other individuals with disabilities, unless an undue burden would result. Physical barriers in existing facilities must be removed if removal is readily achievable; if not readily achievable, alternative methods to provide service or access, if they are readily achievable, must be provided. All new construction and alterations to public accommodations must be accessible. Regulated by the Attorney General.

TITLE IV: TELECOMMUNICATIONS

Companies or businesses offering telephone service to the general public must offer telephone relay services to individuals who use telecommunication devices for the deaf (TDDs) or similar devices. Regulated by the Federal Communications Commission.

the ADA. Graduates of many professional education programs have limited knowledge of the ADA; this limits their ability to educate others or serve as advocates for persons with disabilities. Minimal research has been performed and published related to the effect or outcomes of the act for employers, persons with disabilities, or society; therefore continued investigation of the values, limitations, costs, enforcement, and awareness of the effects of the ADA on society seems warranted.

self-study ACTIVITIES

- State the purpose of the ADA.
- List and describe the major theme of Titles I through IV of the ADA.
- Describe how you could serve as a consultant to an employer to assist with compliance for Titles I and III of the ADA.
- Visit several workplaces or businesses and identify structural architectural barriers; explain how they could be eliminated or modified to comply with Title III of the ADA.
- Outline activities an employer could perform to become prepared to employ persons with disabilities.
- Propose three or four topics related to the ADA that would be appropriate for investigation and research.

problem SOLVING

1. You and an OT are scheduled to perform an assessment of a patient's home. The person will use a wheelchair for mobility indefinitely. What preparatory activities would you perform and with whom would you perform them? What areas should be assessed during the site visit?
2. You have been delegated the responsibility for assessing the workspace at the reception desk for a new employee who is a wheelchair user. What aspects of the office and areas of the facility should be evaluated?

Bibliography

Ability You Can Bank On: President's Committee on Employment of People with Disabilities: Education Kit 2000. Washington, DC: U.S. Government Printing Office, 2000.

Accurso F: *Clinical Trials and Studies, Airway Secretion Clearance in CF.* Denver, CO: University of Colorado, Cystic Fibrosis Foundation, www.cff.org, 2001.

ADA Title I Technical Assistance Manual. Washington, DC: U.S. Equal Employment Opportunity Commission, 1992.

Adaptable Housing. Washington, DC: U.S. Department of Housing and Urban Development, 1992.

Adult Basic Life Support. *Journal of the American Medical Association* 268(16):2184-2198, 1992.

American Red Cross: *Community First Aid and Safety.* St. Louis: Mosby, 1993.

Americans With Disabilities Act Accessibility Requirements. Washington, DC: U.S. Architectural and Transportation Barriers Compliance Board, 1991.

Amundsen LR: Assessing Exercise Tolerance: A Review. *Physical Therapy* 59(5):534-537, 1979.

Apts D, Blankenship K: *The American Back School Manual.* Ashland, KY: American Back School, 1980.

Atlas of Orthotics, American Academy of Orthopedic Surgeons. St. Louis: Mosby, 1975.

Back Owner's Manual. Daly City, CA: Physicians Art Service, 1991.

Back Pain. San Bruno, CA: Krames Communications, 1986.

Back Tips for Health Care Providers. San Bruno, CA: Krames Communications, 1987.

Barrier-Free House Plans. Des Plaines, IL: Professional Builder, 1995.

Benner TF: *Personal Communication, Rehabilitation Team Leader.* Columbus, OH: The Ohio State University, University Medical Center, 2001.

Bergen A, Colongelo C: *Evaluating the Environment: Problem Solving Worksheet.* Camarillo, CA: Everest & Jennings, 1984.

Bergstrom N, Bennett MA, Carlson CE, et al.: *Treatment of Pressure Ulcers.* Clinical Practice Guideline, No. 15. AHCPR Publication No. 95-0652. Rockville, MD: U.S. Department of Health and Human Services. Public Health Service, Agency for Health Care and Research, 1994.

Birdsall C: How Accurate Are Your Blood Pressures? *American Journal of Nursing* 84(11):1414, 1984.

Blood Borne Infections: A Practical Guide to OSHA Compliance. Arlington, TX: Johnson & Johnson Medical, 1992.

Body Substance Precautions in Schools: Recommendations. Columbus, OH: The Ohio Department of Health, 1991.

Bohannon RW: Horizontal Transfers Between Adjacent Surfaces: Forces Required Using Different Methods. *Archives of Physical Medicine and Rehabilitation* 90:851-853, 1999.

Bohannon RW: Reducing the Burden of Patient Handling. *Advance for Physical Therapists and PT Assistants* 13(4):45-46, 2002.

Bonewit K: *Clinical Procedures for Medical Assistants.* 3rd edition. Philadelphia: W.B. Saunders, 1990.

Borg G: *Borg's Perceived Exertion and Pain Scale: Human Kinetics,* Champaign, IL: Human Kinetics, 1998.

Brennan MJ, Miller LT: Overview of Treatment Options and Review of Current Role and Use of Compression Garments, Intermittent Pumps, and Exercise in the Management of Lymphedema. American Cancer Society Lymphedema Workshop. *Supplement to Cancer* Aug. 20, 1998.

Brown V, Graf S: Lecture notes and handouts. Columbus, OH: Physical Therapy Division, School of Allied Medical Professions, The Ohio State University, 1985.

Calloway SD: *New HCFA Regulations on Patient Rights, What Every Hospital Should Know.* Columbus, OH: Mt. Carmel College of Nursing, 1999.

Cardiopulmonary Resuscitation. Dallas, TX: American Heart Association, 1987.

Care and Service. *Wheelchair Prescriptions,* Booklet No. 4. Camarillo, CA: Everest & Jennings, 1983.

Carr J, Shepherd R: *A Motor Relearning Program for Stroke.* 2nd edition. Rockville, MD: Aspen Publishing, 1987.

Case-Smith J: *Practical Aspects of Using Outcomes Measures.* Model Program for Linking Allied Health Education, Research and Practice: Columbus, OH: 1996.

Castile R, Tice J, Flucke R, Filbrun D, Varekojis S, McCoy K: *Comparison of Three Sputum Clearance Methods in In-Patients with Cystic Fibrosis.* Abstract presented in 20th Annual North American Cystic Fibrosis Conference. Montreal, Quebec, Canada: 1998.

Choosing a Wheelchair System. *Journal of Rehabilitation Research and Development* 3(suppl 2):1990.

City of Sacramento: *Disability Etiquette, Americans With Disability Act, Accessibility Information, Disability Etiquette.* ADA Information home page. www.cityofsacramento.gov, 2001.

City of San Antonio: *Disability Etiquette Handbook, City of San Antonio Planning Department, Disability Access Office.* City Services home page. www.cityofsanantonio.gov, 2001.

Clarkson HM, Gilewich GB: *Musculoskeletal Assessment.* Baltimore, MD: Williams & Wilkins, 1989.

Code of Federal Regulations: *28CFR Part 36: Nondiscrimination on the Basis of Disability by Public Accommodations and in Commercial Facilities.* Washington, DC: U.S. Government Printing Office, 1994.

Connolly JB: A New Breed of Consultant. *Clinical Management* 12:72-80, 1992.

Connolly JB: Understanding the ADA. *Clinical Management* 12:40-45, 1992.

Cooper RA, Gonzalez J, Lawrence B, Rentschler A, Boninger ML, Van Sickle DP: Performance of Selected Lightweight Wheelchairs on ANSI/RESNA Tests. *Archives of Physical Medicine and Rehabilitation* 78(10):1138-1144, 1997.

Cooper RA, Schmeler M, Cooper R, Thorman T, Boninger ML: Light Touch. *Advance for Physical Therapists and PT Assistants* 13(4):9-10, 2002.

Cooper RA: *Wheelchairs: A Guide to Selection and Configuration.* New York: Demos Medical Publishers, 1998.

Coruth F, Thompson F: *Transfer and Lifting Techniques for Extended Care.* Vancouver, BC: Evergreen Press, 1983.

Danger Signs and Symptoms: Clinical Skillbuilders. Springhouse, PA: Springhouse Corporation, 1990.

Daniels L, Worthingham C: *Muscle Testing: Techniques of Manual Examination.* 5th edition. Philadelphia: W.B. Saunders, 1986.

Domenico RL, Ziegler WZ: *Practical Rehabilitation Techniques for Geriatric Aides.* Rockville, MD: Aspen Publishing, 1989.

Downie PA: *Cash's Textbook of Chest, Heart and Vascular Disorders for Physiotherapists.* 3rd edition. Philadelphia: J.B. Lippincott, 1995.

Duff JF: *Youth Sports Injuries.* New York, NY: Macmillan, 1992.

Emergencies. Springhouse, PA: Springhouse Corporation, 1985.

Emergency Procedures: Clinical Skillbuilders. Springhouse, PA: Springhouse Corporation, 1991.

Erdos EE, Steinheiser JM: *Basic Intravenous Therapy.* Seminar proceedings. Cleveland, OH: NCS Health Care, Inc., 1992.

Fahland B, Grendahl BA: *Wheelchair Selection: More Than Choosing a Chair with Wheels.* Minneapolis, MN: American Rehabilitation Foundation, 1967.

First Aid for Choking. Dallas, TX: American Heart Association, 1988.

Fit Back Workout. San Bruno, CA: Krames Communications, 1990.

Freed M, Hofkosh J, Kaplan L, Neuhauser C: Choosing Ambulatory Aids. *Patient Care* 15:20-35, 1987.

Freed M, Hofkosh J, Kaplan L, Neuhauser C: Using Ambulatory Aids. *Patient Care* 21(16):36-46, 1987.

Frownfelter D, Dean E, editors. *Principles and Practice of Cardiopulmonary Physical Therapy.* 3rd edition. St. Louis: Mosby, 1996.

Garner JS, Hospital Infection Control Practices Advisory Committee: *Guidelines for Isolation Precautions in Hospitals.* Atlanta, GA: Centers for Disease Control and Prevention, 1996.

Garner JS, Hospital Infection Control Practices Advisory Committee: *Health Topics A-Z, Healthcare Quality Promotion: Major Healthcare Guidelines, Isolation*. www.cdc.gov, 1996.

Garritan S, Jones P, Kornberg T, Parkin C: Laboratory Values in the Intensive Care Unit. *Acute Care Perspectives* Winter 1995.

Ghasemi Z, Martin T: The Role of the Physical Therapist in the Intensive Care Unit. *Acute Care Perspectives* Winter 1995.

Gomella LG, editor: *Clinician's Pocket Reference*. 6th edition. Norwalk, CT: Appleton & Lange, 1989.

Grevelding P, Bohannon RW: Reduced Push Forces Accompany Device Use During Sliding Transfers of Seated Subjects. *Journal of Rehabilitation Research and Development* 38:135-139, 2001.

Guide to Physical Therapist Practice. *Physical Therapy* 81(1):2001.

Guidelines for Documentation. Presented to nursing personnel at Rosegate Convalescent Center. Columbus, OH, 1991.

Guidelines for Exposure Determination and Prevention. Cincinnati-Dayton, OH: Association for Practitioners in Infection Control, 1992.

Guidelines for Prevention of Transmission of Human Immunodeficiency Virus and Hepatitis B Virus to Health Care and Public Safety Workers. *MMWR* 38(5-6):3-37, 1989.

Hamilton HK, editor: *Nursing Procedures*. Springhouse, PA: Intermed Communications, 1983.

Hay WW Jr, Hayward AR, Levin MJ, Sondheimer JM: *Current Pediatric Diagnosis and Treatment*. 14th edition. Stamford, CT: Appleton & Lange, 1999.

Heiss DG: *Personal Communication*. Columbus, OH: Physical Therapy Division, School of Allied Medical Professions, The Ohio State University, October 2000.

High Blood Pressure. New York, NY: American Heart Association, 1969.

Hill PH et al.: *Making Decisions*. Reading, MA: Addison-Wesley, 1979.

Hollis M: *Safe Lifting for Patient Care*. 2nd edition. Oxford, England: Blackwell Scientific Publications, 1985.

Homnick DN, White F, DeCastro, C: Comparison of Effects on an Intrapulmonary Percussive Ventilator to Standard Aerosol and Chest Physiotherapy in Treatment of Cystic Fibrosis. *Pediatric Pulmonology* 20:50-55, 1995.

Hoppenfeld S: *Physical Examination of the Spine and Extremities*. New York, NY: Appleton-Century-Crofts, 1976.

Hospital Infection Control. In *Employee Orientation Notebook*. Columbus, OH: Riverside Methodist Hospital, 1992.

Hsiang SM, Brogmus GE, Courtney TK: Low Back Pain (LBP) and Lifting Techniques: A Review. *International Journal of Industrial Ergonomics* 19: 59-74, 1997.

Jacox A et al.: *Management of Cancer Pain*. Clinical Guideline No. 9. AHCPR Publication No. 94-0592. Rockville, MD: Agency for Health Care Policy and Research, U.S. Department of Health and Human Services, Public Health Service, 1994.

Jobst-Custom Graduated Compression Supports Measuring and Fitting Manual. Charlotte, NC: Jobst.

Kasner OL, Rodeheaver GT, Sibbold RG, co-editors: *Chronic Wound Care: A Clinical Source Book for Health Care Professionals*. Wayne, PA: HMP Communications, 2001.

Kendall FP, McCreary EK: *Muscle Testing and Function*. 3rd edition. Baltimore, MD: Williams & Wilkins, 1983.

Kendall K: Evolution of Sacred Heart Hospital's Wound Assessment Sheet. *Acute Care Perspectives* (Newsletter of the Acute Care/Hospital Clinical Practice Section, American Physical Therapy Association, Pompton Plains, NJ) Summer:6-8, 1995.

Kennedy KL: *Wound Caring*. Eau Claire, WI: Professional Education Systems, Inc., 1997.

Kennedy KL: *Wound Caring*. Seminar. Columbus, OH, 1997.

Kenney WL: *ASCM's Guidelines for Exercise Testing and Prescription*. 5th edition. Baltimore, MD: Williams & Wilkins, 1995.

Kettenbach G: *Writing S.O.A.P. Notes*. Philadelphia: F.A. Davis, 1990.

Kisner C, Colby LA: *Therapeutic Exercise: Foundations and Techniques*. 3rd edition. Philadelphia: F.A. Davis, 1996.

Koblenzer L, Gyuricza B: *Nursing Concepts and Procedures Relevant to Physical Therapy*. Cleveland, OH: Physical Therapy Department, Department of Health Sciences, Cleveland State University, 1982.

Kulich P: *Personal Communication*. Columbus, OH: Infection Control Practitioner, Department of Epidemiology, The Ohio State University Medical Center, April 2001.

Kumar V, Cotran RS, Robbin SL: *Basic Pathology*. 5th edition. Philadelphia: W.B. Saunders, 1992.

Lehmkuhl LD, Smith LK: *Brunnstrom's Clinical Kinesiology*. 4th edition. Philadelphia: F.A. Davis, 1983.

LePostollec M: The Benefits of Lymphedema Certification. *Advance for Physical Therapists and PT Assistants* 11(18):36-38, 2000.

Lewis C: Wheelchair Use for the Older Patient. *Physical Therapy Forum* 11(23):4-7, 1992.

Lewis LV: *Fundamental Skills in Patient Care*. Philadelphia: J.B. Lippincott, 1976.

Magee DJ: *Orthopedic Physical Assessment*. 2nd edition. Philadelphia: W.B. Saunders, 1992.

Manworren R: *Personal Communication*. Dallas, TX: Director, Pain Assessment Department, Children's Medical Center, 2001.

McArdle WD, Katch FI, Katch VL: *Essentials of Exercise Physiology*. 4th edition. Philadelphia: Lea & Febiger, 1994.

McCash T: *Procedures for the ADA*. Dublin, OH: Meacham & Apel Architects Inc., 1991.

McCulloch JM, Kloth LC, Feddar JA: *Wound Healing Alternatives in Management*. 2nd edition. Philadelphia: F.A. Davis, 1995.

McCulloch JM, Kloth LC: Decision Point: Wound Dressings. *PT Magazine of Physical Therapy* 4(5):52-62, 1996.

McGill SM, Norman RW: Low Back Biomechanics in Industry: The Prevention of Injury through Safer Lifting. Current Issues in Biomechanics. *Human Kinetics* 69-120, 1993.

McGill SM: Low Back Exercises: Evidence for Improving Exercise Regimens. *Physical Therapy* 78(7):754-765, 1998.

McGill SM: The Biomechanics of Low Back Injury: Implications on Current Practice in Industry and the Clinic. *Journal of Biomechanics* 30(5):465-475, 1997.

Measuring Blood Pressure: A Guide for Paramedical Personnel. West Point, PA: Merck, Sharp & Dohme.

Measuring the Patient. Wheelchair Prescriptions. Booklet No. 1. Camarillo, CA: Everest & Jennings, 1983.

Meyer K: *Ten Commandments for Communicating with Persons with Disabilities*. Axis Center for Public Awareness of People with Disabilities: Columbus, OH.

Minor SD, Minor MA: *Patient Care Skills*. 4th edition. Stamford, CT: Appleton & Lange, 1999.

Mirone JA: Understanding the Americans with Disabilities Act. *Healthcare Trends Transactions* 4:36-38, 1993.

Morey S: *Pressure Ulcer Wound Care*. Presented at Ohio Physical Therapy Association, April 17, 1997, Columbus, OH, 1997.

Murdock KR: ICU Paraphernalia: Physical Therapy Implications. *Acute Care Perspectives* Winter 1995.

Najdeski P: Crutch Measurement from the Sitting Position. *Physical Therapy* 57(7):826-827, 1977.

National Kidney Foundation: *New Guidelines For Dialysis Care*. www.kidney/general/news/dial.cfm, 2001.

National Pressure Ulcer Advisory Panel: *A Selected Bibliography: Pressure Ulcer Assessment, Prevention and Treatment*. Buffalo, NY: National Pressure Ulcer Advisory Panel, 1995.

Nettina SM: *The Lippincott Manual of Nursing Practice*, 6th edition. Philadelphia: J.B. Lippincott, 1996.

Norkin C, Levangie P: *Joint Structure and Function: A Comprehensive Analysis*. 2nd edition. Philadelphia: F.A. Davis, 1990.

Nursing Photobook Annual. Springhouse, PA: Springhouse Corporation, 1987.

O'Sullivan SB, Schmitz TJ: *Physical Rehabilitation: Assessment and Treatment*. 3rd edition. Philadelphia: F.A. Davis, 1994.

O'Toole M, editor: *Miller-Keane Encyclopedia and Dictionary of Medicine, Nursing, and Allied Health*. 5th edition. Philadelphia: W.B. Saunders, 1992.

Occupational Safety and Health Administration, Department of Labor: Occupational Exposure to Bloodborne Pathogens: Final Rule. *Federal Register* December 6, 1991.

Ohio Hospital Association: Occupational Exposure to Bloodborne Pathogens: OSHA's Final Rule. *OHA Bulletin* December 20, 1991.

Okamoto GA, Phillips TJ, editors: *Physical Medicine and Rehabilitation*. Philadelphia: W.B. Saunders, 1984.

Palmer ML, Toms J: *Manual for Functional Training*. 3rd edition. Philadelphia: F.A. Davis, 1992.

Palmer ML: Gross Muscle Testing. *Clinical Management* 5(4):18-24, 1985.

Perry AG, Potter PA: *Clinical Nursing Skills and Techniques*. 2nd edition. St. Louis: Mosby, 1990.

Person First. Columbus, OH: AXIS Center for Public Awareness of People with Disabilities, 1995.

Petrek JA, Heelan MC: *Incidence of Breast Carcinoma-Related Lymphedema*. American Cancer Society Lymphedema Workshop. Supplement to *Cancer* August 20, 1998.

Polich S, Faynoor SM: Interpreting Lab Test Values. *PT Magazine of Physical Therapy* 4:76-88, 1996.

Pollack RA, Saunders HD, Melnik MS: *Your Healthy Back, Supervisors Handbook*. Chaska, MN: The Saunders Group, 1991.

Poor Posture Hurts. San Bruno, CA: Krames Communications, 1986.

President's Committee on Employment of People with Disabilities: Washington, DC 20004-1107.

Product Report: Wheelchairs. Washington, DC: American Association of Retired Persons, 1990.

Project Action. Washington, DC: National Easter Seal Society.

Project ADA. Chicago, IL: National Easter Seal Society.

Pronsati, MP: Ergonomics: Designing Jobs to Fit the Worker, *Advance for Physical Therapists and PT Assistants* 1(19):1,18,19, 1990.

Purtilo R: *Health Professional and Patient Interaction*. 4th edition. Philadelphia: W.B. Saunders, 1990.

Rantz MF, Courtial D: *Lifting, Moving and Transferring Patients*. 2nd edition. St. Louis: Mosby, 1981.

Recommendations for Human Blood Pressure Determination by Sphygmomanometers. Dallas, TX: American Heart Association, 1984.

Recommendations for prevention of HIV Transmission in Health Care Settings. MMWR, 36(2S): 377-382, 387-388, 1987.

Restraint and Seclusion: All Your Questions Answered. 1999 Joint Commission Videoconference Series. Includes material from Vencor Hospital. San Diego, CA: Joint Commission on Accreditation of Healthcare Organizations, 1999.

Rinehart-Ayers ME: *Conservative Approaches to Lymphedema Treatment*. American Cancer Society Lymphedema Workshop. Supplement to *Cancer* August 20, 1998.

Rules and Regulations: Occupational Safety and Health Act. *Federal Register* 56(235):64, 175, 182, 1991.

Rules and Regulations: Patient's Rights: Interim Trial Rule. *Federal Register* 64(127):36070-36089, 1999.

Safety and Handling. Wheelchair Prescriptions. Booklet No. 3. Camarillo, CA: Everest & Jennings, 1983.

Saunders HD: *For Your Back, A Self-Help Manual*. Minneapolis, MN: Viking Press, 1985.

Scott R, Cooperman J: Legal and Ethical Practice Issues in Physical Therapy. Presented at Ohio Physical Therapy Association, April 16, 1997. Columbus, OH, 1997.

Scully RM, Barnes MR, editors: *Physical Therapy*. Philadelphia: J.B. Lippincott, 1989.

Sussman C, Bates-Jensen BM: *Wound Care: A Collaborative Practice Manual for Physical Therapists and Nurses*. Gaithersburg, MD: Aspen Publishing, 1998.

Swanson MA: *Crutches on the Go*. Bellevue, WA: Medic Publications, 1974.

Taylor DL: *Personal Communication*. Columbus, OH: Infection Control Practitioner, Department of Epidemiology, The Ohio State University Medical Center, April 2001.

Taylor PM, Taylor DK, editors: *Conquering Athletic Injuries*. Champaign, IL: Leisure Press, 1988.

Techniques for Moving Patients. Deerfield, MA: Dray Publications.

The Accessible Housing Design File. Florence, KY: Barrier Free Environments, Inc.

The ADA: An Easy Checklist. Chicago, IL: National Easter Seal Society.

The Agency for Health Care Policy and Research: *Quick Reference Guide*. Silver Springs, MD: The Agency, 1994.

The Association for Hospitals and Health Systems: New Medicare Conditions of Participation Take Effect August 2, 1999. *OHA Bulletin* 99-042: 1-5, Columbus, OH: The Association, 1999.

The Association for Hospitals and Health Systems: OHA Responds to HCFA's New Rule on Restraint and Seclusion Use. *OHA Bulletin* 99-055:1-5, Columbus, OH: The Association, 1999.

Thiadens SRJ: Advances in the Management of Lymphedema, *Perspectives in Plastic Surgery* 4(1):181-197, 1990.

Umiker W: *Management Skills for the New Health Care Supervisor*. Rockville, MD: Aspen Publications, 1988.

Umphred DA, editor: *Neurological Rehabilitation*. 2nd edition. St. Louis: Mosby, 1990.

Update: Universal Precautions for Prevention of Transmission of Human Immunodeficiency Virus, Hepatitis B Virus and Other Bloodborne Pathogens in Health-Care Settings. MMWR, 37(24):377-382.

Voss DE, Ionta MK, Myers BJ: *Proprioceptive Neuromuscular Facilitation*. 3rd edition. Philadelphia: Harper & Row, 1985.

Weiss M: *Class Notes and Handouts*. Columbus, OH: Physical Therapy Division, School of Allied Medical Professions, The Ohio State University, 1975.

Weiss M: *Class Notes and Handouts*. Canton, OH: Stark Technical College, 1982.

What Everyone Should Know About Diabetes. Greenfield, MA: Channing L. Bete Company, 1994, Revised February, 2001.

Wheelchair Selection. Wheelchair Prescriptions. Booklet No. 2. Camarillo, CA: Everest & Jennings, 1983.

Wilson AB Jr: *Wheelchairs: A Prescription Guide*. Charlottesville, VA: Rehabilitation Press, 1986.

Wolf SL: *Clinical Decision Making in Physical Therapy*. Philadelphia: F.A. Davis, 1985.

Wood EC, Becker PD: *Beard's Massage*. 4th edition. Philadelphia: W.B. Saunders, 1990.

Wood LA, editor: *Nursing Skills for Allied Health Services*. 3 vols. Philadelphia: W.B. Saunders, 1975.

Index

T